SECOND EDITION

AMERICAN CANCER SOCIETY

COMPLETE GUIDE TO

Complementary & Alternative Cancer Therapies

SECOND EDITION

AMERICAN CANCER SOCIETY

COMPLETE GUIDE TO Complementary & Alternative Cancer Therapies

SENIOR CONTRIBUTING EDITORS

Terri Ades, MS, FNP-BC, AOCN

Rick Alteri, MD

Ted Gansler, MD

Patricia Yeargin, MN, MPH, RN

EDITORS

Jill Russell, Editor

Amy Rovere, Editorial Assistant

Foreword

David Rosenthal, MD

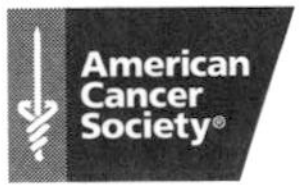

Published by the American Cancer Society / Health Promotions
250 Williams Street NW, Atlanta, Georgia 30303-1002 USA

Printed in the United States of America
Design and composition by LaShae V. Ortiz

5 4 3 2 1 09 10 11 12 13

Library of Congress Cataloging-in-Publication Data

American Cancer Society complete guide to complementary & alternative cancer therapies / from the experts at the American Cancer Society. —2nd ed.
p. cm.
Rev. ed. of: American Cancer Society's complementary and alternative cancer methods handbook. c2002.
Includes bibliographical references and index.
ISBN-13: 978-0-944235-71-3 (pbk. : alk. paper)
ISBN-10: 0-944235-71-9 (pbk. : alk. paper)
1. Cancer—Alternative treatment—Handbooks, manuals, etc.
I. American Cancer Society.
II. American Cancer Society's complementary and alternative cancer methods handbook. c2002.
III. Title: Complete guide to complementary and alternative cancer therapies.
RC271.A62A46 2009
616.99'406—dc22 2008030017

AMERICAN CANCER SOCIETY
Strategic Director, Content: Chuck Westbrook
Director, Book Publishing: Len Boswell
Book Marketing/Rights Manager: Candace Magee
Managing Editor, Books: Rebecca Teaff, MA
Books Editor: Jill Russell
Book Publishing Coordinator: Vanika Jordan, MSPub
Editorial Assistant, Books: Amy Rovere

Quantity discounts on bulk purchases of this book are available. Book excerpts can also be created to fit specific needs. For information, please contact the American Cancer Society, Health Promotions Publishing, 250 Williams Street NW, Atlanta, GA 30303-1002, or send an e-mail to **trade.sales@cancer.org.**

A NOTE TO THE READER

This information represents the views of the doctors and nurses serving on the American Cancer Society's Cancer Information Database Editorial Board. These views are based on their interpretation of studies published in medical journals, as well as their own professional experience.

The treatment information in this book is not official policy of the Society and is not intended as medical advice to replace the expertise and judgment of your cancer care team. It is intended to help you and your family make informed decisions, together with your doctor.

If you are considering a complementary or alternative treatment for your cancer, please consult with your doctor first.

For more information about cancer, contact your American Cancer Society at **800-ACS-2345** or **www.cancer.org**. For updates on the therapies discussed in this book, go to **www.cancer.org/cam**.

Reviewers

Debra Barton RN, PhD, AOCN
Associate Professor, Oncology
Mayo Clinic College of Medicine
Symptom Management Research
Rochester, MN

Lorenzo Cohen, PhD
Associate Professor
Department of Behavioral Science
Director, Integrative Medicine Program, Division of Cancer Medicine
Section Chief, Integrative Medicine, Dept. of General Oncology
The University of Texas M. D. Anderson Cancer Center
Houston, TX

Susan Decristofaro, RN, MS, OCN
Director, Patient Family Education
Dana-Farber Cancer Institute
Boston, MA

Gary Deng, MD, PhD
Assistant Member
Integrative Medicine Service
Memorial Sloan-Kettering Cancer Center
New York, NY

Tieraona Low Dog, MD
Director of the Fellowship
Arizona Center for Integrative Medicine
Clinical Assistant Professor
Department of Medicine
University of Arizona Health Sciences Center
Tucson, AZ

Cynthia D. Myers, PhD, LMT
Director, Integrative Medicine Program
Moffitt Cancer Center and Research Institute
Tampa, FL

Briane Pinkson, LPN, LMT
Healing Arts Practitioner
Department of Palliative Care
Dartmouth Hitchcock Medical Center
Lebanon, NH

Cheryl L. Rock, PhD, RD
Professor
Department of Family and Preventive Medicine
School of Medicine
University of California, San Diego
La Jolla, CA

David Rosenthal, MD
Director, Harvard University Health Services
Professor of Medicine and Henry K. Oliver Professor of Hygiene, Harvard Medical School
Medical Director, Leonard P. Zakim Center for Integrative Therapies, Dana-Farber Cancer Institute (Boston)
Cambridge, MA

Heather S. Shaw, MD
Assistant Professor of Medicine
Multidisciplinary Breast Program
Duke University Medical Center
Durham, NC

Michael Stefanek, PhD
Vice President, Behavioral Research
Director, Behavioral Research Center
American Cancer Society
Atlanta, GA

Andrew Vickers, PhD
Associate Attending Research Methodologist
Department of Epidemiology and Biostatistics
Memorial Sloan-Kettering Cancer Center
New York, NY

Contributors, First Edition

Much of the information in this book was based on content from the first edition, which was created with the assistance of the contributors below.

Stuart J. Birkby
Dorothy Breckner
Katherine Bruss, PsyD
Lynne Camoosa
Carol Carter
Jeff Clements
Suzy Crawford
Dennis Connaughton
Peter Dakutis
Steve Frandzel
Tom Gryczan, MS
Melissa Kulick, PhD
Steve Lewis
Jennifer Miller
Christina Salter, MA
Ryan Siemers, MPH
Leah Tuzzio

ABBREVIATED TABLE OF CONTENTS

CONTENTS

FOREWORD

Much has changed in the nine years since the first edition of the *American Cancer Society's Guide to Complementary and Alternative Cancer Methods* was published. Substantially more scientific research is available about complementary and alternative methods (CAM) and their benefit, or lack thereof, for cancer patients. It is estimated that patients are spending tens of billions of dollars annually on CAM treatments. In fact, CAM has become so accepted in mainstream cancer care that many large cancer centers are opening integrative oncology programs—programs aimed at education, research, and clinical investigation of complementary and alternative therapies alongside conventional ones.

Despite advancements in science and greater application of complementary and alternative therapies, understanding the basic tenets and terminology of CAM remains as valid and important as ever. New therapies are continually being introduced into medicine, and public access to information about them is greater than ever before. However, some of these treatments have not been thoroughly tested and, in fact, may be harmful. So, how should one navigate and evaluate the constant sea of information and claims?

Informed, authoritative sources within the medical community should address any new claims regarding CAM, and that is the primary reason for publishing this new edition. Experts at the American Cancer Society, along with many thought leaders in the field of CAM have analyzed the most recent research and claims surrounding alternative and complementary treatments. In this new edition, they share important facts regarding what has been proven or disproven in the field during the last decade.

When the first edition of this book was published, CAM topics were rarely discussed with treating physicians. But with the development of integrative oncology centers and increasing positive results from outcome studies, doctors tend to be much more accepting of complementary therapies. That being said, there is an important caveat surrounding this book: It is crucial that patients share with their doctors, specialists, and oncologists what they are doing for their health in addition to taking prescribed medications—whether it be nutritional supplements, massage, artwork, counseling, or meditation. Information about all aspects of your health should be shared with your doctor. Your doctor and other decision makers on your team can provide optimal assistance to you only when they are aware of all the resources you are using.

The goal of the American Cancer Society is to ensure that people have access to the best and most accurate health information available. Cancer patients and their caregivers will find this book to be a reliable and valuable guide for making informed decisions about their health.

David Rosenthal, MD
Director, Harvard University Health Services
Professor of Medicine and Henry K. Oliver Professor of Hygiene, Harvard Medical School
Medical Director, Leonard P. Zakim Center for Integrative Therapies, Dana-Farber Cancer Institute

INTRODUCTION

There is no doubt that complementary and alternative methods (also known as complementary and alternative medicine or CAM) are tremendously popular in the United States and in many other parts of the world. Speaking with your friends about health concerns, reading newspaper and magazine articles and advertisements, browsing the Internet, or perusing the shelves of your local pharmacy or health food store, you are constantly reminded that these approaches to health are extensively promoted and widely used.

Many cancer patients may be reluctant to talk with their doctors about complementary or alternative therapies. We encourage you to talk openly with your health care providers about any therapy—conventional, complementary, or alternative—you are considering. Open, trusting, noncritical communication is essential in making wise health care decisions. Discussing treatment options openly with your health care providers will help ensure that you select the methods most likely to be safe and effective and avoid methods that are dangerous, likely to interfere with conventional treatments, or ineffective.

This book reflects the American Cancer Society's commitment to providing comprehensive information to empower patients and the public in making informed decisions about the use of conventional methods as well as CAM in cancer prevention and treatment and in optimizing quality of life for cancer survivors. Since its inception in 1913, the Society has taken on the task of educating the public about cancer and about the safety and effectiveness of cancer treatment. Early in its existence, the Society expressed concern over dubious claims of "cancer cures" and began gathering information on these therapies. In the 1950s, as the organization became increasingly concerned with the exploitation of people with cancer—especially those in the advanced phases of illness—we began to publish information about specific claims, as well as the criteria for assessing the value or merit of particular cancer treatments or diagnostic tests.

In the spirit of our longstanding ACS mission—to educate, advocate, research, and serve—the *American Cancer Society Complete Guide to Complementary & Alternative Cancer Therapies, Second Edition* was born. This book will serve as a comprehensive guide to the wide variety of methods available. Each entry provides critical information such as proponents' claims, what the method involves, historical background, recent research findings, and side effects and complications. The latest complementary and alternative treatment methods are included, as well as those that have been used for many years. This second edition has been updated with the latest research in the field of integrative oncology, as well as an expanded glossary and resource list.

Although the overall format and style of the first and second editions of this book are quite similar, the content is substantially different. The reason is the tremendous explosion of interest in CAM and the progress that has resulted from the application of mainstream scientific methods to studying the basis and effectiveness of many complementary approaches. According to results of the 2002 National Health Interview Survey, 36 percent of U.S. adults had used some form of complementary or alternative medicine (CAM) during the past year. When megavitamins and nonpharmacologic methods such as prayer for health were included as part of CAM, that percentage rose to 62 percent. An American Cancer Society study published in 2008 concluded that as many as 61 percent of the cancer survivors surveyed used some type of CAM. If prayer for health was excluded, the percentage who had used CAM was still 44 percent.

According to the National Center for Complementary and Alternative Medicine (NCCAM), Americans spent an estimated $36 to $47 billion on complementary and alternative treatment methods during 1997. Although this is the most current estimate based on data from government surveys, it is extremely likely that we are currently spending far more.

The field of CAM has grown and matured greatly during the past couple of decades, and its importance is now widely acknowledged by the general public and mainstream health care providers and researchers. A search of the MEDLINE database—the National Library of Medicine's database of articles published in life sciences and biomedical journals—using the terms "alternative medicine", "complementary medicine", or "complementary therapies" found 127 articles published in 1991, the year Congress authorized creation of the Office of Alternative Medicine (OAM) as a part of the National Institutes of Health. By 2007, that number had increased to 848. Although these numbers may not include all the published research in the field, they clearly reflect the rapid growth of this field of study. In addition to government organizations such as the OAM (later expanded and renamed the National Center for Complementary and Alternative Medicine), the Office of Dietary Supplements, and the Office of Cancer Complementary Medicine, there are now a number of professional organizations (such as the Society of Integrative Oncology) dedicated to the scientific study of CAM. Access to complementary care has also changed; most national and regional cancer centers now have integrative oncology clinics in which care is provided collaboratively by a team that includes mainstream oncologists, nurses, acupuncturists, massage therapists, art and music therapists, and other complementary practitioners.

Looking back at our first edition, the main messages were warnings about unproven alternative therapies and cautious optimism regarding some complementary methods, based largely on a few preliminary studies. Eight years later, our concern regarding alternative therapies remains unchanged, but we are very pleased that the evidence of benefits from some complementary therapies is becoming much clearer.

As in our first edition, this second edition aims to provide readers with a reliable guide to selecting and using treatment methods wisely. Through objective information based on scientific evidence from peer-reviewed medical literature, readers may evaluate the evidence and make informed choices—together with their doctors—about complementary therapies.

This book is also designed to provide some clarity in the sea of information about complementary and alternative medicine. Patients should always seek information from unbiased and reliable sources. These can be medical professionals, print publications from reputable sources, or online resources, among others. In Chapter 10 we provide some resources for information about cancer and complementary and alternative methods, as well as some characteristics of reliable, ethical Web sites.

Individuals with cancer have the right to decide what treatment is best for them, and moreover, they have the right to accurate and reliable information about the treatments available. The decision to use alternative or complementary methods is an important one. This book will aid patients in making informed and safe decisions.

For additional information, support, or referrals to resources in your community, please call the American Cancer Society at **800-ACS-2345** or visit our Web site at **www.cancer.org**.

References

Barnes PM, Powell-Briner E, McFann K, Nahin RL. Complementary and alternative medicine use among adults: United States, 2002. *CDC Advance Data Report #343*. 2004.

Gansler T, Kaw C, Crammer C, Smith T. A population-based study of prevalence of complementary methods use by cancer survivors: a report from the American Cancer Society's studies of cancer survivors. *Cancer*. 2008;113:1048-1057.

Office of Cancer Complementary and Alternative Medicine Web site. http://www.cancer.gov/CAM/. Accessed October 8, 2008.

Office of Dietary Supplements Web site. http://ods.od.nih.gov/. Accessed October 8, 2008.

Society of Integrative Oncology Web site. http://www.integrativeonc.org/. Accessed October 8, 2008.

The use of complementary and alternative medicine in the United States. National Center for Complementary and Alternative Medicine Web site. http://nccam.nih.gov/news/camsurvey_fs1.htm#. Updated May 2007. Accessed October 8, 2008.

Chapter One

How to Use this Book

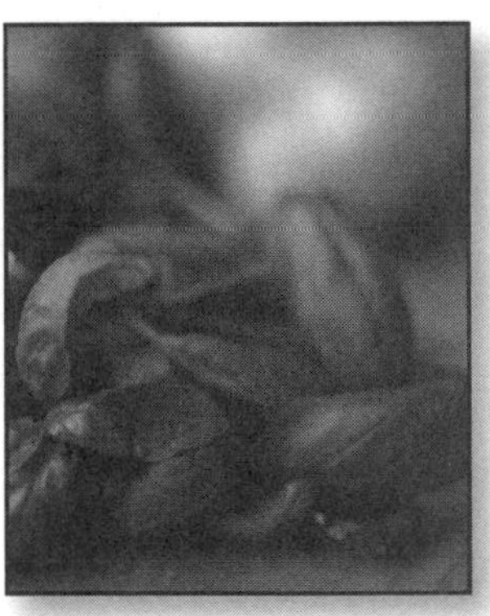

IF YOU ARE READING THIS BOOK, it is probably because you or someone you care about has received a cancer diagnosis or is concerned about cancer. You or your loved one may have received advice and treatment from doctors, nurses, and other conventional health care providers. But you may be wondering if there is anything else you can do to feel better and improve your health.

If you have been thinking about trying a complementary or alternative therapy, you are not alone. Interest in this field has grown enormously, especially during the past decade. Americans spend billions of dollars on complementary and alternative therapies for a wide variety of diseases, ailments, and medical complaints, including cancer. The growing popularity of complementary and alternative therapies has had an enormous impact on every aspect of health care in the United States, Europe, and elsewhere in the developed world. The rise of complementary and alternative medicine has had a particular influence on people with cancer. While accurate figures are difficult to obtain, it is estimated that about half of all people living with cancer have sought some type of complementary or alternative therapy.

The next chapter will present some concepts and terminology to help you understand the field of complementary and alternative medicine and the types of research that scientists use to evaluate safety and effectiveness. We give an overview of how drugs and dietary supplements are regulated and marketed. We will suggest some general approaches to help you decide what might work for you and give tips for talking with your regular doctor and finding and choosing a complementary health care provider. And in Chapters 5 through 9, we will present information on common and not-so-common complementary and alternative methods of cancer care. Methods included in the book have been promoted for conditions related to cancer, its consequences, or effects related to treatment. The information is collected from many sources and distilled into a concise format that we hope you will find helpful.

Therapies are organized into the five categories listed below and listed alphabetically within each chapter. Methods have been categorized based on similar characteristics and how the treatment is administered or performed.

Chapter 5. Mind, Body, and Spirit Therapies: This chapter includes methods that focus on the connections between the mind, body, and spirit, and their powers for healing.
Chapter 6. Manual Healing and Physical Touch Therapies: This chapter includes treatment methods that involve touching, manipulation, or movement of the body. These techniques are based on the idea that problems in one part of the body often affect other parts of the body.
Chapter 7. Herb, Vitamin, and Mineral Therapies: This chapter contains plant-derived preparations, vitamins, and minerals that are used for therapeutic purposes. It is noted when chemicals extracted from plants are used rather than parts of the plant itself.

Chapter 8. Diet and Nutrition Therapies: This chapter includes dietary approaches and nutritional programs related to prevention and treatment.
Chapter 9. Pharmacologic and Biologic Therapies: This chapter provides information about substances that are synthesized and produced from chemicals or concentrated from plants or other living things.

Chapter 10 lists some resources to assist you in finding other reliable sources of information. In addition, the glossary (starting on page 847) defines many of the terms used throughout the book.

This book is intended to serve as a reference, not to be read from beginning to end. However, we recommend that you read the next few chapters first, particularly if you are unfamiliar with complementary and alternative therapies. Much of the first four chapters is intended to help you evaluate the information to follow.

If you do not find a particular therapy in the section you would expect, please consult the index (starting on page 869) to see if it is included elsewhere. In some cases, methods have been grouped together into broader categories that you may not immediately consider. If an entire chapter interests you, you may want to read through all of the entries contained in that chapter to gain a better understanding of that area of complementary or alternative care. Some methods contain only a few lines or short paragraphs because information on the therapy is limited or it is not widely available. In these cases, there was not enough scientific information to evaluate the evidence, so only a brief description is provided.

Sample Book Entry

All of the entries in Chapters 5–9 follow the same format, allowing a consistent presentation of information so the content can be quickly accessed from entry to entry.

How is it promoted for use?

This section discusses advocates' claims about the effectiveness of the therapy and their theories about how the method works. Claims about the method's value for conditions other than cancer may also be included.

What does it involve?

This section covers what the treatment method involves, how often it is administered, and in what forms the treatment is provided.

What is the history behind it?

This section explores the background of how, when, and by whom the method was developed.

What is the evidence?

This section explores the latest scientific research on each treatment method, as well as general conclusions about the effectiveness of the method based on scientific data.

Are there any possible problems or complications?

This section notes anything people should be aware of or concerned about, such as side effects, drug interactions, reports of death, or other adverse reactions.

References

A reference list of the resources used to compile each entry, specifically the most important information sources, can be found here. Readers may use this reference list and the resource guide in Chapter 10 to obtain more information. This list does not necessarily include every scientific journal article on a topic or all Web sites promoting a method. Doing so would increase the length of the book by several times. Instead, we have chosen the information sources we consider most useful, relevant, and reliable.

Complementary and alternative medicine includes a wide variety of therapies and types of care. Some have been shown to help relieve symptoms and improve quality of life. Others can be harmful. In addition, there is an immense amount of information available about complementary and alternative therapies—some legitimate, and some not.

Perhaps more than in any other aspect of wellness and health, choices about complementary and alternative care can be very personal. Your choices can be strongly influenced by your beliefs and values. This book offers information and tools to help anyone interested in nonconventional methods evaluate the information and evidence available. It will not tell you what to do or not do. Instead, our hope is that this guide can assist you in making informed choices about whether complementary or alternative care is right for you.

References

Are you considering using CAM? National Center for Complementary and Alternative Medicine Web site. http://nccam.nih.gov/health/decisions/index.htm. Accessed June 5, 2008.

Cassileth B. Why integrative oncology? Complementary therapies are increasingly becoming part of mainstream care. *Oncology (Williston Park)*. 2006;20:1302.

Cassileth BR, Vickers AJ. High prevalence of complementary and alternative medicine use among cancer patients: implications for research and clinical care. *J Clin Oncol.* 2005;23:2590-2592. Epub 2005 Feb 22.
Comment in:
J Clin Oncol. 2005;23:2645-2654.

Complementary and alternative methods for cancer management. American Cancer Society Web site. http://www.cancer.org/docroot/ETO/content/ETO_5_1_Introduction.asp. Accessed June 2, 2008.

Deng G, Cassileth BR. To what extent do cancer patients use complementary and alternative medicine? *Nat Clin Pract Oncol.* 2005;2:496-497.

What is CAM? National Center for Complementary and Alternative Medicine Web site. http://nccam.nih.gov/health/whatiscam/. Accessed May 30, 2008.

Chapter Two

Defining and Evaluating Complementary and Alternative Therapies

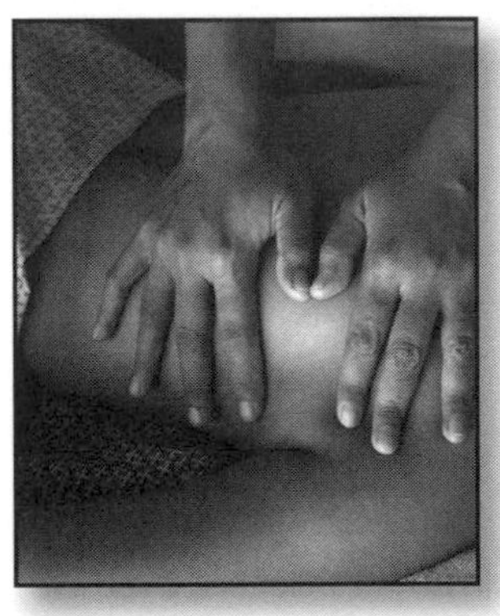

YOU WILL ENCOUNTER MANY TERMS IN THIS BOOK—some new, some familiar. The two most common words are *complementary* and *alternative*, but there are many other terms with which you should become familiar. This chapter introduces a vocabulary of complementary and alternative therapies and discusses how research is used to evaluate therapies' safety and effectiveness. Becoming comfortable with some of these terms and concepts will help you evaluate the descriptions of therapies later in the book. The more you understand, the better equipped you will be to evaluate information and make informed choices about your care.

How Complementary and Alternative Therapies Differ

The words *complementary* and *alternative* are often used interchangeably; however, there are important distinctions between the two terms.

Complementary therapies are those that patients use **along with** conventional medicine. Many of these therapies have been shown to help relieve symptoms and improve quality of life by lessening the side effects of conventional treatments or providing psychological and physical benefits to the patient.

Alternative therapies are unproven treatments that patients use **instead of** conventional therapy in an attempt to prevent, lessen, or cure disease. Alternative therapies may be harmful and, because they are used instead of conventional medicine, may delay treatments that are proven to be helpful.

Until the late 1990s, the term alternative was generally used to describe most of the therapies that are not part of conventional medicine. When the National Institutes of Health (NIH) established a special department to evaluate complementary and alternative therapies, it was originally named the Office of Alternative Medicine (OAM). In 1999, recognizing the distinction between complementary and alternative therapies, the NIH renamed the office the National Center for Complementary and Alternative Medicine (NCCAM). This terminology is also reflected in the name of the National Cancer Institute's Office of Cancer Complementary and Alternative Medicine (OCCAM), which was created in 1998.

The boundaries between complementary, alternative, and conventional methods are not always sharply defined and sometimes depend on the situation in which the treatment is used as much as the treatment itself. For example, scientifically conducted clinical trials have shown that arsenic trioxide is an effective drug for some forms of leukemia, so its use for promyelocytic leukemia would be considered conventional. Homeopathic practitioners may recommend highly diluted arsenic solutions for diarrhea, asthma, or anxiety, and use of arsenic in this context together with conventional medicine would be considered complementary. If an alternative practitioner recommended a homeopathic arsenic solution as the main treatment for lung cancer and advised the patient to avoid any conventional therapy, that would be alternative medicine.

Living With Evidence, Odds, and Uncertainty

Every day, we all make innumerable small decisions. In making these decisions, we use information, experience, and knowledge to estimate likely outcomes of our options. If we're planning to spend time outdoors, we may think about the possibility of rain. You might check the weather forecast in your newspaper or on the Internet. If the forecast shows a 100 percent chance of thunderstorms, most people will bring an umbrella. If the chance of precipitation is 0 percent, most people will not.

But what would you do if the probability of rain was 20 percent? Or 50 percent? If you are like most people, your answer will be, "It depends." It depends on your individual circumstances: where you are going, how you will get there, and what you are wearing, to name a few.

Similarly, decisions about medical care, particularly about complementary and alternative therapies, are individual and depend on many things: your body, your illness, your prognosis, your beliefs and values, and the available information about the safety and effectiveness of any treatment. In this chapter, we will help you understand various kinds of scientific evidence. In other chapters, we will review the evidence relevant to various complementary and alternative therapies. But every person is different, and choices about health care should reflect that.

Commonly Used Terms

The many different terms used to describe cancer treatments can be confusing. Here are some definitions of commonly used terms.

- **Proven or conventional treatments** are evidence-based, mainstream, or standard medical treatments that have been tested following a strict set of research guidelines and found to be safe and effective. Articles detailing such research have been published in peer-reviewed medical journals—meaning that other physicians or scientists in the field evaluate the quality of the research study and decide whether the results will be published. Conventional drugs are approved by the U.S. Food and Drug Administration (FDA). The FDA does not need to approve surgical procedures or radiation protocols, although it does approve the medical devices used in surgery or radiation therapy.
- **Investigational treatments** are therapies currently being studied in a clinical trial. Clinical trials—research involving human subjects—determine whether a new treatment is effective and safe for patients. Before a drug or other treatment can be used regularly to treat patients, it is carefully studied and tested, first in the laboratory or in animals. After these studies are completed and the therapy is found safe and promising, it is then tested in clinical trials. If the therapy is found to be safe and effective, the FDA may approve it for regular use. Only then does the drug or therapy become part of the standard, conventional treatment.

- The term **complementary** is used to describe supportive methods that complement, or add to, conventional treatments. Examples might include meditation to reduce stress, peppermint or ginger tea for nausea, and guided imagery to help relieve stress and pain during medical procedures. Complementary methods help control symptoms and improve well-being.
- **Integrative therapy** is a term now frequently used to describe the combined use of evidence-based proven therapies and complementary therapies. You have likely heard the term integrative oncology. Integrative medicine services are becoming part of cancer centers across the country.
- The terms **unproven** and **untested** can be confusing because they are sometimes used to refer to treatments that have little basis in scientific fact, while they may also refer to treatments or tests that are under investigation. In general, there is not adequate scientific evidence to support the use of unproven or untested treatments.
- **Alternative treatments** are used instead of conventional treatments. They are either unproven because they have not been scientifically tested, or they have been disproved, that is, they have been tested and found to be ineffective. They may cause the patient to suffer because they are not helpful, cause delays in curative therapy, or actually are harmful.
- **Quackery** refers to the promotion of methods that claim to prevent, diagnose, or cure cancer; however, they are known to be false or are unproven and likely to be false. These methods are often based on theories of disease and treatment that are contrary to conventional scientific ideas, and they may use patient testimonials as evidence of their effectiveness and safety. Many times, the treatment is claimed to be effective against other diseases as well as cancer.
- **Unconventional** is a term used to cover all types of complementary and alternative treatments that fall outside the definition of proven, conventional therapies.
- **Nontraditional** is used in the same way as unconventional to describe complementary and alternative therapies. However, some therapies that seem "nontraditional" to modern American or European physicians may have been used in certain cultures for thousands of years, such as traditional Chinese medicine or traditional Native American medicine. These medicines are often used in complementary or alternative therapies.
- **Questionable treatments** are those that are unproven or untested therapies.

A Scientific View of Cancer

The beginning of the twentieth century is widely viewed by medical historians as the turning point in cancer treatment. There was important progress in understanding, preventing, and treating cancer before that time, of course, but progress has greatly accelerated in the past hundred years. Researchers and physicians began sharing knowledge with each other more than ever, and medical institutions became centers of research.

During the early years of cancer research, scientists began to realize that the disease had no one single cause. Cancer is many diseases with many causes. Scientists also began investigating various treatment methods in the hope of finding ways to treat cancer that were safe and effective.

Today, researchers continue to search for causes of cancer and strive to find new and better ways to prevent, diagnose, treat, and, in some cases, even cure the disease. What's different, however, is how they go about their work.

Most of what we know about cancer is the result of research, defined as a trained inquiry or experiment that follows what is known as the scientific method. Scientists ask a question, design experiments to answer that question, collect data, interpret the results, and apply those results to treat disease and improve health care.

According to the NCCAM, complementary and alternative medicine should be investigated by the same rigorous scientific methods used in conventional medicine. Substantial progress has been made in recent years to make the field of integrative oncology much more scientifically rigorous than it had been. This is an approach strongly supported by the American Cancer Society, the National Cancer Institute, and a growing number of complementary and conventional health care providers and researchers.

Types of Scientific Studies and Evidence

Many different types and levels of scientific studies and evidence are relevant to complementary, alternative, and conventional cancer care. The sections on specific therapies in this book discuss the types and results of these studies, as well as other evidence or claims used by marketers to promote their products. The terms below can help the reader put that information into perspective.

In vitro research studies human or animal cells growing in laboratory dishes or flasks. The term *in vitro* originates from the Latin words for "in glass," although most modern laboratories now use plastic flasks. This type of research is sometimes referred to as laboratory or test-tube studies.

In vivo research is research focused within the living body of laboratory animals or humans. The Latin literally translates as "in life."

Clinical research is research on humans. Specifically, it is the study of methods for treating, preventing, or diagnosing health problems in humans. Clinical research studies in which one or more health care methods are given to participants according to a predetermined plan are called **clinical trials**. Clinical trials are also called intervention studies, because the researchers systematically intervene by influencing the participants' use of medications, foods, supplements, or anything else that is expected to influence their health. There are several phases of clinical trials, which provide different kinds of information. Other terms may be used in varying combinations to describe clinical trials:

- A **randomized** study is one in which the method of assigning treatment ensures that each participant has an equal chance of being assigned to either the treatment or control group.
- A **blind** study is one in which the participants do not know which treatment they are receiving. This helps to avoid the "placebo effect" whereby some participants' perceptions of the treatment are influenced by their expectations regarding its effectiveness.
- In a **double-blind** study, neither the subjects nor the investigators are aware of who is receiving which treatment, nor are others associated with the study, such as monitors or statisticians. This study design helps avoid the placebo effect as well as biases in clinical observations caused by the researchers' expectations about the treatment.
- A **controlled** study is an experiment or clinical trial that includes a comparison, or control, group. An **uncontrolled** study, therefore, would be a study without a control group. The control group helps ensure that the variable being studied is actually responsible for any resulting effect.

See pages 16–21 for more information on clinical trials.

Observational studies are studies in which individuals are observed or certain outcomes are measured. No attempt is made to affect the outcome. For example, an observational study may compare health outcomes (longevity, likelihood of a cancer occurrence, quality of life, etc.) of people who regularly use a particular dietary supplement with those who do not. In these studies, the researchers do not tell the participants whether to use the supplement—rather, they observe which patients used the supplement and determine whether there was any statistical association with health outcomes. There are several types of observational studies, each with certain advantages and disadvantages. The three main types of observational studies are *ecologic studies*, *case-control studies*, and *cohort studies*. For researchers who are evaluating the strength of evidence from studies, knowing the type of observational study helps them recognize potential weaknesses in the evidence.

- **Ecologic studies** compare potential risk factors and protective factors among groups of people. For example, an ecologic study comparing people in the United States and China, overall, would report a lower risk for most types of cancer in China. The limitation of such studies is that they do not tell us which differences between the two populations were responsible. Was it because Chinese people exercise more, eat less meat, weigh less, use certain herbs, practice tai chi, or have some genetic differences? These questions can be answered only by other kinds of studies. An ecologic study might also report a statistical link between populations that consume more of a particular food or supplement per capita and the risk for a certain disease. But this information still does not tell us whether the people consuming the highest levels of the food or supplement are the ones with the lowest (or highest) disease risk.

- **Case-control studies** start by identifying two groups of people: "cases" are people with a particular health outcome (such as diagnosis of a certain form of cancer), and "controls" are people without that outcome. The second step is asking people in both groups about their past exposures to potential risk factors and protective factors. Unlike ecologic studies, in which statistics compare the population's average exposures and outcomes, case-control studies collect and analyze data about individuals, which is a big advantage. The main disadvantage of case-control studies is that people's recollections of past exposures may not be very accurate.
- **Cohort studies** begin with a large group of volunteers who provide information about potential risk factors and protective factors. Researchers then check the volunteers' health outcomes periodically to look for statistical links between exposures and health outcomes. These studies are considered the strongest type of observational study.

Review studies combine and analyze findings from several other studies. In some cases, they compare and discuss the finding of prior studies. In **meta-analyses**, the researchers use statistical methods to combine the results of individual studies into one giant study.

Epidemiologic research provides information about health and disease in populations. Many of these studies evaluate statistical associations between risk factors or protective factors and various health problems. Observational studies are the most common type of epidemiologic research. Technically, clinical trials are also a type of epidemiologic research, but when most researchers refer to epidemiologic studies, they usually mean observational studies.

In Vitro and Animal Research

Much of what is known about human physiology, such as how different organs function in the body, is based on in vitro and animal research studies. There is virtually no area of medicine that has not benefited enormously from appropriate laboratory studies. Examples include the development of antibiotics, organ transplantation, the development of hepatitis and polio vaccines, and nearly all cancer treatments.

In early phases of research, experiments may be primarily "test-tube" studies, which typically involve examination of isolated cells. New techniques involving human cell and tissue cultures continue to be developed. But treatments must also be tested on living organisms that are made of interrelated organs to identify and evaluate proper doses and possible side effects in humans.

Animal research is crucial for understanding many of the biological processes involved in cancer. Research with animals allows scientists to identify cancer-causing substances and the dietary factors that inhibit or encourage the growth of cancer. They can also study the effectiveness of new drugs and surgical techniques, new ways to deliver radiation treatment, and other new treatments. Computer models cannot reliably predict how drugs will affect organ systems, that is, how the body will metabolize and clear both the drug and its metabolic product from the system and whether the drug will actually have the power to produce the desired effect.

In addition, all drugs must first be tested for safety in animals before they can be tested with reasonable assurance of safety in humans. New chemicals and occupational exposures are also most accurately tested for safety risk in animals.

All institutions that conduct animal research are required to comply with the federal Animal Welfare Act, which was amended in 1985 through The Improved Standards for Laboratory Animals Act. Among other regulations, the law provides that procedures are conducted under supervision of a licensed veterinarian and sets out requirements for sanitation, housing, ventilation, adequate exercise, and minimizing pain and distress. In addition, any institution receiving federal funding for animal research must have an Institutional Animal Care and Use Committee (IACUC). The IACUC must include at least one veterinarian with training in laboratory animal science and expertise in the relevant species, at least one practicing research scientist, and at least one person who is not affiliated with the institution to represent community interests in the proper care and use of animals. Research institutions also have their own review boards, which monitor all experiments using animals.

Limits of Observational Epidemiologic Research

In the field of cancer, epidemiologists observe how many people have cancer, who gets specific types of cancer, and what factors (such as environment, job hazards, family history and inherited genes, smoking, and diet) play a part in the development of cancer. Epidemiologic research is the source of many of our ideas about what causes cancer, what determines high risk for development of cancer, and how cancer can be prevented.

Epidemiologic studies can point to an association between a factor and a disease. These studies do not provide conclusive evidence of cause and effect. For example, epidemiologic studies show that a diet high in fruits and vegetables is associated with a lower risk for several forms of cancer, as well as heart disease. To learn more about how these foods benefit health or prevent cancer, researchers conduct laboratory experiments on animals or isolated cells. To confirm any cause and effect relationship with greater certainty, they must conduct clinical trials in which volunteers are randomly assigned to continue their usual diet or to change their diet to one higher in fruits or vegetables.

You may be wondering why a clinical trial is important if an observational study already reported lower cancer risk among people who eat plenty of vegetables. Well, what if it turned out that, on average, people who eat vegetables are less likely to smoke cigarettes and more likely to exercise? How would we know whether the apparent good health of vegetable eaters is due to their diet or their tendency to exercise more and smoke less? Epidemiologists can adjust for the influence of multiple factors. However, it is impossible to prove conclusively through this type of study that vegetables are the key factor. There could be an unknown characteristic of people who like vegetables that might be the key to avoiding cancer. This is the reason randomized clinical trials are considered more convincing than observational studies. Although clinical trials are ideal for studying ways to prevent or treat cancer, it would be unethical to conduct a clinical trial in which some volunteers were assigned to receive a substance suspected of causing cancer.

Let's return to our vegetable example for a moment. It turns out that nearly all of the evidence regarding vegetables and prevention of cancer comes from observational studies. This is simply a topic that has not been adequately studied in clinical trials. Left with evidence that is good but not perfect, we need to weigh the benefits, risks, and costs. You might not love okra or brussels sprouts, but it is likely that there are at least a few vegetables you enjoy. Vegetables are extremely safe, and they tend to be inexpensive. So, despite imperfect evidence, it is very reasonable to recommend a diet high in vegetables.

Although observational epidemiologic research is most often used to study risk factors, it can also be used to help evaluate conventional, complementary, or alternative treatments. If an observational study suggested that people who took a new chemotherapy drug lived, on average, 20 percent longer than people who had no treatment, how convinced would you be? You might wonder whether people also took other treatments that made a difference in their outcomes. If the new drug had substantial side effects, you might want to see the results of a randomized clinical trial before making a decision. Most doctors would. And the FDA would require further study to be sure of the drug's benefit before approving the drug for clinical use.

Clinical Trials

Advances in medicine and science are the result of new ideas and approaches developed through laboratory and clinical research. New cancer treatments must prove to be safe and effective in scientific studies with a certain number of patients before they can be made widely available. These studies must withstand critical review by other scientists (known as peer review) in order to be published in peer-reviewed medical and scientific journals.

A clinical trial is done only when there is some reason to believe that the treatment being studied may be valuable to the patient. Treatments used in clinical trials are often found to have real benefits. Researchers conduct studies of new treatments to answer the following questions:

Is the treatment helpful?
How does this new type of treatment work?
Does it work better than other treatments already available?
What side effects does the treatment cause?
Are the side effects greater or less than with the standard treatment?
Do the benefits outweigh the side effects?
In which patients is the treatment most likely to be helpful?

Types of clinical trials: There are three phases of clinical trials in which a treatment is studied before it is eligible for approval by the FDA. Clinical trials can still be used to learn about the safety and effectiveness of many complementary therapies, even though those therapies are not subject to the same FDA regulations as drugs.

Phase I clinical trials: The purpose of a phase I study is to find the best way to give a new treatment and how much of it can be given safely. The cancer care team watches patients carefully for any harmful side effects. The treatment has been well tested in laboratory and animal studies, but the side effects in patients are not completely known. Researchers conducting the clinical trial start by giving very low doses of the drug or dietary supplement to the first patients and increasing the dose for later groups of patients until side effects appear. Although doctors are hoping to help patients, the main purpose of a phase I study is to test the safety of the drug.

Phase II clinical trials: Phase II studies are designed to see whether the treatment works. Patients are usually given the highest dose that does not cause severe side effects (determined from the phase I study) and closely observed for an effect on the cancer. The cancer care team also looks for side effects.

Phase III clinical trials: Phase III studies involve large numbers of patients—often several hundred. One group (the control group) receives the standard, or most accepted, treatment. The other group receives the new treatment. All patients in phase III studies are closely watched. The study will be stopped if the side effects of the new treatment are too severe or if one group has much better results than the other.

Relevance of clinical trial phases to complementary and alternative medicine: Most complementary mind–body methods are extremely safe. So, there is no need for a phase I study to determine how many hours of meditation or music therapy people can tolerate. At the other extreme, some alternative biologic therapies are no less toxic than chemotherapy, so phase I studies are necessary. Even though the details of clinical trials for evaluating drugs and complementary methods may differ a little, the basic principles are the same.

Informed Consent

An important part of clinical trials is a process called informed consent. In general, informed consent means that a physician or nurse must assure that the patient has been informed of the treatment or procedure and obtain the patient's signed consent before beginning diagnosis or treatment. In some cases, even a simple blood test or an injection requires written permission from the patient. In addition, medical care cannot begin unless the patient gives consent, as long as the patient is mentally and physically able to discuss his condition. If the patient is a minor, has a serious mental disability, or cannot communicate consent, then the parents, legal guardian, or person authorized by the court (usually a close family member who has reason to know what the patient would want) must give consent.

Informed consent laws apply to physicians and, increasingly, to nurses, and they vary from state to state. Some states have very specific laws governing particular situations (e.g., the issues of treatment for breast cancer or for clinical trials). Some states call only for "reasonable" information, while others require "full and complete disclosure." The patient gives consent by signing a document that names the procedures to be performed. The language of the document may be very general, stating only that the patient has been informed of the risks of the treatment and what other treatments are available, or it may be very specific, outlining in detail what the risks and other options are. The patient may be signing for one specific procedure or may give blanket approval for any procedures the health provider deems necessary.

The Placebo Effect

Placebos are sometimes used in clinical trials to test new medications or new treatments. A placebo is a substance or other kind of treatment that is designed to resemble the therapy, but is actually inactive (such as a sugar pill). Placebos are sometimes called sham treatments. Even though placebos lack chemical or other value in and of themselves, they have a very real effect in 30 to 40 percent of patients.

In order to study the benefit of a new treatment, a placebo is sometimes used to compare the new treatment's effect against no treatment. Half the people in the study are given the actual medication, and the other half receive a placebo or the current conventional treatment. A placebo is given only when there is no useful conventional treatment. If any treatments are available that might help a patient, these will be given instead of a placebo. The placebo looks, tastes, or feels just like the actual treatment. In a blind controlled study, the subjects do not know which treatment they are receiving. In a double-blind controlled study, neither the subjects nor the investigators know who receives which treatment. People who receive the placebo in medical studies play an important role because their reactions provide a baseline against which the effect of the treatment being tested can be accurately measured.

Because people do not know when they are taking a placebo, and because they believe in the treatment and in their physicians, three or four out of every ten persons will react to the placebo as though it were the active treatment. Their pain will lessen, or they will generally feel better. This change in signs or symptoms as a result of receiving a placebo is called a placebo response. Placebos can be so effective that they can actually produce unwanted side effects, including headaches, nervousness, nausea, and constipation.

A "placebo effect" is a change in a sign or symptom as a result of the placebo or patient–physician interaction. A placebo effect can occur without the presence of a placebo. The relationship between a physician and patient can have a significant effect on the patient's symptoms. This effect occurs because the patient believes in the substance, the treatment, or the physician. The patient's mind somehow influences other physiologic systems in his or her body. Those systems act to bring about helpful results.

There is no question that the placebo effect is real. It has been the subject of many careful scientific tests. There is solid evidence that the mind can have a direct effect on the physical sensations we feel in our bodies.

Scientific evidence suggests that some aspects of the placebo effect may be due to the release of endorphins in the brain. Endorphins are the body's own morphine-like painkillers. However, science is just beginning to learn exactly how the placebo effect occurs. Some scientists believe the effectiveness of some complementary and alternative therapies may be a placebo effect. The patient believed in the treatment and wanted it to work, and so it did.

The importance of the placebo effect can depend on the type of treatment being studied and its expected outcome and side effects. It is particularly important for self-reported symptoms like pain, anxiety, or nausea. For studies in which tumor regression is the main outcome, placebos are still used even though the placebo is expected to have minimal, if any, effect on cancer growth.

Anecdotal Reports

Anecdotal stories from people who claim that a complementary or alternative method cured their disease can be quite powerful, especially for people with cancer. In recent years, a number of complementary and alternative methods for treating cancer have gained widespread attention, often on the basis of anecdotal reports and testimonial stories.

Television news shows, magazines, and even product advertisements frequently carry compelling stories about people with cancer who turned to a complementary or alternative method after a conventional treatment did not work or who used an alternative method instead of conventional treatment. Because the person is alive to tell his or her story and appears to be healthy, it is implied that the complementary or alternative treatment is safe and effective, even if there is no scientific evidence to support the claim.

In the case of anecdotal reports or personal testimonials about complementary or alternative methods, it is important to remember that if something sounds too good to be true, it usually is. Sometimes the person providing the testimonial never had a biopsy to prove he or she actually had cancer. A lump caused by a noncancerous condition may go away on its own shortly after the patient is treated with an alternative therapy. If the patient mistakenly believes the lump was cancerous, he will probably incorrectly attribute its disappearance to the treatment. In other cases, people treated with both conventional and complementary therapy may attribute benefit to the complementary therapy when the conventional treatment was really what helped them.

Some people with cancer die sooner than expected and some live longer, independent of the treatment they receive. If a person seems to be surviving longer than one would expect based on his or her type and stage of cancer, it might be a result of treatment. It might also be because that person is one of the fortunate individuals who, for reasons not well understood by scientists, does better than expected. Let's consider a scenario of one hundred people with a form of cancer for which the average survival is three years after diagnosis. Of these, most will survive between one and five years after diagnosis. Some will live less than one year, and a few may live longer than five years. If one of the lucky people who survived six or seven years used a particular complementary or alternative method, he or she might attribute that good fortune to the treatment. If the person's testimonial is used in marketing the treatment, viewers might incorrectly assume that the case is typical of patients using that method. In other words, for every claim of benefit, there may be many patients who get worse but are not around to tell their stories.

Of course, the same problem could also apply to conventional treatments. The difference is that conventional treatments should not be promoted by patient testimonials. Rather, doctors evaluate conventional treatments by reading reports of clinical trial results in peer-reviewed medical journals, and these reports should include detailed statistical information on patient outcomes.

Best Case Series

Despite cautions about patient testimonials, publication of carefully documented cases of people whose response to complementary or alternative treatments is better than expected can be a valuable step toward scientific evaluation of that treatment. A common first step in evaluating an alternative therapy is collection of a best case series. The alternative provider reviews medical records of patients he or she treated, in order to identify patients whose outcomes are much better than expected. Ideally, these records should also be reviewed by a conventional cancer researcher to assure that the initial diagnosis and stage is accurate and that the tumor response is well documented. If no such cases are found, then there is little reason to continue further research on that method. If statistical methods indicate that some patients treated with that method really lived longer than would otherwise be expected, then the method might be considered promising enough to be evaluated in a randomized clinical trial. Even though a best case series might be encouraging enough to justify further research, conventional clinicians would not consider a best case series convincing enough to recommend using the treatment in practice.

If you are considering a nonconventional treatment, it is important to gather as much information as possible so that you can evaluate a given treatment's effectiveness and safety. Look for information from reputable, credible sources on its potential benefits and risks. Find out what scientific studies have been done. Complementary and alternative therapies should be evaluated by the same rigorous scientific standards as those used in conventional medicine.

In addition, any decisions about medical treatment should be made with the guidance of a health care provider. Chapter 4 will give some suggestions for speaking with your primary care provider about choosing complementary health care.

References

Arsenicum. Herbs 2000 Web site. http://www.herbs2000.com/homeopathy/arsenicum.htm. Accessed June 2, 2008.

Clinical trials: what you need to know. American Cancer Society Web site. http://www.cancer.org/docroot/ETO/content/ETO_6_3_Clinical_Trials_-_Patient_Participation.asp. Accessed June 2, 2008.

Complementary and alternative methods for cancer management. American Cancer Society Web site. http://www.cancer.org/docroot/ETO/content/ETO_5_1_Introduction.asp. Accessed June 2, 2008.

Detailed guide: cancer (general information). American Cancer Society Web site. http://www.cancer.org/docroot/CRI/CRI_2_3x.asp?dt=72. Accessed June 2, 2008.

Hede K. Chinese folk treatment reveals power of arsenic to treat cancer, new studies under way. *J Natl Cancer Inst.* 2007;99:667-668.

Hrobjartsson A, Gotzsche PC. Is the placebo powerless? Systematic review with 52 new randomized trials comparing placebo with no treatment. *J Intern Med.* 2004;256:91-100.
Comment in:
J Intern Med. 2005;257:394; author reply 395-396.

Informed consent. American Cancer Society Web site. http://www.cancer.org/docroot/ETO/content/ETO_1_2X_Informed_Consent.asp. Accessed June 2, 2008.

Kaptchuk TJ. The placebo effect in alternative medicine: can the performance of a healing ritual have clinical significance? *Ann Intern Med.* 2002;136:817-825.

Kushi LH, Byers T, Doyle C, Bandera EV, McCullough M, McTiernan A, Gansler T, Andrews KS, Thun MJ; American Cancer Society 2006 Nutrition and Physical Activity Guidelines Advisory Committee. American Cancer Society guidelines on nutrition and physical activity for cancer prevention: reducing the risk of cancer with healthy food choices and physical activity. *CA Cancer J Clin.* 2006;56:254-281.

Launso L, Drageset BJ, Fonnebo V, Jacobson JS, Haahr N, White JD, Salamonsen A, Horneber M, Egeland E. Exceptional disease courses after the use of CAM: selection, registration, medical assessment, and research. An international perspective. *J Altern Complement Med.* 2006;12:607-613.

Link J, Haggard R, Kelly K, Forrer D. Placebo/nocebo symptom reporting in a sham herbal supplement trial. *Eval Health Prof.* 2006;29:394-406.

Nahin RL. Use of the best case series to evaluate complementary and alternative therapies for cancer: a systematic review. *Semin Oncol.* 2002;29:552-562.

NCI CAM history and the role of OCCAM. National Cancer Institute Web site. http://www.cancer.gov/cam/cam_at_nci.html. Accessed June 2, 2008.

The NIH almanac: National Center For Complementary and Alternative Medicine. National Institutes of Health Web site. http://www.nih.gov/about/almanac/organization/NCCAM.htm. Accessed June 2, 2008.

Placebo effect. American Cancer Society Web site. http://www.cancer.org/docroot/ETO/content/ETO_5_3x_Placebo_Effect.asp. Accessed June 2, 2008.

US Congress, Office of Technology Assessment. *Unconventional Cancer Treatments: OTA-H-405*. Washington, DC: US Government Printing Office; 1990.

Vickers AJ. How to design a phase I trial of an anticancer botanical. *J Soc Integr Oncol.* 2006;4:46-51.

Vickers AJ. Message to complementary and alternative medicine: evidence is a better friend than power. *BMC Complement Altern Med.* 2001;1:1. Epub 2001 May 1.

Vickers AJ. Which botanicals or other unconventional anticancer agents should we take to clinical trial? *J Soc Integr Oncol.* 2007;5:125-129.

Vickers AJ, de Craen AJ. Why use placebos in clinical trials? A narrative review of the methodological literature. *J Clin Epidemiol.* 2000;53:157-161.

Vickers AJ, Kuo J, Cassileth BR. Unconventional anticancer agents: a systematic review of clinical trials. *J Clin Oncol.* 2006;24:136-140.

What is CAM? National Center for Complementary and Alternative Medicine Web site. http://nccam.nih.gov/health/whatiscam/. Accessed May 30, 2008.

Chapter Three

Regulation of Drugs and Dietary Supplements

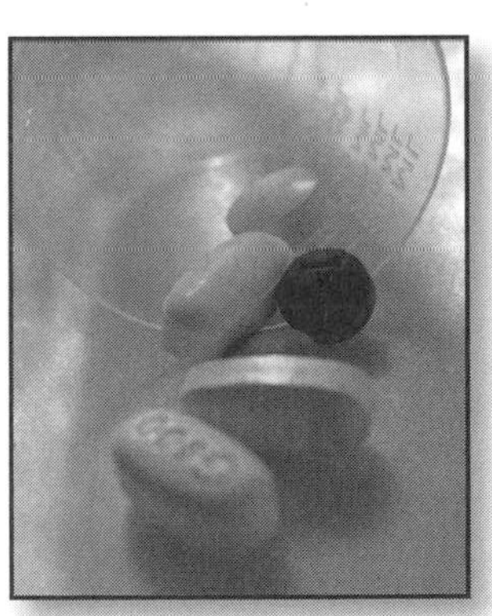

GOVERNMENT AGENCIES INFLUENCE the quality of health care in many ways. One of the most important is their influence on which products can be legally sold as drugs or dietary supplements. In this chapter, we will review some of the differences in the regulation of conventional drugs compared with that of dietary supplements. Learning more about regulatory issues can help you make informed decisions about choosing therapies, as well as providers to administer the therapies.

The History of Drug Regulation in the United States

In 1937, more than one hundred people, mostly children, died after taking Elixir Sulfanilamide, the drinkable form of a sulfa antibiotic medicine. The liquid base of Elixir Sulfanilamide was diethylene glycol, a poisonous substance that can cause kidney failure and death. Manufactured in Tennessee and sold throughout the United States, this liquid sulfa drug had never been tested for safety. By law it did not have to be tested, because at that time there were no government regulations requiring safety tests for drugs sold in the United States.

The Food and Drugs Act of 1906, the first comprehensive law governing food and drugs, had been passed in reaction to risky and misleading practices in the food and drug industries. However, it governed only the misbranding of drugs and the adulteration of food and drug products. While it mandated that drug companies disclose the contents of their products, it did not require that drugs be tested for safety, nor did it require drug companies to report information about the safety and effectiveness of drugs.

Largely as a result of the liquid sulfa disaster, Congress passed the Federal Food, Drug, and Cosmetic Act of 1938 (FDC Act). This act required that drug manufacturers establish the safety of any product that was to be marketed across state lines. It also banned false and misleading labels on food, drugs, and medical devices. Unfortunately, any drug already on the market was exempt from the new law. Manufacturers, therefore, did not have to prove the safety of existing products, which remained for sale to unknowing consumers.

Another major public health crisis convinced Congress that even tighter regulation was required to protect the American public. Thalidomide, a drug manufactured in Germany, was widely distributed in Europe in the late 1950s and early 1960s as a sedative and anti-nausea medication. Of the many pregnant women who took it, nearly four of ten delivered disfigured babies. The babies were born with deformed limbs or stumps where arms and legs should have been. The resulting publicity was worldwide, as were demands for protection against harmful drug products.

Tennessee's popular Senator Estes Kefauver led the way, chairing a committee to investigate the American pharmaceutical industry. The resulting Kefauver Harris Amendments, or the Drug Amendments Act of 1962, required that any drug marketed in the

United States be proven safe and effective for its stated purpose. The U.S. Food and Drug Administration (FDA) was given the authority to enforce the regulations and serve as a watchdog over the drug industry. This law amended the FDC Act and applied to any new drug and any drug sold after 1938.

However, thousands of drugs were already available for sale over the counter throughout the United States. In response to the Drug Amendments of 1962, the FDA established the Drug Efficacy Study Implementation (DESI) program. The DESI program reviewed the drug products approved between 1938 and 1962 for effectiveness. As a result of this two-decades-long process, more than 3,400 drugs with over 16,000 separate therapeutic claims were evaluated by using the criteria of "substantial evidence" for effectiveness. In September 1981, regulatory action had been taken on 90 percent of all DESI products. By 1984, final action had been taken on 3,443 products. Of those, 2,225 were found to be effective, 1,051 were found not effective, and 167 were pending.

Drug Development in the United States

In the decades following the 1962 Drug Amendments, the FDA refined the regulatory process for drug development and the marketing of foods in the United States. Drugs and foods are regulated in different ways by the FDA. Under the FDC Act, drugs must be shown to be both safe and effective before they are marketed to the public. The law specifies that a new drug cannot be approved by the FDA unless there is "substantial evidence" from well-controlled studies that it is safe and effective to diagnose, treat, cure, or prevent a specific disease or medical condition. Studies must be conducted by qualified experts who, on the basis of the data, can fairly and responsibly conclude that the drug will do as claimed when used as prescribed, recommended, or suggested in the labeling or proposed labeling.

Animal studies are required before the drug can be tested in humans. To conduct a clinical research study on an unapproved drug, a company or individual researcher must submit to the FDA an Investigational New Drug Application (NDA). If the application meets the FDA's requirements, experimental clinical research can begin. Small clinical trials are usually done initially to determine a safe dose to be used in later studies. Then one or more large, randomized clinical trials are conducted to demonstrate the drug's safety and effectiveness for its intended use. The FDA must review these studies and decide whether to authorize the use of the drug. The FDA has the authority to prohibit interstate marketing of unsafe or ineffective drugs and to sanction manufacturers, promoters, and distributors who violate the law.

The law is designed to protect the consumer by making sure that a high standard of evidence has been met. Anecdotal evidence, or testimonials, from physicians or patients who have used the drug under study is not enough to meet the FDA's definition of safety and effectiveness. Ruling in a case involving the FDC Act, one judge put it this way:

> *It is simply not enough to show that some people, even experts, have a belief in safety and effectiveness. A reasonable number of Americans will sincerely attest to the worth of almost any product or even idea. To remove the aberrations in uniformity, which can result from a well staged "swearing match," the law requires more. Indeed, it has been heretofore held that the purpose of the normal inquiry is not to determine safety and effectiveness at all, but to ascertain the drug's general reputation in the scientific community for such characteristics. It is certain that a conflicting reputation is insufficient to establish general recognition. Therefore, what is required is more than belief, even by an expert; it is a general recognition based upon substantial scientific evidence as delineated in the regulatory guidelines.* (United States v. Articles of Food and Drug, 1974)

The FDC Act recognizes that there are different levels of acceptable risk for drugs that have a benefit in treating severe illnesses such as cancer. However, the benefits must outweigh the risks. For example, some cancer drugs have side effects so serious that the FDA would not approve them for use in treating less severe illnesses. Side effects that are permitted for a chemotherapy drug would clearly be unacceptable for a drug to treat the common cold. But because the drugs' benefits to cancer patients are considered greater than the risks, the FDA has approved the drugs for that use.

The FDC Act also allows drugs that are being studied in clinical trials, but are not yet approved by the FDA, to be made available to certain patients who have life-threatening or other serious diseases that may be helped by the drug. The purpose of this rule is "to facilitate the availability of promising new drugs to desperately ill patients as early in the drug development process as possible, before general marketing begins, and to obtain additional data on the drug's safety and effectiveness" (US Department of Health and Human Services, 2008). The rule permits eligible patients not enrolled in the clinical trials to receive drugs that are in phase III clinical trials (the final stage of study) or, under certain circumstances, even drugs in phase II of trials. The FDA requires manufacturers and researchers to provide a treatment protocol and experimental data on the drug before it grants approval. This is referred to as emergency, or compassionate, use of an investigational drug.

When the FDA finally approves a drug for marketing, it approves the product for specific uses that were studied in the clinical trials. The approved indications for use must appear on the printed materials packaged with the drug, along with the appropriate dose, how and when it should be administered, information on adverse reactions experienced during the drug's development, and any warning statements or contraindications for use. However, health professionals may prescribe the drug for other medical conditions if, in their professional opinion, the medical situation warrants it. This practice is referred to as off-label use of a drug. It is done when there is sufficient scientific evidence to believe the drug will be effective in treating the unapproved conditions.

Regulation of Food and Dietary Supplements

The regulations for food safety differ significantly from those for drugs. The category of foods includes conventional foods (such as cheese, processed foods, chewing gum, tea, and sodas), food additives (anything added to conventional foods, including spices, flavors, colors, and preservatives), "Foods for Special Dietary Uses" (such as infant formula and medical diets), and dietary supplements.

Foods are required to be properly labeled and not adulterated or misbranded. Food labels also must follow a specific format that provides nutrient content information for the consumer. The Nutrition Labeling and Education Act (NLEA) of 1990 authorized foods to carry nutrient content claims ("contains calcium," "fat free," or "lite") and health claims. Health claims (for example, "folate may reduce the chance of pregnant women delivering an infant with neural tube defects") must be supported by evidence that is under "significant substantial agreement." These claims generally require information from in vitro, animal, and clinical studies to be submitted to the FDA, and the FDA must approve claims before the product is marketed.

In addition, a key part of ensuring the safety of foods is that any new food additive must be preapproved by the FDA. This means it must satisfy requirements of scientific testing to ensure its safety before it can be used.

How the Regulation of Dietary Supplements Has Changed

Dietary supplements have received a tremendous amount of attention over the past two decades. Dietary supplements are sold in grocery stores, health food shops, drug stores, national discount chain stores, mail-order catalogs, and through television programs, the Internet, and direct sales. But what exactly is a dietary supplement?

For many years, most people (including most health care professionals) thought of dietary supplements as products intended to provide essential nutrients, such as vitamins, minerals, and protein. For example, if you thought you weren't getting enough vitamins from conventional foods, you might supplement your diet with vitamin pills, which would be an example of a dietary supplement. In fact, vitamins are still the type of supplement purchased most in this country.

In 1994 Congress passed the Dietary Supplement Health and Education Act (DSHEA).

DSHEA broadened the definition of a dietary supplement, changing it to "… a product (other than tobacco) that is intended to supplement the diet that bears or contains one or more of the following dietary ingredients: a vitamin, a mineral, an herb or other botanical, an amino acid [the individual building blocks of protein], a dietary substance for use by man to supplement the diet by increasing the total daily intake, or a concentrate, metabolite, constituent, extract, or combinations of these ingredients" (US Food and Drug Administration Web site, 1995). This broadened definition includes ordinary multivitamins (which consist of essential substances that are part of a usual diet), as well as products like shark cartilage extract or echinacea (purple coneflower) that are not ordinarily considered essential nutrients or typical foods.

The change in definition was not the result of a scientific consensus of biological or chemical similarity among vitamin C, shark cartilage, and purple coneflower. Rather, this is a legal definition, by which Congress was instructing the FDA in how to regulate these products.

As a result of the DSHEA, ingredients used in dietary supplements are no longer subject to the premarket safety evaluations required of other new food ingredients, such as "food additives," or for new uses of old food ingredients. However, they must meet the requirements of other safety provisions.

The DSHEA amends the adulteration provisions of the FDC Act. Under the DSHEA, a dietary supplement is impure if it or one of its ingredients presents "a significant or unreasonable risk of illness or injury" (FDA Web site, 1995) when used as directed on the label or under normal conditions of use. A dietary supplement that contains an additional "new dietary ingredient" is said to be impure when there is inadequate information to ensure the new ingredient will not cause a significant or unreasonable risk for illness or injury. Supplement manufacturers must notify the FDA at least seventy-five days before marketing products containing new dietary ingredients and provide the agency with safety documentation for those ingredients.

Any interested party, including a manufacturer of a dietary supplement, may petition the FDA to issue an order prescribing the conditions of use under which a new dietary ingredient will reasonably be expected to be safe. The Secretary of the Department of Health and Human Services may also declare that a dietary supplement or dietary ingredient poses an imminent hazard to public health or safety. However, as with any other food product, it is the manufacturer's responsibility to ensure that the dietary supplement is safe and labeled accurately and truthfully before marketing.

Botanicals as Medicines

The term dietary supplement also includes botanical products. Botanicals include products such as garlic, ginger, ginkgo biloba, St. John's wort, and echinacea. A nationwide survey conducted by the Centers for Disease Control and Prevention in 2002 found that about 19 percent of

31,044 adults surveyed used natural products (mostly botanicals) as complementary or alternative medicine. Botanicals have a long history of use in virtually every ancient culture. In many developing areas of the world, herbal remedies are the only medicines available to treat ailments of all kinds.

In the earliest days, herbs were sometimes chosen for medicinal purposes by what is now called the doctrine of signatures. If a plant's leaf was heart shaped, for example, it would be used to treat heart ailments. If its flower was red, it would be used to treat blood problems, and so on. Today, of course, we know that the chemical makeup of some herbs, not their shape or color, makes them useful as a medication. Indeed, many chemicals taken from herbs have become modern drugs. At the beginning of the twentieth century, the majority of the drugs used in the United States were from natural sources, including plants.

Botanicals may be whole plants or plant parts, including roots, stems, flowers, leaves, pollen, and juices. The term herbal refers specifically to the leafy part of a plant. Botanicals are made up of many chemicals, some helpful and others dangerous. Researchers and manufacturers who develop and produce conventional drugs from plant sources seek to isolate the beneficial substances so the patient can avoid any harmful ones initially present in the plant material.

Botanicals are regulated by their "intended use," as determined from their label and labeling. This means that the manufacturer's intent is determined through the claims made (or not made) about the product. Products that are intended to prevent or treat disease are classified as drugs. Cascara and Senna are examples of over-the-counter botanical drugs that were on the market prior to the 1938 FDC Act. Others are licensed biological products, such as allergenic vaccines. Still others are sold as devices, such as adhesives, poultices, and dental materials.

Botanicals are mostly sold as drugs in countries other than the United States. Although some countries have different regulatory requirements for botanicals that have been used traditionally as drugs in that country (such as in Traditional Chinese Medicine), newer botanicals are often required to undergo the same rigorous testing as other types of drugs. In some countries, health professionals are trained in prescribing botanicals.

In the United States, botanicals are mostly sold as foods or dietary supplements and are often self-prescribed by consumers, some of whom are poorly informed regarding safety, effectiveness, and potential interactions with other supplements or conventional drugs.

Manufacturers are required to state on the label the part of the plant the ingredient comes from and list the ingredients in descending order of strength and by the ingredient's common name. Dietary ingredients that are not present in significant amounts do not need to be listed. Manufacturers must also put the company's name, address, product batch and lot numbers, and expiration date on the label. Different parts of a plant and different preparation methods can have different effects. For example, dandelion root is a laxative, while dandelion leaves contain a diuretic. Consumers should read the product label to make sure they know the specific forms of the botanicals they're purchasing.

How Dietary Supplements Can Be Marketed

Under the DSHEA, retailers and distributors of dietary supplements are permitted to make certain materials available to help inform consumers about the supplements' health-related benefits. The materials must be created by a third party and must meet certain guidelines. They cannot be false or misleading and cannot promote a specific brand of supplement. The literature must be displayed separately from the dietary supplements themselves and cannot have other information attached, such as product promotional literature.

The labeling of the dietary supplements themselves can bear four types of claims: nutritional claims, claims of well-being, health claims, and structure or function claims. Dietary supplements cannot claim to diagnose, prevent, treat, or cure a specific disease. If a label on a dietary supplement does make such a claim, such as "cures cancer," the product is being sold illegally as a drug.

Nutritional claims are statements about the effects of dietary supplements, vitamins, and minerals on known nutrient deficiency diseases (for example, "vitamin C prevents scurvy"). These statements are permissible as long as the statements disclose the prevalence of the disease in the United States. Such claims do not have to be preapproved by the FDA.

Claims of *well-being* are just that: they are claims such as "makes you feel better." These claims also are not preapproved by the agency.

Products may carry *health claims,* which mean that the product reduces risk for some health problems. Such claims do require testing and approval by the FDA.

The most controversial and confusing is the claim that a dietary supplement or ingredient can affect the *structure* or *function* of the body. Manufacturers are allowed to describe the product's effects on the mechanism of action ("works as an antioxidant"), cellular structure ("helps membrane stability"), the body's physiology ("promotes normal urinary flow"), or chemical or laboratory parameters ("supports normal blood glucose"). The rule permits claims of maintenance ("maintains a healthy circulatory system"), other nondisease claims ("helps you relax"), and claims for common conditions and symptoms related to life stages, such as for symptoms of premenstrual syndrome, menopause, adolescence, and aging. Serious conditions associated with aging (such as osteoporosis), menopause, and adolescence are treated as diseases, and are outside the scope of what a dietary supplement can claim to treat.

It is easy for consumers to misunderstand or misinterpret structure or function claims. Many people assume that a statement such as "maintains a healthy prostate gland" means the product has been proven to prevent or relieve prostate diseases such as prostate cancer. In fact, no such evidence is required of the company selling a supplement bearing this information on its packaging.

In the case of claims of well-being, nutritional claims, and structure–function claims, manufacturers must include a disclaimer on the label: *"This statement has not been evaluated by the Food and Drug Administration. This product is not intended to diagnose, treat, cure, or prevent any disease."* The claims on the label, claims in all other materials accompanying the product, and all advertising and promotion must be "truthful and not misleading."

Regarding effectiveness, only those drug products that are approved for safety and effectiveness can claim effectiveness. Some drugs, such as homeopathic drugs and drugs that were on the U.S. market prior to the 1938 FDC Act, are not approved for safety or effectiveness. Whereas these drugs may carry drug claims, they cannot be advertised as being approved for safety and effectiveness. The term effectiveness does not generally apply to food products, even though some dietary supplements, such as essential vitamins and minerals, may be effective in preventing deficiencies. Even health claims are usually couched in terms of prevention or risk reduction, rather than effectiveness. The Federal Trade Commission (FTC) requires proof in the form of adequate scientific studies before a drug can claim to be effective.

Signs of Possible Fraudulent Products

- The supplement is promoted with terms such as miracle cure, breakthrough, or new discovery.
- The supplement is claimed to have benefits but no side effects.
- Proponents claim the supplement can be used for a wide variety of unrelated illnesses.
- Claims that the treatment is safe and effective are based solely on testimonials.
- The treatment is supposedly based on a secret ingredient or method.

The Issue of Quality Control

In an industry with rapidly growing numbers of products, there is high potential for a dietary supplement to lack quality control in manufacturing. The FDA, for example, found that some manufacturers were buying plant ingredients without testing to be sure what they ordered was what they received and that the ingredients were free of contaminants.

A number of studies undertaken since the DSHEA was passed in 1994 have documented serious lapses in quality of dietary supplements. Analyses of some supplements have shown that the amount of key ingredient they contain may be far less or far more than the amount promised on the label. Some were found to contain prescription drugs or toxic substances not disclosed on the label. In other cases, herbs were misidentified and mislabeled, so that consumers expecting one herb actually received a different one. In one study of sixty-four ginseng products on the market, researchers found that 60 percent of these products contained cheaper herbs and were so watered down that they were virtually worthless. Quality deficiencies have led to well-documented cases of illness and even death in some cases.

Labeling regulations enacted on March 23, 1999, require the proper identification of ingredients contained in a product. However, if a product is considerably less expensive than a competing brand, it should be suspect and has probably been made with inferior ingredients.

The U.S. Pharmacopeia (USP) establishes standards for the strength, quality, and purity of drugs and dietary supplements for human and veterinary use. The USP works closely with the FDA, the pharmaceutical industry, and health care professionals to create reliable standards for drugs, vitamins and minerals, and herbal products. The standards focus on strength, quality, purity, packaging, and labeling. A USP notation on the label of a dietary supplement indicates that the product complies with standards established by the USP.

In addition to changing the way dietary supplements were regulated, the 1994 DSHEA authorized the FDA to regulate dietary supplement quality. Development of these regulations—called Good Manufacturing Practices (GMPs)—has been a very lengthy process. The FDA released a proposal for dietary supplement GMPs in 2003, and in June 2007, the interim final rules were announced. After a period of public feedback and any resulting revisions, the final standards began to be phased in 2008. Large companies that manufacture dietary supplements were required to follow the rules by June 2008. Medium-sized companies are given an extra year, and small companies get an extra two years before adopting the new GMPs.

According to the FDA, the purpose of the GMPs is "...to ensure that dietary supplements do NOT have wrong ingredients, too much or too little of a dietary ingredient, improper packaging, improper labeling, contamination problems due to natural toxins, bacteria, pesticides, glass, lead, or other substances" (Food and Drug Administration Web site, 2007).

The GMPs scheduled to take effect by 2010 include provisions related to the design and construction of physical plants, cleaning, proper manufacturing operations, quality control procedures, testing final products or incoming and in-process materials, handling consumer complaints, and maintaining records.

Assessing Dietary Supplement Safety

There are differences in how safety is defined for drugs as compared with dietary supplements. A drug is essentially considered unsafe until the company selling the drug can prove to the FDA that it is safe and medically useful. This requirement is imposed on the pharmaceutical industry to help protect patients from unsafe and ineffective drugs.

In contrast, dietary supplements are assumed safe for the general population's use. The regulatory term for this concept is "Generally Recognized as Safe" or "GRAS." Under the 1994

DSHEA, "safe" means that the ingredients in a dietary supplement do not present a "significant or unreasonable risk" of causing illness or injury when the supplement is used as directed on the label or under normal conditions of use if there are no directions on the label.

The assessment of dietary supplement safety, however, is not straightforward. For approved drugs, the manufacturer is required by the FDC Act to report all adverse events (AEs). An adverse event is any negative experience in a person using the product, including new or worsening symptoms. For foods and dietary supplements, AE reporting by manufacturers has been voluntary and not a requirement. If a supplement manufacturer learned of serious or even fatal adverse effects in people using its product, it was not required to notify the FDA. If the FDA has good reason to be concerned about a product's safety, it can obtain such reports by suing the supplement manufacturer. In several such cases, court records have documented examples in which a supplement manufacturer was aware of deadly adverse events but continued to sell the product and provided no warning to the public, health care providers, or the government.

Consumers and health professionals are encouraged to report AEs to the MedWatch program (see page 39), but studies suggest that only a small fraction are reported. And whereas the FDA can assess the AEs reported to the MedWatch program, there is no information as to how many individuals may have purchased the product and what their experience was—information that is available for prescription drugs. For example, if there are ten reports of adverse events for a particular dietary supplement, it is unknown if the event occurred in ten of one hundred or ten of one million users.

The FDA has taken steps to improve this situation, however. Starting in 2008, the supplement industry has been required to report all serious adverse events. And as discussed earlier, the Good Manufacturing Practices, or GMPs, for the supplement industry began to be implemented in 2008.

Although the new regulations will unquestionably improve the safety of these products, consumers should realize that there is still a big difference between safety regulations for dietary supplements and drugs. The new GMPs will, for example, help keep supplements free from dangerous levels of pesticides, lead, and bacteria. But there is still no requirement for the supplement industry to conduct clinical studies to test the safety of their products.

Balancing Consumer Choice and Protection

In recent years, a number of legal challenges have been launched in the courts on behalf of people with cancer with regard to laws and regulations designed to protect patients from untested drugs. These cases charge that the laws actually limit cancer patients' access to complementary and alternative treatments and deny the patients freedom of choice in medical care. There are two opposing forces at work: those who defend the laws as consumer protection and those who want to change the laws to allow consumers greater access to complementary and alternative products. Balancing choice with protection poses difficult challenges. It can also be difficult to know whether current regulations reflect the wishes of the American public. A nationwide survey conducted during the late 1990s found that 80 percent of those surveyed supported "giving the FDA authority to allow new supplements to be sold only if the safety of the supplements has been tested by the FDA" (*Arch Intern Med.* 2001;161:809) but only 37 percent believed that supplements are adequately tested.

We are currently in a "let the buyer beware" mode when it comes to nutritional dietary supplements and herbal products. To this day, there is no requirement for proof of safety, accurate labeling, or proof of a health benefit for dietary supplements sold in the United States. Congress has seen the need to protect the public against harmful prescription medications, but this protection is not extended to dietary supplements sold directly to consumers.

While some members of Congress viewed the DSHEA as an opportunity to pass such protective legislation, a multimillion-dollar effort by the dietary supplement industry resulted in a scaled-down law. That legislation protected thousands of vitamins, herbs, minerals, and other food supplements already on the market from being reviewed. The regulation gives the FDA permission to stop production of a product only when the FDA proves that the product is dangerous to the health of Americans. Manufacturers still are not required to show that their products are safe or effective prior to marketing.

While Congress has limited the FDA's regulatory power over the dietary supplement industry, other government agencies administer laws that apply to the sale of nutritional supplements and herbal remedies. The U.S. Postal Service controls products marketed through the mail. From time to time, it has challenged products accompanied by remarkable claims of cures for cancer and other diseases. The FTC regulates the advertising of food, cosmetics, nonprescription products, and some other health-related goods and services that are sold across state lines. Internet marketing is also regulated by the FTC. In addition to the federal government, individual states have regulatory powers through licensing laws. State boards can regulate the practice of the healing arts, including the licensing and scope of practice for health professionals, conventional practitioners, and "alternative" practitioners. A few states have new laws regulating alternative and complementary therapies and their use by physicians.

But the public still has limited protection against the marketing of products that often promise much and produce little if any benefit. Indeed, some products marketed in health food stores have recently been removed from shelves only after serious harm and even death from those products were reported.

Until Congress passes useful legislation, the challenge to consumers is to determine which products are safe and which are not. The American Cancer Society advises people living with cancer and other health care consumers to read labels carefully and consult with physicians before buying herbal medicines and food supplements. Just because a product is labeled "natural" does not mean that it is safe.

Using Dietary Supplements Safely

Thousands of complaints of adverse effects of herbs have been reported to the FDA, and there have been hundreds of deaths reported from the use of botanicals. Many botanicals contain ingredients that can cause side effects, hazardous drug interactions, and allergic reactions. For example, ginkgo biloba, garlic, feverfew, vitamin E, and ginger can all thin blood; if they are consumed by people who are also taking blood-thinning drugs such as warfarin, heparin, or aspirin, these dietary supplements may cause excessive bleeding. St. John's wort has recently been found to interfere with some prescription drugs, such as irinotecan, indinavir, digoxin, warfarin, and cyclosporine, as well as some birth control pills and antidepressants. Taking combinations of dietary supplements could be even more dangerous, as that can magnify the effect of a single dietary supplement. In addition, if someone who is using medication to control diabetes takes ginseng supplements, his or her blood sugar levels may fall dangerously low.

The possibility of drug–supplement interactions is so high that many cancer experts recommend that patients avoid taking dietary supplements while undergoing chemotherapy. The same advice holds for patients receiving radiation therapy because some dietary supplements make the skin sensitive to light and cause severe reactions to radiation. A number of ingredients in supplements can produce severe changes in blood pressure and other dangerous interactions with anesthetics and, therefore, should not be taken before surgery. In fact, the American Society of Anesthesiologists advises that patients stop taking herbal medications at least two to three weeks before surgery to allow enough time for the herbals to clear from the body. Patients who do not have enough time to stop taking herbal medicines before surgery should bring the product to the hospital to show the anesthesiologist.

The effects of dietary supplements also depend on the dose of the herb or vitamin. In this case, more is not better. The idea that if a little amount of a vitamin or mineral is good, then a megadose ought to do wonders is not valid. Orthomolecular therapy, the idea of using huge doses of vitamins to attack disease, is not supported by the vast majority of scientific research on this topic. In fact, large doses of some vitamins can have serious toxic effects. Recent studies have suggested that high doses of beta carotene may increase the risk for lung cancer among smokers and that vitamin E supplements may increase the risk for lung cancer and heart disease. Antioxidants may interact adversely with some chemotherapy drugs, although no definitive studies have been done on the long-term effects of combining chemotherapy drugs and antioxidants in humans.

Many people are still convinced that megadoses of vitamin C can cure colds, although many good scientific studies have disproven that idea. One should be forewarned that megadoses of nutrients to treat or prevent illness can be harmful, even toxic. Megadoses of the fat-soluble vitamins A, D, and K can easily reach toxic levels.

Because botanicals have an impact on a variety of systems in the human body, they present a potential danger by affecting the way drugs exert their activity on the body, either by increasing the drug's activity or by blocking it. Drug companies do not usually conduct research on such supplement–drug interactions, and herb manufacturers generally do not have the resources or the desire to do that type of research. So consumers themselves must search out information about possibly dangerous interactions.

Buyer Beware

Consumers should be aware of the ingredients in herbal medicines and dietary supplements they take. To help protect consumers, the FDA recommends that consumers consider these suggestions:

- Look for products with the USP notation, indicating that the manufacturer of the product followed standards set by the U.S. Pharmacopoeia in formulating the product.
- Realize that the use of the term "natural" on an herbal product is no guarantee that the product is safe. Poisonous mushrooms, for example, are natural but not safe.
- Take into account the name and reputation of the manufacturer or distributor. Herbal products and other dietary supplements made by nationally known food or drug manufacturers are more likely to have been made under tight quality controls because these companies have a reputation to uphold.
- Write to the manufacturer for more information than is included on the label of the supplement. Ask about the company's manufacturing practices and the quality-control conditions under which the product was made.

Guidelines for the Safe Use of Dietary Supplements

Rule One: Investigate before you buy or use. There are many resources in libraries and on the Internet. However, much of this information is produced by promoters and can contain biased or incorrect information. Rely on materials from trained experts or government agencies.

Rule Two: Check with your physician before you try a dietary supplement. While your physician might or might not be thoroughly versed in all the products available, he or she can prevent you from making a dangerous mistake.

Rule Three: Do not take any self-prescribed remedy instead of the medicine prescribed by your physician without discussing it with him or her first.

Rule Four: Introduce one product at a time. Be alert to any negative effects you experience while taking the product. Any product that produces a rash, sleeplessness, restlessness, anxiety, gastrointestinal disturbances (nausea, vomiting, diarrhea, or constipation), or severe headache should immediately be stopped and the reaction should be reported to your physician.

Rule Five: During pregnancy or if you are breastfeeding, avoid any dietary supplements not prescribed by a licensed physician. Few, if any, of these products have been studied for safety, and their effects on a growing fetus are largely unknown.

Rule Six: Do not depend on any nonprescription product to cure cancer or any other serious disease. Regardless of the claims you may hear, if it sounds too good to be true, it probably is.

Rule Seven: Never give a product to a child under the age of eighteen without consulting your physician. A child's body metabolizes nutrients and drugs differently from an adult's body, and the effects of many products in children are not known.

Rule Eight: Always follow the dosage recommendations on the label. Overdose can be deadly. Do not take a dietary supplement for any longer than experts recommend.

Rule Nine: Try to avoid mixtures. The more ingredients, the greater the possibility for harmful effects.

Reporting Adverse Reactions

Health care consumers have an obligation to share information about any adverse reactions they may have when taking dietary supplements. If you or someone in your family suffers serious harm or illness that you think is related to the use of a supplement, first call your physician or other health care provider. In addition to providing treatment, your physician can report the adverse reaction to the FDA by calling **800-FDA-1088** or going to the FDA's MedWatch Web site at **www.fda.gov/medwatch/report/hcp.htm**. You may also call the toll-free number yourself or go to the consumer page on the MedWatch Web site at **www.fda.gov/medwatch/report/consumer/consumer.htm**. In addition to reporting the adverse reaction to the FDA, you should notify the manufacturer of the product listed on the label and the store where you bought the product. When reporting to the FDA, you will be asked to provide several pieces of information:

- the name, address, and telephone number of the person who got sick
- the name and address of the physician who provided medical care
- a description of the problem
- the name of the product and the name of the store where it was purchased

The MedWatch program is designed to gather information about and monitor medical products that cause serious adverse events. The FDA considers an adverse event serious if it causes death, a life-threatening situation, admission to a hospital or a longer-than-expected hospital stay, permanent disability, a birth defect, or medical or surgical care to prevent permanent impairment or damage.

In 1993, the FDA established the Special Nutritionals Adverse Event Monitoring System. The system maintains computer records of adverse events associated with the use of dietary supplements, infant formulas, and medical foods. MedWatch is one source of reports on adverse reactions to these special nutritionals. Other sources are letters and phone calls from consumers and health care professionals; FDA field offices; and other federal, state, and local public health agencies.

References

Anesthesiologists warn: if you're taking herbal products, tell your doctor before surgery. American Society of Anesthesiologists Web site. http://www.asahq.org/patientEducation/herbal.htm. Accessed April 20, 2008. Content no longer available.

Ang-Lee MK, Moss J, Yuan CS. Herbal medicines and perioperative care. *JAMA*. 2001;286:208-216.

Anthony S. Combating deception in dietary supplement advertising. Federal Trade Commission Web site. http://www.ftc.gov/speeches/anthony/dssp2.shtm. Accessed June 3, 2008.

Bjelakovic G, Gluud C. Surviving antioxidant supplements. *J Natl Cancer Inst.* 2007;99:742-743.

Bjelakovic G, Nikolova D, Lotte Gluud L, Simonetti RG, Gluud C. Mortality in randomized trials of antioxidant supplements for primary and secondary prevention. *JAMA.* 2007;297:842-857.

Bjelakovic G, Nikolova D, Simonetti RG, Gluud C. Antioxidant supplements for prevention of gastrointestinal cancers: a systematic review and meta-analysis. *Lancet.* 2004;364:1219-1228.

Blendon RJ, DesRoches CM, Benson JM, Brodie M, Altman D. Americans' views of the use and regulation of dietary supplements. *Arch Intern Med.* 2001;161:805-810.

Borchers AT, Hagie F, Keen CL, Gershwin ME. The history and contemporary challenges of the U.S. Food and Drug Administration. *Clin Ther.* 2007;29:1-16.

Botanical dietary supplements: background information. Office of Dietary Supplements Web site. http://ods.od.nih.gov/factsheets/BotanicalBackground.asp. Accessed June 3, 2008.

Center for Food Safety and Applied Nutrition. Dietary supplement current good manufacturing practices (CGMPs) and interim final rule (IFR) facts. June 25, 2007. US Food and Drug Administration Web site. http://www.cfsan.fda.gov/~dms/dscgmps6.html. Accessed June 3, 2008.

Center for Food Safety and Applied Nutrition. Dietary Supplement Health and Education Act of 1994. December 1, 1995. US Food and Drug Administration Web site. http://www.cfsan.fda.gov/~dms/dietsupp.html. Accessed June 3, 2008.

Consumer update: final rule promotes safe use of dietary supplements. June 22, 2007. US Food and Drug Administration Web site. http://www.fda.gov/consumer/updates/dietarysupps062207.html. Accessed June 3, 2008.

FDA history. US Food and Drug Administration Web site. http://www.fda.gov/oc/history/default.htm. Accessed June 3, 2008.

Fontanarosa PB, Rennie D, DeAngelis CD. The need for regulation of dietary supplements—lessons from ephedra. *JAMA.* 2003;289:1568-1570. Epub 2003 Mar 10.

Hamilton D. A brief history of the Center for Drug Evaluation and Research. US Food and Drug Administration Web site. http://www.fda.gov/cder/about/history/Histext.htm. Accessed June 5, 2008.

Kaye AD, Kucera I, Sabar R. Perioperative anesthesia clinical considerations of alternative medicines. *Anesthesiol Clin North America.* 2004;22:125-139.

Kurtzweil P. An FDA guide to dietary supplements. US Food and Drug Administration Web site. http://www.fda.gov/fdac/features/1998/598_guid.html. Accessed June 3, 2008.

Labriola D, Livingston R. Possible interactions between dietary antioxidants and chemotherapy. *Oncology (Williston Park).* 1999;13:1003-1008; discussion 1008, 1011-1012.

Melethil S. Proposed rule: current good manufacturing practice in manufacturing, packing, or holding dietary ingredients and dietary supplements. *Life Sci.* 2006;78:2049-2053. Epub 2006 Mar 3.

Selected recent court decisions: third-party reimbursement-Laetrile treatment-Free v. Travelers Insurance Co. *Am J Law Med.* 1983;9:103-116.

Slatore CG, Littman AJ, Au DH, Satia JA, White E. Long-term use of supplemental multivitamins, vitamin C, vitamin E, and folate does not reduce the risk of lung cancer. *Am J Respir Crit Care Med.* 2008;177:524-530.

Sparreboom A, Cox MC, Acharya MR, Figg WD. Herbal remedies in the United States: potential adverse interactions with anticancer agents. *J Clin Oncol.* 2004;22:2489-2503.

United States v. Articles of Food and Drug, 372 F. Supp. 915, 920-921 (N.D.Ga. 1974).

US Congress, Office of Technology Assessment. *Unconventional Cancer Treatments: OTA-H-405.* Washington, DC: US Government Printing Office; 1990.

US Department of Health and Human Services. Treatment use of an investigational new drug. 21CFR312.34. http://www.accessdata.fda.gov/scripts/cdrh/cfdocs/cfcfr/CFRSearch.cfm?FR=312.34. Revised April 1, 2008. Accessed November 6, 2008.

The use of complementary and alternative medicine in the United States. National Center for Complementary and Alternative Medicine Web site. http://nccam.nih.gov/news/camsurvey_fs1.htm#domain. Accessed June 3, 2008.

Chapter Four

Guidelines for Using Complementary and Alternative Therapies

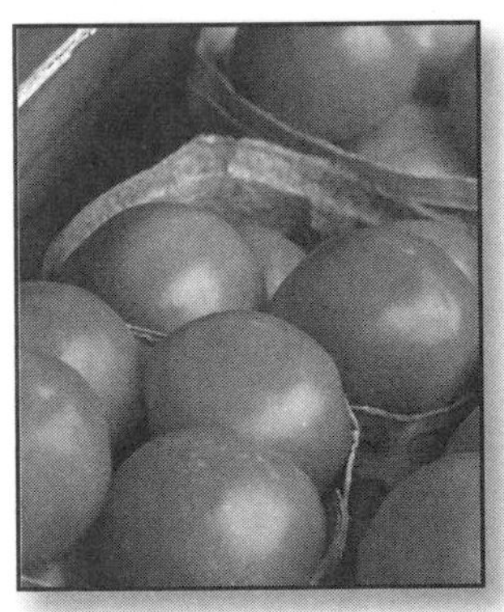

ISN'T THE MOST OBVIOUS WISH OF ALL PEOPLE with cancer to have their cancer disappear permanently and for their health to return to what it was before diagnosis? Sometimes this is possible. There have been substantial advances in conventional cancer care during the past few decades, and more people are cured every year. But conventional oncology is still far from perfect. And conventional treatments often involve temporary or permanent side effects.

Are there any complementary methods that could improve your odds of cure, help you live longer, or keep cancer from recurring? According to some recent studies, a healthful diet and being physically active might help some forms of cancer from recurring, though most of the research so far is on breast cancer and colon cancer. A few supplements might also help. For example, preliminary studies suggest that flaxseed can slow the growth of prostate cancer.

There is very little evidence that most of the therapies described in this book will help you live longer. This does not mean that some aren't worth trying, especially if they are safe and affordable. But the main reason to consider complementary methods is that they might help you feel better. They might help relieve some symptoms or help you cope with them and improve your overall physical, emotional, or spiritual health.

Some proponents of alternative therapies claim that they can cure cancer. Unfortunately, most such claims are untrue. Even in those cases where not enough is known to definitively state that the claims are false, they are very unlikely to be true.

Why We Don't Believe in Alternative Cures

Some people believe that the "medical establishment," including the American Cancer Society, is hiding an alternative cancer cure. This is not the case. Check the obituary section of any newspaper, university alumni magazine, or medical journal, and you will find doctors, including oncologists, who died of cancer. Overall, cancer does not develop in doctors quite as often as it occurs in people in other occupations because doctors are less likely to smoke. But you don't have to look very hard to find reports of oncologists who died of cancer. Their parents, spouses, and children also die of cancer. Do you really believe that all those oncologists would be willing to sacrifice their lives and the lives of their loved ones when they could have been cured by one of the alternative therapies that are easily found on the Internet?

Many people with cancer *are* cured. Some forms of cancer, such as childhood leukemia, some forms of lymphoma, and testicular cancer, are more responsive to available conventional treatment and more likely to be cured. Cancer is not a single disease, so there is no single cure, nor is there likely to be one. Cancer is actually a group of related diseases. Similarly, there are many, many infectious diseases. Some are curable with antibiotics, some are preventable with vaccines, and some are neither preventable nor curable. And, every year, treatment is improved and the prognosis improves for more kinds of infections and more kinds of cancer.

But, some people say, what would the American Cancer Society and the National Cancer Institute do if there really was a cure for cancer? Think of the March of Dimes, which originally collected money for research on a polio vaccine. After a vaccine was developed and shown to be effective, the March of Dimes turned their attention to preventing birth defects and premature birth.

In addition, the American Cancer Society pays a great deal of attention to the prevention of cancer. So, why would we be trying to prevent cancer at the same time we're hiding the cure?

Some people believe that even if the medical establishment is not really hiding "the alternative cure," it is too narrow-minded to recognize that the cure exists. Some doctors do find it difficult to believe that a useful treatment could start anywhere other than in a conventional research laboratory. But more and more doctors and researchers are open to the scientific and fair testing of alternative and complementary treatments. More research grants than ever before are now available for research into these treatments from the National Center for Complementary and Alternative Medicine, the National Cancer Institute, and other sources. The most important reason for not believing claims of alternative cures is that there is no convincing evidence.

Medical treatments are assumed to be ineffective until they are proved to be useful. The vast majority of new drugs developed in research laboratories turn out to be useless for treating cancer in humans. That is why oncologists are so focused on results of rigorously conducted clinical trials. They do not prescribe drugs just because a drug company claims they are useful; those claims have to be proven in studies that are supervised and reviewed by leading oncologists. The same standard applies to alternative therapies. Patient anecdotes, marketing brochures, and testimonials are not convincing evidence.

Occasionally, unconventional treatments are tested in a clinical trial and turn out to be effective. Let's consider arsenic, a toxic metal used historically for many diseases by both Western and Asian clinicians. Use of arsenic in Western medicine for infections was replaced by antibiotics many decades ago. Not long ago, some Chinese doctors recalled that a form of arsenic was used in traditional Chinese medicine for cancer, and they thought it would be useful in treating leukemia. In collaboration with international colleagues, they tested arsenic trioxide against cancer cells in the laboratory, in animals, and in clinical trials. It was useful against a form of leukemia called promyelocytic leukemia and has become an accepted part of conventional care for that disease.

Some advocates of alternative therapies claim that conventional oncologists reject plant-based or natural therapies and prefer synthetic chemicals. There are actually a number of chemotherapy drugs that were first isolated from plants or are chemically modified from compounds found in plants: vincristine and vinblastine from periwinkle, paclitaxel and docetaxel from yew trees, and etoposide from mayapples. Not long ago, screening plants, molds, and other living things for anticancer compounds was one of the main strategies for finding new chemotherapy drugs, and this work still continues. There is less random testing than there once was, but many integrative oncology researchers are now focusing on plants that were used in traditional medical systems.

Most oncologists are open to any new ideas for ways to fight cancer, as long as there is credible scientific evidence. Alternative providers should therefore cooperate with researchers to test their treatments.

Questions to Ask About Complementary or Alternative Methods

Many people with cancer use one or more complementary or alternative therapies. The challenge for you is to decide what is best suited to your medical situation and, equally important, to your values and beliefs. Asking yourself, your conventional health care providers, and your complementary or alternative care providers these questions can help you understand your motives for considering the method and weigh the evidence that the method will meet your needs against the risks and costs.

As you are reading about unconventional therapies, make a list of those that interest you. You will need to evaluate these therapies and determine whether they are a good match for your needs and can help you reach your goals. Here are some questions to help you:

- What claims are made for the treatment? That it can relieve symptoms or side effects? That it can improve general health or wellness? Be very suspicious of claims that any unconventional treatment can cure cancer. Claims that a treatment can cure all cancers or that it can cure cancer and other difficult-to-treat diseases (including chronic fatigue, multiple sclerosis, AIDS, etc.) are certain to be fraudulent.
- What are the credentials of the individuals supporting the treatment? Are they recognized experts in the field of cancer and complementary medicine? Are the findings published in trustworthy medical journals, where articles are peer-reviewed by other scientists in the same field and determined to be accurate and valuable?
- How is information about the therapy communicated? Is it promoted only in the mass media? Be suspicious if it is promoted only in books, magazines, and television and radio talk shows without simultaneous presentation of scientific studies in a trustworthy medical journal.
- Is the method widely available for use within the health care community? Once a treatment is found to be useful, it will be widely adopted by other qualified professionals. Beware of treatments available only in one clinic, especially if that clinic is located in a country with more lax patient protection laws and regulations than those in the United

States or the European Union.

- What is known about the safety of the therapy? Could it be harmful or might it interact adversely with conventional treatments or with other complementary therapies? This question is particularly important with regard to dietary supplements.

Considering Evidence for Complementary Therapies

The more you know about the benefits and risks of any therapy, the more able you will be to decide whether it is right for you. In Chapter 2, we talked about the types of evidence oncologists use to make decisions about conventional therapies. Because by definition alternative therapies are used instead of conventional care, they must be assessed by the same standards of evidence.

Some doctors feel that the same standards should also be applied to complementary methods. In other words, no method, either conventional or complementary, is worth considering until there is convincing evidence, such as clinical trial results, showing that it is useful. Most oncologists recognize, however, that there is a difference between having an operation or starting a new chemotherapy drug and having a therapeutic massage or participating in art therapy sessions. Until there is more research on complementary therapies, patients and doctors must base decisions on limited evidence. In most cases, a combination of basic understanding of the complementary method, together with some common sense, can help you make a sensible decision on whether the balance of benefit, risk, and cost is a favorable one.

Regulation of Complementary and Alternative Medical Practitioners

CAM practitioners generally operate under one of three areas of regulation: licensure, certification, or registration. **Licensure** is a process by which a government agency regulates a profession and grants an individual permission to engage in the profession. Licensing is the result of either local or state legislative action. In order to obtain a license in a particular profession, the individual must meet the requirements dictated by the law and attain the degree of competency required by the licensing agency. There are substantial differences among states as to which complementary and alternative professionals must be licensed and what training and examinations are required for licensure.

Whereas licensure is required in order to practice a profession, **certification** and **registration** are voluntary. Many practitioners of complementary and alternative therapies prefer not to be licensed, and standards among professions vary widely.

The requirements necessary to obtain certification are typically less stringent than those required for licensing, and these requirements vary, depending on the profession and certifying agency. Certification is nearly always offered by private organizations not associated with the local or state government.

The requirements for registration are usually even less stringent than certification and generally require the registrant to meet various criteria. Registration may be offered by private organizations or government agencies, and requirements vary depending on the agency.

All fifty states now license chiropractors, who must complete a four-year program of education and pass a national board examination.

Traditional Chinese Medicine practitioners are trained as acupuncturists (a three-year degree) or as Oriental Medicine practitioners (a four-year degree); both are able to practice acupuncture and herbal medicine. The United States' national professional organization for acupuncturists, the National Certification Commission for Acupuncture and Oriental Medicine, offers a certification process that is required prior to licensing in most states.

Naturopathic physicians are trained via a four-year curriculum, followed by a residency. Education for naturopathic physicians includes clinical science courses, as well as a wide array of CAM modalities, including hydrotherapy, herbal medicine, homeopathy, Oriental medicine, Ayurveda, and diet or nutritional therapy. As of April 2008, fourteen states, the District of Columbia, and the U.S. territories of Puerto Rico and the U.S. Virgin Islands had licensing laws for naturopathic physicians.

Many university-affiliated medical centers or medical schools have instituted centers for integrative medicine. Many universities have internal committees that create credentialing and practice standards for practitioners of complementary and alternative therapies. Western medical physicians do not have to be separately licensed (in addition to their medical license) in order to practice acupuncture or any other complementary or alternative therapy, but they do undergo credentialing by the clinical leadership at cancer centers or hospitals and can have an expanded scope of service.

Sources of Information About Complementary Care Providers

The following guidelines and questions are here to help you select the best practitioner for you.

- Call a national trade association and find the complementary care providers in your geographic area. Most professionals, such as acupuncturists, naturopaths, and chiropractors, as well as physicians and nurses, belong to a national association related to their profession. Trade associations typically offer membership and various benefits to members of a given profession, including ongoing education within the specific field. Trade associations will not usually recommend practitioners, but they can provide a list of licensed practitioners located near your home. Simply having a license does not mean someone is the right practitioner for you, but you should be cautious about someone who does not have a license in fields where such licenses are expected.

- Ask your conventional medical providers for referrals. Many conventional physicians and nurses support the use of complementary therapies and may know of practitioners who are popular with their patients. If you are being treated for an illness or disease, ask your medical provider about any complementary practitioners that have been found helpful and reliable by others with a similar diagnosis.
- Visit the integrative oncology department of a major cancer center. Many cancer centers have programs of complementary care and can recommend practitioners on their staff or who are affiliated in some way with the cancer center. These providers are likely to have experience with the needs of people with cancer and in coordinating care with conventional clinicians.
- Speak with someone who has or has had similar health care goals. If your goal is to manage, alleviate, or combat disease or disease symptoms, speak with someone with a similar goal. Support groups can be a good source of information. Keep in mind that information from other patients may not be completely accurate or may not apply to your medical situation.

Talking with Your Physician About Complementary Therapies

If you are already using a complementary therapy, tell your physician. Although people may be reluctant to share their complementary interests with their physicians, it could be dangerous to the health of the person with cancer to withhold that information. Many people believe that herbs and other complementary therapies are natural and, therefore, harmless. However, herbal products and other dietary supplements could interact with medications (either prescription or nonprescription), or they may have negative effects when taken alone.

If your physician knows about any complementary therapies you are using and writes that information in your medical record, he or she will be able to watch for potential drug interactions and/or harmful side effects.

If you are considering using complementary therapies, here are some tips for discussion with your physician:

- Educate yourself first. Before beginning a conversation with your physician, do some research and find out as much as you can about the complementary or alternative method you wish to discuss.
- Before beginning any therapy, tell your physician you are thinking about a

complementary therapy, but you want to make sure it does not interfere with the treatment he or she prescribes.

- Ask questions. It can be helpful to write down a list of questions for the physician and bring in any literature you want to discuss. Let your physician know you are an educated consumer; even though you may be apprehensive about what you are facing, you are seeking as much information as you can.
- Let your physician know you want him or her to be a supportive partner in your education and treatment process.
- If you have more than one physician or health care provider, let all of them know about the CAM therapies you are using. This will help each provider design the safest and most comprehensive treatment plan for you.

Insurance Coverage

In response to growing patient demand for complementary and alternative therapies, more and more health insurance companies are beginning to cover at least some of the costs of some complementary and alternative therapies and the services of some alternative practitioners. A 2004 survey of employer-sponsored health plans reported that 87 percent of individuals had chiropractic coverage and 47 percent had acupuncture coverage. Not all health insurance plans offer this type of coverage, however. The types of complementary and alternative therapies that might be covered are chiropractic services, acupuncture, massage therapy, biofeedback, and naturopathy.

The trend toward greater insurance coverage is also fueled by efforts on the part of managed care companies to control costs. Complementary and alternative therapies represent at least a potential cost saving for insurers, although actual cost effectiveness studies are generally lacking. Naturopaths, acupuncturists, chiropractors, and other complementary and alternative therapists rely heavily on herbs and other dietary supplements to treat illnesses and medical complaints, and supplements are considered by some to be less costly than conventional drugs.

Among insurers and managed care companies that do offer coverage for nontraditional treatments, the amount of coverage varies widely. Some health maintenance organizations (HMOs) offer complementary and alternative methods as discounted services similar to the reduced-rate services offered for plastic surgery, eye care, and other services not fully covered by the HMO. Other managed care providers and insurers offer complementary and alternative methods as a carved-out benefit, for which the insured pays a premium. Other HMOs and managed care groups are adding alternative providers to their provider teams. And a growing number offer complementary services as a core benefit.

Since 1996, Washington state has required that private health insurance carriers cover licensed complementary and alternative medicine providers. A 2006 study evaluating how insured people in Washington state used complementary and alternative medicine found that the number of people using these benefits was substantial, while the effect on insurance expenditures was modest.

Whereas insurance coverage for at least some of the costs of complementary and alternative methods is expanding, most of the costs are still paid out-of-pocket by consumers. Insurers, including Medicare, tend to grant coverage for treatments that they consider reasonable and necessary or medically necessary. To qualify, the treatment must be shown to be safe and effective. Complementary methods, such as meditation, biofeedback, acupuncture, and hypnosis, may be covered because companies believe there is sufficient scientific evidence to indicate that these therapies help reduce pain and some other side effects of treatment. Insurers generally will not cover unproven therapies, however.

As more controlled clinical trials are conducted to demonstrate the safety and effectiveness or danger and ineffectiveness of various complementary and alternative methods of cancer management, the safe and effective therapies will become part of conventional medicine and qualify for insurance coverage.

In the meantime, learn about what is covered through your insurance before you seek treatment from a complementary medicine provider. Read your plan, and if anything is unclear, contact the insurance company. These are some questions you might consider asking a representative from your insurance company:

- Is this treatment covered by my insurance?
- Does the treatment need to be preauthorized, prescribed, or ordered through a referral?
- Do I need to see a provider from within my network for the treatment to be covered?
- Is there a limit to the number of visits I can make or the amount my plan will cover?
- What will I pay out-of-pocket for this service?

As with all other areas of your cancer care, it is recommended that you keep thorough records of all contacts you have with the insurance company should any conflicts or disputes about treatment arise.

More information about complementary and alternative treatment is available on the Web site of the National Center for Complementary and Alternative Medicine at http://nccam.nih.gov/ or through the American Cancer Society's toll-free number **(800-ACS-2345)** or Web site **(www.cancer.org)**.

References

About us. March of Dimes Web site. http://www.marchofdimes.com/789_821.asp. Accessed June 3, 2008.

American Association of Naturopathic Physicians Web site. http://www.naturopathic.org/. Accessed June 3, 2008.

American Chiropractic Association Web site. http://www.amerchiro.org/index.cfm. Accessed June 3, 2008.

Beyerstein BL. Distinguishing science from pseudoscience. The Centre for Curriculum and Professional Development. Simon Fraser University Web site. http://www.sfu.ca/~beyerste/research/articles/02Sciencevs Pseudoscience.pdf. Published July 1995. Revised October 1996. Accessed June 3, 2008.

Cassileth BR. The Integrative Medicine Service at Memorial Sloan-Kettering Cancer Center. *Semin Oncol.* 2002;29:585-588.

Chiropractic regulatory boards. Federation of Chiropractic Licensing Boards Web site. http://www.fclb.org/boards.htm. Accessed June 3, 2008.

Claxton G, Gil I, Finder B, Holve E, Gabel J, Pickreign J, Whitmore H, Hawkins S, Fahlman C. Employer health benefits: 2004 annual survey. Menlo Park, CA: Kaiser Family Foundation and the Health Research and Educational Trust; September 2004. Kaiser Family Foundation Web site. http://www.kff.org/insurance/7148/upload/2004-Employer-Health-Benefits-Survey-Full-Report.pdf. Accessed June 5, 2008.

Complementary and alternative methods for cancer management. American Cancer Society Web site. http://www.cancer.org/docroot/ETO/content/ETO_5_1_Introduction.asp. Accessed June 3, 2008.

Demark-Wahnefried W, Price DT, Polascik TJ, Robertson CN, Anderson EE, Paulson DF, Walther PJ, Gannon M, Vollmer RT. Pilot study of dietary fat restriction and flaxseed supplementation in men with prostate cancer before surgery: exploring the effects on hormonal levels, prostate-specific antigen, and histopathologic features. *Urology.* 2001;58:47-52.

Ernst E, Cassileth BR. How useful are unconventional cancer treatments? *Eur J Cancer.* 1999;35:1608-1613.

Hede K, Chinese folk treatment reveals power of arsenic to treat cancer, new studies under way. *J Natl Cancer Inst.* 2007;99:667-668.

Kurtzweil P. How to spot health fraud. *FDA Consumer: The Magazine of the US Food and Drug Administration.* 1999;33. US Food and Drug Administration Web site. http://www.fda.gov/fdac/features/1999/699_fraud.html. Accessed June 3, 2008.

Lafferty WE, Tyree PT, Bellas AS, Watts CA, Lind BK, Sherman KJ, Cherkin DC, Grembowski DE. Insurance coverage and subsequent utilization of complementary and alternative medicine providers. *Am J Manag Care.* 2006;12:397-404.

Mann J. Natural products in cancer chemotherapy: past, present and future. *Nat Rev Cancer.* 2002;2:143-148.

Meyerhardt JA, Giovannucci EL, Holmes MD, Chan AT, Chan JA, Colditz GA, Fuchs CS. Physical activity and survival after colorectal cancer diagnosis. *J Clin Oncol.* 2006;24:3527-3534. Epub 2006 Jul 5.

National Certification Commission for Acupuncture and Oriental Medicine Web site. http://www.nccaom.org/index.html. Accessed June 3, 2008.

National Institutes of Health, National Center for Complementary and Alternative Medicine. *About Clinical Trials and Complementary and Alternative Medicine.* Bethesda, MD: National Center for Complementary and Alternative Medicine; 2006. NCCAM Publication No. D338.

Richardson MA, Sanders T, Palmer JL, Greisinger A, Singletary SE. Complementary/alternative medicine use in a comprehensive cancer center and the implications for oncology. *J Clin Oncol.* 2000;18:2505-2514.

Risberg T, Vickers A, Bremnes RM, Wist EA, Kaasa S, Cassileth BR. Does use of alternative medicine predict survival from cancer? *Eur J Cancer.* 2003;39:372-377.
Comment in:
Eur J Cancer. 2003;39:1642; author reply 1643.

Sipkoff M. Steadily, plans increase coverage of unorthodox medical therapies. *Managed Care.* 2005;14:59-60.

US Congress, Office of Technology Assessment. *Unconventional Cancer Treatments: OTA-H-405.* Washington, DC: US Government Printing Office; 1990.

Vickers AJ, Kuo J, Cassileth BR. Unconventional anticancer agents: a systematic review of clinical trials. *J Clin Oncol.* 2006;24:136-140.

Chapter Five

Mind, Body, and Spirit Therapies

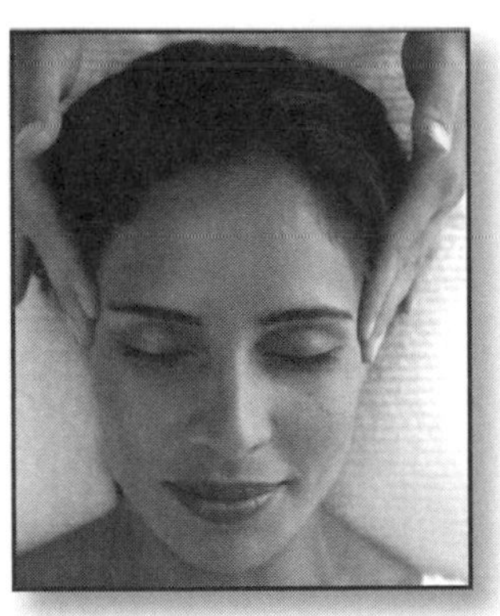

AROMATHERAPY

Other common name(s): holistic aromatherapy, aromatic medicine
Scientific/medical name(s): none

Description

Aromatherapy is the use of fragrant substances, called essential oils, to alter mood or improve health. These highly concentrated aromatic substances are either inhaled or applied to the skin. Essential oils are distilled from plants, and approximately forty are commonly used in aromatherapy; among the most popular are lavender, rosemary, eucalyptus, chamomile, marjoram, jasmine, peppermint, lemon, ylang ylang, and geranium.

Overview

Available scientific evidence does not support claims that aromatherapy is effective in preventing or treating cancer, but its use may enhance quality of life. Early clinical trials suggest aromatherapy may have some benefit as a complementary treatment in reducing stress, pain, nausea, and depression.

How is it promoted for use?

Aromatherapy is promoted as a natural way to help patients cope with stress, chronic pain, nausea, and depression and to produce a feeling of well-being. Proponents also claim aromatherapy can help relieve bacterial infections; stimulate the immune system; fight colds, flu, and sore throats; improve urine production; increase circulation; and cure cystitis, herpes simplex, acne, headaches, indigestion, premenstrual syndrome, muscle tension, and even cancer. Fragrances from different oils are promoted to have specific health benefits. For example, lavender oil is promoted to relieve muscle tension, anxiety, and insomnia.

There are different ideas as to how aromatherapy may work. Scent receptors in the nose are known to send chemical messages through the olfactory nerve to the brain's limbic region, which influences emotional responses, heart rate, blood pressure, and respiration. Some proponents say these connections explain the effects of essential oils' smells. The effects may partly depend on a person's previous associations or recalled experiences with a particular scent. Others say the oils are absorbed directly into the system through the skin.

What does it involve?

Aromatherapy is either self-administered or administered by a practitioner. Many aromatherapists in the United States are trained as massage therapists, psychologists, social workers, or chiropractors and use the oils as part of their practices.

The essential oils can be used individually or in combination and may be inhaled or applied to the skin. For inhalation, a few drops of the essential oil are placed in steaming water, atomizers, or humidifiers that are used to spread the water vapor and oil combination throughout the room. Sometimes the oils are placed in a heatproof dish over a candle or other flame to diffuse the scent.

Essential oils can be applied to the skin during massage, or they can be added to bathwater. For application to the skin, the oils are combined with another substance (a carrier), usually vegetable oil. Some essential oils can sometimes be used directly on the skin. Oils may also be used to make salves, creams, and compresses. Some people also apply drops of certain essential oils to their pillows.

What is the history behind it?

Use of aromatic, perfumed oils dates back thousands of years to ancient Egypt, China, and India. In Egypt, such oils were used after bathing and for embalming mummies. Thousands of years ago the Chinese compiled an encyclopedia of information on the uses of plants, herbs, and different types of wood. In ancient India, aromatic massage was part of Ayurvedic medicine. In addition, the Greeks and Romans used fragrant oils for both medicinal and cosmetic purposes. However, it was the medieval physician Avicenna who first extracted these oils from plants.

René Maurice Gattefossé, a French chemist, originated modern aromatherapy and even the term itself. After burning his hand in a laboratory accident, he used lavender oil to soothe the pain. His hand healed quickly with no scar, and he attributed this outcome to the lavender oil. He published his first thesis, titled "Aromatherapie," in 1928 and published a book under the same title in 1937. Aromatherapy was revived in the 1960s by French homeopaths Dr. and Mme. Maury. In the 1980s, aromatherapy began to grow in popularity in the United States. It is fairly well established in England, France, Switzerland, and New Zealand.

What is the evidence?

Available scientific evidence does not support claims that aromatherapy cures or prevents disease; however, a few clinical studies suggest aromatherapy may be a helpful complementary therapy. In Britain, there are reports of the successful use of aromatherapy massage in people with cancer to reduce anxiety, depression, tension, and pain. However, some studies show no difference in outcome between massage with aromatherapy oils and massage without them. There are also reports that breathing the vapors of peppermint, ginger, and cardamom oil seems to relieve the nausea caused by chemotherapy and radiation. However, these claims are not supported by available scientific evidence. Laboratory studies suggest that the oils can affect organ function, although whether this can be useful is not yet clear.

Clinical research on aromatherapy is in its infancy. Early trials suggest aromatherapy may help patients cope with chronic pain, stress, nausea, and depression.

In one controlled clinical trial, inhaling the vapors from black pepper extract reduced the craving for tobacco and improved participants' moods. In a second controlled trial, the use of citrus fragrance by twelve depressed patients made it possible to reduce the amount of antidepressant medicine they needed.

Another study of aromatherapy suggested that the scent changed a person's memory of pain, even though the patient's perception of the severity of the pain while it was happening did not change. There was no difference between the aromatherapy group's and control group's pain ratings during a procedure, but after the fact, the aromatherapy group reported that the event was less distressing overall than did the control group.

There is also some evidence that the power of suggestion may explain at least part of the effect of aromatherapy. For example, in one study, the salt-water placebo was just as effective in reducing nausea as the essential oil. In another study, the oils were more likely to produce the effect about which the subjects were told, regardless of whether it was the normally predicted effect. Several controlled studies using essential oils have shown no measurable effect.

In a randomized clinical trial, a daily scalp massage with essential oils was shown to be a safe and effective treatment for hair loss resulting from *alopecia areata*, a condition in which the patient's immune system damages the hair follicles. This treatment has not been evaluated as a treatment for hair loss related to cancer treatments. Other laboratory and animal studies have looked at the ability of essential oils to kill or control certain germs and viruses when the oil is placed in direct contact with the germ.

Are there any possible problems or complications?

Aromatherapy is generally safe. However, essential oils usually should not be taken internally, as many of them are poisonous. Some oils can cause an allergic reaction. Some may cause irritation if applied undiluted to the skin. Aromatherapy oils have been reported as causing headaches, nausea, and allergic reactions.

Relying on this type of treatment alone and avoiding or delaying conventional medical care for cancer may have serious health consequences.

References

Anderson LA, Gross JB. Aromatherapy with peppermint, isopropyl alcohol, or placebo is equally effective in relieving postoperative nausea. *J Perianesth Nurs.* 2004;19:29-35.

Buckle J. Use of aromatherapy as a complementary treatment for chronic pain. *Altern Ther Health Med.* 1999;5:42-51.

Campenni CE, Crawley EJ, Meier ME. Role of suggestion in odor-induced mood change. *Psychol Rep.* 2004;94:1127-1136.

Cawthorn A. A review of the literature surrounding the research into aromatherapy. *Complement Ther Nurs Midwifery.* 1995;1:118-120.

Cerrato PL. Aromatherapy: is it for real? *RN.* 1998;61:51-52.

Ernst E, ed. *The Desktop Guide to Complementary and Alternative Medicine: An Evidence-Based Approach.* New York: Mosby; 2001.

Fellowes D, Barnes K, Wilkinson S. Aromatherapy and massage for symptom relief in patients with cancer. *Cochrane Database Syst Rev.* 2004;(2):CD002287.

Gedney JJ, Glover TL, Fillingim RB. Sensory and affective pain discrimination after inhalation of essential oils. *Psychosom Med.* 2004;66:599-606.

Hay IC, Jamieson M, Ormerod AD. Randomized trial of aromatherapy. Successful treatment for alopecia areata. *Arch Dermatol.* 1998;134:1349-1352.

Komori T, Fujiwara R, Tanida M, Nomura J, Yokoyama MM. Effects of citrus fragrance on immune function and depressive states. *Neuroimmunomodulation.* 1995;2:174-180.

Nelson NJ. Scents or nonsense: aromatherapy's benefits still subject to debate. *J Natl Cancer Inst.* 1997;89:1334-1336.

Rose JE, Behm FM. Inhalation of vapor from black pepper extract reduces smoking withdrawal symptoms. *Drug Alcohol Depend.* 1994;34:225-229.

Soden K, Vincent K, Craske S, Lucas C, Ashley S. A randomized controlled trial of aromatherapy massage in a hospice setting. *Palliat Med.* 2004;18:87-92.

ART THERAPY

Other common name(s): creative arts therapy, expressive arts therapy
Scientific/medical name(s): none

Description

Art therapy is used to help people manage physical and emotional problems by using creative activities to express emotions. It provides a way for people to come to terms with emotional conflicts, increase self-awareness, and express unspoken and often unconscious concerns about their illness and their lives. "Expressive arts therapy" or "creative arts therapy" may also include the use of dance and movement, drama, poetry, and photography, as well as more traditional art methods.

Overview

Many clinicians have observed and documented significant benefits among people who have used art therapy. Art therapy has not been studied scientifically to find out whether it has value for people with cancer.

How is it promoted for use?

Art therapy is based on the idea that the creative act can be healing. According to practitioners, called art therapists, it helps people express hidden emotions; reduces stress, fear, and anxiety; and provides a sense of freedom. Many art therapists also believe the act of creation influences brain wave patterns and the chemicals released by the brain.

Art therapy has been used with bone marrow transplant patients, people with eating disorders, emotionally impaired young people, disabled people, the chronically ill, chemically addicted individuals, sexually abused adolescents, caregivers of cancer patients, and others. Art therapy may also be used to engage and distract patients whose illnesses or treatments cause pain.

Artwork may also be used as a diagnostic tool, particularly with children, who often have trouble talking about painful events or emotions. Art therapists say that often children can express difficult emotions or relay information about traumatic times in their lives more easily through drawings than through conventional therapy.

What does it involve?

People involved in art therapy are given the tools they need to produce paintings, drawings, sculptures, and many other types of artwork. Art therapists work with patients individually or in groups. The job of the art therapist is to help patients express themselves through their creations and to talk to patients about their emotions and concerns as they relate to their art. For example, an art therapist may encourage a person with cancer to create an image of himself or herself with cancer, and in this way express feelings about the disease that may be hard to talk about or may be unconscious.

In another form of art therapy, patients look at pieces of art, often in photographs, and then talk with a therapist about what they have seen. A caregiver or family member can also gather artwork in the form of photographs, books, or prints, and give the patient a chance to look at and enjoy the art.

Many medical centers and hospitals include art therapy as part of inpatient care. It can be practiced in many other settings, such as schools, psychiatric centers, drug and alcohol rehabilitation programs, prisons, day care treatment programs, nursing homes, hospices, patients' homes, and art studios.

What is the history behind it?

The connection between art and mental health was first recognized in the late 1800s. In 1922, a book titled *Artistry of the Mentally Ill* aroused interest in the subject and caused the medical community to examine the diagnostic value of patients' creations. Some practitioners realized that art might be valuable for rehabilitating patients with mental illness.

In the 1940s, ideas from psychoanalysis and art were combined to develop art as a tool to help patients release unconscious thoughts. Patients' creations began to be considered as a type of symbolic speech. In 1958, at the National Institute of Mental Health, an artist named Hana Kwiatkowska translated her knowledge as an artist into the field of family work and introduced methods of evaluation and treatment techniques using art therapy.

In 1969, the American Art Therapy Association was established. The organization now has more than forty-five hundred members and, along with the Art Therapy Credentials Board, sets standards for art therapists and educates the public about the field. Registered art therapists must have graduate degree training and a background in studio arts and therapy techniques. More recently, several groups specializing in various kinds of art therapy and expressive art therapies in general have been established.

What is the evidence?

Numerous case studies have reported that art therapy benefits patients with both emotional and physical illnesses. Case studies have involved many areas, including burn recovery in adolescents and young children, eating disorders, emotional impairment in young children, reading performance, childhood grief, and sexual abuse in adolescents. Studies of adults using art therapy have included adults or families in bereavement, patients and family members dealing with addictions, and patients who have undergone bone marrow transplants, among others. Some of the potential uses of art therapy to be researched include reducing anxiety levels, improving recovery times, decreasing hospital stays, improving communication and social function, and controlling pain.

Are there any possible problems or complications?

Art therapy is considered safe when conducted by a skilled therapist. It may be useful as a complementary therapy to help people with cancer deal with their emotions. Although uncomfortable feelings may be stirred up at times, this is considered part of the healing process.

Relying on this type of treatment alone and avoiding or delaying conventional medical care for cancer may have serious health consequences.

References

Expressive arts therapy. Arts in Therapy Network Web site. http://www.artsintherapy.com/whatis.asp?id=269. Accessed May 30, 2008.

Kirk K, McManus M. Containing families' grief: therapeutic group work in a hospice setting. *Int J Palliat Nurs.* 2002;8:470-480.

The National Expressive Therapy Association Web site. http://www.geocities.com/SoHo/museum/5408/index.html. Accessed May 30, 2008.

National Institutes of Health. *Alternative Medicine: Expanding Medical Horizons: A Report to the National Institutes of Health on Alternative Medical Systems and Practices in the United States.* Washington, DC: US Government Printing Office; 1994. NIH publication 94-066.

Noice H, Noice T, Staines G. A short-term intervention to enhance cognitive and affective functioning in older adults. *J Aging Health.* 2004;16:562-585.

Walsh SM, Martin SC, Schmidt LA. Testing the efficacy of a creative-arts intervention with family caregivers of patients with cancer. *J Nurs Scholarsh.* 2004;36:214-219.

AYURVEDA

Other common name(s): Ayurvedic medicine
Scientific/medical name(s): none

Description

Ayurveda is an ancient Indian system of medicine. It follows an integrated approach to the prevention and treatment of illness and tries to maintain or reestablish harmony between the mind, body, and forces of nature. It combines a number of approaches, such as changes in lifestyle, herbal remedies, exercise, and meditation, to strengthen and purify the body and mind and increase spiritual awareness.

Overview

Ayurveda is one of several ancient Asian healing systems that have recently gained popularity in the West. While the effectiveness of many aspects of Ayurveda has not been scientifically proven, early research suggests certain components may offer potential therapeutic value.

How is it promoted for use?

A central idea in Ayurveda is that illness results when a person's physical, emotional, and spiritual forces are out of balance with each other and with the natural environment. Those who practice Ayurveda claim that certain combinations of methods, matched to a patient's unique physical and emotional needs and personal medical history, increase physical vitality, foster spiritual well-being, bring people into harmony with the world, and even prevent and cure disease.

According to Ayurvedic theory, all diseases and other health problems result from imbalances in the body's fundamental forces and disharmony with the natural environment. One of the primary goals of Ayurveda is to restore this balance and invigorate the body's biological and spiritual forces. Practitioners of Ayurveda use a combination of therapies to restore physical and spiritual harmony by balancing energy forces.

What does it involve?

Practitioners of Ayurveda may combine dietary programs, herbal remedies, intestinal cleansing preparations, yoga, meditation, massage, breathing exercises, and visual imagery to treat their patients. Ayurvedic herbal preparations often consist of complex mixtures of plants. An estimated 1,250 plants are used by practitioners. Some of the more controversial and less common practices of Ayurveda include bloodletting, bowel purging, and inducing vomiting.

To diagnose illness, Ayurveda practitioners closely observe a patient's tongue, nails, lips, and the body's nine "doors": the two eyes, two ears, two nostrils, mouth, genitalia, and anus. They also listen carefully to the lungs and observe the pulse at length, then take a detailed history of the patient's life and health. Through these observations, practitioners claim to evaluate a patient's doshas, or primary life forces.

According to Ayurveda practitioners, balancing a person's doshas not only enables the various organs of the body to work together, it also establishes a person's connection to the environment and the cosmos. Practitioners claim that each person is dominated by one of three doshas but is influenced to some extent by all three. The dominant dosha describes an individual's physical, emotional, and spiritual characteristics as well as his or her daily habits and lifestyle.

When planning a course of treatment, Ayurveda practitioners take into account the state of a patient's doshas and the complex relationship between the doshas and other factors such as emotions, illness, physical activity, lifestyle, diet, relationships with other people, and even the four seasons and the time of day. Practitioners strive to harmonize all of these factors so that their patients can attain health and well-being.

What is the history behind it?

Ayurveda is thought to have appeared in India more than five thousand years ago. It emerged from an ancient body of knowledge called the *Vedas*. In fact, veda is the Sanskrit word for knowledge. From these Vedas, India developed its moral, religious, cultural, and medical codes.

Many of the beliefs and practices of Ayurveda are similar to those of ancient Chinese medicine.

In India today, Ayurveda practitioners are trained in state-recognized programs. Some of these practitioners are now practicing and teaching Ayurveda in the United States. There are several Ayurvedic clinics in North America.

What is the evidence?

Although Ayurveda has been largely untested by Western researchers, there is a growing interest in integrating some parts of the system into modern medical practice. Some early studies suggest that Ayurveda may have potential therapeutic value.

According to a report of a panel convened by the National Institutes of Health (NIH), one clinical study showed that in 79 percent of cases, the health of patients with various chronic diseases improved measurably after Ayurvedic treatment. Laboratory and clinical studies have suggested that some Ayurvedic herbal preparations may have the potential to prevent and treat certain types of cancer, including breast, lung, and colon cancer. Randomized clinical trials in humans are needed to make conclusions about the role of Ayurveda in cancer prevention and treatment. The National Cancer Institute (NCI) has added several Ayurvedic herbal compounds to its list of potential cancer treatment agents and has funded a series of laboratory studies to evaluate two Ayurvedic herbal remedies (called MAK-4 and MAK-5). The decision to fund the further research was based on preliminary laboratory studies indicating that the two medicines significantly inhibited growth of cancer cells taken from human and rat tumors. To date, there are no reports of tests of these two herbal remedies in humans.

In a controlled clinical trial of cancer patients in India, researchers found an Ayurvedic herbal mixture was just as effective as a conventional laxative for relieving constipation caused by opioid pain medicine. In another controlled clinical trial, Ayurveda was found to be an effective treatment for patients with Parkinson's disease. Many other individual herbs and spices used in Ayurveda are being studied in the laboratory or in animals. Some are already being tested in human clinical trials to find out whether they can be used to treat or prevent cancer. (For more information, see individual herbs, such as "Turmeric," page 514, "Garlic," page 611, and "Gotu Kola," page 382.)

Are there any possible problems or complications?

Some aspects of Ayurveda, such as bloodletting and inducing vomiting, can be harmful. Many people with cancer already have low blood cell counts as a result of the disease itself, and removing additional blood can worsen fatigue and other symptoms. Inducing vomiting can cause imbalances of electrolytes (salt and minerals) in the blood. In addition, the potential interactions between Ayurvedic herbal preparations and conventional drugs and other herbs should be taken into consideration. Some of these combinations may be dangerous. Always tell your doctor and pharmacist about any herbs you are taking. Ayurveda should be delivered by a trained therapist.

There have been reports of contamination with lead, mercury, and arsenic in some Ayurvedic herbal preparations sold in U.S. markets. Several cases of lead poisoning occurred between 2000 and 2003, with patients suffering nausea, vomiting, abdominal pain, and/or anemia.

Relying on this type of treatment alone and delaying or avoiding conventional medical care for cancer may have serious health consequences.

These substances may have not been thoroughly tested to find out how they interact with medicines, foods, or dietary supplements. Even though some reports of interactions and harmful effects may be published, full studies of interactions and effects are not often available. Because of these limitations, any information on ill effects and interactions should be considered incomplete.

References

Aggarwal BB, Ichikawa H, Garodia P, Weerasinghe P, Sethi G, Bhatt ID, Pandey MK, Shishodia S, Nair MG. From traditional Ayurvedic medicine to modern medicine: identification of therapeutic targets for suppression of inflammation and cancer. *Expert Opin Ther Targets.* 2006;10:87-118.

Centers for Disease Control and Prevention. Lead poisoning associated with Ayurvedic medications—five states, 2000-2003. *MMWR.* 2004;53:582-584.

Dev S. Ancient-modern concordance in Ayurvedic plants: some examples. *Environ Health Perspect.* 1999;107:783-789.

HP-200 in Parkinson's Disease Study Group. An alternative medicine treatment for Parkinson's disease: results of a multicenter clinical trial. *J Altern Complement Med.* 1995;1:249-255.

National Institutes of Health. *Alternative Medicine: Expanding Medical Horizons: A Report to the National Institutes of Health on Alternative Medical Systems and Practices in the United States.* Washington, DC: US Government Printing Office; 1994. NIH publication 94-066.

Ramesh PR, Kumar KS, Rajagopal MR, Balachandran P, Warrier PK. Managing morphine-induced constipation: a controlled comparison of an Ayurvedic formulation and senna. *J Pain Symptom Manage.* 1998;16:240-244.

Saper RB, Kales SN, Paquin J, Burns MJ, Eisenberg DM, Davis RB, Phillips RS. Heavy metal content of Ayurvedic herbal medicine products. *JAMA.* 2004;292:2868-2873.

Thatte UM, Rege NN, Phatak SD, Dahanukar SA. The flip side of Ayurveda. *J Postgrad Med.* 1993;39:179-182.

BIOENERGETICS

Other common name(s): bioenergetic therapy, bioenergetic medicine, bioenergetic analysis
Scientific/medical name(s): none

Description

Bioenergetics is a complementary therapy that involves psychotherapy, relaxation techniques, and gentle touch to relieve muscle tension. The term "bioenergetic" is sometimes used in describing other types of complementary therapies that do not use the techniques described here. The term is also used by scientists to talk about cellular energy.

Overview

Available scientific evidence does not support claims that bioenergetics therapy is effective in treating cancer; however, some patients report it is useful as a relaxation method.

How is it promoted for use?

Supporters of bioenergetics believe the body "records" negative emotional reactions and stores them in the form of muscle tension and stiffness, poor posture, and low energy levels. To release these trapped emotions and return the body and mind to a balanced, healthy, peaceful state, patients must first release muscle tension and correct physical imbalances. Proponents further claim that bioenergetics can offer relief from the side effects of cancer treatment and even strengthen the body's ability to fight disease.

Bioenergetics practitioners claim they can "read" a patient's muscular movements, tone of voice, breathing, posture, and emotions to determine his or her physical and psychological problems. They also believe disease is a part of the life process, and serious illnesses (including cancer) are symptoms of underlying imbalances caused by factors such as poor diet, exposure to toxins, genetic history, and repressed emotions. They claim that by balancing electrical and energy disturbances within the patient and eliminating toxins, the body will heal itself (see "Electromagnetic Therapy," page 194).

What does it involve?

Bioenergetics therapists use a combination of psychotherapy, gentle body movements, massage, deep breathing, and exercises that involve crying, screaming, and kicking in an effort to help patients "release" their emotional memories. The therapy may also include aspects of traditional Chinese medicine, biofeedback, herbal medicine, homeopathy, acupuncture, and nutrition.

What is the history behind it?

Bioenergetics was developed by psychiatrist Alexander Lowen, MD, in the 1950s. He based his work on Reichian therapy, a practice developed by Wilhelm Reich, MD, that theorized that a person's repressed emotions are transformed into muscle tension and rigidity, what Dr. Reich called "body armor." Dr. Lowen, who first earned a law degree in New York, became a therapist under Dr. Reich's training and then completed medical school at the University of Geneva in Switzerland. In 1956, Dr. Lowen created the Institute for Bioenergetic Analysis.

What is the evidence?

Some patients may feel more relaxed and at ease after a bioenergetics therapy session. However, available scientific evidence does not support bioenergetics as a useful treatment for cancer or any other disease. Since it is usually practiced by psychotherapists, it is difficult to evaluate apart from the psychotherapy itself.

Are there any possible problems or complications?

People with cancer and chronic conditions such as arthritis and heart disease should talk to their doctor before using any type of therapy that involves herbs or manipulation of joints and muscles. Treatment should be given by a skilled professional psychotherapist.

Relying on this type of treatment alone and avoiding or delaying conventional medical care for cancer may have serious health consequences.

References

Bioenergetic analysis. New York Society for Bioenergetic Analysis Web site.http://www.bioenergetics-nyc.org/. Accessed May 23, 2008.

Cassileth B. *The Alternative Medicine Handbook: The Complete Reference Guide to Alternative and Complementary Therapies*. New York: W.W. Norton; 1998.

National Institutes of Health. *Alternative Medicine: Expanding Medical Horizons: A Report to the National Institutes of Health on Alternative Medical Systems and Practices in the United States*. Washington, DC: US Government Printing Office; 1994. NIH publication 94-066.

What is bioenergetic analysis? International Institute for Bioenergetic Analysis Web site. http://www.bioenergetic-therapy.com/iibamain/about/1frm_about.htm. Accessed May 23, 2008.

BIOFEEDBACK

Other common name(s): none
Scientific/medical name(s): none

Description

Biofeedback is a treatment method that uses monitoring devices to help people consciously control physical processes that are usually controlled automatically, such as heart rate, blood pressure, temperature, sweating, and muscle tension.

Overview

Biofeedback is one of several relaxation methods that were evaluated and found to be of possible benefit by an independent panel convened by the National Institutes of Health (NIH). The panel found it a somewhat useful complementary therapy for treating chronic pain. The panel also found that, while biofeedback might help with some sleep problems (such as insomnia), its effect on how long it took to fall asleep and total sleep time were uncertain. Available scientific evidence does not support claims that biofeedback can influence the development or progression of cancer; however, it can help to improve quality of life for some people with cancer.

How is it promoted for use?

Biofeedback is promoted to help a person regulate specific body functions. Proponents say that by helping a patient change his or her heart rate, skin temperature, breathing rate, muscle tension and other such activity in the body, biofeedback can reduce stress and muscle tension from a number of causes. It can promote relaxation, help correct urinary incontinence, and treat migraines and less serious headaches. It is also promoted to help some people with Raynaud's disease (problems of blood circulation that make the fingers and toes feel very cold, numb, or even painful) increase the temperature of their hands and toes. Through generating a greater awareness of bodily functions, it can help a person regulate or alter other physical functions that may be causing discomfort. Biofeedback is also said to be useful in retraining muscles after injury, or in teaching muscles to take over for other muscles that can no longer perform as needed.

What does it involve?

Monitoring devices are used to amplify physical processes that are hard to detect without help. This information is then "fed back" in the form of a continuous signal (such as a tone or image readout). The person can adjust his or her thinking, emotional state, or other mental processes to focus on changing the signal and controlling his or her bodily functions.

For example, under the guidance of a biofeedback therapist, the patient concentrates on changing a specific physical process, such as heart rate, temperature, perspiration, blood flow, brain activity, or muscle tension. A monitor connected via electrodes to the patient's skin measures changes in the function the patient is trying to alter. Tones or images produced by the monitor inform the patient when he or she achieves the desired result. The process is repeated as often as necessary until the patient can reliably use conscious thought to change physical functions. After this is learned, the biofeedback equipment is no longer needed, although some patients return to have their condition monitored and repeat their biofeedback sessions.

There are at least five different ways to measure bodily functions for biofeedback purposes:

- An electromyogram (EMG) measures the electrical activity of muscles. It is used in conventional medicine to diagnose a variety of nerve and muscle diseases and in biofeedback to help heal muscle injuries and relieve chronic pain and some types of incontinence.
- Thermal biofeedback provides information about skin temperature, which is a good indicator of blood flow. Several health problems, such as migraine headaches, Raynaud's disease, anxiety, and high blood pressure, are related to blood flow.
- Electrodermal activity (EDA) shows changes in perspiration rate, which is an indicator of anxiety.
- Finger pulse measurements are used to reflect high blood pressure, heartbeat irregularities, and anxiety.
- Breathing rate is also monitored. This measurement is used in the treatment of asthma and hyperventilation and to promote relaxation.

Biofeedback is often a matter of trial and error as patients learn to adjust their thinking and connect changes in thought, breathing, posture, and muscle tension with changes in physical functions that are usually controlled unconsciously.

What is the history behind it?

For centuries, followers of ancient Eastern practices such as meditation and yoga have claimed they could control physical processes usually considered beyond the power of conscious thought. Studies on how biofeedback works were not conducted until the 1970s. Originally, it was used by counselors, psychologists, and other mental health professionals. Today, physicians and other health care professionals in the United States use biofeedback as a complementary therapy to promote relaxation and treat headaches, migraines, and insomnia.

What is the evidence?

Although biofeedback has no direct effect on the development or progress of cancer, it can improve quality of life for some people with cancer. Research has found that biofeedback can be helpful for patients in regaining urinary and bowel control after surgery. A recent study looked at 125 men who were having surgery for prostate cancer. Of those who had biofeedback training to learn bladder control exercises before surgery, 6 percent still had urine leakage six months after surgery. Of the men who did not have the biofeedback training, nearly 20 percent had leakage six months after surgery.

In another clinical trial, relaxation therapy was more effective than biofeedback in reducing some side effects of chemotherapy. Biofeedback is often used with relaxation for the best results.

After looking at data on biofeedback, an NIH panel found the method is moderately effective for relieving many types of chronic pain, particularly tension headaches. Its benefit was less clear for sleep problems, since its effect on how long it took to fall asleep and how long a person stayed asleep was uncertain. The panel also found that biofeedback was better than relaxation therapy for treating migraine headaches. The effects of biofeedback vary significantly from person to person. Small studies have suggested that biofeedback may be used to improve circulation in people with diabetes and to improve migraine headaches in children.

Are there any possible problems or complications?

Biofeedback is thought to be a safe technique. It is noninvasive and requires little effort. There have been occasional reports of dizziness, anxiety, disorientation, and a sensation of floating, which may be emotionally upsetting to some people. Biofeedback requires a trained and certified professional to manage equipment, interpret changes, and monitor the patient. Battery-operated devices sold for home use have not been found to be reliable.

Relying on this type of treatment alone and avoiding or delaying conventional medical care for cancer may have serious health consequences.

References

Astin JA, Shapiro SL, Eisenberg DM, Forys KL. Mind-body medicine: state of the science, implications for practice. *J Am Board Fam Pract.* 2003;16:131-147.

Burgio KL, Goode PS, Urban DA, Umlauf MG, Locher JL, Bueschen A, Redden DT. Preoperative biofeedback assisted behavioral training to decrease post-prostatectomy incontinence: a randomized, controlled trial. *J Urol.* 2006;175:196-201.

Burish TG, Jenkins RA. Effectiveness of biofeedback and relaxation training in reducing the side effects of cancer chemotherapy. *Health Psychol.* 1992;11:17-23.

Cassileth B. *The Alternative Medicine Handbook: The Complete Reference Guide to Alternative and Complementary Therapies*. New York: W.W. Norton; 1998.

Ernst E, ed. *The Desktop Guide to Complementary and Alternative Medicine: An Evidence-Based Approach*. New York: Mosby; 2001.

Fiero PL, Galper DI, Cox DJ, Phillips LH II, Fryburg DA. Thermal biofeedback and lower extremity blood flow in adults with diabetes: is neuropathy a limiting factor? *Appl Psychophysiol Biofeedback*. 2003;28:193-203.

Mathewson-Chapman M. Pelvic muscle exercise/biofeedback for urinary incontinence after prostatectomy: an education program. *J Cancer Educ*. 1997;12:218-223.

Mind-body medicine: an overview. National Center for Complementary and Alternative Medicine Web site. http://nccam.nih.gov/health/backgrounds/mindbody.htm. Accessed June 12, 2008.

NIH Technology Assessment Panel. Integration of behavioral and relaxation approaches into the treatment of chronic pain and insomnia. *JAMA*. 1996;276:313-318.

Pain control: a guide for people with cancer and their families. National Cancer Institute Web site. http://www.cancer.gov/cancertopics/paincontrol. Accessed June 12, 2008.

Scharff L, Marcus DA, Masek BJ. A controlled study of minimal-contact thermal biofeedback treatment in children with migraine. *J Pediatr Psychol*. 2002;27:109-119.

BREATHWORK

Other common name(s): none
Scientific/medical name(s): none

Description

Breathwork is a general term used to describe a variety of conscious breathing techniques that are used in many relaxation exercises and spiritual healing methods.

Overview

Available scientific evidence does not support claims for improving health; however, breathwork may help in relaxation and stress reduction.

How is it promoted for use?

Focused deep-breathing exercises, such as exaggerating the way you naturally inhale and exhale, are said to promote relaxation, awareness, and emotional release. Shallow breathing can be a symptom of stress or anxiety. The goal in breathwork is usually to take long, deep breaths. These breaths are said to be "cleansing" in that they free the body and mind from restrictions and release toxins that work against a healthy state.

What does it involve?

There are many types of breathwork and practitioners. Depending on the type of breathwork, the person usually lies down. Each session can last for an hour or more. Breathwork may be done as part of a group or in one-on-one sessions. Music may be included. Effects may include sleepiness; tingling in the hands, feet, or face; and a sense of altered consciousness that can be distressing to some. Unpleasant feelings that surface are "breathed through" to free up energy from the repressed emotions.

What is the history behind it?

Breathwork is a part of ancient meditation practices including yoga. It has also been adapted in modern times to include many different types of breathwork.

What is the evidence?

Available scientific evidence does not support claims that breathwork can improve health. There are indications that it may help in relaxation and stress reduction.

Are there any possible problems or complications?

Breathwork is considered safe as long as it is done with a skilled practitioner. Some people may find the effects distressing. Relying on this type of treatment alone and avoiding or delaying conventional medical care for cancer may have serious health consequences.

References

Kane P. What is breathwork? Relationship Transformations Web site. http://www.rebirthing.com/pages/breathwork.html. Accessed May 23, 2008.

Radiance breathwork. Holistic Healing Web site. http://www.holisticmed.com/inner/breath/radiance.html. Accessed May 23, 2008.

Raso J. The expanded dictionary of metaphysical healthcare, alternative medicine, paranormal healing, and related methods. Quackwatch Web site. http://www.quackwatch.org/01QuackeryRelatedTopics/dictionary/md00.html. Accessed May 28, 2008.

What is holotropic breathwork? Grof Transpersonal Training, Inc. Web site. http://www.holotropic.com/about.shtml. Accessed May 23, 2008.

CRYSTALS

Other common name(s): crystal healing
Scientific/medical name(s): none

Description

Crystals such as quartz, malachite, amethyst, and other gemstones are used for the purposes of healing physical and emotional conditions.

Overview

Available scientific evidence does not support the idea that crystals are effective in treating cancer or any other disease. However, there are individual reports that crystals can be used as a method to promote relaxation and relieve stress.

How is it promoted for use?

Crystals are thought to focus or otherwise transform energy to stimulate healing. Specific crystals are suggested to treat a wide variety of physical and emotional conditions including bursitis, headaches, indigestion, insomnia, hemorrhages, rheumatism, thrombosis, forgetfulness, anxiety, depression, Parkinson's disease, blindness, and cancer. Some people claim certain gemstones or crystals carry special energy that can be transferred to people to provide protection against disease, restore health, and provide spiritual guidance.

Most supporters do not claim stones or crystals can cure illness directly. They say certain stones and crystals emit vibrations that can correct underlying problems, although some crystal healers say that they are used only as adjuncts to other types of healing. It is thought that illness occurs when an individual is misaligned with the divine energy or light that is believed to be the foundation of all creation. The application of stones or crystals within specific energy centers, called chakras, draws light and color into the body's aura. This creates a flow of energy that promotes healing by clearing, balancing, and reenergizing the body's energy fields.

What does it involve?

Crystal therapists are said to intuitively locate "blockages" of energy in the body's aura. They then place stones or crystals on specific parts of the body. Different types and colors of stones or crystals are promoted to have different healing powers. For example, amethysts are thought to calm the mind and uplift the spirit, sapphires are thought to help hearing and mental clarity, and rubies are thought to cleanse the blood and foster courage. Each one is chosen based on the individual's needs and energy fields.

Some people carry crystals in their pockets, wear them on a chain, put them in bath water, or place them in their homes to bring the power of healing within reach. Crystals are sometimes used with other methods such as acupuncture, meditation, and polarity therapy (see pages 156, 105, and 235 for more information).

What is the history behind it?

The use of crystals for healing dates back to the ancient Greeks and Indians, who believed there were large gems that gave light to another world under the known world. Some ancient cultures believed that spirits lived inside crystals. They also thought crystals created and gave off light. Crystals remain popular among some alternative therapy proponents today.

What is the evidence?

Available scientific evidence does not support the idea that crystals are useful in promoting healing. Some crystals have the ability to bend or refract light, which creates a rainbow effect. Phosphorescent crystals can hold light for a short period of time, but they do not have their own energy source or special powers. Some people believe that crystals or gemstones are helpful as a complementary treatment to promote relaxation and reduce stress. This may occur as a result of the "placebo effect," in which believing that something can or will happen produces a positive result.

Are there any possible problems or complications?

Crystals are thought to be relatively safe. However, relying on this type of treatment alone and avoiding or delaying conventional medical care for cancer may have serious health consequences.

References

Beyerstein BL. Distinguishing science from pseudoscience. Prepared for The Centre for Curriculum and Professional Development. Simon Fraser University Web site. http://www.sfu.ca/~beyerste/research/articles/02Sciencevs Pseudoscience.pdf. Published July 1995. Revised October 1996. Accessed May 23, 2008.

Healing with crystals. Mystical Soup Web site. http://mysticalsoup.com/crystals.html Accessed March 20, 2007. Site now discontinued.

Maasdijk H. Crystal healing. Complementary Healthcare Information Service UK Web site. http://www.chisuk.org.uk/articles/result.php?key=132. Accessed May 23, 2008.

Raso J. The expanded dictionary of metaphysical healthcare, alternative medicine, paranormal healing, and related methods. Quackwatch Web site. http://www.quackwatch.org/01QuackeryRelatedTopics/dictionary/md00.html. Accessed May 28, 2008.

CURANDERISMO

Other common name(s): Latin American healing, Latin American folk medicine, curandismo
Scientific/medical name(s): none

Description

Curanderismo is a form of folk healing that includes various techniques such as prayer, herbal medicine, healing rituals, spiritualism, massage, and psychic healing. It is a system of traditional beliefs that are common in Hispanic-American communities, particularly in the southwestern United States.

Overview

Available scientific evidence does not support the idea that curanderismo is effective in treating cancer or any other disease. However, there are some individual reports that curanderismo helps to improve symptoms, reduce pain, and relieve stress.

How is it promoted for use?

While some aspects of curanderismo, such as using folk remedies for minor illness, are practiced at home, many people seek out specially trained folk healers called *curanderos* (male healers) or *curanderas* (female healers). Curanderos' knowledge of healing may be passed down from close relatives or learned through apprenticeships with experienced healers. In some cases, their healing powers may be described as a divine gift received later in life. Most curanderos say that their ability to heal involves divine energy being channeled through their bodies.

In addition to the curanderos, there are *yerberos* (herbalists), *parteras* (midwives), and *sobadors* or *sobadoras* (who use massage, bone manipulation, acupressure, etc.), each of whom treat more specific or limited problems. All of these healers may use herbs in addition to their other treatment methods. Most of these healers do not charge for their services, but they may accept donations.

Proponents claim curanderismo can be used to treat a wide range of social, spiritual, psychological, or physical problems, including headache, gastrointestinal distress, back pain, and fever as well as anxiety, irritability, fatigue, and depression. Bad luck, marital discord, and illnesses caused by "loss of spirit" may be treated by curanderos or curanderas. Treatment may involve physical, spiritual, and mental approaches.

Practitioners believe good health is achieved by maintaining a balance of hot and cold. In order to treat a person, curanderos often classify that person's physical activities, food intake, drug consumption, and illnesses as hot or cold and treat the person to restore balance. Proponents also claim folk illnesses such as *mal de ojo* (the evil eye), *susto* (fright), and *empacho* (blockage of the digestive tract) can be treated by curanderismo. In these cases, the curandero may perform *barridas* (ritual cleansing) to rebalance the body and soul of the sick person.

What does it involve?

Curanderismo techniques can involve the use of herbs, massage, manipulation of body parts, spiritual rituals, and prayer—either in combination or by themselves. The healing often involves others in the family and community.

The treatments given by curanderos can vary widely depending upon the nature of the illness or complaint. For physical illnesses, herbal mixtures, poultices, or teas are often recommended. One cure for a headache is to place a slice of raw potato over each temple. Dandruff is treated by rinsing hair with juice from the olivera plant, a type of cactus. To reduce the size of an overly large "energy field," the curandero may beat the air around the patient's head with a large feather, then roll an egg around the patient's face before cracking it open into a glass.

What is the history behind it?

Curanderismo evolved from the culture that grew out of the Spanish colonization of Mexico hundreds of years ago. It takes its name from the Spanish word *curar*, meaning "to heal." The tradition combines aspects of both Catholicism and the traditional folk medicine of the natives of Latin America.

Today, it is practiced in several Latin American countries as well as in the United States. Because of its long history of cultural connection, curanderismo remains popular among some Mexican-American communities as an alternative form of medicine. Curanderismo has remained popular among some of these communities because it offers a spiritual treatment for problems that conventional medicine does not recognize, such as evil spirits. Also, many people have turned to curanderismo after conventional treatments have failed to cure their disease or because they do not trust conventional methods.

What is the evidence?

Available scientific evidence does not support any claims that curanderismo cures cancer or any other disease. However, some people report it helps to reduce pain, relieve stress, and promote spiritual peace. A study in 1977 that looked at the relationship between Mexican-American populations and folk medicine suggested that conventional medicine look more closely at curanderismo. Researchers proposed that a better understanding of folk medicine, including curanderismo, might help physicians treat patients more effectively and understand patients' fears and beliefs. A more recent study found that patients often seek treatment by curanderos alongside conventional medical treatment.

Are there any possible problems or complications?

Treatment by curanderos may involve taking unregulated herbs, some of which may have harmful effects. In addition, the potential interactions between herbal preparations and conventional drugs and other herbs should be considered. Some of these combinations may be dangerous. Always tell your doctor and pharmacist about any herbs you are taking.

Relying on this type of treatment alone and avoiding or delaying conventional medical care for cancer may have serious health consequences.

These substances may have not been thoroughly tested to find out how they interact with medicines, foods, or dietary supplements. Even though some reports of interactions and harmful effects may be published, full studies of interactions and effects are not often available. Because of these limitations, any information on ill effects and interactions should be considered incomplete.

References

Alegria D, Guerra E, Martinez C Jr, Meyer GG. El hospital invisible. A study of curanderismo. *Arch Gen Psychiatry.* 1977;34:1354-1357.

Allen H. Folk healer discusses art of 'curanderismo.' *Yale Daily News Online.* Yale Daily News Web site. http://www.yaledailynews.com/. Accessed December 11, 1999. Content no longer available.

Cosentino BW. Harmony and healing: the practices of curanderismo. Swedish Medical Center Web site. http://www.swedish.org/16379.cfm?InFrame. Accessed March 20, 2007. Content no longer available.

Graham J. Curanderismo. Handbook of Texas Online. Texas State Historical Association Web site. http://www.tshaonline.org/handbook/online/articles/CC/sdc1.html. Accessed May 23, 2008.

Liñan L. Curanderismo: holistic healing. Denver Public Schools Web site. http://www.dpsk12.org/programs/almaproject/pdf/Curanderismo.pdf. Accessed May 23, 2008.

National Institutes of Health. *Alternative Medicine: Expanding Medical Horizons: A Report to the National Institutes of Health on Alternative Medical Systems and Practices in the United States.* Washington, DC: US Government Printing Office; 1994. NIH publication 94-066.

Ness RC, Wintrob RM. Folk healing: a description and synthesis. *Am J Psychiatry.* 1981;138:1477-1481.

CYMATIC THERAPY

Other common name(s): cymatherapy
Scientific/medical names(s): none

Description

Cymatic therapy is a form of sound therapy. Cymatics refers to the effect of sound waves on matter, and cymatic therapy presumes that sound can have similar effects on the body.

Overview

Available scientific evidence does not support the claim that cymatics can have a healing effect.

How is it promoted for use?

According to practitioners, illness occurs when the rhythms of the heart, brain, and other organs are not working harmoniously. Proponents say that the sound waves promote a healing environment for the body's cells, restoring the body's rhythms and boosting the immune system.

What does it involve?

During treatment, computerized instruments are used to transmit sound waves through the skin, either directed toward the diseased organ or transmitted along the acupuncture meridians. The practitioner selects frequencies that are similar to those that are normally emitted by the healthy body part. The signals passed through these cymatic devices are supposed to restore synchronous rhythms and boost the body's regulatory and immune systems. In some of the newer cymatic devices, a magnetic field has been added to oscillate along with the sound waves.

What is the history behind it?

Cymatic therapy was developed in the 1960s by Sir Peter Guy Manners, MD, DO, PhD, of England. It is based on the work of Hans Jenny, who coined the term "cymatics" in the mid-twentieth century.

What is the evidence?

Practitioners of cymatic therapy believe that sound waves can rearrange molecules in the body. Although the sound waves do not directly heal, proponents say that the waves promote a healing environment for the body's cells. Available scientific evidence does not support this claim.

Are there any possible problems or complications?

Cymatic therapy is safe as long as it is done by a skilled practitioner. Relying on this type of treatment alone and avoiding or delaying conventional medical care for cancer may have serious health consequences.

References

Helwig D. Cymatic therapy. In: Krapp K, Longe J, eds. *The Gale Encyclopedia of Alternative Medicine*. Farmington Hills, MI: Gale Group; 2001.

Raphael A. Cymatics today with Elizabeth Colorio. *Spirit of Ma'at*. 2002;3. Spirit of Ma'at Web site. http://www.spiritofmaat.com/archive/oct3/colorio.htm. Accessed May 23, 2008.

DANCE THERAPY

Other common name(s): movement therapy
Scientific/medical names(s): none

Description

Dance therapy is the therapeutic use of movement to improve the mental and physical well-being of a person. It focuses on the connection between the mind and body to promote health and healing. Dance therapy can be considered an expressive therapy.

Overview

Few scientific studies have been done to evaluate the effects of dance therapy on health, prevention, and recovery from illness. Clinical reports suggest dance therapy may be effective in improving self-esteem and reducing stress. As a form of exercise, dance therapy can be useful for both physical and emotional aspects of quality of life.

How is it promoted for use?

Dance therapy is offered as a health promotion service for healthy people and as a complementary method of reducing the stress of caregivers and people with cancer and other chronic illnesses. Physically, dance therapy can provide exercise, improve mobility and muscle coordination, and reduce muscle tension. Emotionally, dance therapy is reported to improve self-awareness, self-confidence, and interpersonal interaction and is an outlet for communicating feelings. Some promoters claim that dance therapy may strengthen the immune system through muscular action and physiological processes and can even help prevent disease.

Dance therapy is based on the belief that the mind and body work together. Through dance, it is thought that people can identify and express their innermost emotions, bringing those feelings to the surface. Some people claim this can create a sense of renewal, unity, and completeness.

What does it involve?

Dance therapists help people develop a nonverbal language that offers information about what is going on in their bodies. The therapist observes a person's movements to make an assessment and then designs a program to help the specific condition. The frequency and level of difficulty of the therapy are usually tailored to meet the needs of the participants.

Dance therapy is used in a variety of settings with people who have social, emotional, cognitive, or physical concerns. It is often used as a part of the recovery process for people with chronic illnesses. Dance therapists work with both individuals and groups, including entire families.

What is the history behind it?

Dance has been an important part of self-expression, ceremonial and religious events, and health in most cultures throughout history. For example, medicine men and women of many Native American tribes used dance as part of their healing rituals. The use of dance as a complement to conventional Western medical therapy began in 1942 through the work of Marian Chace. She was asked to work at St. Elizabeth's Hospital in Washington, D.C., after psychiatrists saw therapeutic benefit in patients who attended her dance classes. Another woman who was a dancer and mime, Trudi Schoop, volunteered to work with patients at a state hospital in California at about that time. In 1956, the American Dance Therapy Association was founded to establish and maintain high standards in the field of dance therapy. There are now more than 1,200 dance therapists in the United States and abroad. In 1993, the Office of Alternative Medicine of the National Institutes of Health provided a research grant to explore dance therapy for people with medical illnesses.

A master's degree is required to be a dance therapist. Beginning-level dance therapists who have at least seven hundred hours of supervised clinical training hold the title of "Dance Therapists Registered" (DTR). The title "Academy of Dance Therapists" (ADTR) is awarded to advanced-level dance therapists who have completed 3,640 hours of supervised clinical work in an agency, institution, or special school with additional supervision from an ADTR.

What is the evidence?

Although individual accounts provide most of the support for the value of dance therapy, a few experimental studies evaluating the effects of dance therapy on health have been published. In one recent study, a group of breast cancer survivors took part in a twelve-week dance therapy and movement class. The women who had dance therapy showed better range of motion in their shoulders than those who had not had the class. The patients' perceptions of their bodies also improved after dance therapy. Clinical reports suggest that dance therapy helps in developing body image; improving self-concept and self-esteem; reducing stress, anxiety, and depression; decreasing isolation, chronic pain, and body tension; and increasing communication skills and feelings of well-being.

Some of the physical motions used in dance therapy can provide the same health benefits produced by other types of exercise. Physical activity is known to increase special neurotransmitter substances in the brain, called endorphins, which create a feeling of well-being. Total body movement also enhances the functions of other body systems, such as the circulatory, respiratory, skeletal, and muscular systems. Regular aerobic exercise helps with glucose metabolism, cardiovascular fitness, and weight control. Dance or movement therapy, when done regularly, can confer the same benefits as other types of exercise. Moderate to vigorous exercise for thirty to forty-five minutes on most days of the week can reduce the risk for heart disease and certain types of cancer. Dance therapy can help people stay physically fit and experience the pleasure of creating rhythmic motions with their bodies. Well-controlled research is needed, however, to confirm the effects of dance therapy on prevention of and recovery from illness.

Are there any possible problems or complications?

People with cancer and chronic conditions such as arthritis and heart disease should talk with their doctors before starting any type of therapy that involves manipulation or movement of joints and muscles. Relying on this type of treatment alone and avoiding or delaying conventional medical care for cancer may have serious health consequences.

References

Cassileth B. *The Alternative Medicine Handbook: The Complete Reference Guide to Alternative and Complementary Therapies*. New York: W.W. Norton; 1998.

Castaneda C. Diabetes control with physical activity and exercise. *Nutr Clin Care*. 2003;6:89-96.

Cohen SO, Walco GA. Dance/movement therapy for children and adolescents with cancer. *Cancer Pract*. 1999;7:34-42.

Dance/movement therapy fact sheet. American Dance Therapy Association Web site. http://www.adta.org/about/factsheet.cfm. Accessed May 23, 2008.

Hanna JL. The power of dance: health and healing. *J Altern Complement Med*. 1995;1:323-331.

Kushi LH, Byers T, Doyle C, Bandera EV, McCullough M, McTiernan A, Gansler T, Andrews KS, Thun MJ; American Cancer Society 2006 Nutrition and Physical Activity Guidelines Advisory Committee. American Cancer Society guidelines on nutrition and physical activity for cancer prevention: reducing the risk of cancer with healthy food choices and physical activity. *CA Cancer J Clin.* 2006;56:254-281.

National Institutes of Health. *Alternative Medicine: Expanding Medical Horizons: A Report to the National Institutes of Health on Alternative Medical Systems and Practices in the United States.* Washington, DC: US Government Printing Office; 1994. NIH publication 94-066.

Sandel SL, Judge JO, Landry N, Faria L, Ouellette R, Majczak M. Dance and movement program improves quality-of-life measures in breast cancer survivors. *Cancer Nurs.* 2005;28:301-309.

FAITH HEALING

Other common name(s): spiritual healing, laying on of hands
Scientific/medical name(s): none

Description

Faith healing is founded on the belief that certain people or places have the ability to cure and heal—that someone or something can eliminate disease or heal injuries through a close connection to a higher power. Faith healing can involve prayer, a visit to a religious shrine, or simply a strong belief in a supreme being.

Overview

Available scientific evidence does not support claims that faith healing can cure cancer or any other disease. Even the "miraculous" cures at the French shrine of Lourdes, after careful study by the Catholic Church, do not outnumber the historical percentage of spontaneous remissions seen among people with cancer. However, faith healing may promote peace of mind, reduce stress, relieve pain and anxiety, and strengthen the will to live.

How is it promoted for use?

According to proponents, there is little that faith healing cannot do. Many religious sects claim faith can cure blindness, deafness, cancer, AIDS, developmental disorders, anemia, arthritis, corns, defective speech, multiple sclerosis, skin rashes, total body paralysis, and various injuries. Christian Scientists, for instance, believe that illness is an illusion that can be healed through prayer, either for oneself or by trained practitioners.

What does it involve?

Faith healing can be practiced near the patient or at a distance from the patient. When practiced from afar, it can involve a single faith healer or a group of people praying for the patient. When near to the patient, as in revivalist tent meetings, the healer often touches, or "lays hands on," the patient while calling on a supreme being. Faith healing can also involve a pilgrimage to a religious shrine, such as the French shrine at Lourdes, in search of a miracle. Christian Scientists train and use their own practitioners to heal sick persons through prayer.

What is the history behind it?

Faith healing is believed to have begun even before the earliest recorded history. In the Bible, both God and holy people are said to have the power to heal. In Medieval times, the Divine Right of Kings was thought to give royalty the ability to heal through touch. Through the years, up to and including the twentieth century, there have been numerous reports of saints performing miracle cures. Today, several religious groups, including Christian Scientists, evangelical Protestants, and some orthodox Jewish sects, practice faith healing.

What is the evidence?

Although it is known that a small percentage of people with cancer experience remissions of their disease that cannot be explained, available scientific evidence does not support claims that faith healing can actually cure physical ailments. When a person believes strongly that a healer can create a cure, a "placebo effect" can occur. The placebo effect can make the person feel better, but it has not been found to induce remission or improve chance of survival. The patient usually credits the improvement in how he or she feels to the healer, even though the perceived improvement occurs because of the patient's belief in the treatment. Taking part in faith healing can evoke the power of suggestion and affirm one's faith in a higher power, which may help promote peace of mind. This may help some people cope more effectively with their illness.

One review published in 1998 looked at 172 cases of deaths among children who had been treated by faith healing instead of conventional methods. These researchers estimated that if conventional treatment had been given, the survival rate for most of these children would have been more than 90 percent, with the remainder of the children also having a good chance of survival. A more recent study found that more than two hundred children had died of treatable illnesses in the United States over the past thirty years because their parents relied on spiritual healing rather than conventional medical treatment.

In addition, at least one study has suggested that adult Christian Scientists, who generally use prayer rather than medical care, have a higher death rate than other people of the same age.

Are there any possible problems or complications?

People who seek help through faith healing and are not cured may have feelings of hopelessness, failure, guilt, worthlessness, and depression. In some groups, the person may be told that his or her faith was not strong enough. The healer and others may hold the person responsible for the failure of their healing. This can alienate and discourage the person who is still sick.

Relying on this type of treatment alone and avoiding or delaying conventional medical care for cancer may have serious health consequences. Death, disability, and other unwanted outcomes have occurred when faith healing was elected instead of medical care for serious injuries or illnesses.

While competent adults may choose faith healing over medical care, communities often become concerned when parents make such choices for their children. This concern has sparked organizations to work toward creating laws to protect children from inappropriate treatment by faith healers.

Finally, a few "faith healers" have been caught using fraud as a way to get others to believe in their methods. These people often solicited large donations or charged money for their healing sessions.

References

Asser SM, Swan R. Child fatalities from religion-motivated medical neglect. *Pediatrics*. 1998;101:625-629.

Barrett S. Some thoughts about faith healing. Quackwatch Web site. http://www.quackwatch.org/dantest/faith.html. Updated July 21, 2000. Accessed May 23, 2008.

The Church of Christ, Scientist (Christian Science). Ontario Consultants on Religious Tolerance Web site. http://www.religioustolerance.org/cr_sci.htm. Accessed May 23, 2008.

Hickey KS, Lyckholm L. Child welfare versus parental autonomy: medical ethics, the law, and faith-based healing. *Theor Med Bioeth*. 2004;25:265-276.

National Institutes of Health. *Alternative Medicine: Expanding Medical Horizons: A Report to the National Institutes of Health on Alternative Medical Systems and Practices in the United States*. Washington, DC: US Government Printing Office; 1994. NIH publication 94-066.

US Congress, Office of Technology Assessment. *Unconventional Cancer Treatments: OTA-H-405*. Washington, DC: US Government Printing Office; 1990.

FENG SHUI

Other common name(s): none
Scientific/medical name(s): none

Description

Feng shui is the ancient Chinese philosophy and art of placing objects, ornaments, furniture, rooms, buildings, and even towns in position so they promote the beneficial flow of vital energy or life force called qi or chi. The words *feng shui* literally mean wind and water.

Overview

The ancient Chinese art of feng shui rests on placement of things so they are in harmony with one another and with the environment. Available scientific evidence does not support claims that feng shui can influence health.

How is it promoted for use?

Proponents of feng shui hold that the same natural elements that form the earth, such as wind and water, can bring healthy energy into homes, buildings, and cities if the placement of these manmade elements permits energy to flow through the environment.

Some also believe that living and work environments that are out of balance may promote disease, including cancer, and prevent those who live in the environment from responding to treatment. Changes in the environment, supporters claim, may help prevent disease and promote healing. For example, simply placing the bed of a person with cancer, or at risk for cancer, in a new position is thought to prevent the development or progression for the disease.

What does it involve?

The idea behind feng shui is to position physical objects to allow people to live in harmony with the environment and the universe. In order to meet this goal, a feng shui practitioner will first study the physical environment outside a person's home to make sure the house is positioned in a way that promotes a positive flow of energy. Next, the inside of the house is reviewed. Furniture may be moved or placed at angles until rooms are more open and free of clutter or obstacles that could hinder energy from flowing around the house. Fountains, plants, or other objects may be added to increase energy in certain areas. Materials and colors are used in certain areas to represent the five elements—wood, fire, earth, metal, and water. A feng shui practitioner will also analyze the electromagnetic energy in a person's home, sometimes using a specialized compass to make sure the energy is balanced in order to promote good health and well-being.

What is the history behind it?

Feng shui has been practiced in China since the Qin Dynasty beginning in about 221 BC. In ancient China, feng shui began as an oral tradition and was taught only to a select few by a master. The techniques were a well-guarded secret.

In 1929, a German baron, Gustave von Pohl, reportedly linked an unusually high cancer rate in the German village of Vilsbiburg to "radiation" coming from geological faults below the city. In 1932, von Pohl published a book called *Earth Currents: Causative Factors of Cancer and Other Diseases*. Currently, some alternative medical practitioners have cited von Pohl's theories as proof that imbalances in the natural energy or magnetic force of a physical area can cause illness. They claim that feng shui can be used to rebalance a physical environment and restore well-being. The philosophy of feng shui has spread to the Western world, where it has become popular for interior and building design.

What is the evidence?

Available scientific evidence does not support claims that feng shui has any effect on cancer or any other disease.

Are there any possible problems or complications?

No adverse effects have been reported with the use of feng shui. Relying on this type of treatment alone and avoiding or delaying conventional medical care for cancer may have serious health consequences.

References

Frequently asked questions about feng shui. Fast Feng Shui Web site. http://www.fastfengshui.com/faqs_about fengshui.htm. Accessed May 23, 2008.

Rossbach S. Feng shui explores relationship between design and health—ancient Chinese art of placement. *Calif Hosp*. 1991;5:29-31.

Von Pohl GF. *Earth Currents: Causative Factor of Cancer and Other Diseases.* Feucht, Germany: Fortschritt fuer alle-Verlag; 1983.

HOLISTIC MEDICINE

Other common name(s): holistic health, holistic care, wholistic health, holism
Scientific/medical name(s): none

Description

Holistic medicine focuses on how the physical, mental, emotional, and spiritual elements of the body are interconnected to maintain wellness, or holistic health. When one part of the body or mind is not working properly, it is believed to affect the whole person. Holistic approaches focus on the whole person rather than just on the illness or part of the body that is not healthy.

Overview

Available scientific evidence does not support claims that holistic medicine, when used without mainstream or conventional medicine, is effective in treating cancer or any other disease. However, many health professionals promote healthy lifestyle habits such as exercising, eating a nutritious diet, not smoking, and managing stress as important in maintaining good health. Holistic methods are becoming more common in mainstream care and may be used as complementary therapy or preventive care.

In mainstream medicine, a holistic approach generally means a more inclusive approach to a person's health, one that includes the patient's social and cultural situation as well as his or her illness. This term holistic is used by doctors to reflect a focus on a person's overall health, a focus that includes prevention, rehabilitation, and other approaches, rather than illness alone. Nurses, for example, may speak of the "biopsychosocial sphere" of a patient. This concept means that a person's health includes the mind, body, and spirit as well as the surrounding culture and environment. This can include one's family situation, housing, employment, insurance, and more, since these all have an impact on the patient and his or her health. If all these factors are taken into account when a person is treated for cancer, it may make treatment easier and improve chances of success.

How is it promoted for use?

Holistic medicine approaches health and disease from several angles. The approach suggests that a person should treat not only the illness but also the whole self to reach a higher level of wellness. For example, practitioners may treat cancer by making dietary and behavioral changes and adding social support groups and counseling. Others may suggest taking botanical supplements and using complementary therapies, such as art therapy, hypnosis, imagery, meditation, psychotherapy, spirituality and prayer, and yoga. These approaches can be used with conventional medical treatments such as chemotherapy, surgery, radiation therapy, and hormone therapy. Combining these different methods can help a person take control of his or her situation and attain a feeling of total wellness—spiritual, physical, and mental.

Some supporters of holistic medicine claim, however, that conventional medicine does not work and that only the holistic approach to cancer and other diseases is effective. They may offer a "cure" based on individual stories of success or personal experiences, which are very hard to prove. Some of the types of cancer that they claim can be cured by holistic methods include cancers of the bone, breast, tongue, liver, lung, throat, skin, testicle, prostate, ovary, uterus, stomach, intestine, colon, brain, pancreas, spleen, kidney, and bladder as well as leukemia, lymphoma, and melanoma.

What does it involve?

The field of holistic medicine is very diverse and broad. Some providers define holistic oncology as including emotional and spiritual care, while others focus on these aspects to the exclusion of the physical. There are many different techniques and approaches in holistic medicine, depending on the practitioner, the person, and the illness. All, however, stress the use of treatments that encourage the body's natural healing system and take into account the person as a whole.

Holistic medicine can involve the use of conventional and alternative therapies but focuses mostly on lifestyle changes. A holistic approach to stomach cancer might include reducing sodium intake, increasing intake of antioxidants through food or vitamins, eliminating *Helicobacter pylori* (a bacterium in the stomach), quitting smoking, improving oral hygiene, avoiding foods that contain genotoxic agents, and increasing the amount of vegetables and fruits consumed.

Holistic medicine can also include natural supplements that cause the same changes as conventional drugs. For instance, synthetic interferon is currently used to treat some people with cancer. A holistic approach might be to take high doses of intravenous vitamin C instead, in an attempt to stimulate the body's production of its own interferon.

The American Holistic Association says that healthy lifestyle habits will improve a person's energy and vitality. Those habits might include exercising, eating a nutritious diet, getting enough sleep, learning how to breathe properly, taking antioxidants and supplements, and using acupuncture, acupressure, healing touch, craniosacral therapy, yoga, qigong, and other methods.

What is the history behind it?

Holistic medicine has its roots in several ancient healing traditions that stress healthy living and being in harmony with nature. Socrates promoted a holistic approach. Plato was another advocate of holism, advising doctors to respect the relationship between mind and body. Hippocrates emphasized the body's ability to heal itself and cautioned doctors not to interfere with that process.

It was not until 1926, however, that Jan Christiaan Smuts coined the term "holism," which gave rise to the more integrated concept of psychosomatic medicine now known as holistic medicine. In the 1970s, holistic became a more common term. Today, holistic medicine is known as an approach to life and health that brings together the physical, mental, and spiritual aspects of a person in order to create a total sense of well-being.

What is the evidence?

Although there has been research on various complementary methods that may be considered part of a holistic approach, scientific research generally does not focus on holistic medicine by itself as a cure for cancer or any other disease. Available scientific evidence does not support the idea that alternative practitioners are more effective than conventional physicians in persuading their patients to improve their lifestyles. Nor have available scientific studies shown that any of these approaches are effective or cost-effective against any disease if holistic methods are used without conventional medical treatment.

Some health care professionals suggest that cancer pain and some side effects of treatment can be managed with a holistic approach that includes the physical, psychological, and spiritual factors involved with each person. Increasingly, the health care team comprises a diverse and varied group of health care professionals. Members of this team are drawn from the specialties of medicine, nursing, surgery, radiation therapy, oncology, psychiatry, psychology, and social work. In addition, the team may call on dietitians, physical therapists, and the clergy for support. Health professionals realize that a person's health depends on the balance of physical, psychological, social, and cultural forces. However, available scientific evidence does not support claims that holistic medicine alone can cure illness.

Are there any possible problems or complications?

Adopting healthy habits related to diet, exercise, and emotional and spiritual well-being is considered important to maintaining good health. In fact, studies have shown that certain dietary changes and regular exercise can reduce your risk for some kinds of cancer. However, relying on healthy habits or holistic measures alone and avoiding or delaying conventional medical care for cancer may have serious health consequences.

These substances may have not been thoroughly tested to find out how they interact with medicines, foods, or dietary supplements. Even though some reports of interactions and harmful effects may be

published, full studies of interactions and effects are not often available. Because of these limitations, any information on ill effects and interactions should be considered incomplete.

References

Barrett S. Be wary of "alternative" health methods. Quackwatch Web site. http://www.quackwatch.org/01QuackeryRelatedTopics/altwary.html. Updated February 10, 2004. Accessed May 23, 2008.

Cancer and the impact of family history. *Network Newsletter*. Spring 2003. The University of Texas M. D. Anderson Cancer Center Web site.http://www.mdanderson.org/publications/network/display.cfm?id=31d5ee07-ba4e-45c8-8a81c1519793162b&pn=8f5f110c-a318-46ea-8d0bd00e7d3770ed&method=displayfull. Accessed May 23, 2008.

Carson JW, Keefe FJ, Lynch TR, Carson KM, Goli V, Fras AM, Thorp SR. Loving-kindness meditation for chronic low back pain: results from a pilot trial. *J Holist Nurs*. 2005;23:287-304.

Curry SJ, Byers T, Hewitt M, eds. National Cancer Policy Board and the Institute of Medicine National Research Council of the National Academies. *Fulfilling the Potential for Cancer Prevention and Early Detection*. Washington, DC: National Academies Press; 2003.

Deming S. Center for Research on Minority Health: working with the community to end health disparities. *OncoLog*. 2003;48:4-6.

Hassed C. Cancer and chronic pain. *Aust Fam Physician*. 1999;28:17-21, 23-24.

Kohara H, Miyauchi T, Suehiro Y, Ueoka H, Takeyama H, Morita T. Combined modality treatment of aromatherapy, footsoak, and reflexology relieves fatigue in patients with cancer. *J Palliat Med*. 2004;7:791-796.

Kushi LH, Byers T, Doyle C, Bandera EV, McCullough M, McTiernan A, Gansler T, Andrews KS, Thun MJ; American Cancer Society 2006 Nutrition and Physical Activity Guidelines Advisory Committee. American Cancer Society guidelines on nutrition and physical activity for cancer prevention: reducing the risk of cancer with healthy food choices and physical activity. *CA Cancer J Clin*. 2006;56:254-281.

National Center for Complementary and Alternative Medicine. March 23-24, 1998: AMPAC Meeting Minutes: IX. Public Comments.

Robins JL, McCain NL, Gray DP, Elswick RK Jr, Walter JM, McDade E. Research on psychoneuroimmunology: tai chi as a stress management approach for individuals with HIV disease. *Appl Nurs Res*. 2006;19:2-9.

HUMOR THERAPY

Other common name(s): laugh therapy
Scientific name(s): none

Description

Humor therapy is the use of humor for the relief of physical or emotional pain and stress. It is used as a complementary method to promote health and cope with illness.

Overview

Although available scientific evidence does not support claims that laughter can cure cancer or any other disease, it can reduce stress and enhance a person's quality of life. Humor has physical effects because it can stimulate the circulatory system, immune system, and other systems in the body.

How is it promoted for use?

Humor therapy is generally used to improve quality of life, provide pain relief, encourage relaxation, and reduce stress. Researchers have described different types of humor. Passive humor results from seeing prepared material, such as watching a funny movie or stand-up comedy or reading an amusing book. Spontaneous or unplanned humor involves finding humor in everyday situations. Being able to find humor in life can be helpful when dealing with cancer.

What does it involve?

The physical effects of laughter on the body include increased breathing, increased oxygen use, short-term changes in hormones and certain neurotransmitters, and increased heart rate. Many hospitals and treatment centers have set up special rooms with humorous materials for the purpose of making people laugh, such as movies, audio recordings, books, games, and puzzles. Many hospitals use volunteers who visit patients for the purpose of making them laugh. Some cancer treatment centers offer humor therapy in addition to standard treatments.

What is the history behind it?

Humor has been used in medicine throughout recorded history. One of the earliest mentions of the health benefits of humor is in the book of Proverbs in the Bible. As early as the thirteenth century, some surgeons used humor to distract patients from the pain of surgery. Humor was also widely used and studied by the medical community in the early twentieth century. In more modern times, the most famous story of humor therapy involved Norman Cousins, then editor of the *Saturday Review*. According to the story, Mr. Cousins cured himself of an unknown illness with a self-invented regimen of laughter and vitamins.

What is the evidence?

Available scientific evidence does not support humor as an effective treatment for cancer or any other disease; however, laughter has many benefits, including positive physical changes and an overall sense of well-being. One study found the use of humor led to an increase in pain tolerance. It is thought laughter causes the release of special neurotransmitter substances in the brain called endorphins, which help control pain. Another study found that neuroendocrine and stress-related hormones decreased during episodes of laughter. These findings provide support for the claim that humor can relieve stress. More studies are needed to clarify the impact of laughter on health.

Are there any possible problems or complications?

Humor therapy is considered safe when used with conventional medical therapy. It can be harmful if used to avoid difficult or delicate issues that are important to you or your family. Laughter can also cause temporary pain after some types of surgery. This improves as the body heals and causes no lasting harm. Relying on this type of treatment alone and avoiding or delaying conventional medical care for cancer may have serious health consequences.

References

Berk LS, Tan SA, Fry WF, Napier BJ, Lee JW, Hubbard RW, Lewis JE, Eby WC. Neuroendocrine and stress hormone changes during mirthful laughter. *Am J Med Sci.* 1989;298:390-396.

Joshua AM, Cotroneo A, Clarke S. Humor and oncology. *J Clin Oncol.* 2005;23:645-648.

Penson RT, Partridge RA, Rudd P, Seiden MV, Nelson JE, Chabner BA, Lynch TJ Jr. Laughter: the best medicine? *Oncologist.* 2005;10:651-660.

Seaward BL. Humor's healing potential. *Health Prog.* 1992;73:66-70.

Weisenberg M, Tepper I, Schwarzwald J. Humor as a cognitive technique for increasing pain tolerance. *Pain.* 1995;63:207-212.

Ziegler J. Immune system may benefit from the ability to laugh. *J Natl Cancer Inst.* 1995;87:342-343.

HYPNOSIS

Other common name(s): hypnotherapy, hypnotic suggestion, self-hypnosis
Scientific/medical name(s): none

Description

Hypnosis is a state of restful alertness during which a person uses deeply focused concentration. The person can be relatively unaware of but not completely blind to his or her surroundings, and he or she may be more open to suggestion. It is considered to be a type of complementary therapy.

Overview

Hypnosis is one of several relaxation methods that was evaluated and found to be of possible benefit by an independent panel convened by the National Institutes of Health (NIH). The panel found it may be useful for treating chronic pain when used with standard medical care. Hypnosis may also be effective in reducing fear and anxiety, reducing the frequency and severity of headaches, and controlling bleeding and pain during dental procedures. Available scientific evidence does not support the idea that hypnosis can influence the development or progression of cancer. However, it may help to improve quality of life for some people with cancer.

How is it promoted for use?

Practitioners say that hypnosis creates a state of deep relaxation, quiets the conscious mind, and leaves the unconscious mind open to suggestions that can help to improve health and lifestyle. People who are hypnotized have selective attention and are able to concentrate intensely on a specific thought, memory, feeling, or sensation while blocking out distractions.

Hypnosis is commonly used to reduce stress and anxiety and create a sense of well-being. It is also promoted to change undesirable behaviors, such as smoking, alcohol dependence, and bedwetting. It is used along with other methods by some mental health professionals to help patients overcome common fears, such as the fear of flying or the fear of meeting new people. Hypnosis is sometimes used to help relieve pain caused by cancer. Supporters generally do not claim that hypnosis can cure cancer or any other disease or that it always attains the desired results. However, they say that it can be a useful addition to conventional therapy for some conditions.

Hypnosis is occasionally used instead of anesthetic drugs during minor surgical and dental procedures and during childbirth. Some supporters also believe hypnosis speeds recovery after operations, can reduce the amount of surgical bleeding, and enhances the body's immune system.

What does it involve?

There are many different hypnotic techniques. One method involves leading patients into a state of hypnosis by talking in gentle, soothing tones and describing images meant to create a sense of relaxation, security, and well-being. People under hypnosis may appear to be asleep, but they are actually in an altered state of concentration and can focus intently when asked to do so by the hypnotherapist. While a patient is under hypnosis, the hypnotherapist may suggest specific outcomes, such as pain control, more peaceful emotions, and less stress, fear, or anxiety.

Contrary to what many believe, people under hypnosis are not under the control of the hypnotherapist. They cannot be made to do something they do not want to do. Quite the opposite is true. Hypnosis is used to help patients gain more control over their behavior, emotions, and even some physical processes that cause problems for them. People cannot be hypnotized unless they wish to be, and not everyone can be put into a hypnotic state. Success depends upon whether the patient is willing and receptive to the idea of hypnosis. Some people can enter into a deeper hypnotic state than others and are said to be more hypnotizable. With training, many people can learn to hypnotize themselves. This is called self-hypnosis or autohypnosis.

What is the history behind it?

Hypnosis and hypnotic suggestion have been a part of healing practices for thousands of years. The word comes from the Greek word *hypnos*, which means sleep. The use of trance-like states and positive suggestion was an important feature of the early Greek healing temples. Variations of those techniques were practiced throughout the ancient world.

Modern hypnosis can be traced back to the German physician Franz Anton Mesmer, who believed that imbalances in magnetic forces in the human body were responsible for illness. Mesmer applied a therapy, which he called mesmerism, involving the use of tranquil gestures and soothing words to relax patients and restore the balance to their magnetic forces. The evolution of Mesmer's ideas and practices led the Scottish neurosurgeon James Braid to coin the term hypnosis in 1842. Called the father of modern hypnotism, Braid rejected Mesmer's theory of magnetic forces and instead ascribed the "mesmeric trance" to a physical process that resulted from prolonged attention to an object of fixation. Sigmund Freud, the father of psychotherapy, found hypnosis useful for treating hysteria, but later abandoned the practice after observing that he stirred up powerful emotions within his patients.

Eventually, the notion of using a state of altered awareness gained greater acceptance in conventional Western medicine. Today, hypnosis is used widely in the United States and other Western countries. People who practice hypnosis are generally licensed and are often trained in several psychological techniques.

What is the evidence?

Many reports demonstrate that hypnosis can help patients reduce blood pressure, stress, anxiety, and pain. Hypnosis can create relaxing brain wave patterns, although reports on how much it helps to change behaviors such as smoking, alcohol consumption, and overeating are mixed. Most researchers who reviewed clinical trials on the use of hypnosis to help people stop smoking found that the evidence did not support its effectiveness.

Hypnosis can be used by therapists as a tool to help eliminate phobias or decrease their strength. Research has also shown that hypnosis can help reduce anticipatory nausea and vomiting. (Anticipatory nausea or vomiting occurs when, after a few doses of chemotherapy have caused nausea or vomiting, some people have nausea or vomiting just *before* the next dose is to be given.) Hypnosis appears less likely to help nausea and vomiting that happen after the chemotherapy dose is given. According to a report from the NIH, there is evidence that hypnosis can help reduce some kinds of cancer pain. In 2006, researchers reviewed studies of children with cancer and found that hypnosis appeared to help reduce pain and distress from medical procedures. In one study published in 2008, giving breast cancer patients a brief hypnosis session before surgery reduced the pain, nausea, fatigue, discomfort, emotional upset, and cost of the procedure.

Another NIH report, which reviewed several scientific studies, showed that women under hypnosis before childbirth had shorter labors and more comfortable deliveries. According to the report, hypnosis may also enhance the immune system. The report looked at one study that found that hypnosis raised the levels of immunoglobulin (an important part of the immune system) in healthy children. Another study found that self-hypnosis led to an increase in white blood cell activity. The NIH report also looked at twelve different controlled studies: One showed that hypnosis reduced the intensity or frequency of migraine headaches in children and teenagers. Another study on chronically ill patients found a 113 percent increase in pain tolerance among highly hypnotizable subjects versus those who were not hypnotized. According to the NIH report, why hypnosis causes these changes is not well understood.

Are there any possible problems or complications?

Hypnosis done under the care of a professionally trained hypnotherapist is generally considered safe when used with standard medical treatment. Emotional distress may happen in some situations. People who have certain types of mental illness should not be hypnotized.

Relying on this type of treatment alone and avoiding or delaying conventional medical care for cancer may have serious health consequences.

References

Astin JA, Shapiro SL, Eisenberg DM, Forys KL. Mind-body medicine: state of the science, implications for practice. *J Am Board Fam Pract.* 2003;16:131-147.

Cassileth B. *The Alternative Medicine Handbook: The Complete Reference Guide to Alternative and Complementary Therapies.* New York: W.W. Norton; 1998.

Hypnotherapy. Aetna InteliHealth Web site.http://www.intelihealth.com/IH/ihtIH/WSIHW000/8513/31455/346706.html?d=dmtContent. Updated March 4, 2002. Accessed May 27, 2008.

Levitan AA. The use of hypnosis with cancer patients. *Psychiatr Med.* 1992;10:119-131.

Montgomery GH, Bovbjerg DH, Schnur JB, David D, Goldfarb A, Weltz CR, Schechter C, Graff-Zivin J, Tatrow K, Price DD, Silverstein JH. A randomized clinical trial of a brief hypnosis intervention to control side effects in breast surgery patients. *J Natl Cancer Inst.* 2007;99:1304-1312.

National Institutes of Health. *Alternative Medicine: Expanding Medical Horizons: A Report to the National Institutes of Health on Alternative Medical Systems and Practices in the United States.* Washington, DC: US Government Printing Office; 1994. NIH publication 94-066.

Newell SA, Sanson-Fisher RW, Savolainen NJ. Systematic review of psychological therapies for cancer patients: overview and recommendations for future research. *J Natl Cancer Inst.* 2002;94:558-584.

NIH Technology Assessment Panel. Integration of behavioral and relaxation approaches into the treatment of chronic pain and insomnia. *JAMA.* 1996;276:313-318.

Okuyemi KS, Nollen NL, Ahluwalia JS. Interventions to facilitate smoking cessation. *Am Fam Physician.* 2006;74:276.

Richardson J, Smith JE, McCall G, Pilkington K. Hypnosis for procedure-related pain and distress in pediatric cancer patients: a systematic review of effectiveness and methodology related to hypnosis interventions. *J Pain Symptom Manage.* 2006;31:70-84.

Villano LM, White AR. Alternative therapies for tobacco dependence. *Med Clin North Am.* 2004;88:1607-1621.

IMAGERY

Other common name(s): guided imagery, visualization
Scientific/medical name(s): none

Description

Imagery involves mental exercises designed to allow the mind to influence the health and well-being of the body. The patient imagines sights, sounds, smells, tastes, or other sensations to create a kind of purposeful daydream. It is used with standard medical treatment in people with cancer and other diseases.

Overview

Available scientific evidence does not support claims that imagery can influence the development or progress of cancer. Imagery can help to reduce stress, anxiety, and depression; manage pain; lower blood pressure; ease some of the side effects of chemotherapy; and create feelings of being in control.

How is it promoted for use?

Imagery is said to be a relaxation technique, similar to meditation and self-hypnosis, that has physical and psychological effects. Promoters claim it can relax the mind and body by decreasing heart rate, lowering blood pressure, and altering brain waves. Some supporters also say that imagery can relieve pain and emotional anxiety, make drugs more effective, and provide emotional insights.

Practitioners use imagery to treat people with phobias and depression, reduce stress, increase motivation, promote relaxation, increase control over one's life, improve communication, and even help people stop smoking. Imagery is also used in biofeedback, hypnosis, and neuro-linguistic programming.

For people with cancer, some supporters of imagery report that it can relieve nausea and vomiting from chemotherapy, relieve stress associated with having cancer, enhance the immune system, help with weight gain, combat depression, and lessen pain.

What does it involve?

There are many different imagery techniques. One popular method is called "palming." It involves placing the palms of your hands over your eyes and imagining a color you associate with anxiety or stress (such as red) and then a color you associate with relaxation or calmness (such as blue). Picturing a calming color is supposed to make you feel relaxed and improve your health and sense of well-being. Other methods use images such as a ball of gentle healing energy forming in your chest and expanding through your body as you breathe. Some techniques involve imagining yourself in a peaceful scene of your own choosing, such as a beach or meadow, with all the sights, sounds, smells, and sensations that complete the experience.

Another common technique is known as guided imagery and involves picturing a specific image or goal and imagining yourself achieving that goal. Athletes use this technique to improve their game. One type of guided therapy used for cancer patients is called the Simonton method, which was developed in the 1970s by O. Carl Simonton, a radiation oncologist, and Stephanie Matthews-Simonton, a psychotherapist. In the Simonton method, people with cancer are asked to imagine their bodies fighting cancer cells and winning the battle. One popular exercise is modeled on the old Pac-Man video game. Patients picture tiny Pac-Man characters eating and destroying tumor cells, just as he destroys his enemies in the game. The Simontons used this method with conventional cancer treatments.

Imagery techniques can be self-taught with the help of one of the many books or audio recordings that have been published on the subject. They can also be practiced under the guidance of a trained therapist. Imagery sessions with a health professional may last twenty to thirty minutes.

What is the history behind it?

Imagery is believed to have been used as a medical therapy for centuries. There is recorded evidence that Tibetan monks in the thirteenth and fourteenth centuries began meditating and imagining that Buddha would cure diseases. Some say the techniques even go back to the ancient Babylonians, Greeks, and Romans. The Simontons popularized imagery therapies in a best-selling 1978 book titled *Getting Well Again*. The book described their experiences in treating cancer patients with imagery and other therapies.

Currently, imagery is used in clinics at medical centers and local hospitals. It is often combined with other behavioral treatments.

What is the evidence?

According to some studies, guided imagery may help reduce some of the side effects of standard cancer treatment. A review of forty-six studies that were conducted from 1966 to 1998 suggested that guided imagery may be helpful in managing stress, anxiety, and depression and in lowering blood pressure, reducing pain, and reducing some side effects of chemotherapy. Another review in 2002 noted that imagery was possibly helpful for anxiety as well as anticipatory nausea and vomiting from chemotherapy. (Anticipatory nausea or vomiting occurs when, after a few doses of chemotherapy have caused nausea or vomiting, some people have nausea or vomiting just *before* the next dose is to be given.) A 2006 review of clinical trials of imagery found that only three studies showed improvement in anxiety and comfort during chemotherapy. Two other studies showed no difference between those who used imagery and those who used other techniques. In addition, a clinical trial involving women with early-stage breast cancer found guided imagery helped to ease anxiety related to radiation therapy, including fears about the equipment, surgical pain, and recurrence of cancer.

Some studies also suggest that imagery can directly affect the immune system. Although one uncontrolled, exploratory study suggested that guided imagery could improve survival for people with cancer, available scientific evidence does not support that these techniques can cure cancer or any other disease. More carefully constructed studies have shown improved quality of life in some patients, but have found no survival advantage for imagery or other psychological techniques.

Overall, imagery is considered one of the more useful psychological measures to reduce some side effects of chemotherapy. Additional systematic, well-designed research on guided imagery would help answer some questions about how it can best be used.

Are there any possible problems or complications?

Imagery techniques are considered safe, especially under the guidance of a trained health professional. They are best used with conventional medical treatment. Relying on this type of treatment alone and avoiding or delaying conventional medical care for cancer may have serious health consequences.

References

Astin JA, Shapiro SL, Eisenberg DM, Forys KL. Mind-body medicine: state of the science, implications for practice. *J Am Board Fam Pract.* 2003;16:131-147.

Barrett S, Herbert V. Questionable cancer therapies. Quackwatch Web site. http://www.quackwatch.org/01QuackeryRelatedTopics/cancer.html. Updated July 6, 2001. Accessed May 23, 2008.

Cassileth B. *The Alternative Medicine Handbook: The Complete Reference Guide to Alternative and Complementary Therapies.* New York: W.W. Norton; 1998.

Eller LS. Guided imagery interventions for symptom management. *Annu Rev Nurs Res.* 1999;17:57-84.

Huebscher R, Shuler P. Mind-body-spirit interventions. In: Huebscher R, Shuler P, eds. *Natural, Alternative, and Complementary Health Care Practices.* St. Louis, MO: Mosby; 2003:762-787.

Kolcaba K, Fox C. The effects of guided imagery on comfort of women with early stage breast cancer undergoing radiation therapy. *Oncol Nurs Forum.* 1999;26:67-72.

National Institutes of Health. *Alternative Medicine: Expanding Medical Horizons: A Report to the National Institutes of Health on Alternative Medical Systems and Practices in the United States.* Washington, DC: US Government Printing Office; 1994. NIH publication 94-066.

Newell SA, Sanson-Fisher RW, Savolainen NJ. Systematic review of psychological therapies for cancer patients: overview and recommendations for future research. *J Natl Cancer Inst.* 2002;94:558-584.

Pain control: a guide for people with cancer and their families. National Cancer Institute Web site. http://www.cancer.gov/cancertopics/paincontrol. Accessed June 12, 2008.

Richardson MA, Post-White J, Grimm EA, Move LA, Singletary SE, Justice B. Coping, life attitudes, and immune responses to imagery and group support after breast cancer treatment. *Altern Ther Health Med.* 1997;3:62-70.

Roffe L, Schmidt K, Ernst E. A systematic review of guided imagery as an adjuvant cancer therapy. *Psychooncology.* 2005;14:607-617.

Spencer JW, Jacobs JJ. *Complementary/Alternative Medicine: An Evidence-Based Approach*. St. Louis, MO: Mosby; 1999.

Walker LG, Walker MB, Ogston K, Heys SD, Ah-See AK, Miller ID, Hucheon AW, Sarkar TK, Eremin O. Psychological, clinical and pathological effects of relaxation training and guided imagery during primary chemotherapy. *Br J Cancer*. 1999;80:262-268.

KIRLIAN PHOTOGRAPHY

Other common name(s): aura photography
Scientific/medical name(s): none

Description

Kirlian photography refers to a type of photographic image made with high voltage. This method is usually used to capture an image of a body part, such as a person's hand.

Overview

Available scientific evidence does not suggest that Kirlian photography is useful in diagnosing cancer or any other disease.

How is it promoted for use?

Supporters of Kirlian photography believe that all physical masses, including humans, give off auras that represent the body's energy fields or life forces. These auras are invisible, believers say, but Kirlian photography can capture them on film. They claim that Kirlian photographs of the human body carry information about the subject's physical, psychological, and psychic states. The various colors and lines of the photographs are said to reflect the subject's mood, personality traits, and health. Supporters of Kirlian photography say that the photographs can be used to diagnose problems with organs (such as kidney disorders), nutritional deficiencies, substance abuse, mental illness, anxiety, confusion, and even cancer.

What does it involve?

Kirlian photography does not actually involve a photographic lens or camera. The machine used to produce a Kirlian photograph consists of a high-voltage electrical source that is attached to a metal plate. A glass plate sits on top of the metal plate, and a piece of photographic paper is laid on top of the glass plate. The object being photographed, such as a hand or foot, is placed directly on the photographic paper. A Kirlian photograph emerges consisting of jagged, colored lines that outline the shape of the photographed object with colors or shadings around it. This image is said to represent an aura, or outline, of the body's life force.

What is the history behind it?

Kirlian photography was developed by a Russian electrician, Semyon Kirlian, and his wife Valentina, in the 1950s. It is based on the theories of Rudolf Steiner, an Austrian philosopher, educator, and artist. In 1978, researchers in Romania claimed that the technique could detect malignant tumors; however, these claims have not been proven.

What is the evidence?

Available scientific evidence does not support the idea that Kirlian photographs can be used to diagnose physical or psychological problems. Research has shown that the images are caused by a variety of factors, none of which are an indication of health problems.

Scientists explain that Kirlian film images reflect differences in skin temperature, the position and pressure of the object on the plate, air temperature, moisture levels, voltage, type of film used, and other factors. Changes in length of exposure and development time can also affect the images captured in the films. Coins and other nonliving objects also appear to have auras when photographed in this manner.

Are there any possible problems or complications?

Kirlian photography is not considered harmful for most people, although pacemakers or implanted cardiac defibrillators may be affected by the electrical field. However, relying on this method alone for diagnosis and avoiding or delaying conventional medical care for cancer may have serious health consequences.

References

Barrett S. Kirlian photography. Quackwatch Web site. http://www.quackwatch.org/01QuackeryRelatedTopics/kirlian.html. Posted June 2, 2001. Accessed May 23, 2008.

Kirlian photography. Aetna InteliHealth Web site. http://www.intelihealth.com/IH/ihtIH/WSIHW000/8513/34968/358832.html. Accessed May 23, 2008.

Stanwick M. Aura photography: mundane physics or diagnostic tool? *Nurs Times*. 1996;92:39-41.

LABYRINTH WALKING

Other common name(s): labyrinths
Scientific/medical name(s): none

Description

Labyrinth walking is a form of meditation that involves walking on labyrinths, winding pathways drawn or laid on the ground. Unlike a maze, a labyrinth has only one path leading in and out, with no intersecting paths or dead ends. There are also lap-sized and smaller versions of labyrinths with grooved paths leading to the center and back out, called finger labyrinths.

Overview

Available evidence does not suggest that labyrinth walking can be used to prevent or treat cancer or other serious diseases. However, it may be helpful as a complementary method to decrease stress and create a state of relaxation.

How is it promoted for use?

Labyrinth walking is generally used as a form of meditation. In fact, it is described by many as walking meditation. People walk through labyrinths to reach any number of goals, such as inner peace, heightened spirituality, personal insight, prayer, relaxation, stress relief, or just "letting go." The labyrinth journey (whether walked or traced with a finger) may represent pilgrimage, the seeking of inner wisdom, and other mysteries.

What does it involve?

Labyrinth walkers follow the labyrinth path from a specified beginning to a well-defined central area and back through the same path to the exit. They might pray, reflect on life, consider a particular problem, let the mind wander, or seek spiritual guidance and unity as they move along the curving trail. Their aim is not to reach the finish, but to become immersed in all aspects of the walk and, potentially, to experience some degree of personal transformation. Labyrinths can be found indoors and outdoors.

Lap or finger labyrinths are generally used for the same purpose. The person can sit down with the portable labyrinth in front of him or her. The eyes may be open or closed as the grooved path is followed with a finger or a stylus.

What is the history behind it?

Labyrinths may date back four thousand years, though their origins are shrouded in mystery. During the Middle Ages, labyrinths were built in a number of large European churches so worshippers could make a symbolic "pilgrimage" to the Holy Land. The labyrinth on the floor of the famous Chartres cathedral in France was built in the year 1220.

Many religious traditions incorporate labyrinths. In Judaism, the Tree of Life, called the Kabbalah, takes the form of an elongated labyrinth. The Hopi medicine wheel is another example of a labyrinth. Labyrinths are being rediscovered and can now be found not only in places of worship but also in retreat centers, hospitals, prisons, parks, airports, and community centers. There are around two thousand permanent labyrinths in the United States alone. Temporary labyrinths may be laid out with stones, tape, fabric, sticks, chalk, plants, and many other materials.

One of the most commonly reproduced labyrinth designs is the eleven-circuit labyrinth, which is named for the eleven circles that must be walked to reach the center. This is the design of the famous labyrinth in the Cathedral of Chartres. Other design types include Classical, Roman, and Contemporary.

What is the evidence?

Available scientific evidence does not suggest that labyrinth walking can be used to treat cancer or any other disease. However, many health care practitioners consider any activity that promotes relaxation and relieves stress beneficial to overall health.

Are there any possible problems or complications?

Labyrinth walking and finger labyrinths are generally considered safe when used with conventional medical treatment. Relying on this type of treatment alone and avoiding or delaying conventional medical care for cancer may have serious health consequences.

References

Artress L. *The Sand Labyrinth: Meditation at your Fingertips*. North Clarendon, VT: Tuttle Publishing: 2000. Grace Cathedral Web site. http://www.gracecathedral.org/enrichment/excerpts/exc_20010328.shtml. Accessed June 12, 2008.

Condren D. Labyrinth walking explores spiritual path to inner peace. *The Buffalo News*. July 11, 1999:1C.

Knight H. The peaceful path: in troubled times, more people turn to labyrinths to walk their worries away. *San Francisco Chronicle*. February 28, 2003. SF Gate Web site. http://www.sfgate.com./cgibin/article.cgi?f=/c/a/2003/02/28/WB186673.DTL. Accessed May 23, 2008.

Saward J. Labyrinth typology. World-Wide Labyrinth Locator Web site. http://wwll.veriditas.labyrinthsociety.org/labyrinth-typology. Accessed May 28, 2008.

Spilner M. Treading ancient paths. *Prevention*. 1997;49:143-146.

MEDITATION

Other common name(s): mindfulness meditation, Transcendental Meditation
Scientific/medical name(s): none

Description

Meditation is a mind-body process that uses concentration or reflection to relax the body and calm the mind. It has been defined as the intentional self-regulation of attention, a mental focus on a particular aspect of one's inner or outer experience.

Overview

Meditation is one of several relaxation methods evaluated and found to be of possible benefit by an independent panel convened by the National Institutes of Health (NIH). The panel found that it might be a useful complementary therapy for treating chronic pain and sleeping problems such as insomnia. Some cancer treatment centers offer meditation or relaxation therapy with standard medical care. Available scientific evidence does not suggest that meditation is effective in treating cancer or any other disease; however, it may help to improve the quality of life for people with cancer.

How is it promoted for use?

The NIH National Center for Complementary and Alternative Medicine reports that regular meditation can reduce chronic pain, anxiety, high blood pressure, cholesterol, substance abuse, post-traumatic stress disorder in Vietnam veterans, and blood cortisol levels that are increased by stress (sometimes called "stress hormones") as well as reducing the use of health care services.

Practitioners also claim meditation improves mood, immune function, and fertility. Supporters further claim meditation increases mental efficiency and alertness and raises self-awareness, all of which contribute to relaxation.

What does it involve?

There are different forms of meditation. Meditation may be done while sitting, but there are also moving forms of meditation, like tai chi, qigong, walking, and the Japanese martial art aikido. One commonly practiced type is Transcendental Meditation, which involves repeating a word or phrase, called a mantra, either silently or aloud. Another is mindfulness meditation, in which a person observes sensations, perceptions, and thoughts without judgment as they arise. There are other types of meditation that focus one's attention through walking or visualizing. Meditations that focus on words or images and do not strive for a state of thoughtless awareness are sometimes called quasimeditative. Meditation can be self-directed or guided by doctors, psychiatrists, other mental health professionals, or yoga masters. It can also be guided by masters from different schools of meditation (for example, Zen meditation, Tibetan meditation, Transcendental Meditation) as well as those from tai chi and martial arts.

Meditation may be done by choosing a quiet place free from distraction, sitting or resting quietly with eyes closed, noticing one's breathing and physical sensations, and letting go of all intruding thoughts. The person may also achieve a relaxed yet alert state by focusing on a pleasant idea or thought or by chanting a phrase or special sound silently or aloud. The ultimate goal of meditation is to separate oneself mentally from the outside world by suspending the usual stream of consciousness. Some practitioners recommend two sessions of fifteen to twenty minutes a day.

What is the history behind it?

Meditation is an important part of ancient Eastern religious practices, particularly in India, China, and Japan, but can be found in all cultures of the world. Meditation began to attract attention in the West in the 1960s when the Indian leader Maharishi Mahesh Yogi brought his method called Transcendental Meditation to the United States. In 1968, a group of practitioners of this method asked a Harvard cardiologist named Herbert Benson to test them on their ability to lower their own blood pressure. There was no change in the practitioners' blood pressure. Benson later developed a popular relaxation technique called the relaxation response. Interest in the use of meditation in the treatment of people with cancer began in the 1970s and early 1980s, when Ainslie Meares, MD, an Australian psychiatrist, studied the use of meditation for enhancing the immune system in order to reduce the size of tumors.

Today, universities and continuing education programs provide training in behavioral medicine, including meditation. Some clinics at major medical centers and local hospitals offer meditation as a form of behavioral medicine.

What is the evidence?

In the last twenty years, meditation has been studied in clinical trials as a way of reducing stress on both the mind and body. Research shows that meditation can help reduce anxiety, stress, blood pressure, chronic pain, and insomnia.

Studies of mindfulness meditation found that it seemed to help with symptoms of anxiety. One controlled study with a group of healthy workers found more brain activity in an area linked to positive emotional states in those who meditated. The same study found that those who meditated had a better immune response to the influenza vaccine than those who did not meditate.

In a controlled study of ninety cancer patients who did mindfulness meditation for seven weeks, 31 percent had fewer symptoms of stress and 67 percent had fewer episodes of mood disturbance than those who did not meditate. Some studies have also suggested that more meditation improves the chance of a positive outcome.

Are there any possible problems or complications?

Most experts agree that the positive effects of meditation outweigh any negative reactions. Complications are rare; however, a small number of people who meditate have become disoriented or anxious and experienced some negative feelings. People with certain types of mental illness may be more likely to have these negative responses. Those with cancer and chronic conditions such as arthritis and heart disease should talk with their doctors before starting any type of meditation that involves movement of joints and muscles, such as qigong or martial arts.

Relying on this type of treatment alone and avoiding or delaying conventional medical care for cancer may have serious health consequences.

References

Astin JA, Shapiro SL, Eisenberg DM, Forys KL. Mind-body medicine: state of the science, implications for practice. *J Am Board Fam Pract.* 2003;16:131-147.

Benson H, Stark M. *Timeless Healing: The Power and Biology of Belief.* New York: Scribner; 1996.

Coker KH. Meditation and prostate cancer: integrating a mind/body intervention with traditional therapies. *Semin Urol Oncol.* 1999;17:111-118.

Davidson RJ, Kabat-Zinn J, Schumacher J, Rosenkranz M, Muller D, Santorelli SF, Uranowski F, Harrington A, Bonus K, Sheridan JF. Alterations in brain and immune function produced by mindfulness meditation. *Psychosom Med.* 2003;65:564-570.

Ernst E, ed. *The Desktop Guide to Complementary and Alternative Medicine: An Evidence-Based Approach.* New York: Mosby; 2001.

Massion AO, Teas J, Hebert JR, Wertheimer MD, Kabat-Zinn J. Meditation, melatonin and breast/prostate cancer: hypothesis and preliminary data. *Med Hypotheses.* 1995;44:39-46.

Meditation. Aetna InteliHealth Web site. http://www.intelihealth.com/IH/ihtIH?d=dmtContent&c=362173&. Accessed May 23, 2008.

Mind-body medicine: an overview. National Center for Complementary and Alternative Medicine Web site. http://nccam.nih.gov/health/backgrounds/mindbody.htm. Accessed June 12, 2008.

National Institutes of Health. *Alternative Medicine: Expanding Medical Horizons: A Report to the National Institutes of Health on Alternative Medical Systems and Practices in the United States.* Washington, DC: US Government Printing Office; 1994. NIH publication 94-066.

Smith JE, Richardson J, Hoffman C, Pilkington K. Mindfulness-based stress reduction as supportive therapy in cancer care: systematic review. *J Adv Nurs.* 2005;52:315-327.
Erratum in:
J Adv Nurs. 2006;53:618.

Speca M, Carlson LE, Goodey E, Angen M. A randomized, wait-list controlled clinical trial: the effect of a mindfulness meditation-based stress reduction program on mood and symptoms of stress in cancer outpatients. *Psychosom Med.* 2000;62:613-622.

Spencer JW, Jacobs JJ. *Complementary/Alternative Medicine: An Evidence-Based Approach.* St. Louis, MO: Mosby;1999.

US Congress, Office of Technology Assessment. *Unconventional Cancer Treatments: OTA-H-405.* Washington, DC: US Government Printing Office; 1990.

Wallace RK, Benson H, Wilson AF. A wakeful hypometabolic physiologic state. *Am J Physiol.* 1971;221:795-799.

MUSIC THERAPY

Other common name(s): none
Scientific/medical name(s): none

Description

Music therapy is the use of music by health care professionals to promote healing and enhance quality of life for their patients. Music therapy may be used to encourage emotional expression, promote social interaction, relieve symptoms, and for other purposes. Music therapists may use active or passive methods with patients, depending on the individual patient's needs and abilities.

Overview

There is some evidence that, when used with conventional treatment, music therapy can help to reduce pain and relieve chemotherapy-induced nausea and vomiting. It may also relieve stress and provide an overall sense of well-being. Some studies have found that music therapy can lower heart rate, blood pressure, and breathing rate.

How is it promoted for use?

Music therapists work with a variety of physical, emotional, and psychological symptoms. Music therapy is often used in cancer treatment to help reduce pain, anxiety, and nausea caused by chemotherapy. Some people believe music therapy may be a beneficial addition to the health care of children with cancer by promoting social interaction and cooperation.

There is evidence that music therapy can reduce high blood pressure, rapid heartbeat, depression, and sleeplessness. There are no claims music therapy can cure cancer or other diseases, but medical experts do believe it can reduce some symptoms, aid healing, improve physical movement, and enrich a patient's quality of life.

What does it involve?

Music therapists design music sessions for individuals and groups based on their needs and tastes. Some aspects of music therapy include making music, listening to music, writing songs, and talking about lyrics. Music therapy may also involve imagery and learning through music. It can be done in different places such as hospitals, cancer centers, hospices, at home, or anywhere people can benefit from its calming or stimulating effects. The patient does not need to have any musical ability to benefit from music therapy.

A related practice called music thanatology is sometimes used at the end of a patient's life to ease the person's passing. It is practiced in homes, hospices, or nursing homes.

What is the history behind it?

Music has been used in medicine for thousands of years. Ancient Greek philosophers believed that music could heal both the body and the soul. Native Americans have used singing and chanting as part of their healing rituals for millennia. The more formal approach to music therapy began in World War II, when U.S. Veterans Administration hospitals began to use music to help treat soldiers suffering from shell shock. In 1944, Michigan State University established the first music therapy degree program in the world.

Today, more than seventy colleges and universities have degree programs that are approved by the American Music Therapy Association. Music therapists must have at least a bachelor's degree, 1,200 hours of clinical training, and one or more internships before they can be certified. There are thousands of professional music therapists working in health care settings in the United States today. They serve as part of cancer-management teams in many hospitals and cancer centers, helping to plan and evaluate treatment. Some music therapy services are covered by health insurance.

What is the evidence?

Scientific studies have shown the value of music therapy on the body, mind, and spirit of children and adults. Researchers have found that music therapy, when used with anti-nausea drugs for patients receiving high-dose chemotherapy, can help ease nausea and vomiting. A number of clinical trials have shown the benefit of music therapy for short-term pain, including pain from cancer. Some studies have suggested that music may help decrease the overall intensity of the patient's experience of pain when used with pain-relieving drugs. Music therapy can also result in a decreased need for pain medicine in some patients, although studies on this topic have shown mixed results.

In hospice patients, one study found that music therapy improved comfort, relaxation, and pain control. Another study found that quality of life improved in cancer patients who received music therapy, even as it declined in those who did not. No differences were seen in survival between the two groups.

A more recent clinical trial looked at the effects of music during the course of several weeks of radiation treatments. The researchers found that while emotional distress (such as anxiety) seemed to be helped at the beginning of treatment, the patients reported that this effect gradually decreased. Music did not appear to help such symptoms as pain, fatigue, and depression over the long term.

Other clinical trials have revealed reductions in heart rate, blood pressure, breathing rate, insomnia, depression, and anxiety with music therapy. No one knows all the ways music can benefit the body, but studies have shown that music can affect brain waves, brain circulation, and stress hormones. These effects are usually seen during and shortly after the music therapy.

Studies have shown that students who take music lessons have improved IQ levels and show improvement in nonmusical abilities as well. Other studies have shown that listening to music composed by Mozart produces a short-term improvement in tasks that use spatial abilities. Studies of brain circulation have shown that people listening to Mozart have more activity in certain areas of the brain. This has been called the "Mozart effect." Although the reasons for this effect are not completely clear, this kind of information supports the idea that music can be used in many helpful ways.

Some clinical trials that involve listening to music have shown no benefit on anxiety during surgical procedures, although one study that allowed patients to choose their own music showed improved anxiety levels. One recent review of studies looked at the effect of music on all types of pain and found a wide variation in its effects. The study authors observed that the best effects were on short-term pain after surgery. It is important to note that not all studies of music use music therapists, who assess the patient's needs, circumstances, and preferences, as well as the different effects of certain types of music. This inconsistency may account for some differences in clinical trial results.

Are there any possible problems or complications?

In general, music therapy done under the care of a professionally trained therapist has a helpful effect and is considered safe when used with standard treatment. Musical intervention by untrained people can be ineffective or can even cause increased stress and discomfort. Relying on this type of treatment alone and avoiding or delaying conventional medical care for cancer may have serious health consequences.

References

Bodner M, Muftuler LT, Nalcioglu O, Shaw GL. FMRI study relevant to the Mozart effect: brain areas involved in spatial-temporal reasoning. *Neurol Res.* 2001;23:683-690.

Cepeda MS, Carr DB, Lau J, Alvarez H. Music for pain relief. *Cochrane Database Syst Rev.* 2006;(2):CD004843.

Clark M, Isaacks-Downton G, Wells N, Redlin-Frazier S, Eck C, Hepworth JT, Chakravarthy B. Use of preferred music to reduce emotional distress and symptom activity during radiation therapy. *J Music Ther.* 2006;43:247-265.

Ezzone S, Baker C, Rosselet R, Terepka E. Music as an adjunct to antiemetic therapy. *Oncol Nurs Forum.* 1998;25:1551-1556.

Hilliard RE. The effects of music therapy on the quality and length of life of people diagnosed with terminal cancer. *J Music Ther.* 2003;40:113-137.

Jausovec N, Habe K. The "Mozart effect": an electroencephalographic analysis employing the methods of induced event-related desynchronization/synchronization and event-related coherence. *Brain Topogr.* 2003;16:73-84.

Krout RE. The effects of single-session music therapy interventions on the observed and self-reported levels of pain control, physical comfort, and relaxation of hospice patients. *Am J Hosp Palliat Care.* 2001;18:383-390.

Lane D. Music therapy: a gift beyond measure. *Oncol Nurs Forum.* 1992;19:863-867.

Lane D. Music therapy: gaining an edge in oncology management. *J Oncol Manag.* 1993;2:42-46.

Pelletier CL. The effect of music on decreasing arousal due to stress: a meta-analysis. *J Music Ther.* 2004;41:192-214.

Phumdoung S, Good M. Music reduces sensation and distress of labor pain. *Pain Manag Nurs.* 2003;4:54-61.

Schellenberg EG. Music and nonmusical abilities. *Ann N Y Acad Sci.* 2001;930:355-371.

Schellenberg EG. Music lessons enhance IQ. *Psychol Sci.* 2004;15:511-514.

Watkins GR. Music therapy: proposed physiological mechanisms and clinical implications. *Clin Nurse Spec.* 1997;11:43-50.

What is music therapy? American Music Therapy Association Web site. http://www.musictherapy.org/. Accessed May 23, 2008.

NATIVE AMERICAN HEALING

Other common name(s): Native American medicine, Indian medicine
Scientific/medical name(s): none

Description

Native American healing is a broad term that includes healing beliefs and practices of hundreds of indigenous tribes of North America. It combines religion, spirituality, herbal medicine, and rituals that are used to treat people with medical and emotional conditions.

Overview

Available scientific evidence does not support claims that Native American healing can cure cancer or any other disease. However, the communal support provided by this approach to health care can have some worthwhile physical, emotional, and spiritual benefits.

How is it promoted for use?

From the Native American perspective, medicine is more about healing the person than curing a disease. Traditional healers aim to "make whole" by restoring well-being and harmonious relationships with the community and the spirit of nature, which is sometimes called God or the Great Mystery. Native American healing is based on the belief that everyone and everything on earth is interconnected, and every person, animal, and plant has a spirit or essence. Even an object, such as a river or rock, and even the earth itself, may be considered to have this kind of spirit.

Native Americans traditionally believe that illness stems from spiritual problems. They also say that diseases are more likely to invade the body of a person who is imbalanced, has negative thinking, or lives an unhealthy lifestyle. Some Native American healers believe that inherited conditions, such as birth defects, are caused by the parents' immoral lifestyles and are not easily treated. Others believe that such conditions reflect a touch from the Creator and may consider them a kind of gift. Native American healing practices aim to find and restore balance and wholeness in a person to restore one to a healthy and spiritually pure state.

Some people believe Native American medicine can help cure physical diseases, injuries, and emotional problems. Some healers claim to have cured conditions such as heart disease, diabetes, thyroid problems, skin rashes, asthma, and cancer.

There are many types of Native American healing practices, and they are promoted to help with a variety of ills. Some of the most common aspects of Native American healing include the use of herbal remedies, purifying rituals, shamanism, and symbolic healing rituals to treat illnesses of both the body and spirit. Herbal remedies are used to treat many physical conditions. Practitioners use purifying rituals to cleanse the body and prepare the person for healing. Shamanism is based on the idea that spirits cause illness, and a Native American healer called a shaman focuses on using spiritual healing powers to treat people. Symbolic healing rituals, which can involve family and friends of the sick person, are used to invoke the spirits to help heal the sick person.

Healers may include shamans, herbalists, spiritual healers, and medicine men or women. Many Native Americans see their healers for spiritual reasons, such as to seek guidance, truth, balance, reassurance, and spiritual well-being, while still using conventional medicine to deal with "white man's illness." However, they believe that the spirit is an inseparable element of healing.

What does it involve?

Native American healing practices vary greatly because there are more than five hundred Native American Nations (commonly called tribes). There are many tribal differences, so it is not surprising that healing rituals and beliefs vary a great deal. The most sacred traditions are still kept secret, passed along from one healer to the next. Because of these factors, information on healing practices is general and somewhat limited.

However, the many types of Native American medicine do have some basic rituals and healing practices in common. Because of Native American tribes' extensive knowledge of herbs, one of the most common forms of Native American healing involves the use of herbal remedies, which can include teas, tinctures, and salves. For example, one remedy for pain uses bark from a willow tree, which contains acetylsalicylic acid, also known as aspirin.

Purifying and cleansing the body is also an important technique used in Native American healing. Sweat lodges (special, darkened enclosures heated with stones from a fire) or special teas that induce vomiting may be used by the healer for this purpose. A practice called smudging, which involves cleansing a place or person with the smoke of sacred plants, can be used to bring about an altered state of consciousness and sensitivity, making a person more open to the healing techniques. Because some illnesses are believed to come from angry spirits, healers may also invoke the healing powers of spirits. They may also use special rituals to try to appease the angered spirits.

Another practice of Native American healing, symbolic healing rituals, can involve whole communities. These rituals use ceremonies that can include chanting, singing, painting bodies, dancing, exorcisms, sand paintings, and even limited use of mind-altering substances to persuade the spirits to heal the sick person. Rituals can last hours or even weeks. These ceremonies are a way of asking for help from the spiritual dimension. Prayer is also an essential part of all Native American healing techniques.

Native American treatment is usually a slow process, spread over a period of days or weeks. It may involve taking time from one's daily activities for reflection, emotional awareness, and meditation. The healer may spend a great deal of time with the person seeking help. Healing is said to take place within the context of the relationship with the healer.

What is the history behind it?

Native American healing has been practiced in North America for up to forty thousand years. It appears to have roots in common with different cultures, such as ancient Ayurvedic (see page 63) and Chinese traditions, but it has also been influenced by the environments in which Native Americans settled and the nature, plants, and animals around them. Other healing practices were influenced over time by the migration of tribes and contact with other tribes along trade routes. The tribes gathered many herbs from the surrounding environment and sometimes traded over long distances.

Many Native medicine practices were driven underground or lost because they were banned or illegal in parts of the United States until 1978, when the American Indian Religious Freedom Act was passed. Even now, there are difficulties with ceremonies and rituals on sacred sites. These activities are sometimes forbidden because the land now serves other purposes. Today, Native American and American Indian community-based medical systems still practice some Native American healing practices and rituals.

What is the evidence?

One clinical trial examined 116 people with a variety of ailments (such as infertility, chest and back pain, asthma, depression, diabetes, and cancer) who were treated with traditional Native American healing. More than 80 percent showed some benefit after a seven- to twenty-eight–day intensive healing experience. Five years later, fifty of the original participants said they were cured of their diseases, while another forty-one said they felt better. Another nine reported no change, five were worse, and two had died. However, the comparison group who received different treatments also showed benefits, and the patients' reports were not verified by doctors. Because of the limitations in this study, it is impossible to draw conclusions about the effectiveness of Native American healing. More clinical studies are needed to confirm the benefits of the specific healing methods.

Although Native American healing has not been proven to cure disease, individual reports suggest that it can reduce pain and stress and improve quality of life. The communal and spiritual support provided by this type of healing could have helpful effects. Prayers, introspection, and meditation can be calming and can help to reduce stress.

Because Native American healing is based on spirituality, there are very few scientific studies to support the validity of the practices. It is hard to study Native American healing in a scientific way because practices differ between various Nations, healers, and illnesses. Many Native Americans do not want their practices studied because they believe sharing such information exploits their culture and weakens their power to heal. Historically, outside society has sometimes misinterpreted Native American cultures and beliefs, which may increase this reluctance.

Are there any possible problems or complications?

Like other complementary therapies, Native American healing practices may be used in relieving certain symptoms of cancer and side effects of cancer treatment. People with cancer and other chronic conditions should talk to their doctors before using purification rituals or herbal remedies. Cleansing rituals may be particularly harmful to people who are already dehydrated or in a weakened state. Relying on this type of treatment alone and avoiding or delaying conventional medical care for cancer may have serious health consequences.

These substances may have not been thoroughly tested to find out how they interact with medicines, foods, or dietary supplements. Even though some reports of interactions and harmful effects may be published, full studies of interactions and effects are not often available. Because of these limitations, any information on ill effects and interactions should be considered incomplete.

References

American Indian Religious Freedom Act, Title 42, Chapter 21, Subchapter 1, USC §1996 (1978). National Park Service Web site. http://www.nps.gov/history/local-law/FHPL_IndianRelFreAct.pdf. Accessed June 5, 2008.

Amor A. Special rapporteur report: religious intolerance in the United States. United Nations Commission on Human Rights Report, 1999. http://daccessdds.un.org/doc/UNDOC/GEN/G98/148/96/PDF/G9814896.pdf. Accessed April 19, 2005. Content no longer available.

Atwood MD. *Spirit Healing: Native American Magic & Medicine.* New York: Sterling Publishing Co; 1991.

Borchers AT, Keen CL, Stern JS, Gershwin ME. Inflammation and Native American medicine: the role of botanicals. *Am J Clin Nutr.* 2000;72:339-347.

Cohen K. Native American medicine. *Altern Ther Health Med.* 1998;4:45-57.
Erratum in:
Altern Ther Health Med. 1999;5:22.

Cohen K. What is Native American medicine? Sacred Earth Circle Web site. http://www.qigonghealing.com/sacred_earth/what.html. Excerpted and adapted from *Honoring the Medicine: The Essential Guide to Native American Healing.* New York: Ballantine Books; 2003. Accessed June 3, 2008.

Johnston L. Native-American medicine. Alternative & Innovative Therapies for Physical Disability Web site. http://www.healingtherapies.info/Native-American%20Medicine.htm. Accessed May 26, 2008.

Marbella AM, Harris MC, Diehr S, Ignace G, Ignace G. Use of Native American healers among Native American patients in an urban Native American health center. *Arch Fam Med* 1998;7:182-185.

Mehl-Medrona LE. Native American medicine in the treatment of chronic illness: developing an integrated program and evaluating its effectiveness. *Altern Ther Health Med.* 1999;5:36-44.

National Institutes of Health. *Alternative Medicine: Expanding Medical Horizons: A Report to the National Institutes of Health on Alternative Medical Systems and Practices in the United States.* Washington, DC: US Government Printing Office; 1994. NIH publication 94-066.

NATUROPATHIC MEDICINE

Other common name(s): naturopathy, natural medicine
Scientific/medical name(s): none

Description

Naturopathic medicine is a complete alternative care system that uses a wide range of approaches such as nutrition, herbs, manipulation of the body, exercise, stress reduction, and acupuncture. Parts of naturopathy are sometimes used with conventional medicine as complementary therapy. Naturopathic medicine is a holistic approach (meaning it is intended to treat the whole person) that tries to enlist the healing power of the body and nature to fight disease.

Overview

Available scientific evidence does not support claims that naturopathic medicine can cure cancer or any other disease, since virtually no studies on naturopathy as a whole have been published. The individual methods used by naturopathic medicine vary in their effectiveness. Homeopathy, for instance, may be of little value. Other naturopathic methods have been shown to help in prevention and symptom management. Examples include diet for lowering the risk for severe illnesses such as heart disease and cancer and acupuncture to reduce pain.

How is it promoted for use?

Supporters claim that naturopathic medicine uses the healing power of nature to maintain and restore health. Their goal is to create a healthy environment inside and outside the body. Supporters claim naturopathic medicine prevents illness because people are taught healthy diets and lifestyles to avoid disease. Treatment is focused on the cause of disease, rather than on the symptoms. Naturopathic doctors may diagnose illness with many of the same methods used in conventional medicine. They use x-rays, laboratory tests, and physical examinations to try to identify the problem. However, naturopathic treatment does not generally use drugs, radiation therapy, or major surgery.

There are three kinds of practitioners who may offer naturopathic treatment. Naturopathic doctors (NDs, who may also call themselves naturopathic physicians) have usually had four years of study in a school of naturopathy. The second group may call themselves naturopaths, although some also call themselves naturopathic doctors. Many naturopaths are self-taught or were apprenticed to another naturopath. They may focus on one or just a few naturopathic methods. The third group consists of chiropractors, massage therapists, dentists, nurses, nutritionists, or doctors who practice under a professional license but include some naturopathic methods in their practice. They may have studied or read on their own or taken courses on naturopathic methods. They use these methods along with their usual treatments.

Naturopathic medicine is promoted for the treatment of conditions such as migraine headaches, chronic lower back pain, enlarged prostate, menopause, AIDS, and cancer. Practitioners claim to use "natural methods" to strengthen the body's ability to heal itself. They believe that this type of care causes fewer side effects and costs less than conventional treatment. However, practitioners often refer complicated cases or people needing major treatment to conventional medical professionals.

What does it involve?

Naturopathic medicine uses many different techniques and methods. Practitioners act mostly as teachers. They decide how to treat a particular patient based on case history, observation, medical records, and previous experience. Naturopathic treatment can include nutritional medicine and fasting; herbs, minerals, and vitamins; homeopathy; Chinese medicine; manipulation of muscles, the spine, and other bones; acupuncture; counseling and hypnotherapy; massage; colonics (enemas); hydrotherapy; hot and cold applications; therapeutic exercise; and some minor surgery. For more information about some of the treatments involved in naturopathic medicine, see the sections on acupuncture, homeopathy, hypnosis, colon therapy, and the information on herb, vitamin, and mineral therapies in Chapter 7.

Counseling or behavioral medicine is an important part of naturopathic medicine. Practitioners are usually trained in counseling, biofeedback, stress reduction, and other means to improve mental health (see "Biofeedback," page 69, and "Psychotherapy," page 123). They may also use other unproven techniques such as ozone therapy for people with cancer and AIDS. These treatments have shown no benefit in curing cancer or other diseases.

Treatment by naturopathic doctors is not covered by many insurance policies, including those offered through Medicare and Tricare. A few states require that treatment by licensed naturopathic doctors be covered by insurance companies. States that license naturopathic doctors as primary care providers may provide coverage on Medicaid programs.

What is the history behind it?

Naturopathic medicine began with Sebastian Kneipp in the 1800s. Kneipp, a German priest, opened a water cure center and developed herbal treatments. Later, a student of Kneipp's, Benedict Lust, opened a water cure institute in New York that used Kneipp's drugless therapies. Lust went on to acquire degrees in osteopathy and chiropractic, homeopathic, and eclectic medicine. In 1902, Lust purchased the rights to naturopathic medicine from another Kneipp student and opened the American Institute of Naturopathy.

By the early 1900s, there were more than twenty schools of naturopathic medicine. With the advances in conventional medicine after World War II, however, interest in naturopathy began to decline. It resurged in the mid-1950s, when the National College of Naturopathic Medicine was founded in Portland, Oregon. In 1968, the U.S. Department of Health, Education, and Welfare issued a report stating that the educational programs for practitioners of naturopathic medicine did not adequately prepare them to make accurate diagnoses or treatment decisions. The report also concluded that naturopathic medicine was not based on widely accepted scientific principles of health, disease, and health care.

The American Naturopathic Medical Association was founded in 1981 and today reports a membership of approximately four thousand people worldwide. The Council on Naturopathic Medical Education (CNME) was approved by the U.S. Secretary of Education in 1987 as an accrediting body for full-time schools. It lost its certification in 2001, but regained it in 2003.

Doctor of Naturopathic Medicine (ND) degrees are offered by four-year graduate-level programs. Naturopathic doctors take some basic science courses and courses on disease prevention, wellness, clinical nutrition, acupuncture, homeopathic medicine, botanical medicine, psychology, and counseling. Naturopathic doctors do not receive residency training. As of this writing, there are four accredited ND programs in the United States, and thirteen states license naturopathic doctors. Some ND degrees are available through nonaccredited correspondence schools.

What is the evidence?

Available scientific evidence does not support claims that naturopathic medicine is effective for most health problems. Most of the claims of effectiveness are based on individual cases, medical records, and summaries of practitioners' clinical experiences. One clinical study that looked at treatment of ear pain in children tested the effectiveness of naturopathic ear drops, anesthetic ear drops, and oral antibiotics. The pain improved over three days in all groups, and the naturopathic drops were slightly more effective than the anesthetic drops. Antibiotics were not helpful and may have slowed recovery, which is in agreement with several other studies and consistent with guidelines of most conventional medical groups, which do not recommend antibiotics for uncomplicated ear pain.

Naturopathic medicine includes several methods, many of which have been shown to vary in effectiveness. Available scientific evidence looking at unproven methods such as homeopathy and colonic irrigation has not shown them to be helpful for cancer or any other disease. Other aspects of naturopathic medicine, like proper diet and nutrition, have been shown to lower the risk for illnesses such as heart disease and cancer. Another component, acupuncture, may help reduce pain. Some aspects of naturopathic medicine may be useful when used with conventional medical treatment.

Are there any possible problems or complications?

Excessive fasting, dietary restrictions, or the use of enemas, which are sometimes components of naturopathic treatment, may be dangerous. Naturopathic treatment may involve taking unregulated herbs, some of which may have harmful effects. In addition, the potential interactions between herbal preparations and conventional drugs and other herbs should be considered. Some of these combinations may be dangerous. Always tell your doctor and pharmacist about any herbs you are taking. Relying on this type of treatment alone and avoiding or delaying conventional medical care for cancer may have serious health consequences.

These substances may have not been thoroughly tested to find out how they interact with medicines, foods, or dietary supplements. Even though some reports of interactions and harmful effects may be published, full studies of interactions and effects are not often available. Because of these limitations, any information on ill effects and interactions should be considered incomplete.

References

Barrett S. A close look at naturopathy. Quackwatch Web site. http://www.quackwatch.org/01QuackeryRelatedTopics/Naturopathy/naturopathy.html. Updated December 23, 2003. Accessed May 27, 2008.

Hugh HJ, Dower C, O'Neil EH. Profile of a Profession: Naturopathic Medicine. San Francisco: Center for the Health Professions, University of California San Francisco, September 2001. The Center for Health Professions, University of California Web site. http://www.futurehealth.ucsf.edu/pdf_files/Naturo2.pdf. Accessed June 12, 2008.

National Institutes of Health. *Alternative Medicine: Expanding Medical Horizons: A Report to the National Institutes of Health on Alternative Medical Systems and Practices in the United States.* Washington, DC: US Government Printing Office; 1994. NIH publication 94-066.

Naturopathic medicine. Bastyr University Web site. http://www.bastyr.edu. Accessed June 12, 2008.

Riley RW. Decision of the Secretary in the matter of the council on naturopathic medical education, US Department of Education, Washington, DC; 2001. http://www.ed-oha.org/secretarycases/2000-06-O.pdf. Accessed June 5, 2008.

Sarrell EM, Cohen HA, Kahan E. Naturopathic treatment for ear pain in children. *J Fam Pract.* 2003;52:673, 676.
Comment to:
Sarrell EM, Cohen HA, Kahan E. Naturopathic treatment for ear pain in children. *Pediatrics.* 2003;111:e574-e579.

Spencer JW, Jacobs JJ. *Complementary/Alternative Medicine: An Evidence-Based Approach.* St. Louis, MO: Mosby; 1999.

Whole medical systems: an overview. National Center for Complementary and Alternative Medicine Web site. http://nccam.nih.gov/health/backgrounds/wholemed.htm. Accessed June 20, 2008.

NEURO-LINGUISTIC PROGRAMMING

Other common name(s): NLP
Scientific/medical name(s): none

Description

Neuro-linguistic programming (NLP) uses a number of techniques or tools to teach people to identify personal goals, change unhelpful beliefs, reach a higher level of achievement, and communicate better with others. Special attention is paid to the relationship between language, thoughts, and behavior.

Overview

Available scientific evidence does not support claims that NLP is effective in treating cancer or any other disease. Some smaller studies have reported positive effects of NLP in such areas as increasing relaxation and treating phobias.

How is it promoted for use?

Practitioners of NLP claim it can be used to identify and change unconscious patterns of thinking and behavior. Some also believe that it can be used to help treat a wide range of physical conditions. They claim NLP can help people with phobias, allergies, arthritis, migraine headaches, Parkinson's disease, AIDS, and cancer.

NLP is based on the belief that the brain (i.e., neuro) controls how the body functions, whereas language (i.e., linguistic) determines how people communicate. "Programming" is used to develop models for interaction.

Proponents of NLP claim that thinking is closely tied to the five senses, that experiences are recreated in memories through the senses, and that these experiences are what limit people's abilities and beliefs. Supporters claim that once people understand that they create their own internal world, they realize they have the power to change their behavior and health. Practitioners claim that people who have problems healing from physical conditions often have negative beliefs about their health.

What does it involve?

NLP practitioners may ask a person questions about specific situations, then analyze eye movements, body posture, voice tone, muscle tension, gestures, and language to understand more about the person's thinking process. These observations are used to learn how the person consciously and unconsciously relates to his or her life and condition, and what limiting beliefs the person may have. Practitioners claim some problems can be cured with one NLP session, although others may require repeated sessions.

What is the history behind it?

In the early 1970s, John Grinder, PhD, and Richard Bandler, PhD, studied the thinking processes, language, and behavioral patterns of several successful people, including Fritz Perls, the father of Gestalt therapy; Virginia Satir, an accomplished family therapist; Milton Erickson, a prominent hypnotherapist; and Gregory Bateson, a well-known anthropologist and author in the field of communication theory. Grinder and Bandler believed that by studying and learning the internal processes of these successful people, they could learn to teach anyone the skills necessary to increase their level of success. Grinder and Bandler made connections between the body language and speaking patterns of these people and related this information to the internal thinking process of each person studied.

They applied what they learned to help people experiencing emotional difficulties by asking those people questions about their problems while observing their body language. Once Grinder and Bandler had identified unconscious patterns, they found the person could be helped to learn new, more useful patterns. Grinder and Bandler created a model based on successful communication patterns, called neuro-linguistic programming.

Today, NLP practitioners can receive training in the process from affiliated organizations such as The Society for Neuro-Linguistic Programming.

What is the evidence?

Although there have been anecdotal and case reports of the effectiveness of NLP, there have been no large-scale randomized clinical trials of the method. One small-scale study found that NLP might be effective in treating phobias. However, a National Research Council committee did not find the theories or practices of NLP to be well founded. Indeed, some studies have found that eye movement, one of the points of analysis included in NLP, is not a consistent marker of type of mental processing. This finding appears to contradict the observations of the NLP founders.

Several reviews of the medical literature have reported there is little or no evidence to support the effectiveness of NLP. A survey of 139 psychologists listed in the National Register of Health Service Providers in Psychology found that the soundness of NLP was questionable. Claims that NLP can help cancer or any other physical illness are not supported by available scientific research. More study is needed to determine whether NLP may help psychological conditions.

Are there any possible problems or complications?

Not all NLP practitioners have a background in physical or mental health, and some may not even be properly trained. Someone without training or experience in the field may not be skilled or sensitive to the needs and issues important to someone living with cancer and could cause psychological harm. Relying on this type of treatment alone and avoiding or delaying conventional medical care for cancer may have serious health consequences.

References

Barrett S. Mental help: procedures to avoid. Quackwatch Web site. http://www.quackwatch.org/01Quackery RelatedTopics/mentserv.html. Updated July 10, 2003. Accessed May 27, 2008.

Beyerstein BL. Brainscams: neuromythologies of the new age. *Intern J Mental Health.* 1990;19:27-36.

Burke DT, Meleger A, Schneider JC, Snyder J, Drovlo AS, Al-Adawi S. Eye-movements and ongoing task processing. *Percept Mot Skills.* 2003;96:1330-1338.

Einspruch EL, Forman BD. Neuro-linguistic programming in the treatment of phobias. *Psych Priv Prac.* 1988;6:91-100.

Sharpley CF. Research findings on neurolinguistic programming: nonsupportive data or an untestable theory? *J Counsel Psych.* 1987;34:103-107.

Starker S, Pankratz L. Soundness of treatment: a survey of psychologists' opinions. *Psychol Rep.* 1996;78:288-290.

Swets JA, Bjork RA. Enhancing human performance: an evaluation of "New Age" techniques considered by the US Army. *Psychol Sci.* 1990;1:85-86.

PSYCHOTHERAPY

Other common name(s):
therapy, counseling, psychological intervention, psychotherapeutic treatment
Scientific/medical name(s): none

Description

Psychotherapy covers a wide range of approaches designed to help people change their ways of thinking, feeling, or behaving.

Overview

Research has shown that psychotherapy may improve a patient's quality of life. It can help reduce anxiety and depression that sometimes occur in people with cancer. It can also help people cope with cancer and the changes in their lives. Psychotherapy has not, however, been demonstrated to increase survival in people with cancer.

How is it promoted for use?

Psychotherapists believe that psychotherapy can help people, including those with cancer, find the inner strength they need to improve their coping skills, allowing them to more fully enjoy their lives. Psychotherapy can be used to help people deal with the diagnosis and treatment of cancer. It can also be useful in overcoming depression and anxiety, which are common in people with cancer.

Psychotherapy is available in many forms. People may seek individual therapy, where there is a one-on-one relationship with a therapist. There are also therapists who work with couples or entire families, in order to help those most affected by the cancer diagnosis. Psychotherapy also may be practiced with groups, in which a number of people meet together to discuss common experiences and issues and to learn specific coping techniques. Unlike self-help groups, psychotherapy groups are offered and managed by a professional therapist.

What does it involve?

There are many different kinds of therapy, from long-term analysis to brief, problem-oriented treatment. Therapy may include looking at emotional experiences, working with coping styles, doing homework assignments, and more.

People can get referrals to therapists by asking members of their health care team or by contacting professional organizations for names of psychotherapists. Oncology units of hospitals sometimes have departments that include therapists.

Most individual psychotherapy is held in the therapist's office. In some situations, it may be done in the hospital or the patient's home. Sessions typically last forty-five to fifty minutes. The number of meetings is decided by the client and therapist. Most meet weekly for a short time, depending on the problem and the client's response to therapy.

There are a wide range of psychotherapy approaches and techniques. These are some examples:

Behavioral Therapy (Behavior Modification)

This therapy focuses on replacing problematic behavior patterns (such as obsessive-compulsive behavior) with more healthy responses. A behavioral therapist may use techniques such as biofeedback and muscle relaxation. This kind of therapy deals only with the symptoms of a problem.

Client-Centered Therapy

This form of therapy focuses on the feelings and current experiences of the individual. The therapist encourages the patient to direct the sessions while providing empathy and support. The goal is to help patients help themselves. The length of this therapy varies.

Body-Oriented Therapy

This kind of therapy is based on the belief that emotions are stored in the body and may be expressed in the form of physical tension and restriction. Breathing techniques, movement, and manual pressure are used to help people release emotions that have built up in the body.

Cognitive Therapy (also called Cognitive-Behavioral Therapy)

Cognitive therapy is directed at changing thoughts and behaviors by addressing the repeated, faulty, negative thoughts that affect behavior. Cognitive therapists help people learn to reprogram harmful internal messages and create a positive internal dialogue. This kind of therapy often includes homework assignments for the patient such as disputing disturbing thoughts, trying different responses to criticism, or making a list of things he or she likes about himself or herself. It also includes different forms of behavioral therapy.

Family/Couples Therapy

Family therapy focuses on relationship patterns. All family members may be involved in therapy sessions. A therapist involved in this type of therapy acts as a facilitator to help the family or couple communicate their feelings more effectively. Although usually short-term, this therapy can last longer depending on the needs of the individuals.

Group Therapy

Group therapy varies widely in size and format, as well as in length. Some groups are small and meet weekly without a scheduled agenda. Others may meet monthly and offer information, teach coping skills, help reduce anxiety, and provide a place to share common concerns and emotional support.

Psychodynamic Therapy

Similar to traditional psychoanalysis, the goal of this form of therapy is to change lifelong personality patterns by uncovering the connections between current emotional reactions and early childhood experiences. This form of therapy is long-term (lasting several years) and focuses on the underlying causes of a problem.

Whatever approach is used, when a person has a serious physical illness such as cancer, the therapy is likely to focus on the emotional stress resulting from the illness. It will also focus on any depression or anxiety and explore past or present issues that may affect the person's adjustment to the illness. The therapist may ask about the person's previous experiences with loss in general and loss related to the current illness.

What is the history behind it?

The influence of personality characteristics on health has been examined for many years. Research conducted by Lawrence LeShan, PhD, during the early 1950s on the relationship between personality characteristics and cancer found that many patients experienced a loss of hope in finding true meaning in their lives well before their cancer diagnoses. Dr. LeShan developed a specific approach to psychotherapy designed to treat people living with cancer. This approach focuses on helping patients use their own inner self-healing abilities to live more fulfilled, enjoyable, and personally meaningful lives.

Over the past twenty years, several books on the role of emotions and behavior in recovery from serious illness have become popular. Books by Norman Cousins, Bernie Siegel, MD, and Carl Simonton, MD, have focused on developing effective coping strategies to manage the feelings of hopelessness, passivity, and depression that can occur with life-threatening illness. Psychological and behavioral methods are now becoming a regular part of cancer treatment.

Psychotherapy is practiced by licensed mental health professionals, including psychologists, psychiatrists, social workers, nurses, counselors, and marriage and family therapists. Specialized training and experience in the issues involved in treating people with cancer is necessary, and some professionals specifically work as psycho-oncologists.

What is the evidence?

Research has consistently shown that psychotherapy can be beneficial to people with cancer in a variety of ways. A psychologist at the University of California School of Medicine in Los Angeles reported in 1999 that behavioral therapy is most useful in managing anxiety related to specific treatment concerns, such as phobic reactions to needles, fears related to surgery or chemotherapy, and claustrophobic feelings during magnetic resonance imaging (MRIs). A 1996 study reported weekly individual cognitive therapy and bimonthly family counseling improved both depression and quality of life of women with nonmetastatic breast cancer. Research has generally shown that psychotherapy can help reduce anxiety and depression in people with cancer, help them make better use of their time, and help them return to work. Psychotherapy can also help people learn to communicate better with their doctors and adhere to medical treatment.

A 2006 study of nearly two hundred women with early-stage breast cancer showed that a ten-week cognitive-behavioral therapy group course helped the women reduce social disruption and improve their outlook, sense of well-being, and ability to relax, even up to one year after the therapy. A similar effect was shown in a 2006 study of men who had been treated for early-stage prostate cancer with surgery or radiation. The group of men who had the ten-week cognitive behavioral therapy stress management course had better quality of life afterward than those who did not.

The National Comprehensive Cancer Network (NCCN), a group of expert cancer treatment centers in the United States, now recommends that all patients with cancer be evaluated for emotional distress. People who are found to have higher distress levels during cancer treatment are referred for counseling or therapy. Psychotherapy has become a standard complementary measure to improve quality of life for people with cancer.

Research has not shown, however, that psychotherapy can prolong the life of cancer patients. Few controlled studies of this nature have been conducted. In 1982, researchers studied 120 end-stage male cancer patients. About half were randomly assigned to a control group and the other half received individual counseling. Whereas those receiving psychotherapy showed improvement on quality of life measures, no difference was found between groups in survival rate after one year. A 1989 study from Stanford University reported a substantial survival benefit among women with metastatic breast cancer who received psychotherapy. However, a later study from the same researcher reported improved quality of life but no difference in survival.

A 2004 analysis pooled the results of several well-designed studies of cancer patients receiving psychotherapy. With more than a thousand patients in the final analysis, no effect was found on survival.

Are there any possible problems or complications?

Psychotherapists vary in the amount of their training and experience in dealing with issues that are important for people with cancer. Difficult personal issues that arise from psychotherapy can also be emotionally upsetting or uncomfortable. Most physicians now view psychotherapy as complementary to standard medical treatment for cancer. Relying on this type of treatment alone and avoiding or delaying conventional medical care for cancer may have serious health consequences.

References

Antoni MH, Lechner SC, Kazi A, Wimberly SR, Sifre T, Urcuyo KR, Glück S, Carver CS. How stress management improves quality of life after treatment for breast cancer. *J Consult Clin Psychol.* 2006;74:1143-1152.

Cassileth BR. The aim of psychotherapeutic intervention in cancer patients. *Support Care Cancer.* 1995;3:267-269.

Chow E, Tsao MN, Harth T. Does psychosocial intervention improve survival in cancer? A meta-analysis. *Palliat Med.* 2004;18:25-31.

Fox BH. The role of psychological factors in cancer incidence and prognosis. *Oncology (Williston Park).* 1995;9:245-253.

Linn MW, Linn BS, Harris R. Effects of counseling for late stage cancer patients. *Cancer.* 1982;49:1048-1055.

Marchioro G, Azzarello G, Checchin F, Perale M, Segati R, Sampognaro E, Rosetti F, Franchin A, Pappagallo GL, Vinante O. The impact of a psychological intervention on quality of life in non-metastatic breast cancer. *Eur J Cancer.* 1996;32A:1612-1615.

NCCN clinical practice guidelines in oncology: distress management. National Comprehensive Cancer Network Web site. http://www.nccn.org/professionals/physician_gls/PDF/distress.pdf. Accessed March 23, 2007.

Penedo FJ, Molton I, Dahn JR, Shen BJ, Kinsinger D, Traeger L, Siegel S, Schneiderman N, Antoni M. A randomized clinical trial of group-based cognitive-behavioral stress management in localized prostate cancer: development of stress management skills improves quality of life and benefit finding. *Ann Behav Med.* 2006;31:261-270.

Sourkes BM, Massie MJ, Holland JC. Psychotherapeutic issues. In: Holland JC, Breitbart W, eds. *Psycho-Oncology.* New York: Oxford University Press; 1998.

Spiegel D. Essentials of psychotherapeutic intervention for cancer patients. *Support Care Cancer.* 1995;3:252-256.

Spiegel D, Butler LD, Giese-Davis J, Koopman C, Miller E, Dimiceli S, Classen CC, Fobair P, Carlson RW, Kraemer HC. Effects of supportive-expressive group therapy on survival of patients with metastatic breast cancer: a randomized prospective trial. *Cancer.* 2007;110:1130-1138.

Wellisch DK. Treating cancer patients: a growing area for psychologists. *The National Psychologist.* May/June;1999: 26-27.

QIGONG

Other common name(s): chi kung
Scientific/medical name(s): none

Description

Qigong is a Chinese system designed to enhance the natural flow of vital energy called qi or chi, pronounced "kee" or "chee," in the body. The process of working toward a regulated, smooth flow of qi is called "gong" (pronounced "kung").

Overview

Qigong can involve meditation, breathing, and movement. Available scientific evidence does not show that qigong is effective in treating cancer or any other disease; however, it may be useful to enhance quality of life.

How is it promoted for use?

People who practice qigong believe disease, injury, and stress can disrupt the vital energy or life force (qi) of the body. By correcting these problems, people can lead healthier, less stressful lives. Qigong is said to strengthen the body or to enhance other conventional health care treatments, not to cure existing disease. Practitioners claim it may be helpful in managing pain and reducing anxiety. There is some limited evidence for these claims.

Some promoters also claim that qigong can help to prevent cancer by improving the oxygen supply to the body and regulating the autonomic nervous system. They further claim qigong can be used to treat stroke, heart and other circulatory diseases, abnormal sex hormone levels, low bone density, and senility. Some even claim they can cure a person with the energy released from their fingertips using external qigong.

What does it involve?

The goal of qigong is to help the flow of energy through the body. There are two forms of qigong: internal and external. Internal qigong consists mainly of meditation, physical movement, and breathing exercises that people can do on their own. External qigong involves skilled masters who claim to use their own qi to help heal other people. The qigong master does not have to touch a person in order to promote healing.

A typical qigong session might have a person sit or stand quietly while thinking about the qi flowing through his or her body and doing breathing and movement exercises at the same time. The breathing and movement used in qigong is slow, focused, and controlled. Qigong can also be used to target specific areas of the body where problems may exist.

Hospitals in China include qigong as part of their health care programs. Only in rural China is it practiced without conventional health care. In the United States, qigong classes are offered for various fees at health clubs, schools, hospitals, YMCAs, and community fitness facilities as part of adult education programs. There are also a number of "qigong institutes" that charge a small fee for classes. Qigong is also taught through videotapes or DVDs and printed materials.

In addition to the type of qigong used for healing, there are two other forms: spiritual qigong, which is used for self-awareness, and martial arts qigong, which is used for self-defense (see "Tai Chi," page 142).

What is the history behind it?

Qigong is a form of traditional Chinese medicine based on the theory of yin and yang, which asserts that there are two opposing but complementary forces in all nonstatic objects and processes. People in China have been practicing qigong for at least 7,000 years to maintain health and achieve long life. Originally, the ancient Chinese realized that certain body movements and mental concentration could adjust and enhance body functions. Qigong techniques even became part of religious rituals.

Over the past few centuries, qigong slowly separated from religious beliefs, and a more conventional form was developed in the 1970s. In the early 1980s, Chinese scientists began scientific investigations of qigong. Hundreds of medical applications were subsequently published in Chinese literature, but many studies only involved a few patients and did not use well-controlled scientific methods. By the 1990s, the Chinese government began to manage qigong and made it an official part of the Chinese health plan.

Today, qigong is widely practiced and studied in China. In the United States, it is used as a form of relaxation and meditation in some health clubs and fitness centers.

What is the evidence?

Whereas some scientists believe that internal qigong may be useful as a form of exercise to help relieve stress, improve coordination, and generally improve a person's quality of life, the idea that qigong can cure cancer is not supported by high-quality clinical trials.

One study published in the United States found that for people with chronic pain, training in internal qigong resulted in a short-term reduction of pain and a long-term reduction in anxiety. However, this was a small study involving only twenty-six patients. A Hong Kong study of people with high blood pressure showed that after twelve weeks of qigong, blood pressure and cholesterol levels were lower. Another study in Korea showed similar effects on blood pressure as well as reduced levels of cortisol (stress hormones). A nonrandomized clinical study from Taiwan reported less psychological distress among chemotherapy patients using qigong. More well-controlled clinical research using larger groups of patients is needed to learn what effect qigong may have in treating various medical conditions.

A review of animal research studies in China reported that external qigong slowed the growth of tumors in mice. Another study found that it did not help reduce signs of pain in rats. Scientific studies of external qigong's effects on humans have not been promising so far.

Are there any possible problems or complications?

Qigong is generally considered safe because of the slow, deliberate movements involved. People who are prone to muscle aches and joint pain may notice these problems if movement or effort is overdone. A small number of people may become disoriented or anxious and experience some negative feelings.

Relying on this type of treatment alone and avoiding or delaying conventional medical care for cancer may have serious health consequences.

References

Barrett S. Be wary of acupuncture, Qigong, and "Chinese medicine." Quackwatch Web site. http://www.quackwatch.org/01QuackeryRelatedTopics/acu.html. Accessed May 23, 2008.

Cassileth B. *The Alternative Medicine Handbook: The Complete Reference Guide to Alternative and Complementary Therapies*. New York: W.W. Norton; 1998.

Eisenberg DM, Kessler RC, Foster C, Norlock FE, Calkins DR, Delbanco TL. Unconventional medicine in the United States. Prevalence, costs, and patterns of use. *N Engl J Med.* 1993;328:246-252.

Lee MS, Chen KW, Sancier KM, Ernst E. Qigong for cancer treatment: a systematic review of controlled clinical trials. *Acta Oncol.* 2007;46:717-722.

Lee MS, Lee MS, Choi ES, Chung HT. Effects of qigong on blood pressure, blood pressure determinants, and ventilatory function in middle-aged patients with essential hypertension. *Am J Chin Med.* 2003;31:489-497.

Lee MS, Lee MS, Kim HJ, Choi ES. Effects of qigong on blood pressure, high-density lipoprotein cholesterol and other lipid levels in essential hypertension patients. *Int J Neurosci.* 2004;114:777-786.

Lee TI, Chen HH, Yeh ML. Effects of chan-chuang qigong on improving symptom and psychological distress in chemotherapy patients. *Am J Chin Med.* 2006;34:37-46.

Qi Gong. Aetna InteliHealth Web site. http://www.intelihealth.com/IH/ihtIH?d=dmtContent&c=358864. Accessed May 23, 2008.

Sancier KM. Medical applications of qigong. *Altern Ther Health Med.* 1996;2:40-46.

Wu WH, Bandilla E, Ciccone DS, Yang J, Cheng SC, Carner N, Wu Y, Shen R. Effects of qigong on late-stage complex regional pain syndrome. *Altern Ther Health Med.* 1999;5:45-54.

Zhang WB, Yu WL, Yang YJ. Absence of an analgesic effect of qigong "external qi" in rats. *Am J Chin Med.* 1998;26:39-46.

SHAMANISM

Other common name(s): shaman, medicine man, shamanka, medicine woman, witch doctor
Scientific/medical name(s): none

Description

Shamanism is the name given to a group of ancient folk medicine practices, all of which use supernatural or spiritual healing. The healing rituals are done by a shaman, a person seen by a people or a tribe as someone with special religious and/or magical powers. Belief that the soul or spirit can leave the body is central to shamanic practice.

Overview

Although stories have existed for centuries and many people around the world continue to practice shamanism today, available scientific evidence does not suggest that it can cure cancer or any other disease. Some key elements of shamanism, such as the use of imagery, have been shown to reduce stress and anxiety.

How is it promoted for use?

Shamanism is based on the belief that healing has a spiritual aspect that must be addressed. People who believe in shamans say that they can heal both the body and soul as well as restore harmony to the community and nature. Shamans claim they communicate with spirits in order to help heal. Some shamans claim they can heal spiritual, psychic, and physical wounds as well as communities and global conditions.

Not all shamans claim the ability to heal every disease. Shamans often work in cultures that include other specialists such as herbalists, diviners, bonesetters, and midwives. Some shamans are very selective in choosing which people they will treat, because if they fail, they may be punished by the tribe. For example, shamans who believe that their brand of healing will not influence the course of cancer may choose not to work with a person who has cancer. Sometimes they prescribe more elaborate rituals to try to address difficult illnesses. At other times, the shaman may pronounce a person incurable.

What does it involve?

The shaman enters a trance, either self-induced or through the aid of hallucinogens or fasting, to determine what is wrong with the patient and what to do about it. The shaman or an assistant may pray, sing, chant, dance, or drum around the patient. Storytelling and other art forms may also be used. During the trance, the shaman's soul is believed to leave the body and travel to the spirit world in a search to help the sick person. In the spirit world, the shaman communicates with the spirits thought to be responsible for the illness. Although the shaman is in a trance, he is still conscious and aware. He or she is able to bargain with the spirits who can help the patient's illness. The shaman returns and shares his or her vision with the sick person.

True shamans must complete rigorous training, especially in the ability to achieve the controlled trance required for communication with the spirits. Shamans work both with individual patients and with groups. In the United States, many Native American healers also practice shamanism, although they are usually called medicine men or medicine women. It is common practice for Native American medicine men or women to conduct healing sessions at night, most often in places with some religious connection or significance.

What is the history behind it?

Shamanism may be the oldest of all healing practices, dating back as far as 40,000 years. It is believed to have begun in the Altai and Ural Mountains of western China and Russia, probably in the form of a religion. In the Tungusu-Manchurian language, the word shaman means "one who knows."

Many early cultures had their own forms of shamanism. These included people on the North American and South American continents and in Asia, India, Africa, the South Pacific, and Australia. Each early culture throughout the world had its own shamans, though not all were called by that name. The shaman, shamanka, or native healer was thought to be the only person in the tribe who could see beyond the everyday world and communicate with the spirits of ancestors, animals, gods, and demons.

Today, shamanism is still practiced as folk medicine in some parts of Europe, Africa, and Asia. Because of increased interest in shamanic traditions, some new age practitioners now claim to be shamans but do not practice within the traditions of any folk or traditional system.

What is the evidence?

There are many stories about the success of shamans throughout history. Most of these stories are not unlike the reports of religious "miracles" at shrines such as Lourdes. Available scientific evidence does not support claims that spirits exist, that a shaman can communicate with and influence them, or that illness is caused by spirits.

Those who accept shamanism believe it works in a spiritual dimension of life that must be cleansed of evil spirits. Available scientific evidence furnishes no proof of shamanic ability to cure disease. Any results are most likely due to the placebo effect, in which believing that something can or will happen creates a positive result. Pain may subside because the patient believes the shaman made it subside.

Some key elements of shamanism, such as the use of imagery, have been shown to reduce stress and anxiety. One researcher at Stanford University reported that some aspects of shamanism might be helpful in changing destructive thought patterns in people with cancer. However, available scientific evidence does not support claims that shamanism is effective in treating cancer or any other disease.

Are there any possible problems or complications?

Shamanism is generally considered safe and may be useful as a complementary approach to help people who have cancer deal with their emotions, certain symptoms of cancer, and the side effects of cancer treatment. However, people who believe in spirits may fear being harmed by them. In addition, some shamans expect the patient to share in taking a hallucinogenic drug, which may be harmful to some people.

It is important to know that some who claim to be shamans are not trained within a folk or traditional system of medicine. Someone without training or experience in the field may not be skilled or sensitive to the needs and issues important to someone living with cancer and could cause psychological harm.

Relying on this type of treatment alone and avoiding or delaying conventional medical care for cancer may have serious health consequences.

References

Anumolu AK, Miller H, Popoola MM, Talley B, Rushing A, et al. Alternative health care systems. In: Huebscher R, Shuler PA, eds. *Natural, Alternative, and Complementary Health Care Practices.* St. Louis, MO: Mosby; 2004:745-751.

Cassileth B. *The Alternative Medicine Handbook: The Complete Reference Guide to Alternative and Complementary Therapies.* New York: W.W. Norton; 1998.

Metzner R. Hallucinogenic drugs and plants in psychotherapy and shamanism. *J Psychoactive Drugs.* 1998;30:333-341.

Money M. Shamanism and complementary therapy. *Complement Ther Nurs Midwifery*. 1997;3:131-135.

National Institutes of Health. *Alternative Medicine: Expanding Medical Horizons: A Report to the National Institutes of Health on Alternative Medical Systems and Practices in the United States*. Washington, DC: US Government Printing Office; 1994. NIH publication 94-066.

Takatoka. False shamans. Manataka American Indian Council Web site. http://www.manataka.org/page23.html. Accessed May 23, 2008.

Vitebsky P. *The Shaman*. New York: Little, Brown and Company; 1995.

SPIRITUALITY AND PRAYER

Other common name(s): religion, spiritual healing
Scientific/medical name(s): none

Description

Spirituality is generally described as an awareness of something greater than the individual self. It is often expressed through religion and/or prayer, although there are many other paths of spiritual pursuit and expression.

Overview

Studies have found spirituality and religion are very important to the quality of life for some people with cancer. Although available research has not supported claims that spirituality can cure cancer or any other disease, the psychological benefits of praying may include reduction of stress and anxiety, promotion of a more positive outlook, and the strengthening of the will to live.

How is it promoted for use?

Proponents of spirituality claim that prayer can decrease the negative effects of disease, speed recovery, and increase the effectiveness of medical treatments. Faith and religious beliefs are also thought to improve coping and provide comfort during illness. Attendance at religious events and services is sometimes linked with improvement of various health conditions such as heart disease, hypertension, stroke, colitis, uterine and other cancers, and overall health status.

Some religious groups, such as Christian Scientists, claim prayer can cure any disease. These groups often rely entirely on prayer in place of conventional medicine. This belief is based on a spiritual rather than a biological explanation of how disease develops. See the section on faith healing on page 83 for more information.

Many people believe the spiritual dimension is important when a person is coping with serious illness. The ability to find meaning in life can be helpful when dealing with cancer, even though it cannot cure the disease. Spirituality may also help us accept death, both our own and the deaths of those we love.

What does it involve?

Spirituality has many forms and can be practiced in many ways. Prayer, for example, may be silent or spoken out loud and can be done alone in any setting or in groups, as in a church or temple. Regular attendance at a church, temple, or mosque may involve prayer that focuses on one's self (called supplication) or on others (called intercessory prayer). In this type of setting, the entire congregation may be asked to pray for a sick person or the person's family.

Some religions set aside certain times of day and days of the week for prayer. Standard prayers written by religious leaders are often memorized and repeated in private sessions and in groups. Prayer is also practiced individually and in informal groups, without a specific religion or denomination, and on no particular schedule. Prayers often ask a higher being for help, understanding, wisdom, or strength in dealing with life's problems.

Spirituality can also be practiced without a formal religion. Meditation, twelve-step work (as practiced in Alcoholics Anonymous and similar groups), and seeking meaning in life all involve spirituality. Even simple practices such as silent observation, listening, or gratitude can become part of an open-ended spirituality that can infuse everyday life. Some people express their spirituality by spending time with nature, doing creative work, or serving others.

Many medical institutions and practitioners include spirituality and prayer as important components of healing. In addition, hospitals have chapels and contracts with ministers, rabbis, clerics, and voluntary organizations to serve their patients' spiritual needs.

What is the history behind it?

Since the beginning of recorded history, all cultures throughout the world have developed systems of religion and spirituality. Earlier religions of ancient Egypt and Greece have given way to more modern religions such as Christianity, Judaism, Hinduism, Islam, and Buddhism.

Within each culture, some form of spirituality and prayer has served as the institutionalized means of seeking assistance from a supreme being or beings perceived as powerful enough to alter nature, health, and disease. Different religions hold different beliefs about a supreme being. Today, spirituality is practiced by billions of people throughout the world, both within and outside the framework of formal religion.

What is the evidence?

Studies done on the impact of prayer and spirituality often focus on the effect of religious beliefs and behavior and the effects of intercessory prayer on health, survival, and quality of life. For many of these studies, results have been mixed. Although some research has found that religious groups with orthodox beliefs and behavior have lower cancer death rates, other studies have not found any health benefits related to religion and survival.

The U.S. Office of Technology Assessment reported that a survey of articles published in the *Journal of Family Practice* over ten years found that 83 percent of studies on religiosity found a positive effect on physical health. Another study of two major psychiatric journals over twelve years found that for the studies that measured religiosity, 92 percent showed a benefit for mental health, 4 percent were neutral, and 4 percent showed harm. Religiosity was measured by participation in religious ceremony, social support, prayer, and belief in a higher being.

An analysis of forty-three studies on people with advanced cancer noted that those who reported spiritual well-being were able to cope more effectively with terminal illnesses and find meaning in their experience. Major themes of spiritual well-being included self-awareness, coping with stress, connectedness with others, faith, empowerment, confidence, and the ability to live with meaning and hope.

Research has also been conducted on the effects of intercessory prayer in coronary care patients. In the late 1980s, a study in San Francisco found that heart patients who were prayed for by others appeared to have fewer complications, although length of hospital stay and death rates did not differ between those who were prayed for and those who were not. A larger study at a Kansas City hospital coronary care unit reported similar findings. Although overall length of hospital stay and time in the critical care unit did not differ between groups, the group that had been prayed for had 11 percent fewer complications. These results suggested that prayer might be helpful when used with conventional medical care, although more research was needed to confirm that finding. The studies drew a great deal of public attention, and several other studies were done to confirm the findings, with mixed results. When a research group reanalyzed fourteen of these studies, they concluded that intercessory prayer had no effect on any medical outcomes.

In a further study, a group of Harvard researchers studied more than 1,800 patients who were undergoing heart surgery in 2006. The patients were randomly assigned to three groups. The first group was told that prayers would be said for them, while the second and third groups were told that they might or might not have prayers said for them. The first and second groups received prayer, and the third group did not. Complications occurred within thirty days for 59 percent of the first group, 52 percent of the second group, and 51 percent of the third group. Prayer did not reduce complications for those who had heart surgery in this large, well-controlled scientific study. At this point, available scientific evidence does not support claims of reduced complications in those who receive prayer.

Are there any possible problems or complications?

Patient consent is important before conducting any activity that may affect health. Those who do not believe in prayer and those who do not wish to be healed are among those who may not want to be the object of intercessory prayer. Relying on this type of treatment alone and avoiding or delaying conventional medical care for cancer may have serious health consequences.

References

Benson H, Dusek JA, Sherwood JB, Lam P, Bethea CF, Carpenter W, Levitsky S, Hill PC, Clem DW Jr, Jain MK, Drumel D, Kopecky SL, Mueller PS, Marek D, Rollins S, Hibberd PL. Study of the Therapeutic Effects of Intercessory Prayer (STEP) in cardiac bypass patients: a multicenter randomized trial of uncertainty and certainty of receiving intercessory prayer. *Am Heart J.* 2006;151:934-942.

Breitbart W. Spirituality and meaning in supportive care: spirituality- and meaning-centered group psychotherapy interventions in advanced cancer. *Support Care Cancer.* 2002;10:272-80. Epub 2001 Aug 28.

Brussat F, Brussat MA. *Spiritual Literacy: Reading the Sacred in Everyday Life.* New York: Simon and Shuster; 1996.

Byrd RC. Positive therapeutic effects of intercessory prayer in a coronary care unit population. *South Med J.* 1988;81:826-829.

Chao CS, Chen CH, Yen M. The essence of spirituality of terminally ill patients. *J Nurs Res.* 2002;10:237-245.

Dwyer JW, Clarke LL, Miller MK. The effect of religious concentration and affiliation on county cancer mortality rates. *J Health Soc Behav.* 1990;31:185-202.

Harris WS, Gowda M, Kolb JW, Strychacz CP, Vacek JL, Jones PG, Forker A, O'Keefe JH, McCallister BD. A randomized, controlled trial of the effects of remote, intercessory prayer on outcomes in patients admitted to the coronary care unit. *Arch Intern Med.* 1999;159:2273-2278.
    Erratum in:
    Arch Intern Med. 2000;160:1878.

Kurtz E, Ketcham K. *Spirituality of Imperfection: Storytelling and the Search for Meaning.* New York; Bantam Books:1993.

Lin HR, Bauer-Wu SM. Psycho-spiritual well-being in patients with advanced cancer: an integrative review of the literature. *J Adv Nurs.* 2003;44:69-80.

Marcus A. Lord, please heal whatshisname: anonymous prayer helps heart patients, study finds. HealthScout Web site. http://www.healthscout.com. Accessed October 15, 1999. Content no longer available.

Masters KS, Spielmans GI, Goodson JT. Are there demonstrable effects of distant intercessory prayer? A meta-analytic review. *Ann Behav Med.* 2006;32:21-26.

Mytko JJ, Knight SJ. Body, mind and spirit: towards the integration of religiosity and spirituality in cancer quality of life research. *Psychooncology*. 1999;8:439-450.

National Institutes of Health. *Alternative Medicine: Expanding Medical Horizons: A Report to the National Institutes of Health on Alternative Medical Systems and Practices in the United States*. Washington, DC: US Government Printing Office; 1994. NIH publication 94-066.

Prayer. Aetna InteliHealth Web site. http://www.intelihealth.com/IH/ihtIH/WSIHW000/8513/34968/360051.html. Accessed May 23, 2008.

Spencer JW, Jacobs JJ. *Complementary/Alternative Medicine: An Evidence-Based Approach*. St. Louis, MO: Mosby; 1999.

US Congress, Office of Technology Assessment. *Unconventional Cancer Treatments: OTA-H-405*. Washington, DC: US Government Printing Office; 1990.

SUPPORT GROUPS

Other common name(s):
group therapy, group psychotherapy, psychosocial interventions, psychosocial treatment
Scientific/medical name(s): none

Description

Support groups present information, provide comfort, teach coping skills, help reduce anxiety, and provide a place for people to share common concerns and emotional support.

Overview

Preliminary research has shown that many support groups can enhance quality of life. Available scientific evidence does not consistently support claims that support groups can actually extend the survival time of people with cancer.

How is it promoted for use?

People who take part in support groups believe that they can live healthier, happier lives if they spend time relating to others. They believe that when relatives and friends lend support, it is easier for people to deal with their health and social problems. Some claim that the bonds formed between members of support groups help them feel stronger. They further claim that sharing feelings and experiences within support groups can reduce stress, fear, and anxiety and help to promote healing.

What does it involve?

Support groups may include education, behavioral training, and group interaction. Behavioral training can involve muscle relaxation or meditation to reduce stress or the effects of chemotherapy or radiation therapy. People with cancer are often encouraged by health care professionals to seek support from groups of people who have direct or indirect experiences with the same type of cancer.

Many different kinds of support groups are available, and they vary in their structure and activities. Some are time-limited, while others are ongoing. Some support groups are made up of people with the same type of cancer, while others include people who are having the same kind of treatment. Support groups are available for patients, family members, and other caregivers of people who have cancer. The format of different groups varies from lectures and discussions to exploration and expression of feelings. Topics discussed in support groups are those of concern to the members and those the group leader thinks are important.

Support groups are different from group therapy. Support groups may be led by survivors, group members, or trained professionals, while therapy groups are always facilitated by licensed counselors such as marriage and family therapists, nurses, psychologists, psychiatrists, and social workers. Group therapy is generally longer, more involved, and focuses on in-depth personal growth, whereas support groups focus on learning to manage current concerns and situations. Most support groups involve little or no cost to the participants, whereas there is usually a fee for group therapy. Support group meetings can be held in hospitals, school classrooms, community centers, office buildings, or in one of the group member's homes.

Support groups can also take place on the Internet, in which case they usually involve interacting with people by sending and receiving messages via computer. These groups vary widely in quality. Some are led by moderators in chat rooms or on e-mail lists, while others are not moderated.

What is the history behind it?

In the late 1970s, a type of therapeutic group meeting called an encounter group became popular, and group-intervention studies began appearing in a variety of science journals. An influential study by Dr. David Spiegel in 1989 reported that group therapy helped women with breast cancer to cope and live longer. The demand for support groups from people who have cancer has grown since then. Today, there are many hospital-based, independent, and national networks of support groups for people with various types of cancer and other diseases, as well as for their families.

What is the evidence?

The scientific community believes that support groups can enhance quality of life for people who have cancer by providing information and support to overcome feelings of aloneness and helplessness that sometimes result from a cancer diagnosis. Research has shown that people with cancer are better able to deal with their disease when supported by others in similar situations.

One clinical trial found that support groups helped in reducing tension, anxiety, fatigue, and confusion. Some research has shown that there is a link between group support and greater tolerance of cancer treatment and treatment compliance. One psychologist found that an educational, supportive intervention resulted in more patients taking their medicines as prescribed, which led to an increase in survival rates.

Overall, research has shown conflicting results about the ability of group participation to extend life. In Dr. Spiegel's 1989 clinical trial, women with metastatic breast cancer lived eighteen months longer if they had taken part in supportive group therapy. However, scientists later realized that his study had used average survival rather than median survival to compare the groups. Average survival can be greatly changed by one early death or one long-term survivor, so it can be quite misleading. Another clinical trial found no significant difference in survival between breast cancer patients who took part in group therapy and those who did not. Yet another clinical trial found that patients with malignant melanoma lived longer if they had taken part in a group psycho-educational course. A 2005 review of four studies of breast cancer patients found no relationship between survival and support groups beyond Dr. Spiegel's study.

One study at the Ontario Cancer Institute found that women with breast cancer who lacked support from families and friends were helped the most by support groups. Researchers at Carnegie Mellon University recently found that educational groups helped women adjust to a diagnosis of early-stage breast cancer. However, they also found there were some negative effects from group discussion. Some of the women in the group who were already getting support at home gained no benefit from the group.

In summary, randomized clinical trials have shown inconsistent effects on survival, but most have shown improved quality of life in support group participants. Although more research is needed to determine what types of groups are most effective for which types of people, support groups may be useful as a complementary therapy for people with cancer and other diseases.

Are there any possible problems or complications?

Support groups vary in quality and focus. People with cancer may find the support group they have joined does not discuss topics of interest to them. Some people may find a support group upsetting because it stirs up too many uncomfortable feelings or because the leader is not skilled enough. Information that is shared in some groups may not always be reliable.

Online support groups should be used with caution. This venue cannot always assure privacy or confidentiality, and the people involved may have no special training or qualifications, especially if the group takes place in an unmonitored chat room.

Relying on this type of treatment alone and avoiding or delaying conventional medical care for cancer may have serious health consequences.

References

Azar B. Does group therapy mean longer life? *APA Monitor.* 1999;30:13-14.

Cunningham AJ, Edmonds CV, Jenkins GP, Pollack H, Lockwood GA, Warr D. A randomized controlled trial of the effects of group psychological therapy on survival in women with metastatic breast cancer. *Psychooncology.* 1998;7:508-517.

Edmonds CV, Lockwood GA, Cunningham AJ. Psychological response to long-term group therapy: a randomized trial with metastatic breast cancer patients. *Psychooncology.* 1999;8:74-91.

Fawzy FI, Fawzy NW, Arndt LA, Pasnau RO. Critical review of psychosocial interventions in cancer care. *Arch Gen Psychiatry.* 1995;52:100-113.

Goodwin PJ. Support groups in advanced breast cancer. *Cancer.* 2005;104:2596-2601.

Helgeson VS, Cohen S, Schulz R, Yasko J. Education and peer discussion group interventions and adjustment to breast cancer. *Arch Gen Psychiatry.* 1999;56:340-347.

Kogon MM, Biswas A, Pearl D, Carlson RW, Spiegel D. Effects of medical and psychotherapeutic treatment on the survival of women with metastatic breast carcinoma. *Cancer.* 1997;80:225-230.

National Institutes of Health. *Alternative Medicine: Expanding Medical Horizons: A Report to the National Institutes of Health on Alternative Medical Systems and Practices in the United States.* Washington, DC: US Government Printing Office; 1994. NIH publication 94-066.

Penson RT, Talsania SH, Chabner BA, Lynch TJ Jr. Help me help you: support groups in cancer therapy. *Oncologist.* 2004:9:217-225.

Richardson JL, Shelton DR, Krailo M, Levine AM. The effect of compliance with treatment on survival among patients with hematologic malignancies. *J Clin Oncol.* 1990;8:356-364.

US Congress, Office of Technology Assessment. *Unconventional Cancer Treatments: OTA-H-405.* Washington, DC: US Government Printing Office; 1990.

Zabalegui A, Sanchez S, Sanchez PD, Juando C. Nursing and cancer support groups. *J Adv Nurs.* 2005;51:369-381.

TAI CHI

Other common name(s):
t'ai chi, tai chi chuan, tai chi chih, tai ji juan, tai ji quan, taijiquan, tai ji, taiji, shadow boxing
Scientific/medical name(s): none

Description

Tai chi is an ancient Chinese martial art that is part of qigong. It is a mind–body, self-healing system that uses movement, meditation, and breathing to improve health and well-being.

Overview

Research has shown tai chi is useful as a form of exercise that can improve posture, balance, muscle mass and tone, flexibility, stamina, and strength in older adults. Tai chi is also recognized as a method to reduce stress that can provide the same cardiovascular benefits as moderate exercise, such as lowered heart rate and blood pressure.

How is it promoted for use?

People who practice the deep breathing and physical movements of tai chi report that it makes them feel more relaxed, younger, and more agile, and that it helps their circulation. The slow, graceful movements of tai chi, accompanied by rhythmic breathing, relax the body as well as the mind. There is also evidence that tai chi is particularly suited for older adults or for others who are not physically strong or healthy.

Supporters claim that tai chi balances the flow of vital energy or life force called qi (or chi), which serves to prevent illness, improve general health, and extend life. It is also based on the theory of yin and yang, which asserts that there are two opposing but complementary forces in all nonstatic objects and processes. Practitioners claim tai chi is designed to balance yin and yang forces to achieve inner harmony.

What does it involve?

Tai chi students begin by learning a series of gentle, deliberate movements, which flow into body positions called forms. Each form contains between twenty to a hundred moves and requires up to twenty minutes to complete. Each form derives its name from nature, with names such as "Wave Hands Like Clouds" or "Grasping the Bird's Tail." In order to balance the yin and yang, movements are practiced in pairs of opposites. For example, a turn to the right follows one to the left. While doing these exercises, the person is urged to pay close attention to his or her breathing, which should be centered in the diaphragm. Tai chi emphasizes technique rather than strength or power, although the slow, precise movements require good muscle control. Meditative concentration is focused on a point just below the navel, from which it is believed qi radiates throughout the body.

Tai chi is taught in many health clubs, schools, and recreational facilities. Practitioners believe that daily practice is needed in order to get the most benefit. Once a person has mastered a form, it can be practiced at home.

What is the history behind it?

Tai chi is based on the philosophy of Taoism, a Chinese belief system first developed in the sixth century BC. Taoism includes beliefs in the existence of qi and the yin and yang. Tai chi began as a martial arts type of qigong and has been practiced as an exercise in China for many centuries.

Tai chi became a sports event in 1990's 11th Asian Games as wushu, a form of tai chi practiced primarily for show or competition. Tai chi has recently gained popularity in the United States and other Western countries as a general exercise technique, especially for older adults. Today, classes, videos, and books on tai chi are widely available.

What is the evidence?

Researchers have focused on studying the benefits of relaxation and exercise that result from practicing tai chi. Clinical trials suggest that tai chi improves posture, balance, flexibility, muscle mass and tone, stamina, and strength in older adults and may help prevent falls and fractures. A small 2006 study compared tai chi with psychosocial therapy in breast cancer survivors. The women in the tai chi group had improved flexibility, strength, and aerobic capacity, whereas the women in the other group had improvements in flexibility only. Another randomized clinical trial of people over age sixty-nine compared results for a group participating in tai chi with those of a group taking part in a stretching exercise class. After six months, the tai chi group had better balance and fewer falls than the stretching group.

Another randomized clinical trial found that tai chi led to a sense of improved well-being in older adults and increased their motivation to continue exercising. When tai chi is used as an exercise, benefits have also been noted for older people with chronic diseases such as arthritis, osteoporosis, chronic obstructive pulmonary disease, and peripheral artery disease. Research has found that tai chi can reduce stress and provide the same cardiovascular benefits as moderate exercise, such as reduced heart rate and blood pressure. In one randomized study, older adults with sleep problems who practiced tai chi were able to fall asleep faster and stay asleep longer than those who did low-impact aerobics.

Available scientific evidence does not support the idea that tai chi can cure cancer or any other disease, although it does suggest it may be helpful when used with conventional treatment.

Are there any possible problems or complications?

Tai chi is considered to be a relatively safe, moderate physical activity, although injuries can happen. As with any form of exercise, it is important to be aware of physical limitations. People with cancer and chronic conditions such as arthritis and heart disease should talk with their doctors before starting any type of therapy that involves movement of joints and muscles.

Relying on this type of treatment alone and avoiding or delaying conventional medical care for cancer may have serious health consequences.

References

Channer KS, Barrow D, Barrow R, Osborne M, Ives G. Changes in haemodynamic parameters following Tai Chi Chuan and aerobic exercise in patients recovering from acute myocardial infarction. *Postgrad Med J.* 1996;72:349-351.

Kutner NG, Barnhart H, Wolf SL, McNeely E, Xu T. Self-report benefits of Tai Chi practice by older adults. *J Gerontol B Psychol Sci Soc Sci.* 1997;52:P242-P246.

Lan C, Lai JS, Wong MK, Yu ML. Cardiorespiratory function, flexibility, and body composition among geriatric Tai Chi Chuan practitioners. *Arch Phys Med Rehabil.* 1996;77:612-616.

Li F, Fisher KJ, Harmer P, Irbe D, Tearse RG, Weimer C. Tai chi and self-rated quality of sleep and daytime sleepiness in older adults: a randomized controlled trial. *J Am Geriatr Soc.* 2004;52:892-900.

Li F, Harmer P, Fisher KJ, McAuley E, Chaumeton N, Eckstrom E, Wilson NL. Tai chi and fall reductions in older adults: a randomized controlled trial. *J Gerontol A Biol Sci Med Sci.* 2005;60:187-194.

Mustian KM, Katula JA, Zhao H. A pilot study to assess the influence of tai chi chuan on functional capacity among breast cancer survivors. *J Support Oncol.* 2006;4:139-145.

Province MA, Hadley EC, Hornbrook MC, Lipsitz LA, Miller JP, Mulrow CD, Ory MG, Sattin RW, Tinetti ME, Wolf SL. The effects of exercise on falls in elderly patients. A preplanned meta-analysis of the FICSIT Trials. Frailty and Injuries: Cooperative Studies of Intervention Techniques. *JAMA.* 1995;273:1341-1347.

Ross MC, Presswalla JL. The therapeutic effects of Tai Chi for the elderly. *J Gerontol Nurs.* 1998;24:45-47.

Schaller KJ. Tai Chi Chih: an exercise option for older adults. *J Gerontol Nurs.* 1996;22:12-17.

Tai chi. Aetna InteliHealth Web site. http://www.intelihealth.com/IH/ihtIH?d=dmtContent&c=358867. Accessed May 23, 2008.

Traditional Chinese medicine: qigong and tai chi. Complementary/Integrative Medicine Education Resources, The University of Texas M. D. Anderson Cancer Center Web site. http://www.mdanderson.org/departments/cimer/display.cfm?id=27b68c52-7868-42a4-96d4c89c3bbd10d0&method=displayfull. Accessed May 23, 2008.

Wolf SL, Barnhart HX, Kutner NG, McNeely E, Coogler C, Xu T. Reducing frailty and falls in older persons: an investigation of Tai Chi and computerized balance training. Atlanta FICSIT Group. Frailty and Injuries: Cooperative Studies of Intervention Techniques. *J Am Geriatr Soc.* 1996; 44:489-497.

Wolfson L, Whipple R, Derby C, Judge J, King M, Amerman P, Schmidt J, Smyers D. Balance and strength training in older adults: intervention gains and Tai Chi maintenance. *J Am Geriatr Soc.* 1996;44:498-506.

YOGA

Other common name(s): hatha yoga
Scientific/medical name(s): none

Description

Yoga is a form of nonaerobic exercise that involves a program of precise posture, breathing exercises, and meditation. In ancient Sanskrit, the word yoga means "union."

Overview

Yoga can be a useful method to help relieve some symptoms of chronic diseases such as cancer, arthritis, and heart disease and can lead to increased relaxation and physical fitness. Available scientific evidence does not support yoga as an effective treatment for cancer or any other disease; however, it may enhance quality of life. Some cancer treatment centers even offer yoga in addition to standard medical treatment.

How is it promoted for use?

Yoga is promoted as a system of personal development. It is a way of life that combines ethical standards, dietary guidelines, physical movements, and meditation to create a union of mind, body, and spirit. Yoga is said to cultivate *prana*, which means vital energy or life force and is similar to qi (or chi) in traditional Chinese medicine. People who practice yoga claim it leads to a state of physical health, relaxation, happiness, peace, and tranquility. There is some evidence that shows that yoga can lower stress, increase strength, and provide a good form of exercise.

Supporters also claim yoga can help eliminate insomnia, increase stamina, and help with smoking cessation. They further claim that the mastery of yoga can give people supernormal mental and physical powers. Yogis, who are masters and teachers of yoga, claim they can obtain heightened senses, overcome hunger and thirst, and develop almost total control over physical processes such as heart rate and breathing.

What does it involve?

There are more than a hundred different types of yoga practiced in the United States today. Most of them are based on hatha yoga, which uses movement, breathing exercises, and meditation to achieve a connection between mind, body, and spirit.

The goal of yoga is perfect concentration to attain Samadhi—pure awareness without mental distractions. Hatha yoga uses forbearance, breath control, withdrawal of senses, attention, concentration, and meditation to attain Samadhi. The three most commonly used aspects of yoga today include the postures of hatha yoga (called *asanas*), the breathing techniques of *pranayama*, and meditation.

Practitioners say yoga should be done at either the beginning or the end of the day. A typical session can last between twenty minutes and an hour. A yoga session starts with the person sitting in an upright position and performing gentle movements, all of which are done very slowly, while taking slow, deep breaths from the abdomen. A session may also include guided relaxation, meditation, and sometimes visualization. It often ends with the chanting of a meaningful word or phrase, called a mantra, to achieve a deeper state of relaxation. Yoga requires several sessions a week in order for a person to become proficient. Yoga can be practiced at home without a teacher or in group classes. Many books and videos on yoga are also available.

What is the history behind it?

First practiced in India more than five thousand years ago, yoga is one of the oldest mind–body health systems in existence. In the United States, yoga was first practiced by the Concord transcendentalists in the 1840s, but it did not become well known until the 1880s, when the English translation of Yoga Sutras was published. This ancient book gave a detailed description of yoga techniques and the quest for Samadhi, which is central to yoga beliefs.

Four traditional yoga paths are meditative (Raja yoga), service (Karma yoga), wisdom (Jnana yoga), and devotional (Bhakti yoga). Hatha yoga is based on a part of Raja yoga and is the best-known form of yoga. In the United States, it is what most people mean when they refer to yoga.

Today, some health plans offer members access to yoga instructors as a form of exercise and relaxation. Health clubs, community centers, adult education centers, and individual teachers offer classes in many subtypes of Hatha yoga, including ananda, ashtanga, bikram, integral, Iyengar, kripalu, and kundalini.

What is the evidence?

Research has shown that yoga can be used to control physical functions such as blood pressure, heart rate, breathing, metabolism, body temperature, brain waves, and skin resistance. This can result in improved physical fitness, lower levels of stress, and increased feelings of relaxation and well-being.

According to a report to the National Institutes of Health, there is also some evidence to suggest yoga may be helpful when used with conventional medical treatment to help relieve some of the symptoms linked to cancer, asthma, diabetes, drug addiction, high blood pressure, heart disease, and migraine headaches. Other studies have shown limited benefit. Yoga may also help to reduce cholesterol levels when used with diet and exercise. Randomized clinical trials have shown that yoga can help relieve the pain of arthritis and may also help anxiety, stress, and depression.

One small clinical trial showed that people with lymphoma reported fewer sleep disturbances, fell asleep more quickly, and slept longer after a seven-week yoga program, compared with patients who did not participate in yoga. However, the patients showed no improvement in depression or fatigue. More well-designed research studies are needed to confirm all of these findings. Recent studies of cancer survivors, especially women who have had breast cancer, suggest yoga may help improve several aspects of quality of life.

Are there any possible problems or complications?

People with cancer and chronic conditions such as arthritis and heart disease should talk to their doctors before starting any type of therapy that involves movement of joints and muscles. Some yoga postures are hard to achieve, and damage can occur from overstretching joints and ligaments. There have been rare reports of damaged nerves or discs in the spine. Rarely, eye damage can occur because of increased pressure in the eyes when doing headstands. This change in pressure can also worsen glaucoma in some people. Blood vessels can sometimes become blocked because of yoga postures, damaging the brain or other parts of the body.

Pregnant women may want to avoid postures that cause pressure on the uterus, such as body twists. People who are sick, dehydrated, or pregnant may be harmed by bikram yoga, which is a vigorous workout practiced in a very warm, humid room (usually between 95° and 105° F).

Relying on this type of treatment alone and avoiding or delaying conventional medical care for cancer may have serious health consequences.

References

About yoga. Asheville Yoga Center Web site. http://www.youryoga.com/ayc/~info.html. Accessed May 23, 2008.

Bower JE, Woolery A, Sternlieb B, Garet D. Yoga for cancer patients and survivors. *Cancer Control.* 2005;12:165-171.

Cohen L, Warneke C, Fouladi RT, Rodriguez MA, Chaoul-Reich A. Psychological adjustment and sleep quality in a randomized trial of the effects of a Tibetan yoga intervention in patients with lymphoma. *Cancer.* 2004;100:2253-2260.

Ernst E, ed. *The Desktop Guide to Complementary and Alternative Medicine: An Evidence-Based Approach.* New York: Mosby; 2001.

Garfinkel MS, Schumacher HR Jr, Husain A, Levy M, Reshetar RA. Evaluation of a yoga based regimen for treatment of osteoarthritis of the hands. *J Rheumatol.* 1994;21:2341-2343.

Garfinkel MS, Singhal A, Katz WA, Allan DA, Reshetar R, Schumacher HR Jr. Yoga-based intervention for carpal tunnel syndrome: a randomized trial. *JAMA.* 1998;280:1601-1603.

McDonald A, Burjan E, Martin S. Yoga for patients and carers in a palliative day care setting. *Int J Palliat Nurs.* 2006;12:519-523.

Moadel AB, Shah C, Wylie-Rosett J, Harris MS, Patel SR, Hall CB, Sparano JA. Randomized controlled trial of yoga among a multiethnic sample of breast cancer patients: effects on quality of life. *J Clin Oncol.* 2007;25:4387-4395.

National Institutes of Health. *Alternative Medicine: Expanding Medical Horizons: A Report to the National Institutes of Health on Alternative Medical Systems and Practices in the United States.* Washington, DC: US Government Printing Office; 1994. NIH publication 94-066.

Taylor E. Yoga and meditation. *Altern Ther Health Med.* 1995;1:77-78.

The tree of classical yoga/Hinduism. Classical Yoga Hindu Academy Web site. http://www.classicalyoga.org/following_were_article_published.htm. Accessed May 23, 2008.

Yoga. Aetna InteliHealth Web site. http://www.intelihealth.com/IH/ihtIH?d=dmtContent&c=358876. Accessed May 23, 2008.

Chapter Six

Manual Healing and Physical Touch Therapies

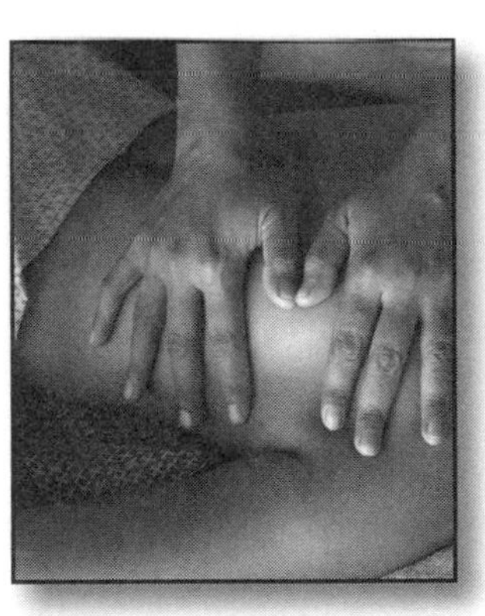

ACUPRESSURE, SHIATSU, AND OTHER ASIAN BODYWORK

Other common names: Tui na, Ohashiatsu, Watsu
Scientific/medical names: none

Description

Bodywork refers to a variety of techniques that touch, manipulate, or otherwise work on the body. Massage and non-Asian types of bodywork are addressed separately (see pages 218 and 167). Acupressure is a form of bodywork based on the Chinese principles of acupuncture. It uses touch or pressure rather than needles. Shiatsu is a Japanese bodywork practice that uses acupressure. Tui na also uses pressure on acupoints, and Ohashiatsu and Watsu are based on the practice of Shiatsu.

Overview

Available scientific evidence does not suggest acupressure and other types of Asian bodywork are effective in treating cancer, but they may be used to enhance quality of life for some patients. There is some evidence from studies with cancer patients that acupressure may be helpful in reducing early nausea related to chemotherapy. Many forms of bodywork may have the potential to help relieve pain and reduce stress, even though the effectiveness of these techniques has not yet been proven scientifically.

How is it promoted for use?

According to the theories and teachings of traditional Chinese medicine, acupoints lie along invisible meridians. There are twelve major meridians in the human body. These meridians are channels for the vital energy or life force called qi (also spelled chi or ki, pronounced "chee" or "kee") that is present in all living things. Meridians also represent an internal system of communication among specific organs or networks of organs. According to traditional Chinese medicine, illness may occur when the energy flow along one or more meridians is blocked or out of balance. Acupressure and other elements of Asian bodywork have the goal of restoring health and balance to the energy flow. Some supporters claim that acupressure can be used to treat the body, mind, emotions, energy field, and spirit.

Some practitioners in the West reject the traditional philosophies of Chinese medicine, believing that any relief given by acupressure and acupuncture is caused by other factors, such as the stimulation of endorphin production. Endorphins are natural substances made by the body that help relieve pain.

What does it involve?

All Asian bodywork uses pressure, soft tissue manipulation, and other techniques to stimulate the acupoints and energy meridians described in traditional Chinese medicine with the goal of balancing energy flow in the body.

Acupressure

Acupressure, also called pressure acupuncture, uses principles of acupuncture based on Chinese medicine. Practitioners use fingers or other body parts and devices to contact or apply pressure to acupoints along the body. Acupressure may also involve stretching, massage, and other methods to balance and restore energy flow in the body. Some people consider acupressure to be a form of acupuncture without needles. There are many different types of acupressure.

Shiatsu

Shiatsu is a Japanese word that literally means "finger pressure." The goal is to improve the body's ability to heal itself and to promote overall health through balancing the flow of qi. Shiatsu consists of touching or pressing on acupoints and energy meridians. Pressure on these vital points is intended to stretch and open pathways for the body's flow of qi. There are a number of subtypes of shiatsu, some of which focus on the use of stretching, special breathing techniques, meditation, and other practices.

Tui Na

Tui na is an older Chinese technique that uses pressure on acupuncture points (acupoints) along with other methods. Tui na has its roots in ancient Chinese medicine and may actually predate the popular practice of acupuncture. Tui na uses the theory of qi described above. Practitioners attempt to free these energy pathways through thirteen basic hand massage techniques, which include manual pushing, pressing, kneading, pulling, rolling, and other techniques on the skin and soft tissue. Practitioners often target the muscles on either side of the spine.

Ohashiatsu

Ohashiatsu is based on the practice of shiatsu. Supporters claim it can achieve balance and harmony by altering the flow of vital energy through the body rather than focusing on any one area. Promoters say it is a "step up" from shiatsu because it offers a more complete experience of healing and personal growth. According to its followers, successful Ohashiatsu sessions depend not only on the technical skill of the practitioner, but also on the feelings of compassion and empathy the practitioner is able to convey. A connection between the giver and receiver of this type of therapy is said to be important to the effectiveness of this practice. Ohashiatsu may also use exercise and meditation to induce a feeling of inner harmony and peace.

Watsu

Watsu, also known as water shiatsu or aquatic shiatsu, is a form of bodywork that is practiced in warm water. A practitioner stretches, cradles, and massages clients while holding them afloat. The goal is to achieve a feeling of peace and to release emotional and physical blockages of the body's energy pathways. Promoters believe that being held and massaged in the water brings the recipient to a deep level of connection and trust, while the warmth of the water brings benefits such as greater freedom of movement. Proponents claim it can speed both physical and emotional healing processes.

What is the history behind it?

Acupressure was used in China as early as 2000 BC. Based on traditional Chinese medicine, it is widely practiced throughout Asia for relaxation, wellness, and treatment of disease. It uses the same energy meridians and acupoints as acupuncture.

Shiatsu came from Japan, but grew out of Tui na and traditional Chinese massage techniques. It was given the name Shiatsu in the early twentieth century to distinguish it from older Japanese massage techniques. It was officially recognized by the Japanese government in 1955. Shiatsu has numerous subtypes and continues to develop.

Tui na is Chinese for "pushing and pulling." It uses acupressure points and emphasizes soft tissue work and realignment. Tui na is a traditional Chinese technique used for health maintenance and to treat pain and illness. It has been practiced for about four thousand years and is used most commonly in Chinese-American communities.

Ohashiatsu was developed in 1974 by a man named Ohashi, shortly after he learned shiatsu. He incorporated the energy principles of shiatsu with an increased emphasis on balancing the body through seitai, a type of stretching. He proposed that the practitioner should be in a state of meditation while working, in order to energize himself or herself, as well as the recipient of the massage. Ohashiatsu calls itself the "touch for peace."

Watsu (also called aquatic shiatsu) was developed about thirty years ago by Harold Dull, who taught Zen Shiatsu. He noted that when shiatsu was practiced in a warm pool, this helped to support the joints and led to greater relaxation.

What is the evidence?

Available scientific evidence does not support use of Asian bodywork to treat cancer. Many people who undergo one or more forms of Asian bodywork say that they feel more relaxed or can move with greater ease or less pain. Some people who have cancer may find that these therapies help to relieve stress, muscle tightness, and certain symptoms of cancer and side effects of treatments over the short term, but evidence is individual or based on very small research studies. Evidence supporting the use of Asian bodywork by cancer patients and survivors comes mainly from anecdotal reports and is related to symptom management and quality of life.

There is some early evidence from small studies with cancer patients suggesting acupressure might be helpful in reducing nausea and vomiting related to chemotherapy. When researchers reviewed these studies, though, it appeared that acupressure mostly helped the nausea that happened right after chemotherapy. Reviewers found that it did not seem to help with vomiting or delayed symptoms.

Very little scientific research has been done to find out what positive effects these treatments can offer, in part due to the challenges of setting up controlled clinical trials. More scientific research is needed to determine the benefits and limitations of acupressure and other forms of Asian bodywork.

Are there any possible problems or complications?

One concern about the use of Asian bodywork for people who have cancer is that tissue manipulation in the area of a tumor could increase the risk that cancer cells will travel to other parts of the body. It may be prudent for cancer patients to avoid massage near tumors and lumps that could be cancerous until this question is clearly answered.

Deep pressure and vigorous bodywork should be avoided during times of active treatment for cancer. People who have cancer that has spread to the bone or who have fragile bones should avoid physical manipulation or deep pressure because of the risk for fracture. Bodywork should be provided by a trained professional with expertise in working safely with people who have cancer and with cancer survivors. Generally, gentle massage and bodywork can be adapted to meet the needs of cancer patients. Patients and caregivers can also be taught to use some acupressure techniques safely.

People with rheumatoid arthritis, cancer that has spread to the bone, spine injuries, osteoporosis, or other bone diseases that could be worsened by physical manipulation should avoid methods that involve body manipulation. People who have cancer and chronic conditions such as arthritis and heart disease should talk to their doctors before having any type of therapy that involves moving joints and muscles.

People with fevers, infections, seizures, or problems with bowel control should not use watsu. Relying on this treatment alone and delaying or avoiding conventional medical care for cancer may have serious health consequences.

References

About shiatsu. Canadian Shiatsu Society of British Columbia Web site. http://www.shiatsupractor.org/aboutshiatsu.html. Accessed May 30, 2008.

Acupressure, shiatsu, tuina. Aetna InteliHealth Web site. http://www.intelihealth.com/IH/ihtIH/WSIHW000/8513/34968/358869.html. Updated July 7, 2005. Accessed May 30, 2008.

Bass SS, Cox CE, Salud CJ, Lyman GH, McCann C, Dupont E, Berman C, Reintgen DS. The effects of postinjection massage on the sensitivity of lymphatic mapping in breast cancer. *J Am Coll Surg.* 2001;192:9-16.

Dibble SL, Chapman J, Mack KA, Shih AS. Acupressure for nausea: results of a pilot study. *Oncol Nurs Forum.* 2000;27:41-47.

Ezzo JM, Richardson MA, Vickers A, Allen C, Dibble SL, Issell BF, Lao L, Pearl M, Ramirez G, Roscoe J, Shen J, Shivnan LC, Streitberger K, Treish I, Zhang G. Acupuncture-point stimulation for chemotherapy-induced nausea or vomiting. *Cochrane Database Syst Rev.* 2006;(2):CD002285.

Kirk L. A brief history of shiatsu. Shiatsu Therapy Association of British Columbia Web site. http://www.shiatsu therapy.ca/shiatsuhistory.htm. Accessed May 30, 2008.

Manipulative & body-based methods: massage & related bodywork detailed scientific review. Complementary/Integrative Medicine Education Resources, The University of Texas M. D. Anderson Cancer Center Web site. http://www.mdanderson.org/departments/CIMER/display.cfm?id=8EBC5A6D-A868-4D4D-AACA6F96F55BFEBC&method=displayFull. Accessed June 2, 2008.

Manipulative and body-based practices: an overview. National Center for Complementary and Alternative Medicine Web site. http://nccam.nih.gov/health/backgrounds/manipulative.htm. Accessed June 2, 2008.

Massage therapy as CAM. National Center for Complementary and Alternative Medicine Web site. http://nccam.nih.gov/health/massage/. Accessed June 2, 2008

Rosser RJ. Sentinel lymph nodes and postinjection massage: it is premature to reject caution. *J Am Coll Surg.* 2001;193:338-339.

Shin YH, Kim TI, Shin MS, Juon HS. Effect of acupressure on nausea and vomiting during chemotherapy cycle for Korean postoperative stomach cancer patients. *Cancer Nurs.* 2004;27:267-274.

What is ohashiatsu? Ohashi Institute Web site. http://www.ohashiatsu.org/Menu/ohashiatsu.html. Accessed May 30, 2008.

ACUPUNCTURE

Other common name(s): acupuncture therapy, sonopuncture, electroacupuncture, Zhenjiu
Scientific/medical name(s): none

Description

Acupuncture is a technique in which very thin needles of varying lengths are inserted through the skin to treat a variety of conditions. There are a number of different acupuncture techniques, including some that use sound waves or tiny electrical charges and that may or may not use actual needles.

Overview

Although available evidence does not suggest acupuncture is effective as a treatment for cancer, clinical studies have found it may help treat nausea caused by chemotherapy drugs and surgical anesthesia. It may also help relieve pain after dental surgery. The technique has been tested on people who are trying to stop addictive behaviors, such as smoking or alcoholism, but reports are mixed. It may be useful for treating headaches, helping in rehabilitation from strokes, and treating a number of musculoskeletal conditions.

How is it promoted for use?

In China, acupuncture is used as an anesthetic during surgery and is believed to have the power to cure diseases and relieve symptoms of illness. According to the theories and teachings of traditional Chinese medicine, acupoints lie along invisible meridians. There are twelve major meridians in the human body, which are said to be channels for the flow of vital energy or life force called qi (also spelled chi or ki, pronounced "chee" or "kee") that is present in all living things. Meridians also represent an internal system of communication between specific organs or networks of organs. According to traditional Chinese medicine, illness may occur when the energy flow along one or more meridians is blocked or out of balance. The goal of acupuncture is to restore health and balance to the energy flow. Supporters claim that acupuncture can be used to treat physical illness, addiction, and mental illness.

Some practitioners in the West reject the traditional philosophies of Chinese medicine, believing that any relief given by acupuncture or acupressure is caused by other factors, such as the stimulation of endorphin production in the body. Endorphins are natural substances made by the body that help relieve pain.

What does it involve?

In traditional acupuncture (sometimes called acupuncture therapy), needles are inserted at specific locations called acupoints in order to restore balance and healthy energy flow to the body. Needles are inserted just deep enough into the skin to keep them from falling out and are usually left in place for a few minutes. Skilled acupuncturists cause virtually no pain. The acupuncturist may twirl the needles or apply heat or a weak electrical current to enhance the effects of the therapy.

Sonopuncture is similar to acupuncture, but needles are not used. Instead, an ultrasound device that transmits sound waves is applied to the body's acupoints. Sonopuncture is sometimes combined with tuning forks and other vibration devices. Proponents claim this approach is useful in treating many of the same disorders as acupuncture.

Electroacupuncture is considered an enhanced version of traditional acupuncture. Electroacupuncture uses tiny electrical charges, with or without needles, to stimulate the same acupoints that are used in traditional acupuncture. Electroacupuncture devices are sometimes promoted for diagnosis or testing.

In acupressure, a popular variation of acupuncture, therapists press on acupoints with their fingers instead of using needles. This technique is used by itself or as part of a system of manual healing such as shiatsu (see page 151).

In other variations of acupuncture, heat, friction, suction, magnets, or laser beams are directed to acupoints. Acupuncture is sometimes used along with less well-known traditional healing techniques, such as moxibustion (page 223) and cupping (page 189). Acupuncture may sometimes be referred to as Zhenjiu, which is the standard Mandarin word for needle.

What is the history behind it?

Acupuncture began more than two thousand years ago and is an important part of traditional Chinese medicine (also called Oriental Medicine). Originally, 365 acupoints were identified, corresponding to the number of days in a year, but gradually, the number of acupoints grew to more than two thousand. Traditional acupuncture needles were made of bone, stone, or metal, including silver and gold. Modern acupuncture needles are made of very thin sterile stainless steel and are disposable. In 1996, the U.S. Food and Drug Administration (FDA) approved the use of acupuncture needles by licensed practitioners. By law, needles must be labeled for one-time use only, to prevent infection and the transmission of germs.

In China, acupuncture is commonly accepted as a treatment for many diseases. Acupuncture has also become quite popular in the United States and Europe, where the technique is mainly used to control pain and relieve symptoms of disease, such as nausea caused by chemotherapy, but not to cure the disease itself. In 2000, there were an estimated eleven thousand licensed acupuncturists in the United States, with the number expected to double by 2010. More than forty states have set up training standards for licensing or certification to practice acupuncture. Medicare does not cover acupuncture, but it is covered by some private health insurance plans and health maintenance organizations. There are about three thousand doctors in the United States who also practice acupuncture.

What is the evidence?

Available scientific evidence does not support claims that acupuncture is effective as a treatment for cancer, but it appears it may be useful as a complementary method for relieving some symptoms related to cancer and other conditions. Acupuncture has been the subject of many clinical studies. A recent analysis of eleven studies looked at the effect of acupuncture in reducing nausea and vomiting related to chemotherapy. The report suggested that acupuncture may reduce the vomiting that occurs shortly after chemotherapy is given, even though it had little effect on nausea. It also did not seem to help with delayed vomiting.

A small clinical trial found that acupuncture helped reduce the number of hot flashes men experienced during hormonal therapy for prostate cancer. There is also some evidence that acupuncture may lessen the need for pain medicines. A study of headache sufferers compared acupuncture with standard medical treatment. Those treated with acupuncture used less pain medicine and missed fewer work days. However, some recent studies of acupuncture have had mixed or uncertain results. Part of the problem is that it can be difficult to come up with a good control procedure—one that convincingly mimics acupuncture—for scientific comparisons.

A number of studies have looked at the effectiveness of acupuncture in helping smokers to quit. Experts reviewed studies in which acupuncture was used to help reduce withdrawal symptoms from quitting smoking. When the studies were analyzed as a group, the evidence suggested that sham acupuncture worked as well as real acupuncture for smoking cessation. Similar results were found when studies of acupuncture for cocaine withdrawal were analyzed.

Although the scientific evidence is not strong, acupuncture may prove to be useful by itself or when combined with mainstream therapies to treat headache, menstrual cramps, tennis elbow, fibromyalgia, myofascial pain, osteoarthritis, lower back pain, carpal tunnel syndrome, and asthma, and to help in the rehabilitation of stroke patients. Further research is needed in these areas.

Controlled clinical studies of electroacupuncture have suggested that it may help some people with pain after surgery, some of the nausea related to chemotherapy, and pain from kidney stones. However, it was found ineffective in a study that compared it with conventional anesthesia during in vitro fertilization.

Are there any possible problems or complications?

When done by a trained professional, acupuncture is generally considered safe. The number of complications reported have been relatively few, but there is a risk that a patient may be harmed if the acupuncturist is not well trained.

Traditional needle acupuncture can cause dizziness, fainting, local internal bleeding, convulsions, hepatitis B, dermatitis, nerve damage, and increased pain. Rarely, punctured lungs have happened, resulting in a few deaths. Traditional acupuncture also poses risks such as infection from contaminated needles or improper delivery of treatment. The risk for infection is much lower now that acupuncturists in the United States use sterile single-use needles.

Those who are taking anticoagulants (blood thinners) may have bleeding problems with traditional needle acupuncture. People with cardiac pacemakers, infusion pumps, or other electrical devices should avoid electroacupuncture.

Relying on this type of treatment alone and avoiding or delaying conventional medical care for cancer may have serious health consequences.

References

Barrett S. Be wary of acupuncture, qigong, and "Chinese medicine." Quackwatch Web site. http://www.quackwatch.org/01QuackeryRelatedTopics/acu.html. Updated December 30, 2007. Accessed May 30, 2008.

Dincer F, Linde K. Sham interventions in randomized clinical trials of acupuncture—a review. *Complement Ther Med.* 2003;11:235-242.

Ernst E, ed. *The Desktop Guide to Complementary and Alternative Medicine: An Evidence-Based Approach.* New York: Mosby; 2001.

Ernst G, Strzyz H, Hagmeister H. Incidence of adverse effects during acupuncture therapy-a multicentre survey. *Complement Ther Med.* 2003;11:93-97.

Ezzo JM, Richardson MA, Vickers A, Allen C, Dibble SL, Issell BF, Lao L, Pearl M, Ramirez G, Roscoe J, Shen J, Shivnan JC, Streitberger K, Treish I, Zhang G. Acupuncture-point stimulation for chemotherapy-induced nausea or vomiting. *Cochrane Database Syst Rev.* 2006;(2):CD002285.

Gates S, Smith LA, Foxcroft DR. Auricular acupuncture for cocaine dependence. *Cochrane Database Syst Rev.* 2006;(1):CD005192.

Gejervall AL, Stener-Victorin E, Möller A, Janson PO, Werner C, Bergh C. Electro-acupuncture versus conventional analgesia: a comparison of pain levels during oocyte aspiration and patients' experiences of well-being after surgery. *Hum Reprod.* 2005;20:728-735. Epub 2004 Dec 17.

Hammar M, Frisk J, Grimås O, Höök M, Spetz AC, Wyon Y. Acupuncture treatment of vasomotor symptoms in men with prostatic carcinoma: a pilot study. *J Urol.* 1999;161:853-856.

He JP, Friedrich M, Ertan AK, Müller K, Schmidt W. Pain-relief and movement improvement by acupuncture after ablation and axillary lymphadenectomy in patients with mammary cancer. *Clin Exp Obstet Gynecol.* 1999;26:81-84.

An introduction to acupuncture. National Center for Complementary and Alternative Medicine Web site. http://nccam.nih.gov/health/acupuncture/. Accessed March 9, 2007.

Kemper KJ, Sarah R, Silver-Highfield E, Xiahos E, Barnes L, Berde C. On pins and needles? Pediatric pain patients' experience with acupuncture. *Pediatrics.* 2000;105;941-947.

Laws and regulations. Acupuncture Web site. http://www.acupuncture.com/statelaws/statelaw.htm. Accessed June 3, 2008.

Membership in the American Academy of Medical Acupuncture. American Academy of Medical Acupuncture Web site. http://www.medicalacupuncture.org/aama_marf/aama_membership.html. Accessed June 3, 2008.

Sherman KJ, Cherkin DC, Eisenberg DM, Erro J, Hrbek A, Deyo RA. The practice of acupuncture: who are the providers and what do they do? *Ann Fam Med.* 2005;3:151-158.

Vickers AJ, Rees RW, Zollman CE, McCarney R, Smith CM, Ellis N, Fisher P, Van Haselen R. Acupuncture for chronic headache in primary care: large, pragmatic, randomised trial. *BMJ.* 2004;328:744. Epub 2004 Mar 15.

White AR, Rampes H, Campbell JL. Acupuncture and related interventions for smoking cessation. *Cochrane Database Syst Rev.* 2006;(1):CD000009.

APPLIED KINESIOLOGY

Other common name(s): muscle testing, manual muscle testing, AK
Scientific/medical name(s): none

Applied kinesiology is different from kinesiology, a field of scientific study of the movements of the human body. Kinesiology is sometimes called academic kinesiology, and, occasionally, applied kinesiology, which can be very confusing. It is important to understand which kind of kinesiology you are considering. The information below refers only to applied kinesiology as a complementary practice, and not to the science of human movement.

Description

Applied kinesiology (AK) is a technique used to diagnose illness or choose treatment by testing muscles for strength and weakness.

Overview

Available scientific evidence does not support the claim that applied kinesiology can diagnose or treat cancer or other illness.

How is it promoted for use?

The basis of applied kinesiology is that any problem with an organ is accompanied by weakness in a corresponding muscle. For instance, a weak muscle in the chest might indicate liver disease, while weakness of the lower back or leg muscles may be the result of lung problems. Practitioners claim that by finding the weak muscle they can identify the underlying illness and make decisions about treatment. They believe that strengthening of the weak muscles shows that the internal organs have strengthened as well.

Applied kinesiology is sometimes used to try to determine whether a particular food or other substance weakens or strengthens the person. The food or substance may be placed under the tongue or held in the hand as a muscle is tested. Applied kinesiology may also be used to check emotional responses to situations or other people. Emotional responses are checked by testing a muscle as the patient imagines being in the situation, says the person's name, or pictures the person nearby.

Applied kinesiologists claim muscle weakness may also be caused by a number of internal energy disruptions, such as nerve damage, poor drainage in the lymph system, reduced blood supply, chemical imbalances, or organ and gland problems. Practitioners may recommend that people confirm the diagnosis with standard diagnostic methods, such as laboratory tests and x-rays.

Applied kinesiology is usually used for evaluation purposes, but claims have been made that after undergoing an AK session, it is possible to observe the "spontaneous remission" of cancer.

What does it involve?

Applied kinesiologists are often chiropractors, but they may also be naturopaths, doctors, nurses, or other health care workers. They assess patients by observing posture, gait, muscle strength, and range of motion and by touching the patient. These observations may be combined with more common methods of diagnosis, such as a health history, a physical examination, and laboratory tests. Practitioners may also test for environmental or food sensitivities.

During the treatment, the patient might be asked to hold a body part in a certain position while the practitioner tries to push it out of that position. The relative strength differences are supposed to help the applied kinesiologist diagnose internal imbalances. The practitioner might also press on key "trigger points" to find out if they cause muscle weakness.

To restore muscle strength, the applied kinesiologist may apply manual stimulation and relaxation techniques to key muscles. The treatment may also include joint manipulation or movement, dietary changes, reflex procedures, manipulation of the head, or other types of treatment.

What is the history behind it?

Applied kinesiology was developed by Michigan chiropractor George J. Goodheart, Jr., in 1964. Dr. Goodheart reported that a patient with an immobile shoulder visited his office. An examination revealed no abnormalities, even though the patient had complained of the problem for more than fifteen years. When Dr. Goodheart pressed on small nodules near the origin of the pain, the muscle strength returned to normal and the shoulder's motion was restored. By "tugging" on particular trigger points, Goodheart claimed he could stimulate muscles to regain lost strength and function. He later incorporated disease diagnosis into his applied kinesiology system.

Today, practitioners who use applied kinesiology include chiropractors, naturopaths, physicians, dentists, nutritionists, physical therapists, massage therapists, and nurse practitioners. Certification to practice as an applied kinesiologist is available from the International College of Applied Kinesiology. To reach the highest level of certification, more than three hundred hours of instruction, several proficiency exams, and submission of original research papers are required. However, this college is not recognized by the Council on Chiropractic Education, the agency recognized by the U.S. Secretary of Education for the accreditation of programs offering the doctor of chiropractic degree. This agency works to ensure the quality of chiropractic education in the United States.

What is the evidence?

A few researchers have investigated kinesiology muscle-testing procedures in controlled clinical studies. The results showed that applied kinesiology was not an accurate diagnostic tool, and that muscle response was not any more useful than random guessing. In fact, one study found that assessments by experienced applied kinesiologists of nutrient status for the same patients varied widely. In addition, when muscle testing was compared with laboratory testing for the nutrients in question, muscle testing did not correlate to laboratory results that showed adequate or deficient nutrients.

A German group of researchers tried applied kinesiology to see if it would be helpful in diagnosing nutritional intolerances in children. Different applied kinesiologists got different results for the same patients, and there was no significant relationship between muscle testing and laboratory tests for these conditions.

More recently, dentists used applied kinesiology to test patients for tolerance to two types of dental material. Each subject's result was recorded. Later, applied kinesiology was used to test the same patients so that neither the tester nor the patients knew which material was being used. The results did not match the previous results any better than random chance, leading the researchers to conclude that the method was not reliable.

Although some claim that research supports applied kinesiology, the studies cited are often about academic kinesiology (the study of human movement), not the practice of applied kinesiology. In addition, a review study of more than fifty research papers published by the International College of Applied Kinesiology found that the studies did not meet basic standards for scientific research.

Some personal accounts of successful applied kinesiology treatments do exist. However, available scientific evidence does not support the use of applied kinesiology to diagnose or cure cancer or any other disease.

Are there any possible problems or complications?

Applied kinesiology procedures are considered relatively safe, although conclusions drawn from them may be incorrect. Treatment that is based on applied kinesiology has occasionally resulted in harm, including at least one death, due to incorrect diagnosis or treatment selection. Relying on this diagnostic method alone and avoiding or delaying conventional medical diagnosis and treatment for cancer may have serious health consequences.

References

Applied kinesiology. WholeHealthMD Web site. http://www.wholehealthmd.com/ME2/dirmod.asp?type=AWHN_Therapies&id=6618ABF7E906482B9BEBCB3619CDD775&tier=2. Updated August 1, 2007. Accessed June 2, 2008.

Barrett S. Applied kinesiology: muscle-testing for "allergies" and "nutrient deficiencies." Quackwatch Web site. http://www.quackwatch.org/01QuackeryRelatedTopics/Tests/ak.html. Updated September 26, 2004. Accessed May 30, 2008.

Haas M, Peterson D, Hoyer D, Ross G. Muscle testing response to provocative vertebral challenge and spinal manipulation: a randomized controlled trial of construct validity. *J Manipulative Physiol Ther.* 1994;17:141-148.

Hyman R. How people are fooled by ideomotor action. Quackwatch Web site. http://www.quackwatch.org/01QuackeryRelatedTopics/ideomotor.html. Posted August 26, 2003. Accessed May 30, 2008. Also available in print at Hyman R. The mischief-making of ideomotor action. *The Scientific Review of Alternative Medicine.* Fall-Winter, 1999.

Jarvis WT. Applied kinesiology. National Council Against Health Fraud Web site. http://www.ncahf.org/articles/a-b/ak.html. Posted December 1, 2000. Accessed May 30, 2008.

Kenney JJ, Clemens R, Forsythe KD. Applied kinesiology unreliable for assessing nutrient status. *J Am Diet Assoc.* 1988;88:698-704.

Klinkoski B, Leboeuf C. A review of the research papers published by the International College of Applied Kinesiology from 1981 to 1987. *J Manipulative Physiol Ther.* 1990;13:190-194.

Pothmann R, von Frankenberg S, Hoicke C, Weingarten H, Lüdtke R. Evaluation of applied kinesiology in nutritional intolerance of childhood [in German]. *Forsch Komplementarmed Klass Naturheilkd.* 2001;8:336-344.

Staehle HJ, Koch MJ, Pioch T. Double-blind study on materials testing with applied kinesiology. *J Dent Res.* 2005;84:1066-1069.

What is applied kinesiology? International College of Applied Kinesiology Web site. http://www.icak.com/about/whatis.shtml. Accessed May 30, 2008.

BIOLOGICAL DENTISTRY

Other common name(s): holistic dentistry
Scientific/medical name(s): none

Description

Biological dentistry is the removal of dental fillings or teeth claimed to contain toxins, which are said to cause systemic diseases or pain.

Overview

Available scientific evidence does not support claims that removing healthy teeth or amalgam fillings can prevent cancer or any other disease. The American Dental Association (ADA) has twice declared that the unnecessary removal of silver amalgam is improper and unethical.

How is it promoted for use?

Practitioners of biological dentistry claim that the mercury in ordinary fillings can escape, travel to distant organs, and contribute to the development of diseases, including cancer. They claim replacing metal fillings with synthetic, nontoxic compounds will eliminate toxins from the body and increase resistance to disease.

Some biological dentists also claim that decaying teeth produce a chemical called dimethyl sulfide, which can cause cancer and other illnesses. They further state that there can be infected cavities within jawbones that are not detectable by x-ray and that must be scraped out, even though there is no visible evidence that the teeth are infected or diseased in any way. They call this condition "cavitational osteopathosis."

Some practitioners claim that each tooth is related to a corresponding organ in the body. Because of this relationship, an unhealthy, misaligned, or filled tooth (which may contain mercury) disturbs the flow of vital energy or life force called qi (or chi) that flows freely through a healthy person. By removing the tooth or filling, or realigning the jaw, practitioners claim they can stop the production of toxins from the mouth and restore the proper flow of energy, resulting in improved health. Some biological dentists say that root canal procedures increase the risk for disease in other parts of the body.

Several Web sites promoting or supporting biological dentistry claim that patients with conditions such as chronic fatigue syndrome, allergies, and thyroid problems improve after their mercury-containing fillings are removed. A Swiss physician claimed that 90 percent of breast cancer patients he treated had dental problems that may have contributed to formation of the disease.

What does it involve?

Biological dentistry involves the removal and replacement of mercury-containing dental fillings with synthetic substitutes. Practitioners approach their patients holistically, meaning they consider the entire body rather than just the illness or diseased area. A biological dentist may also prescribe other remedies or diets, claiming that they can detoxify the body and strengthen the immune system. Biological dentistry can also involve oral acupuncture, surgical scraping, chelation therapy, neural therapy, laser therapy, and "mouth balancing," which is an attempt to improve structural deformities in the mouth and jaw.

What is the history behind it?

Dentists have used silver amalgam, which contains about 50 percent mercury, to fill cavities for more than 160 years. A German physician, Dr. Josef Issels, was among the first to state that toxins from dental fillings could harm a person's overall health, and that root canal procedures posed the threat of infection to various organ systems. Dr. Issels also claimed there was a connection between the growth of tumors and the presence of dental toxins. He stated that 98 percent of his adult patients with cancer had from two to ten teeth that had undergone root canal procedures. Such teeth, he believed, must be removed in order to decrease the level of toxicity in the body.

In 1999, a practitioner who removed fillings containing mercury was placed on probation by his state's Board of Dental Examiners for five years. They ruled on the basis of extensive complaints from patients who claimed their health and safety had been compromised. A few years earlier, a group of patients filed a lawsuit against several practitioners of biological dentistry, claiming that perfectly healthy teeth had been removed without any improvement in health.

What is the evidence?

Typical dental fillings contain metals such as mercury, copper, and silver, but there is no solid evidence showing that the presence of these metals in teeth causes disease in other parts of the body. The clinical studies that have been published in peer-reviewed conventional medical journals found no link between mercury-containing fillings and the development of cancer and other diseases. The amount of mercury absorbed by the body from amalgams is so small it is considered harmless. A study of U.S. dentists found that dentists themselves have higher mercury levels in their bodies than patients with mercury-containing fillings, because of daily exposure at work. However, the dentists showed the same disease patterns as everyone else and actually outlived nondentists by about three years. A 1998 study concluded "there was no clear evidence that dental radiography or amalgam fillings is related to the development of tumors of the [central nervous system]" (*Oral Oncol.* 1998;34:265). Another study found there was no connection between amalgam fillings, cardiovascular disease, diabetes, cancer, or early death.

In 1987, the American Dental Association declared that removing perfectly good fillings (even if they contained mercury) is unethical, and this position was reaffirmed in 2002. They stated that the use of dental amalgam was reviewed and found to be safe. National Institutes of Health experts also concluded there was no evidence to support the idea that dental fillings caused serious health problems. The U.S. Food and Drug Administration has conducted long-term investigations into amalgam safety and continues to conclude that it is safe. In 2006, an independent panel generally agreed that there is no evidence that dental amalgams cause health problems in most people. However, the panel did have concerns about the lack of knowledge about possible effects of dental amalgam on people who are very sensitive to mercury, such as pregnant women and small children. Some dentists prefer to use other types of filling materials for pregnant women and small children because of concern over the slight possibility of harm during periods of rapid growth.

Some people do, however, have metal allergies that can lead to problems in the mouth if they have metal fillings. In a few people, certain kinds of mouth sores or spots, called contact lesions or oral lichen planus, will develop. These are linked to direct contact with metal fillings. One study found that replacing the fillings that were touching the lesions helped most of them to heal. Some people respond similarly to metals in dentures and bridgework.

Are there any possible problems or complications?

Most dentists and other health experts believe the removal of healthy teeth or fillings is improper and unethical and should be avoided. Removal of teeth that show no infection or abnormality usually results in restricted food choices and poorer nutrition, even if the teeth are replaced with bridges or dentures.

Relying on this treatment alone and avoiding or delaying conventional medical care for cancer may have serious health consequences.

References

ADA Council on Scientific Affairs. Dental amalgam: update on safety concerns. *J Am Dent Assoc.* 1998;129:494-503.

Ahlqwist M, Bengtsson C, Lapidus L. Number of amalgam fillings in relation to cardiovascular disease, diabetes, cancer and early death in Swedish women. *Community Dent Oral Epidemiol.* 1993;21:40-44.

Bratel J, Hakeberg M, Jontell M. Effect of replacement of dental amalgam on oral lichenoid reactions. *J Dent.* 1996;24:41-45.

Dodes JE, Barrett S. A critical look at cavitational osteopathosis, NICO, and "biological dentistry." Quackwatch Web site. http://www.quackwatch.org/01QuackeryRelatedTopics/cavitation.html. Accessed May 30, 2008.

Effects and side-effects of dental restorative materials. National Institutes of Health Technology Assessment Conference. Bethesda, MD: August 26–28, 1991. *Adv Dent Res.* 1992;6:1-144.

Issa Y, Brunton PA, Glenny AM, Duxbury AJ. Healing of oral lichenoid lesions after replacing amalgam restorations: a systematic review. *Oral Surg Oral Med Oral Pathol Oral Radiol Endod.* 2004;98:553-565.

McComb D. Occupational exposure to mercury in dentistry and dentist mortality. *J Can Dent Assoc.* 1997;63:372-376.

Questions and answers on dental amalgams. Center for Devices and Radiologic Health Consumer Services, US Food and Drug Administration Web site. http://www.fda.gov/cdrh/consumer/amalgams.html. Updated October 31, 2006. Accessed June 3, 2008.

Rodvall Y, Ahlbom A, Pershagen G, Nylander M, Spännare B. Dental radiography after 25 years, amalgam fillings and tumours of the central nervous system. *Oral Oncol.* 1998;34:265-269.

Trans-agency Working Group on the Health Effects of Dental Amalgam. Executive summary, review and analysis of the literature on the health effects of dental amalgams. Life Sciences Research Office Web site. http://www.lsro.org/amalgam/frames_amalgam_report.html. Accessed June 4, 2008.

BODYWORK

Other common name(s): Rolfing, Feldenkrais Method, Alexander Technique, Trager Approach

Scientific/medical name(s): none

Description

Bodywork refers to a variety of physically oriented techniques. Some forms of bodywork involve hands-on manipulation of joints or soft tissue, realigning the body, and correcting posture imbalances. Others focus on increasing a person's awareness of his or her own body through gentle, deliberate movement and breathing exercises.

Overview

Available scientific evidence does not support bodywork as a means of treating cancer, but it may be used to enhance quality of life. There are individual reports that certain forms of bodywork may be used along with medical treatment to help relieve symptoms and reduce stress, although the effectiveness of bodywork techniques has not yet been proven scientifically.

How is it promoted for use?

Various forms of bodywork are generally promoted to relieve pain, reduce stress, soothe injured muscles, stimulate blood and lymphatic circulation, and promote relaxation. Some practitioners also claim that through bodywork, their patients become more comfortable with their bodies by learning how to move more freely, gracefully, and efficiently.

A few practitioners claim bodywork can be used to treat many conditions, including cancer, circulation problems, colic, depression, headaches, heart problems, high blood pressure, hyperactivity, insomnia, sinus infections, and tension.

What does it involve?

Rolfing

Rolfing Structural Integration, or Rolfing, is a form of deep bodywork in which Rolfers (the name given to practitioners) use their fingers, hands, elbows, and knees to place pressure on connective tissue. Their goal is to promote proper alignment by releasing constriction and making movement easier. Some people find Rolfing painful.

The Feldenkrais Method

The Feldenkrais Method involves a slow and gentle sequence of movements to help people develop a heightened awareness of their bodies, improve mobility, and break habits of poor posture and inefficient motion that can cause pain and discomfort.

The Alexander Technique

The Alexander Technique involves gently mobilizing parts of a patient's body that appear to be strained. Therapists also explain how to relax and move the body properly. The technique is designed to improve the mechanical relationships among body parts and to align the head, neck, torso, and spine.

The Trager Approach

The Trager Approach uses gentle, rhythmical touch combined with movement exercises. The therapist feels how the client is holding his or her body and then applies various rocking, pulling, and rotational movements to the head, neck, torso, arms, and legs. Practitioners ask their clients to focus on the lightness and ease of movement.

What is the history behind it?

Rolfing Structural Integration was developed in the 1930s by Ida Rolf, PhD, who believed that humans function most efficiently and comfortably when key parts of the body, such as the head, torso, pelvis, and legs, are properly aligned. Different versions of Rolfing have since been developed, such as Aston Patterning and Hellerwork.

The Feldenkrais Method was developed during the first half of the twentieth century by physicist Moshe Feldenkrais. A sports injury early in his life caused chronic pain and led Feldenkrais to explore unconventional methods of healing. He "re-educated" himself to walk again without pain using this method.

The Alexander Technique was developed by Frederick Matthias Alexander in the late 1800s. Alexander was an actor who kept losing his voice. He learned that he habitually moved his head back and down when he spoke, which caused him to suck in his breath and tense up his throat. Using this technique, he developed a method of breathing to alter this old habit and recovered his voice.

The Trager Approach was developed in 1927 by Milton Trager, MD. Dr. Trager was born with a spinal deformity, but he overcame his handicap and became a dancer and gymnast. The physical movements of his therapy are intended not only to improve mobility and promote relaxation but also to alter deep-seated thought patterns, which Dr. Trager believed were responsible for many physical problems.

There are many other types of bodywork practiced today, including massage, reflexology, the Rubenfeld Synergy Method, the Rosen Method, and different types of Asian bodywork.

What is the evidence?

Many people who have undergone one or more of these forms of bodywork report they feel more relaxed or can move with greater ease or less pain. Very little scientific research has been done to find out what positive effects these treatments can offer, in part because of the challenges of setting up controlled scientific clinical trials of bodywork. The consensus of available evidence does not support claims that any bodywork techniques are effective in treating cancer.

Are there any possible problems or complications?

One concern for people who have cancer is that tissue manipulation in the area of a tumor could increase the risk that cancer cells will travel to other parts of the body. It may be prudent for people with cancer to avoid massage near tumors and lumps that could be cancerous until this question is clearly answered.

Rolfing can involve deep manipulation of soft tissues, which is a concern during active cancer treatment. The Alexander Technique requires a great deal of commitment and practice from the student, and this may be an issue for patients if they are fatigued or feeling poorly. The rocking movement of the Trager Approach may worsen nausea.

People with rheumatoid arthritis, cancer that has spread to the bone, spinal injuries, osteoporosis, or other bone diseases that could be worsened by physical manipulation should avoid physical manipulation or deep pressure. Manipulation of a bone in an area where cancer has metastasized could result in a bone fracture. Also, people who have had radiation therapy may find even light touch on the treatment area to be uncomfortable. People with cancer and chronic conditions such as arthritis and heart disease should consult their physicians before undergoing any type of therapy that involves manipulation of joints and muscles. Generally, gentle bodywork can be adapted to meet the needs of cancer patients.

It is important for people with cancer to let their health care providers know they are receiving bodywork. Bodywork should be provided by a trained professional with expertise in working safely with people who have cancer and with cancer survivors. Relying on this treatment alone and delaying or avoiding conventional medical care for cancer may have serious health consequences.

References

Bass SS, Cox CE, Salud CJ, Lyman GH, McCann C, Dupont E, Berman C, Reintgen DS. The effects of postinjection massage on the sensitivity of lymphatic mapping in breast cancer. *J Am Coll Surg.* 2001;192:9-16.

Bower PJ, Rubik B, Weiss SJ, Starr C. Manual therapy: hands-on healing; use of hands in alternative medicine. *Patient Care.* 1997;31:69-90.

Burke C, Macnish S, Saunders J, Gallini A, Warne I, Downing J. The development of a massage service for cancer patients. *Clin Oncol (R Coll Radiol).* 1994;6:381-384.

Ernst E, ed. *The Desktop Guide to Complementary and Alternative Medicine: An Evidence-Based Approach.* New York: Mosby; 2001.

Gam AN, Warming S, Larsen LH, Jensen B, Høydalsmo O, Allon I, Andersen B, Gøtzsche NE, Petersen M, Mathiesen B. Treatment of myofascial trigger-points with ultrasound combined with massage and exercise—a randomized controlled trial. *Pain.* 1998;77:73-79.

Jones TA. Rolfing. *Phys Med Rehabil Clin N Am.* 2004;15:799-809, vi.

Manipulative & body-based methods: massage & related bodywork detailed scientific review. Complementary/ Integrative Medicine Education Resources, The University of Texas M. D. Anderson Cancer Center Web site.

http://www.mdanderson.org/departments/CIMER/display.cfm?id=8EBC5A6D-A868-4D4D-AACA6F96F55BF EBC&method=displayFull. Accessed June 2, 2008.

Manipulative and body-based practices: an overview. National Center for Complementary and Alternative Medicine Web site. http://nccam.nih.gov/health/backgrounds/manipulative.htm. Accessed May 30, 2008.

Mehling WE, DiBlasi Z, Hecht F. Bias control in trials of bodywork: a review of methodological issues. *J Altern Complement Med.* 2005;11:333-342.

Rosser RJ. Sentinel lymph nodes and postinjection massage: it is premature to reject caution. *J Am Coll Surg.* 2001;193:338-339.

CANCER SALVES

Other common name(s):
black salve, escharotics, escharotic therapy, botanical salve, Curaderm, Cansema
Scientific/medical name(s): none

Description

Cancer salves are pastes, salves, or poultices applied to skin tumors or the skin over internal tumor sites. There are many variations in the formulas, which can contain up to ten ingredients or more. They may be mixed in bases of olive oil, beeswax, or pine tar. Ingredients may include chaparral *(Larrea tridentata)*, bloodroot *(Sanguinaria canadensis)*, DMSO (dimethyl sulfoxide), chickweed *(Stellaria media)*, Indian tobacco *(Lobelia inflata)*, comfrey *(Symphytum officinale)*, myrrh *(Commiphora myrrha)*, marshmallow *(Althaea officinalis)*, mullein *(Verbascum thapsus)*, and other herbs, oils, and chemicals.

Overview

Available scientific evidence does not support claims that salves are effective in treating cancer or tumors. In fact, some ingredients may cause great harm to the body. There have been numerous reports of severe burns and permanent scarring from some of these salves.

How is it promoted for use?

Practitioners claim that cancer salves have the power to kill cancer cells or draw them out of the body and that salves can cure any type of cancer. Some of the companies that sell cancer salves claim their products can heal cancer without the need for conventional treatments such as surgery, chemotherapy, or radiation therapy. One manufacturer has claimed the company's salves are successful at curing from 75 percent to 80 percent of cancer cases, and even 99 percent of one type of skin cancer. Other proponents claim their cancer salves have antitumor properties that cause no damage to healthy skin.

One salve called Curaderm is promoted as a cure for three types of skin growths: solar keratosis, basal cell carcinoma, and squamous cell carcinoma. Promoters claim it will not leave scars or harm normal skin. The cream contains solasodine glycosides, which are chemicals derived from Sodom's apple *(Solanum sodomaeum)*, also called devil's apple and kangaroo apple. It also contains an aspirin-related compound that is normally used to treat warts. Supporters do not claim the salve is effective against melanoma, the most serious type of skin cancer. Curaderm is not approved by the U.S. Food and Drug Administration (FDA).

What does it involve?

For skin cancers, the salves are rubbed directly onto the tumor. For other types of cancers, the salves are rubbed on the skin over the internal location of the tumor. Because the salves are widely available, some people apply them at home, while others receive salve treatments from naturopaths (see "Naturopathic Medicine," page 116).

Nearly all cancer salves fall into a category of naturopathic medicine called "escharotics." An escharotic is a corrosive substance that creates an eschar, a dark, thick, crust of dead skin and tissue. Eschars often form after a person has been burned by heat or caustic chemicals.

What is the history behind it?

The use of cancer salves to cure disease dates back centuries, perhaps even to ancient Egypt. The use of salves to cure cancer became fairly common in the eighteenth and nineteenth centuries. One eighteenth-century English cancer surgeon, Dr. Richard Guy, used a black salve to treat dozens of cancer patients, particularly those with breast cancer. His claims of a high success rate were never verified. A later physician, Dr. Eli G. Jones, claimed he had miraculous results curing cancer patients using a salve made of figwort syrup. Many homegrown salve recipes have been handed down through families for generations.

More recently, salves have been sold by phone, via mail order, and over the Internet. Books and Web sites also offer formulas for salves that can be made at home. Some of these vendors claim that doctors or the FDA try to prevent them from sharing information on their treatments. In fact, the FDA forbids statements that a treatment can prevent or cure cancer if scientific studies have not shown that to be true. Some vendors continue to make such statements anyway.

What is the evidence?

Although the Curaderm Web site reports that clinical trials have been done in humans, this claim refers to uncontrolled trials or studies that have not been published in conventional medical journals. Further clinical trials are needed to determine whether this preparation has any role in the treatment of non-melanoma skin cancer.

Otherwise, claims that cancer salves cure cancer are based on anecdotal reports and testimonials. There have been no controlled clinical studies of cancer salves published in the medical literature, and available scientific evidence does not support claims that cancer salves can cure cancer or any other disease.

Are there any possible problems or complications?

There have been numerous reports of severe scarring and burns from the use of cancer salves. Some have been severe enough to require reconstructive surgery. One report involving Curaderm states that, while the cream appeared to make a basal cell carcinoma go away, a later biopsy revealed that there were cancer cells left underneath the surface of the skin. In another case of salve treatment, the cancer initially appeared to have "healed" but later recurred in tissues underneath the original tumor, presumably because the cancer was never completely cured. As a result, the cancer had to be removed by a much more extensive operation than would have been required if standard treatment had been used initially.

The FDA does not regulate cancer salves, although it sometimes becomes involved when individuals or companies make unsubstantiated or unproven health claims. The contents of different cancer salves vary and can contain potentially dangerous substances. Women who are pregnant or breastfeeding may cause harm to their infants as well if medicines or herbs are absorbed through the skin. Using salves while delaying or avoiding standard medical treatment for cancer may have serious health consequences.

References

Barrett S. Don't use corrosive cancer salves (escharotics). Quackwatch Web site. http://www.quackwatch.org/01QuackeryRelatedTopics/Cancer/eschar.html. Updated June 2, 2008. Accessed June 12, 2008.

Cham BE, Daunter B, Evans RA. Topical treatment of malignant and premalignant skin lesions by very low concentrations of a standard mixture (BEC) of solasodine glycosides. *Cancer Lett.* 1991;59:183-192.

Jarvis WT. How quackery harms cancer patients. Quackwatch Web site. http://www.quackwatch.org/01QuackeryRelatedTopics/harmquack.html. Accessed May 30, 2008.

McDaniel S, Goldman GD. Consequences of using escharotic agents as primary treatment for nonmelanoma skin cancer. *Arch Dermatol.* 2002;138:1593-1596.

Morris CA, Avorn J. Internet marketing of herbal products. *JAMA.* 2003;290:1505-1509.

Moss R. *Herbs Against Cancer: History and Controversy.* New York: Equinox Press; 1998.

Office of Criminal Investigations, US Food and Drug Administration. Fiscal year 2004 report. US Food and Drug Administration Web site. http://www.fda.gov/ora/about/enf_story2004_archive/ch6/default.pdf. Accessed June 3, 2008.

Osswald SS, Elston DM, Farley MF, Alberti JG, Cordero SC, Kalasinsky VF. Self-treatment of a basal cell carcinoma with "black and yellow salve". *J Am Acad Dermatol.* 2005;53:509-511.

CASTOR OIL

Other common name(s): castor, castor bean, palma christi, Mexico seed, oil plant, mole bean
Scientific/medical name(s): *Ricinus communis*

Description

Castor oil is extracted from the seeds of *Ricinus communis*, an herb native to Africa and India. For the use described in this section, castor oil is applied to the skin rather than swallowed.

Overview

Available scientific evidence does not support claims that applying castor oil to the skin (called topical use) is effective in preventing or treating cancer. However, castor oil is used in mainstream medicine as a way to deliver chemotherapy drugs to cancerous tumors.

How is it promoted for use?

Castor oil, taken by mouth, is used as a laxative in conventional medicine. It may also be used to treat some eye irritations and skin conditions and is used in mainstream medicine to deliver chemotherapy drugs to cancerous tumors.

Naturopathic practitioners and some others claim that castor oil boosts the immune system by increasing the numbers of white blood cells, which help the body fight infection, and other immune cells. Some also claim that castor oil helps dissolve cysts, warts, and tumors and softens bunions and corns. Other claims for castor oil include treating lymphoma, bacterial and viral diseases (including human immunodeficiency virus), arthritis, skin and hair conditions, eye irritations, diseases of the colon and gallbladder, bursitis, multiple sclerosis, and Parkinson's disease.

What does it involve?

Treatment involves massaging castor oil into the body or using a warm or hot castor oil pack or compress. The castor oil is massaged along the problem region, spine, abdomen, and sites (or pathway) of lymphatic drainage. If a compress is used, the warm castor oil pack is placed over the affected joint or organ and left in place for up to an hour. Promoters say application of castor oil should continue until the problem is healed.

What is the history behind it?

Ancient Egyptians were the first to record the use of castor oil for medicinal purposes, and since then it has been used by many cultures as a folk medicine. Castor oil was reportedly used as a medicine during the early Middle Ages in Europe. In his *Encyclopedia of Healing*, Edgar Cayce claimed that castor oil helped to heal the lymphatic tissue in the small intestines, thus increasing absorption of fatty acids and allowing for tissue growth and repair. Most of the plants used in producing castor oil are now grown in India and Brazil.

What is the evidence?

Available scientific evidence does not support claims that the application of castor oil to the skin cures cancer or any other disease. Castor oil is taken by mouth in conventional medicine as a laxative and used as an eye drop to treat some eye irritations. It is also an ingredient in some hair conditioners and skin products. Available scientific evidence does not support any other claims.

Oncologists now use castor oil as a vehicle for delivering some chemotherapy drugs to cancerous tumors. A special formula of castor oil called Cremophor EL is used as a carrier for paclitaxel, a drug used to treat metastatic breast cancer and other tumors. Unfortunately, the vehicle sometimes causes problems of its own, including allergic reactions. This side effect has prompted a search for substitute carriers.

Researchers at Texas Tech University, Harvard University, the National Cancer Institute, and other institutions are studying ricin, a strong poison produced by the castor bean. Early clinical trials indicate that when combined with an antibody to shield other cells from the poison, ricin may shrink tumors in lymphoma patients. Ricin has recently been recognized as a possible bioterror agent, since inhaling or swallowing small amounts can cause severe illness and death.

Are there any possible problems or complications?

Castor oil is considered safe in proper doses for conventional uses as a laxative. However, side effects can include abdominal pain or cramping, colic, nausea, vomiting, and diarrhea. Long-term use of castor oil can lead to fluid and electrolyte loss. Women who are pregnant or breastfeeding should not use castor oil, nor should people with intestinal blockage, acute inflammatory intestinal disease, appendicitis, or abdominal pain. Medicines that are dissolved in or based on castor oil compounds can cause allergic reactions.

Castor beans are extremely poisonous and can kill people or animals if chewed or swallowed. Also, handling the seeds can lead to allergic reactions.

Relying on this treatment alone and delaying or avoiding conventional medical care for cancer may have serious health consequences.

This product is sold as a dietary supplement in the United States. Unlike companies that produce drugs (which must provide the FDA with results of detailed testing showing their product is safe and effective before the drug is approved for sale), the companies that make supplements do not have to show evidence of safety or health benefits to the FDA before selling their products. Supplement products without any reliable scientific evidence of health benefits may still be sold as long as the companies selling them do not claim the supplements can prevent, treat, or cure any specific disease. Some such products may not contain the amount of the herb or substance that is written on the label, and some may include other substances (contaminants). Though the FDA has written new rules to improve the quality of manufacturing processes for dietary supplements and the accurate listing of supplement ingredients, these rules do not take full effect until 2010. The new rules also do not address the safety of supplement ingredients or their effects on health when proper manufacturing techniques are used.

Most such supplements have not been tested to find out if they interact with medicines, foods, or other herbs and supplements. Even though some reports of interactions and harmful effects may be published, full studies of interactions and effects are not often available. Because of these limitations, any information on ill effects and interactions should be considered incomplete.

References

Belson MG, Schier JG, Patel MM. Case definitions for chemical poisoning. *MMWR Recomm Rep.* 2005; 54;1-24.

Bown D. *Encyclopedia of Herbs & Their Uses.* New York: DK Publishing Inc; 1995.

Fetrow CW, Avila JR. *Professional's Handbook of Complementary & Alternative Medicines.* Springhouse, PA: Springhouse Corp; 1999.

Fjällskog ML, Frii L, Bergh J. Paclitaxel-induced cytotoxicity—the effects of cremophor EL (castor oil) on two human breast cancer cell lines with acquired multidrug resistant phenotype and induced expression of the permeability glycoprotein. *Eur J Cancer.* 1994;30A:687-690.

Gruenwald J. *PDR for Herbal Medicines.* 3rd ed. Montvale, NJ: Thomson PDR; 2004.

Henderson CW. Researchers know beans about cancer research. *Cancer Weekly.* 1998. http://www.newsrx.com/newsletters/Cancer-Weekly/1998-11-02/1998110233329CW.html. Published November 2, 1998. Accessed June 19, 2008.

Price KS, Castells MC. Taxol reactions. *Allergy Asthma Proc.* 2002;23:205-208.

Rischin D, Webster LK, Millward MJ, Linahan BM, Toner GC, Woollett AM, Morton CG, Bishop JF. Cremophor pharmacokinetics in patients receiving 3-, 6-, and 24-hour infusions of paclitaxel. *J Natl Cancer Inst.* 1996;88:1297-1301.

CHIROPRACTIC

Other common name(s): chiropractic techniques, spinal manipulation
Scientific/medical name(s): none

Description

Chiropractic is a health care system that focuses on the relationship between the body's skeletal and muscular structure and its functions. Treatment often involves manipulating the bones of the spine to correct medical problems. Other methods may also be used.

Overview

Available scientific evidence does not support claims that chiropractic treatment cures cancer or any other life-threatening illness. However, chiropractic treatment has been shown to be effective in treating lower back pain and other pain caused by muscle or bone problems. It can also promote relaxation and stress reduction.

How is it promoted for use?

Chiropractic is most commonly used for back pain and other pain from muscle or bone problems. However, some chiropractors claim to be able to treat health problems such as heart disease, epilepsy, impotence, and allergies. They claim the spine plays a vital role in nearly all health problems.

The basic concept of chiropractic is that illness stems from underlying "subluxations," or spinal bones that are slightly out of place. These are thought to affect the nerve bundles as they branch off the spinal cord. Chiropractors do not treat the illness directly. Instead, they seek to correct the spine-related cause.

Chiropractic is based on the idea that the human body has the ability to heal itself, and that the body always seeks to maintain a balance among its systems and organs. Practitioners claim this is achieved through the nervous system. Illness is thought to result from a compression of the nerves from muscle spasm or abnormal position of the joints. Chiropractors claim manipulating the spine can correct compressed nerves and other unnatural relationships between bones and nerves.

What does it involve?

The chiropractor first diagnoses the person's ailment through a personal interview, examination, and x-rays of the spine. The person's flexibility and posture also may be examined. Electrical activity of the nerves and muscles may be measured. The exam is designed to pinpoint the source of the symptoms. For example, if a person complains of a pain in the shoulder, the chiropractor may search for the cause of the pain in the spinal column. Then the chiropractor will try to restore proper alignment and nerve function by adjusting the bones of the spine, called the vertebrae.

The patient usually lies down on a special treatment table. The chiropractor stands by the table and uses hands, elbows, and specially designed equipment to adjust and align the bones of the spine. Some chiropractors may also use heat, ice, electrical current, massage, vibration, traction, and other methods. They may prescribe exercises to correct health problems, especially those that involve the skeletal and nervous systems.

What is the history behind it?

Chiropractic comes from the Greek words *cheir* ("hands") and *praktikos* ("efficient"). It was practiced by priest healers in ancient Egypt and for centuries by Asian healers. Modern chiropractic was founded by Daniel D. Palmer, a grocer and magnetic healer. Palmer applied his knowledge to a man who had lost his hearing in the 1890s. The man remembered that something had "popped" in his back just before his hearing loss. Palmer saw that a vertebra was out of place and was able to thrust it back. After this, the man's hearing was restored. Although Palmer wasn't the first to use this technique, he was the first to use the vertebrae's bony bumps as levers to shift their position. Palmer founded the first chiropractic school in 1897. In the three decades that followed, other chiropractic colleges were opened and a variety of concepts developed regarding how to approach the practice of chiropractic.

Chiropractic colleges require at least four years of academic and professional training. The Council on Chiropractic Education establishes accreditation criteria for education. Around sixty thousand licensed chiropractors were practicing in the United States as of 2005; the number is projected to reach about one hundred thousand by the year 2010.

What is the evidence?

Many studies have suggested chiropractic is effective in treating lower back pain and other pain due to muscle or bone problems. However, one study showed that people with scoliosis, a condition in which the spine curves abnormally, did no better when treated by chiropractors.

Chiropractic has been studied for many conditions and is thought to be helpful mainly for muscle and bone problems. Unfortunately, the research methods used in studies of chiropractic have often not met scientific standards for clinical research well enough to prove that there is a relationship between chiropractic treatment and the outcome. Researchers looking at the overall quality of studies found weaknesses in the way they were conducted and interpreted. Because of these weaknesses, most studies cannot be used to reach strong conclusions.

Some evidence does suggest that tension headaches may respond to chiropractic treatment. Studies of chiropractic treatment for migraine headaches, however, have mostly shown little benefit. One exception is a recent randomized, controlled trial of people with frequent migraine headaches. The results suggested that those who received chiropractic care had less frequent and less severe headaches over several months of follow-up. They also required less pain medicine than those who were not treated with chiropractic.

Are there any possible problems or complications?

Chiropractic is considered fairly safe. However, there have been some reported cases of paralysis, blindness, and, in rare cases, death following chiropractic care. There have also been reports of misdiagnoses of patients' conditions, resulting in delayed medical care and worse outcomes. In several people with cancer, paralysis of the legs and full-body paralysis developed after manipulation of the spine when cancer had spread to and weakened the bones.

People with bleeding problems or those taking blood-thinning medications may have a higher risk for stroke caused by manipulation of the spine. People with cancer and chronic conditions such as arthritis, heart disease, and weakened bones should talk to their doctors before having any type of therapy that involves manipulation of joints and muscles. Relying on this treatment alone and delaying or avoiding conventional medical care for cancer may have serious health consequences.

References

Abenhaim L, Bergeron AM. Twenty years of randomized clinical trials of manipulative therapy for back pain: a review. *Clin Invest Med.* 1992;15:527-535.

Agency for Health Care Policy and Research. Acute pain management: operative or medical procedures and trauma. Rockville, MD; Agency for Health Care Policy and Research, Public Health Service, US Department of Health and Human Services; 1992. Publication AHCPR 92-0032.

Canter PH, Ernst E. Sources of bias in reviews of spinal manipulation for back pain. *Wien Klin Wochenschr.* 2005;117:333-341.

Cassileth B. *The Alternative Medicine Handbook: The Complete Reference Guide to Alternative and Complementary Therapies.* New York: W.W. Norton; 1998.

Chiropractic, spinal manipulative therapy, spinal manipulation. Aetna InteliHealth Web site. http://www.intelihealth.com/IH/ihtIH?d=dmtContent&c=368023. Accessed June 2, 2008.

Coulter ID, Shekelle PG. Supply, distribution, and utilization of chiropractors in the United States. In: *Chiropractic in the United States: Training, Practice, and Research.* Rockville, MD: Agency for Health Care Policy and Research, Public Health Service, US Department of Health and Human Services; 1997. Publication No. 98-N002.

Ernst E. Ophthalmological adverse effects of (chiropractic) upper spinal manipulation: evidence from recent case reports. *Acta Ophthalmol Scand.* 2005;83:581-585.

National Institutes of Health. *Alternative Medicine: Expanding Medical Horizons: A Report to the National Institutes of Health on Alternative Medical Systems and Practices in the United States.* Washington, DC: US Government Printing Office; 1994. NIH publication 94-066.

Lantz CA, Chen J. Effect of chiropractic intervention on small scoliotic curves in younger subjects: a time-series cohort design. *J Manipulative Physiol Ther.* 2001;24:385-393.

Shekelle PG, Adams AH, Chassin MR, Hurwitz EL, Brook RH. Spinal manipulation for low-back pain. *Ann Intern Med.* 1992;117:590-598.

Spencer JW, Jacobs JJ. *Complementary/Alternative Medicine: An Evidence-Based Approach.* St. Louis, MO: Mosby; 1999.

Tuchin PJ, Pollard H, Bonello R. A randomized controlled trial of chiropractic spinal manipulative therapy for migraine. *J Manipulative Physiol Ther.* 2000;23:91-95.

van Tulder MW, Furlan AD, Gagnier JJ. Complementary and alternative therapies for low back pain. *Best Pract Res Clin Rheumatol.* 2005;19:639-654.

Wang CC, Kuo JR, Chio CC, Tsai TC. Acute paraplegia following chiropractic therapy. *J Clin Neurosci.* 2006;13:578-581.

COLD LASER THERAPY

Other common name(s): low-level laser therapy, low-power laser therapy, low-intensity laser, low-energy laser therapy, photobiomodulation, laser biostimulation

This method should not be confused with conventional laser surgery, which is used as a proven treatment for some cancers. Hot lasers may be used to shrink or destroy tumors on the skin or on the surfaces of internal organs. They are sometimes used to remove colon polyps or tumors that are blocking the windpipe, colon, or stomach. They can help relieve symptoms of cancer, such as bleeding. Laser surgery for cancer is usually combined with other treatments such as conventional surgery, chemotherapy, or radiation therapy.

Description

The term cold laser refers to the use of low-intensity laser light. Proponents claim that cold laser therapy can reduce pain and inflammation.

Overview

The term LASER stands for "light amplification by stimulated emission of radiation." Laser light is different from regular light. The light from the sun or from a light bulb has many wavelengths (colors) and spreads out in all directions. Laser light, on the other hand, has one wavelength and moves in a single direction. There are many kinds of lasers, which produce light of different wavelengths and with different amounts of energy, and some of these are used for scientific, industrial, and medical purposes. For example, high-energy lasers are often used in conventional surgery.

Cold lasers use very-low-energy beams that do not destroy cells or tissues. There is some evidence suggesting cold lasers may alter the function of cells in ways that are currently not completely understood and that these devices may have a role in treating some types of pain. There is mixed evidence regarding prevention and treatment of mouth sores due to conventional cancer treatment. Claims that cold lasers are useful for many other conditions are still not supported by reliable clinical evidence, and more research is needed.

How is it promoted for use?

Cold laser therapy is promoted as a treatment for pain, inflammation, wound healing, arthritis, weight loss, temporomandibular (jaw) joint problems, and cellulite reduction. Some providers advertise that cold lasers can help with herpes infections, high blood pressure, wrinkles, and cerebral palsy. Some cold laser therapy providers advertise this method as a way to help people quit smoking, and some television stations have reported this claim as news. The treatment is claimed to relax the smoker by releasing endorphins, naturally occurring pain relief substances in the body, to simulate the effects of nicotine in the brain. Some claim that the treatment balances the body's energy to relieve the addiction. Other proposed ways in which cold lasers might work include stimulating nerve cells, altering cellular metabolism, stimulating the immune system, and activating microcirculation (small blood vessels).

What does it involve?

Treatments are given in a provider's office or other outpatient setting. Typical lasers used in conventional medicine use high-energy beams that heat and vaporize diseased tissue. Cold lasers use beams with less than one-thousandth the energy of a medical laser and therefore do not destroy cells by heating them.

Beams from cold lasers are generally used directly on or over the affected area. Cold lasers are also sometimes used for acupuncture, using laser beams to stimulate the body's acupoints rather than needles (see "Acupuncture," page 156). This treatment regimen appeals to some people who want acupuncture but who fear needles.

What is the history behind it?

Soon after the first working laser was developed in 1960, researchers began studying its possible uses in medicine. In 1961, lasers were first used in conventional medicine to treat a type of skin discoloration and to repair detached retinas. The first report of cold laser therapy was in 1967.

What is the evidence?

There is a great deal of variation in the types of lasers that are used and how they are used. Some devices do not have the output that they promise, and others are little more than light-emitting diodes (LED lights). The U.S. Food and Drug Administration (FDA) forbids statements that a treatment can help or cure diseases if scientific studies have not found it to be true. It has warned at least one seller of low-level lasers to stop making such claims.

No results of clinical trials on the use of cold lasers as a cancer treatment have been published in peer-reviewed medical journals. Several clinical trials have studied cold lasers for relief of some side effects of cancer treatment, especially for mouth sores caused by chemotherapy and/or radiation therapy. Results have been mixed. Some studies reported less pain or faster healing, and others found no benefit.

The situation is similar for most other uses of cold laser therapy. Relatively few clinical trials have been conducted. Most involved small numbers of patients, and many were designed or conducted in ways that might limit the reliability of their results. Many systematic reviews have concluded that while there is some preliminary evidence of benefit for some conditions, the scarcity of evidence from high-quality clinical trials precludes confident conclusions about the value of this treatment.

Despite claims of success by some cold laser therapy providers, available scientific evidence does not support claims that this treatment is an effective method of helping people stop smoking.

Some well-controlled scientific studies are under way; if these studies show positive results, certain types of cold laser treatment may eventually become part of conventional medical care.

Are there any possible problems or complications?

Cold laser therapy is thought to be safe when used properly. One 2005 review article suggested that cold lasers should not be used over the location of a malignant tumor, in people with epilepsy, over the thyroid gland, on the abdomen during pregnancy, in people with light hypersensitivity, and in people with blood clots in deep veins of the legs.

Others suggest that children should not have cold laser therapy near the ends of growing bones and that cold lasers should not be used by pregnant women at all, as their effects on a growing fetus are unknown. Talk to your doctor if you are considering this treatment.

Relying on this treatment alone and delaying or avoiding conventional medical care for cancer may have serious health consequences.

References

American Cancer Society. Lasers in cancer treatment. American Cancer Society Web site. http://www.cancer.org/docroot/ETO/content/ETO_1_2x_Lasers_In_Cancer_Treatment.asp. Accessed October 8, 2008.

Arora H, Pai KM, Maiya A, Vidyasagar MS, Rajeev A. Efficacy of He-Ne Laser in the prevention and treatment of radiotherapy-induced oral mucositis in oral cancer patients. *Oral Surg Oral Med Oral Pathol Oral Radiol Endod.* 2008;105:180-186, 186.e1.

Cigna Healthcare coverage position. Cigna Healthcare Web site. http://www.cigna.com/customer_care/healthcare_professional/coverage_positions/medical/mm_0115_coveragepositioncriteria_lowlevel_laser_therapy.pdf. Revised July 15, 2008. Accessed October 8, 2008.

Cold laser therapy: a treatment option for knee pain? Mayo Clinic Web site. http://www.mayoclinic.com/health/cold-laser-therapy/AN01677. Updated November 6, 2007. Accessed October 8, 2008.

Cruz LB, Ribeiro AS, Rech A, Rosa LG, Castro CG Jr, Brunetto AL. Influence of low-energy laser in the prevention of oral mucositis in children with cancer receiving chemotherapy. *Pediatr Blood Cancer.* 2007;48:435-440.

Emshoff R, Bosch R, Pumpel E, Schoning H, Strobl H. Low-level laser therapy for treatment of temporomandibular joint pain: a double-blind and placebo-controlled trial. *Oral Surg Oral Med Oral Pathol Oral Radiol Endod.* 2008;105:452-456.

Energy medicine: an overview. National Center for Complementary and Alternative Medicine Web site. http://nccam.nih.gov/health/backgrounds/energymed.htm. Accessed March 29, 2007.

Laser facts. Center for Devices and Radiologic Health Consumer Services, US Food and Drug Administration Web site. http://www.fda.gov/cdrh/consumer/laserfacts.html. Accessed May 30, 2008.

Lasers in cancer treatment: questions and answers. National Cancer Institute Web site. http://www.cancer.gov/cancertopics/factsheet/Therapy/lasers. Updated August 10, 2004. Accessed May 30, 2008.

The lower level laser therapy LLLT Internet guide. Swedish Laser Medical Society Web site. http://www.laser.nu/lllt/LLLT_critic2_on_critics.htm. Accessed May 30, 2008. Excerpted from Tunér J, Hode L. *Low Level Laser Therapy: Clinical Practice and Scientific Background.* Grängesberg, Sweden: Prima Books; 1999.

Moshkovska T, Mayberry J. It is time to test low level laser therapy in Great Britain. *Postgrad Med J.* 2005;81:436–441.

Rindge D. Laser acupuncture. *Acupuncture Today.* 2005;06(5). Acupuncture Today Web site.http://www.acupuncturetoday.com/mpacms/at/article.php?id=30129. Accessed June 3, 2008.

Schubert MM, Eduardo FP, Guthrie KA, Franquin JC, Bensadoun RJ, Migliorati CA, Lloid CM, Eduardo CP, Walter NF, Marques MM, Hamdi M. A phase III randomized double-blind placebo-controlled clinical trial to determine the efficacy of low level laser therapy for the prevention of oral mucositis in patients undergoing hematopoietic cell transplantation. *Support Care Cancer.* 2007;15:1145-1154.

Tunér J. Low level lasers in dentistry. Swedish Laser Medical Society Web site. http://www.laser.nu/lllt/Laser_therapy_%20in_dentistry.htm. Accessed May 30, 2008.

White AR, Rampes H, Campbell JL. Acupuncture and related interventions for smoking cessation. *Cochrane Database Syst Rev.* 2006;(1):CD000009.

COLON THERAPY

Other common name(s): colonic irrigation, high colonic, detoxification therapy, colon hydrotherapy, coffee enemas, enema irrigation, hydro-colon therapy, high enema
Scientific/medical name(s): none

Description

Colon therapy is the cleansing of the large intestine (colon) through the administration of water, herbal solutions, enzymes, or other substances such as coffee.

Overview

Available scientific evidence does not support claims that colon therapy is effective in treating cancer or any other disease. Colon therapy can be dangerous and can cause infection or death.

How is it promoted for use?

Proponents of colon therapy consider it to be a method of detoxifying the body through the removal of accumulated waste from the colon. Because they claim detoxification increases the efficiency of the body's natural healing abilities, it is sometimes promoted as a treatment for illness. It is often promoted as a general preventive health measure or as part of a routine internal hygiene regimen.

Coffee enemas have been promoted as part of several controversial cancer treatment regimens. People who promote the use of coffee enemas to detoxify the body claim that an "unpoisoned" body or a "clean" colon has the ability to recognize and destroy cancer cells. Practitioners claim coffee enemas can stimulate the liver and gallbladder into releasing toxins and flushing them from the body, allowing the body's immune system to battle malignant cells.

What does it involve?

Colon therapy is given by a colonic hygienist or colon therapist, through the use of plastic tubes inserted through the rectum and into the colon. A machine or gravity-driven pump sends large quantities of liquid (up to twenty gallons) into the large intestine. In contrast, regular enemas only flush out the rectum, and generally use about a quart of fluid. After filling the colon with water, the therapist massages the abdomen to help the removal of waste material from the colon wall, and then fluid and waste are carried out of the body through another tube. The procedure is generally repeated several times, and the average session lasts from forty-five to sixty minutes. Coffee enemas may be included in the treatment program.

What is the history behind it?

As far back as the ancient Egyptians, enemas and other "cleansing rituals" were commonly used to rid the body of toxic waste products believed to cause disease and death. In the nineteenth century, proponents described the large intestine as a sewage system and claimed stagnation caused toxins to form and be absorbed by the body, which led to the theory of "autointoxication." Laxatives, purges, and enemas were routinely recommended to prevent the accumulation of waste.

Colon therapy became very popular in the United States in the 1920s and 1930s, when irrigation machines were commonly found in hospitals and physicians' offices. Although the procedure became less popular when advances in science and medicine did not support its founding theory, colon therapy has recently shown an increase in popularity.

In 1985, the California Department of Health Services issued a statement that listed some of the potential hazards of colon therapy, including infection and death from contaminated equipment, death from electrolyte depletion, and perforation of the intestinal wall leading to life-threatening infection or death. The U.S. Food and Drug Administration (FDA) considers colonic irrigation machines to be Class III devices, which means they cannot be legally marketed except for medically needed colon cleansing (such as before an x-ray or endoscope exam). The FDA forbids practitioners and sellers from making claims that have not been proven in scientific studies about their services. The FDA has warned several companies to stop making such claims. No colonic irrigation machine or system has been approved for routine use.

What is the evidence?

Available scientific evidence does not support the claims on which colon therapy is based. It is known that most digestive processes take place in the small intestine, where nutrients are absorbed into the body. What remains enters the large intestine, where it passes to the rectum for elimination after water and minerals are extracted. Available scientific evidence does not support the premise that toxins accumulate on intestinal walls or that toxicity results from poor elimination of waste from the colon.

Are there any possible problems or complications?

The machines used for colon therapy are illegal unless used during conventional medical treatment. Colon therapy can be dangerous. Illness and even deaths have resulted from contaminated equipment, electrolyte imbalance, or perforation of intestinal walls. People with diverticulitis, ulcerative colitis, Crohn's disease, severe hemorrhoids, rectal or colon tumors, or who are recovering from bowel surgery may be at higher risk of bowel injury. People with kidney or heart failure may be more likely to experience fluid overload or electrolyte imbalances. In addition, many substances can be absorbed into the body from the colon walls and cause toxic or allergic reactions. Colon therapy can also cause discomfort and cramps. Relying on this type of treatment alone and avoiding or delaying conventional medical care for cancer may have serious health consequences.

References

Barrett S. Gastrointestinal quackery: colonics, laxatives, and more. Quackwatch Web site. http://www.quackwatch.org/01QuackeryRelatedTopics/gastro.html. Accessed May 30, 2008.

Brown BT. Treating cancer with coffee enemas and diet. *JAMA.* 1993;269:1635-1636.

Cassileth B. *The Alternative Medicine Handbook: The Complete Reference Guide to Alternative and Complementary Therapies.* New York: W.W. Norton; 1998.

Centers for Disease Control (CDC). Amebiasis associated with colonic irrigation—Colorado. *MMWR Morb Mortal Wkly Rep.* 1981;30:101-102.

Colonic irrigation. Aetna InteliHealth Web site. http://www.intelihealth.com/IH/ihtIH/WSIHW000/8513/34968/358752.html. Accessed June 2, 2008.

Eisele JW, Reay DT. Deaths related to coffee enemas. *JAMA.* 1980;244:1608-1609.

Ernst E. Colonic irrigation and the theory of autointoxication: a triumph of ignorance over science. *J Clin Gastroenterol.* 1997;24:196-198.

Green S. A critique of the rationale for cancer treatment with coffee enemas and diet. *JAMA.* 1992;268:3224-3227.

CRANIOSACRAL THERAPY

Other common name(s):
cranial balancing, cranial osteopathy, cranial sacral manipulation, craniopathy
Scientific/medical name(s): none

Description

Craniosacral therapy involves the gentle massage of bones in the skull (including the face and mouth), spine, and pelvis to ease stress in the body and improve physical movement.

Overview

Available scientific evidence does not support claims that craniosacral therapy is effective in treating cancer or any other disease. However, it may help some people with cancer feel more relaxed. The gentle, hands-on method is noninvasive and may offer some relief for symptoms of stress, headaches, and muscle tension.

How is it promoted for use?

Craniosacral therapy is a variation of chiropractic and osteopathic medicine (see "Chiropractic," page 177, and "Osteopathy," page 231). Supporters claim that gentle massage of the bones of the head, spine, and pelvis increases the flow of cerebrospinal fluid, which can cure any number of ailments. Craniosacral therapists say that there is a link between the fluid in the head and the sacrum (the base of the lower back) and that the rhythm of the fluid that flows between these areas can be detected like a pulse. They say craniosacral therapy normalizes, balances, and eliminates blockages in various systems throughout the body. They claim that with obstructions removed, the body can function in a healthy manner.

Promoters claim this therapy can be used to help relieve headaches; neck and back pain; problems with the temporomandibular joint (the hinge of the jaw, sometimes called the TMJ); chronic fatigue; poor coordination; eye problems; depression; hyperactivity; attention deficit disorder; problems with the central nervous system, the immune system, and the endocrine system; and many other conditions.

Practitioners also claim the birthing process can have a negative effect on growth of the cartilage and membranes surrounding an infant's skull, and they offer this treatment to fix this problem.

What does it involve?

Craniosacral therapy is usually performed by osteopaths, chiropractors, or massage therapists. The treatment involves either gentle massage or manipulation to the bones of the skull. Sessions last from thirty minutes to an hour.

What is the history behind it?

Dr. William G. Sutherland developed cranial osteopathy in the early 1930s. John E. Upledger, DO, developed craniosacral therapy, a derivative of Sutherland's work, in the 1970s. Upledger opened the Upledger Institute of Florida in the 1980s, where thousands of health care professionals attend his program every year to learn about releasing stresses in the skull and the membranes surrounding the brain.

What is the evidence?

The theoretical basis of craniosacral therapy is inconsistent with mainstream scientific concepts of anatomy and physiology of the skull, brain, and spinal fluid circulation. There are only anecdotal reports of successful treatment with craniosacral therapy. Some patients report that it helps to reduce stress, tension, and headaches. However, there have been few well-controlled clinical studies of this method. A 1994 report to the National Institutes of Health stated that successes have not been documented in formal studies.

Researchers have tested the ability of craniosacral therapists to detect and count the rhythmic cranial impulse, an important part of the therapy. Numerous therapists assessed the same patients at the same time, without comparing notes. The therapists' counts did not match, which suggests that the measures are not reliable. In addition, the British Columbia Office of Health Technology Assessment conducted a wide-ranging search for solid information on craniosacral therapy and found no evidence to support the claims made about it.

Are there any possible problems or complications?

Craniosacral therapy should not be used in children under age two because the bones of the skull are not fully developed. In one very small study, several adults with head injuries had worse symptoms after starting craniosacral therapy. People who have cancer and chronic conditions such as arthritis and heart disease should talk to their doctors before starting any type of therapy that involves manipulation of joints and muscles. Relying on this treatment alone and delaying or avoiding conventional medical care for cancer may have serious health consequences.

References

Barrett S. Dubious aspects of osteopathy. Quackwatch Web site. http://www.quackwatch.org/04ConsumerEducation/QA/osteo.html. Updated August 18, 2003. Accessed May 30, 2008.

Barrett S. Why craniosacral therapy is silly. Quackwatch Web site. http://www.quackwatch.org/01QuackeryRelatedTopics/cranial.html. Updated September 21, 2004. Accessed May 30, 2008.

Cassileth B. *The Alternative Medicine Handbook: The Complete Reference Guide to Alternative and Complementary Therapies.* New York: W.W. Norton; 1998.

Craniosacral therapy. Aetna InteliHealth Web site. http://www.intelihealth.com/IH/ihtIH/WSIHW000/8513/34968/358810.html. Accessed June 2, 2008.

Green CJ, Martin CW, Bassett K, Kazanjian A. A systematic review and critical appraisal of the scientific evidence on craniosacral therapy. British Columbia Office of Health Technology Assessment, Centre for Health Services and Policy Research. University of British Columbia Web site. http://www.chspr.ubc.ca/files/publications/1999/bco99-01J_cranio.pdf. Accessed May 30, 2008.

Greenman PE, McPartland JM. Cranial findings and iatrogenesis from craniosacral manipulation in patients with traumatic brain syndrome. *J Am Osteopath Assoc.* 1995;95:182-188;191-192.

Moran RW, Gibbons P. Intraexaminer and interexaminer reliability for palpation of the cranial rhythmic impulse at the head and sacrum. *J Manipulative Physiol Ther.* 2001;24:183-190.

National Institutes of Health. *Alternative Medicine: Expanding Medical Horizons: A Report to the National Institutes of Health on Alternative Medical Systems and Practices in the United States.* Washington, DC: US Government Printing Office; 1994. NIH publication 94-066.

Rogers JS, Witt PL, Gross MT, Hacke JD, Genova PA. Simultaneous palpation of the craniosacral rate at the head and feet: intrarater and interrater reliability and rate comparisons. *Phys Ther.* 1998;78:1175-1185.

CUPPING

Other common name(s): fire cupping, body vacuuming, the horn method
Scientific/medical name(s): none

Description

Cupping involves warming the air inside a glass, metal, wooden, or bamboo cup and inverting it over a part of the body to treat various health conditions.

Overview

Cupping is based on traditional Chinese medicine. Available scientific evidence does not support claims that cupping has any health benefits.

How is it promoted for use?

Cupping is a practice of Chinese medicine recommended mainly for treating bronchial congestion, arthritis, and pain. It is also promoted to ease depression and reduce swelling. Cupping is supposed to realign and balance the flow of one's vital energy or life force, called qi or chi, pronounced "kee" or "chee." In the presence of illness or injury, proponents say, the qi is disturbed, and there may be too much or too little at certain points in the body. The practitioner diagnoses any imbalances in the qi and attempts to restore them. Although not widely used as an alternative method of treatment for cancer, some practitioners may use it to rebalance energy in the body that has been blocked by tumors.

What does it involve?

A flammable substance, such as alcohol, herbs, or paper, is placed in a cup made of glass, metal, wood, or bamboo. The material inside the cup is set on fire. As the fire goes out, the cup is placed upside down over qi pathways, places on the body that, according to traditional Chinese medicine, are linked to the patient's illness. The cup is usually left in place for five to ten minutes.

As the air inside the jar cools, it creates a vacuum, which causes the skin to rise. This is thought to open up the skin's pores and create a route for toxins to escape the body. The skin under the cup reddens as blood vessels expand. In a more modern version of cupping, a rubber pump attached to the jar is used to create the vacuum.

In "wet" cupping, the skin is punctured before treatment. When the cup is applied, blood flows out of the punctures and is said to remove harmful substances and toxins from the body. In "dry" cupping, the skin is left intact. Some practitioners sterilize the cups in an autoclave, a device that uses steam under pressure to sterilize medical instruments by heating the cups to more than 250° F.

What is the history behind it?

Cupping is an ancient component of Chinese medicine. It is also a well-known folk remedy in Vietnam and other Asian countries. Besides "fire" cupping, other methods include acupuncture cupping, water cupping, and air-pump cupping.

What is the evidence?

Available scientific evidence does not support cupping as a cure for cancer or any other disease. Reports of successful treatment with cupping are mainly anecdotal rather than from research studies.

Are there any possible problems or complications?

Cupping is considered relatively safe. However, the treatment may be slightly painful or even cause burns. Cupping leaves purplish marks on the skin, which usually heal after several days. It can also cause swelling due to the buildup of excess fluid around the cupped area. Relying on this treatment alone and delaying or avoiding conventional medical care for cancer may have serious health consequences.

References

Cassileth B. *The Alternative Medicine Handbook: The Complete Reference Guide to Alternative and Complementary Therapies*. New York: W.W. Norton; 1998.

Raso J. The expanded dictionary of metaphysical healthcare, alternative medicine, paranormal healing, and related methods. Quackwatch Web site. http://www.quackwatch.org/01QuackeryRelatedTopics/dictionary/md00.html. Accessed May 30, 2008.

Sagi A, Ben-Meir P, Bibi C. Burn hazard from cupping—an ancient universal medication still in practice. *Burns Incl Therm Inj*. 1988;14:323-325.

Tierra L. Barefoot doctor healing techniques. Planet Herbs Web site. http://www.planetherbs.com/articles/barefoot.html. Accessed May 30, 2008. Also available in print at: Tierra L. *The Herbs of Life*. Berkeley, CA: Crossing Press; 1992.

ELECTRODERMAL SCREENING

Other common name(s):
EAV (electroacupuncture according to Voll), bioelectric functional diagnosis, Vegatesting
Scientific/medical name(s): none

Electrodermal screening is different from electrical impedance scanning, in which an electrical current is sent through deep body tissues to detect changes due to cancer. The U.S. Food and Drug Administration has reviewed electrical impedance scanning and allowed it to go into clinical trials to determine whether it can help to diagnose breast cancer.

Description

Electrodermal screening is used to diagnose disease by measuring the skin's electrical resistance. The purpose is to detect energy imbalances along invisible lines along the body called meridians.

Overview

Available scientific evidence does not support electrodermal diagnosis as a method that can diagnose, cure, or otherwise help people with cancer.

How is it promoted for use?

Proponents claim the devices can help detect energy imbalances in the body, help with the selection of treatments, measure the progress of therapy, and even detect disease before it becomes apparent. They claim that some of the devices can be used to find allergies, organ weakness, parasites, heavy metal intoxication, dietary intolerances, pesticide burden, nutrient deficiencies, and more.

What does it involve?

This kind of testing may be done by a homeopath, acupuncturist, naturopath, chiropractor, or other practitioner. The testing device sends a tiny electrical current, too small to be detected by the patient, through a probe. The patient holds a probe in one hand, while a second probe is touched to another part of the body. This completes a low-voltage electrical circuit, and a computer screen or a needle on a gauge reads out a number between 0 and 100. This process may be repeated at many different places on the skin. These numbers are used to decide if the patient's energy is out of balance.

If the patient is being tested for a type of treatment, samples of various remedies may be tried as the probe is touched to the problem area. Remedies may include homeopathic liquids and dietary or vitamin supplements. Different substances are tested until one is found that "balances" the energy disturbance.

What is the history behind it?

Electrodermal screening has its earliest roots in what was called galvanic skin testing. The galvanic skin response, a method of measuring the electrical resistance of the skin, was discovered in the early 1900s. Galvanic skin testing detects sweat on the skin, and more sweat produces better electrical conduction.

In the 1950s, a West German physician and acupuncturist named Reinhold Voll combined acupuncture theory with galvanic skin response technology. He tested the skin along various points with particular attention to the acupuncture meridians (see page 156). This is how galvanic skin response testing became known as electrodermal screening.

The first device for electrodermal screening was called the Vegatest, followed by the Vegatest II. Later versions have been called Accupath 1000, Biotron, Computron, Dermatron, DiagnoMètre, Eclosion, Elast, Interro, LISTEN System, MORA, Natrix Physiofeedback

System, Omega AcuBase, OmegaVision, Orion System, Prophyle, Punctos III, and Vitel 618, among others. Because the devices are simple to make, new brands and different-looking devices are created often.

Changes in galvanic skin response are still sometimes used in mental health research studies or to detect hot flashes in menopausal women. Galvanic skin response changes are also still used in lie-detector tests, along with several other measures such as pulse, breathing, and blood pressure. For most purposes, this method has been replaced with more advanced types of testing.

What is the evidence?

Available scientific evidence does not support electrodermal screening (galvanic skin response) as a reliable aid in diagnosis or treatment of cancer or other illness.

The FDA requires that any device used to diagnose or treat disease be proven effective before it can be marketed. None of these devices has earned FDA approval for diagnostic use, although several are registered as "galvanic skin response detection devices." The FDA has warned several manufacturers to stop making false claims about diagnosis and has banned some devices from being imported. Various licensing boards in the United States have disciplined licensed practitioners who have used electrodermal screening for diagnosis or treatment selection. In spite of these efforts, the devices are still frequently advertised and promoted as diagnostic tools.

Are there any possible problems or complications?

Electrodermal screening itself is relatively safe, although people with implanted pacemakers should avoid electrical current. However, misdiagnosis and improper treatment may cause problems. For example, people have had healthy teeth removed based on recommendations from this type of screening. One man was told he did not have cancer when, in fact, he did. His treatment was delayed for several months because of misinformation.

Relying on this diagnostic method alone while avoiding or delaying conventional diagnosis and medical care for cancer may have serious health consequences.

References

Barrett S. Quack "electrodiagnostic" devices. Quackwatch Web site. http://www.quackwatch.org/01QuackeryRelatedTopics/electro.html. Revised September 5, 2007. Accessed May 30, 2008.

Carpenter JS, Monahan PO, Azzouz F. Accuracy of subjective hot flush reports compared with continuous sternal skin conductance monitoring. *Obstet Gynecol.* 2004;104:1322-1326.

Ernst E, ed. *The Desktop Guide to Complementary and Alternative Medicine: An Evidence-Based Approach.* New York: Mosby; 2001.

Research on sensing human affect. Affective Computing Web site. http://affect.media.mit.edu/areas.php?id=sensing. Accessed June 2, 2008.

Semizzi M, Senna G, Crivellaro M, Rapacioli G, Passalacqua G, Canonica WG, Bellavite P. A double-blind, placebo-controlled study on the diagnostic accuracy of an electrodermal test in allergic subjects. *Clin Exp Allergy.* 2002;32:928-932.

Stojadinovic A, Nissan A, Gallimidi Z, Lenington S, Logan W, Zuley M, Yeshaya A, Shimonov M, Melloul M, Fields S, Allweis T, Ginor R, Gur D, Shriver CD. Electrical impedance scanning for the early detection of breast cancer in young women: preliminary results of a multicenter prospective clinical trial. *J Clin Oncol.* 2005;23:2703-2715.

US Food and Drug Administration. FDA guidance document for galvanic skin response measurement devices. Device Watch Web site. http://www.devicewatch.org/reg/gsr.shtml. Accessed June 20, 2008.

ELECTROMAGNETIC THERAPY

Other common name(s):
BioResonance Tumor Therapy, Cell Com system, Rife machine, zapping machine, electromagnetism, bioelectricity, magnetic field therapy, bioelectromagnetics, bioenergy therapy, black boxes, energy medicine, electronic devices, electrical devices
Scientific/medical name(s): none

Description

Electromagnetic therapy involves the use of energy to diagnose or treat disease. Electromagnetic energy includes electricity, microwaves, radio waves, and infrared rays, as well as electrically generated magnetic fields. Although light is also a type of electromagnetic energy, light therapy is addressed in a separate section on page 210.

Overview

Some electronic devices are approved for medical use, such as the electroencephalogram (EEG), electrocardiogram (EKG), and transcutaneous electrical nerve stimulation units (TENS; see page 252). Such devices are used to diagnose nervous system and heart problems and to treat pain by interfering with nerve conduction of pain impulses. However, many of the alternative electronic devices promoted to cure disease have not been scientifically proven to be effective.

How is it promoted for use?

Many types of electromagnetic devices have been promoted as part of this therapy. Some of the specific ones discussed in this section are some of the most common or best known. In general, practitioners of electromagnetic therapy claim that when electromagnetic frequencies or energy fields within the body go out of balance, disease and illness occur. They claim that these imbalances disrupt the body's chemical makeup. By applying electromagnetic energy from outside the body, usually with electronic devices, practitioners claim they can correct the imbalances in the body. Practitioners claim that these methods can treat ulcers, headaches, burns, chronic pain, nerve disorders, spinal cord injuries, diabetes, gum infections, asthma, bronchitis, arthritis, cerebral palsy, heart disease, and cancer.

Practitioners of BioResonance Tumor Therapy (a kind of electromagnetic treatment) use an electronic device they claim results in the self-destruction of tumor cells by "energizing the *p53* gene." Practitioners say it cures cancer in 80 percent of cases. There is no description of precisely how this is accomplished.

Proponents of an electronic device called the Cell Com system claim it regulates the chemical and electrical communication between cells. Proponents claim it can be used to relieve pain caused by cancer and for fighting recurrent infections, asthma, bronchitis, and arthritis. They further claim the device can stop the growth of cancer cells.

Practitioners claim the Rife machine, another electronic device, can diagnose and eliminate diseases, including cancer, by tuning into electrical impulses given off by diseased tissue. The Rife machine then directs energy of the same frequency back at the diseased tissue. Promoters claim that the device kills microorganisms that cause disease.

Another electronic device that has been promoted to cure cancer is the zapping machine. Based on the claim that cancer is related to parasites, promoters say it kills the parasites that cause cancer.

What does it involve?

Electromagnetic therapy is claimed to use electromagnetic, microwave, or infrared energy to diagnose or treat an illness by detecting and correcting imbalances in the body's energy fields. Electronic devices that emit some form of low-voltage electrical current or radio frequency are often involved. Magnets and other unconventional treatments may also be a part of electromagnetic and energy field therapy. The most commonly used electronic devices are listed below.

BioResonance Tumor Therapy

This method uses a small electronic device to create vibrations that are supposed to "re-enliven" the *p53* gene in order to cure cancer. While the *p53* gene is often defective in cancerous tissues, available scientific evidence does not support claims that it can be electronically repaired. Some reports estimate that the course of therapy can last up to six weeks.

Cell Com System

This device reportedly transmits low-voltage electricity through electrodes placed on the hands and feet in order to regulate communication between cells in the body.

Rife Machine

Also called frequency therapy, frequency generator, and Rife frequency generator, the Rife machine is used to direct electrical impulses at the feet to break up the supposed accumulated deposits of toxins at nerve endings. During treatment, the patient places his or her feet in a plastic box attached to the Rife unit.

Zapping Machine

A zapping machine is a small, battery-powered device that produces a low-frequency electrical current. Wires connected to copper tubes transmit the electricity to patients.

What is the history behind it?

The effects of magnetism and energy forces have been studied since the time of the Greek and Roman empires. Chinese medicine uses one of the oldest energy-based systems of healing. Traditional Chinese medicine is based on the concept of qi (or chi), which is thought to be the vital energy or life force that flows throughout the body. The concept of life force is also a central aspect of Indian medical beliefs.

In modern times, the discovery of electricity brought about the promotion of electromagnetic treatments. The use of different forms of electrical devices and frequency generators in medicine has intrigued practitioners and patients for generations. Since the mid-1800s, countless electronic machines have been applied to a long list of ailments. Most of these devices have never been proven effective. In some cases, their use has resulted in serious injury or even death. However, some electromagnetic and electrical technologies have become mainstays of modern medical practice, such as diagnostic x-rays, radiation therapy, magnetic resonance imaging (MRI), and cardiac pacemakers.

An early use of electromagnetic therapy came in the late 1800s when Albert Abrams, MD, developed a number of devices he claimed could detect the frequencies of diseased tissue and heal the underlying imbalances. Dr. Abrams and his colleagues were never able to prove his devices were effective, and investigators from *Scientific American* magazine reported in 1924 that the device did not correctly diagnose any of six specimens. The idea that disease can be diagnosed and treated by tuning in to radio-like frequencies has also been called radionics.

Dozens of similar unconventional and unproven electronic devices have been made and marketed over the years. BioResonance Tumor Therapy, the Cell Com system, the Rife machine, and the zapping machine are four popular systems on the market today.

BioResonance Tumor Therapy was developed by Martin Keymer, a German biophysicist, who claims the therapy is rooted in the age-old idea that it is possible to tap into the vital energy that flows throughout the body. A clinic offering the therapy, which opened in Tijuana, Mexico, in 1998, has been the subject of a great deal of controversy. The Cell Com system, which is said to increase communication between cells, was invented by a Danish acupuncturist named Hugo Nielsen. The Rife machine (or Rife frequency generator) was created by Royal Raymond Rife, an American who asserted that cancer was caused by bacteria. The machine supposedly emitted radio waves at the same frequency as those discharged by offending bacteria. According to Rife, the radio waves created vibrations that "shattered" the bacteria.

The most widely marketed zapping machine today is the Zapper, designed by Hulda Clark, PhD, a physiologist with no formal clinical medical training. She currently uses her device to treat patients with cancer, AIDS, and other diseases in a Tijuana, Mexico medical clinic.

Electronic devices and other frequency generators are available through a number of companies. Treatment programs that incorporate the devices are offered in Mexican and Canadian clinics. Practitioners do not need a license to conduct frequency therapy in the United States.

The U.S. Food and Drug Administration (FDA) has not approved any alternative electronic devices promoted to cure illness and does not recognize any frequency generator as a legitimate medical device. It has, however, launched an investigation into the industry.

What is the evidence?

There is no relationship between conventional medical uses of electromagnetic energy and the alternative devices or methods that use externally applied electrical forces. Available scientific evidence does not support claims that these alternative electrical devices are effective in diagnosing or treating cancer or any other disease.

Science has established that electrical and magnetic energies exist in the human body. Electrical energy is used by physicians to restart the heart after heart attacks and is even applied to promote bone growth. Some accepted electrical devices commonly used in hospitals include EEGs to measure electrical activity in the brain and EKGs to measure electrical patterns of heartbeats. However, low-level radio waves or tiny electrical impulses are not strong enough to produce a significant effect on the body. There is no evidence that the radio waves produced by these devices can destroy bacteria or any living cells. Microwaves, another form of electromagnetic therapy, are used in some cancer treatment centers to heat and destroy tumor cells. High-energy radio waves can also be used to "cook" cancer cells, a process called radiofrequency ablation.

In addition, powerful electromagnetic fields (stronger and of a different type than those produced by radionic devices) may be able to change the responses of certain cells in the body. Early evidence suggests that these electromagnetic fields may help broken bones that are not healing well. Some researchers have reported that pulsed electromagnetic stimulation may reduce frequency of migraine headaches, although larger studies are needed to prove any benefit. Some early studies found that electromagnetic energy may reduce some kinds of pain, although the methods and results still need to be checked by others to learn whether they hold true. One review analyzed two studies and found that electromagnetic treatment did not seem to help heal bedsores. Scientific studies are looking at whether these powerful electromagnetic fields may help with other problems. These studies are done only in carefully controlled research settings. If they show benefit, it is possible that electromagnets may be used in conventional medicine in the future.

Are there any possible problems or complications?

Untested, unproven electrical devices may pose some risk. There have been reports of injuries due to faulty electrical wiring, power surges during lightning storms, and misuse of equipment. People with pacemakers, defibrillators, or insulin pumps should avoid exposure to electric current and magnetic fields, including electromagnets. Relying on this type of treatment alone and avoiding or delaying conventional medical care for cancer may have serious health consequences.

References

American Cancer Society. Questionable methods of cancer management: electronic devices. *CA Cancer J Clin.* 1994;44:115-127.

Barrett S. James Gary Davidson and the Monterrey Wellness Center. Quackwatch Web site. http://www.quackwatch.org/01QuackeryRelatedTopics/Cancer/davidson.html. Updated September 13, 2002. Accessed May 30, 2008.

Cassileth B. *The Alternative Medicine Handbook: The Complete Reference Guide to Alternative and Complementary Therapies.* New York: W.W. Norton; 1998.

Lescarboura AC. Our Abrams verdict: the electronic reactions of Abrams and electronic medicine in general found utterly worthless. *Scientific American.* 1924;131:158-159.

Manesh AO, Flemming K, Cullum N, Ravaghi H. Electromagnetic therapy for treating pressure ulcers. *Cochrane Database Syst Rev.* 2006;(2):CD002930.

National Institutes of Health. *Alternative Medicine: Expanding Medical Horizons: A Report to the National Institutes of Health on Alternative Medical Systems and Practices in the United States.* Washington, DC: US Government Printing Office; 1994. NIH publication 94-066.

Questions and answers about using magnets to treat pain. National Center for Complementary and Alternative Medicine Web site. http://nccam.nih.gov/health/magnet/magnet.htm. Accessed March 29, 2007.

Rubik B. Energy medicine and the unifying concept of information. *Altern Ther Health Med.* 1995;1:34-39.

Sherman RA, Acosta NM, Robson L. Treatment of migraine with pulsing electromagnetic fields: a double-blind, placebo-controlled study. *Headache.* 1999;39:567-575.

HEAT THERAPY

Other common name(s): hyperthermia, heat treatment, thermotherapy, thermal therapy
Scientific/medical name(s): none

Heat therapy as an alternative practice is different from "hyperthermia" as used in conventional clinical trials for treatment of cancer. Both types of heat therapy are discussed here.

Description

Heat therapy involves exposing part or all of the body to increased temperatures, often to enhance other forms of therapy, such as radiation and chemotherapy. Heat may be applied to affected parts of the body along with other treatments to help relieve certain kinds of pain or a few types of infections. Heat therapy may also involve injecting substances, such as DNP (chemical name 2-4-dinitrophenol), to cause a fever (see also "Coley Toxins," page 725).

Overview

Local and regional heat therapy is being studied as part of conventional treatment for some types of cancer. Heat therapy is currently being investigated, and clinical trials are studying its use alone and in combination with radiation therapy and chemotherapy. More research is needed to determine the full benefits of heat therapy in cancer treatment. The use of heat therapy for cancer treatment outside clinical trials remains questionable and is considered an alternative treatment. There are some serious complications associated with whole-body heat therapy.

The injection of unproven substances such as DNP to cause "intracellular hyperthermia" (see page 200) and fever has caused deaths. Available scientific evidence has not supported claims that this is a useful treatment for cancer.

How is it promoted for use?

There is some evidence that local and regional heat therapy may help stop cancer growth. In some cases, increasing temperature by several degrees may increase the effectiveness of radiation therapy and chemotherapy. One possible reason for this effect is that poor supply of blood and oxygen in some types of tumor cells make them resistant to chemotherapy and radiation. Heat therapy seems to help by increasing blood flow and improving the oxygen supply to the tumor, which can make the cancer cells more responsive to these medical treatments. Local and regional heat therapy is being studied as a way to improve delivery of certain drugs to the cancer.

Conventional medicine also uses lasers, radiofrequency devices, and other methods for raising temperature of tissues high enough to kill or, in some cases, even vaporize diseased tissue. Although these methods use heat, they are not considered forms of hyperthermia.

Proponents of the alternative use of heat therapy claim that it reduces or even eliminates the need for conventional treatment. They say it decreases the number of invading organisms so the immune system can handle them, acting much like a fever helping the body fight off disease.

What does it involve?

Three major types of heat therapy are being investigated by medical researchers: local, regional, and whole-body.

- Local heat therapy involves applying heat to a very small area, such as a tumor. The area may be heated externally, with high-frequency waves, or internally, using sterile probes (thin, heated wires or hollow tubes filled with warm implanted microwave antennae) and radiofrequency electrodes. The temperature of the tumor becomes high enough to rapidly kill its cells.
- In regional heat therapy, an organ or limb is heated. One method, called perfusion, involves removing the patient's blood, heating it, and then pumping it into a region to heat the region internally.
- Whole-body heat therapy is used to treat metastatic cancer (cancer that has spread). It involves the use of warm blankets, hot wax, inductive coils (similar to those used in electric blankets), or thermal chambers (similar to large incubators).

In mainstream medicine, heat is sometimes applied to the outside of the body to help relieve stiffness and pain from arthritis or other muscle and joint problems. This method may involve warm compresses, warm baths, melted paraffin, or other techniques. Heat is sometimes used with conventional therapy to help treat certain skin infections or inflammation. Warm soaks, warm compresses, and other means may be used to heat the affected area. Some of these methods are used in treatment centers, while others can be used at home.

Intracellular hyperthermia is an alternative therapy that involves the injection of a substance called DNP to produce fever. It may be used along with other types of treatment in nontraditional treatment settings.

What is the history behind it?

The first documented use of heat treatment dates back to 400 BC with Hippocrates. In 500 BC, the Greek physician Parmenides believed that if he could create fever, he could cure all illness. The early Romans used elaborate heat baths, and Native Americans have used sweat lodges in cleansing practices for centuries.

The first scientific study of heat therapy began in 1866, when M. Busch, a German physician, described a patient with a neck sarcoma that disappeared after he experienced a high fever. Similar reports were made by others twenty years later. In 1893, F. Westermark, a Swedish gynecologist, administered bacterial toxins extracted from Streptococcus and *Serratia marcescens* to cause fever, and used a coil containing hot water as a localized source of heat to treat uterine tumors. Reports followed of tumors responding to both localized and whole-body heat therapy treatments. However, the scientific evidence was weak and interest soon faded.

In the 1960s, a series of biochemical studies involving the effects of elevated temperature on normal and malignant cells were conducted using rodent cells. Based on their observations, researchers concluded that cancer cells were more sensitive to heat than normal cells. However, studies have since shown that there is little or no difference between cancer cells and normal cells in terms of their response to heat alone.

What is the evidence?

In a technique called radiofrequency ablation, very high temperatures can be used to kill cancer cells directly, but the heat is carefully controlled and precisely targeted to avoid damaging normal tissues. Radiofrequency ablation uses much higher temperatures than hyperthermia and uses electrodes to heat and destroy the cancer.

The temperatures normally used for hyperthermia (up to 113° F) are usually not hot enough to kill cancer cells unless used along with radiation therapy or chemotherapy. Many laboratory and clinical studies have shown that heat therapy can enhance the effectiveness of radiation therapy in local and regional tumor control. It can also make chemotherapy more effective for some cancers. Whole-body heat therapy is currently being studied as a method to treat illnesses that are spread throughout the body.

More research is under way on different types of chemotherapy that can be used with local and regional heat therapy as well as whole-body heat therapy. While hyperthermia is a promising way to improve cancer treatment, it is largely an experimental technique at this time and is not commonly used. Many clinical trials of hyperthermia are being done to try to find the best way to use this technique. Current studies are looking at its usefulness in treating many types of cancer.

Local heat is also applied to certain areas of the body in conventional medicine. It has been shown in clinical studies to help relieve symptoms such as arthritis pain for a short time. Its use in other medical conditions, such as small skin infections, may help speed healing. There is less high-quality evidence available on the effect of heat on infections.

There is also an unproven treatment called intracellular hyperthermia, which is based on the theory that injection of a substance called DNP into the body heats cells from the inside out. Available scientific evidence does not support these claims. The injected substance is known to be dangerous and has caused deaths.

Are there any possible problems or complications?

Heat therapy can cause internal bleeding. The high death rate and labor-intensive methods associated with whole-body heat therapy have also caused concerns. Heat therapy should only be given under careful supervision by qualified physicians. Most normal tissues are not harmed during physician-administered hyperthermia if the temperature stays below 113° F. However, the heat can be uneven, and some areas of the body can be exposed to greater heat, resulting in burns, blisters, or pain.

Heat should be used with caution in people who have anemia, heart disease, diabetes, seizure disorders, or tuberculosis, as well as in women who are pregnant and people who are sensitive to the effects of heat. Hot compresses or soaks used to help treat skin infections can spread germs to others if the container or compress is not thoroughly cleaned after use. Talk with your doctor about how to best protect others if heat is recommended for an infection. "Intracellular hyperthermia" using DNP has caused a number of deaths. DNP has long been banned by the FDA.

Relying on this type of treatment alone and avoiding or delaying conventional medical care for cancer may have serious health consequences.

References

Barrett S. Stay away from Nicholas Bachynsky and intra-cellular hyperthermia (ICHT). Quackwatch Web site. http://www.quackwatch.org/01QuackeryRelatedTopics/Cancer/ icht.html. Accessed May 30, 2008.

Dewhirst MW, Jones E, Samulski T, Vujaskovic Z, Li CY, Prosnitz L. Hyperthermia. In: Kufe DW, Bast RC, Hait WN, Hong WK, Pollock RE, Weichselbaum RR, Holland JF, Frei E, eds. *Cancer Medicine 7*. Hamilton, Ontario: BC Decker; 2006:549-561.

Hyperthermia in cancer treatment: questions and answers. National Cancer Institute Web site. http://www.cancer.gov/cancertopics/factsheet/Therapy/hyperthermia. Updated August 12, 2004. Accessed February 21, 2007.

Katschinski DM, Wiedemann GJ, Mentzel M, Mulkerin DL, Touhidi R, Robins HI. Optimization of chemotherapy administration for clinical 41.8 degrees C whole body hyperthermia. *Cancer Lett.* 1997;115: 195-199.

Nakamura Y, Xu X, Saito Y, Tateishi T, Takahashi T, Kawachi Y, Otsuka F. Deep cutaneous infection by *Fusarium solani* in a healthy child: successful treatment with local heat therapy. *J Am Acad Dermatol.* 2007;56:873-877. Epub 2006 Dec 4.

Robins HI, Rushing D, Kutz M, Tutsch KD, Tiggelaar CL, Paul D, Spriggs D, Kraemer C, Gillis W, Feierabend C, Arzoomanian RZ, Longo W, Alberti D, d'Oleire F, Qu RP, Wilding G, Stewart JA. Phase I clinical trial of melphalan and 41.8 degrees C whole-body hyperthermia in cancer patients. *J Clin Oncol.* 1997;15:158-164.

Robinson V, Brosseau L, Casimiro L, Judd M, Shea B, Wells G, Tugwell P. Thermotherapy for treating rheumatoid arthritis. *Cochrane Database Syst Rev.* 2002;(2):CD002826.

US Congress, Office of Technology Assessment. *Unconventional Cancer Treatments: OTA-H-405.* Washington, DC: US Government Printing Office; 1990.

van der Zee J. Heating the patient: a promising approach? *Ann Oncol.* 2002;13:1173-1184.

Wust P, Hildebrandt B, Sreenivasa G, Rau B, Gellermann J, Riess H, Felix R, Schlag PM. Hyperthermia in combined treatment of cancer. *Lancet Oncol.* 2002;3:487-497.

HYDROTHERAPY

Other common name(s): water therapy, balneotherapy, hydrothermal therapy
Scientific/medical name(s): none

Description

Hydrotherapy is the use of water as a medical treatment, either internally or externally.

Overview

Hydrotherapy has been proven effective in various ways. It is used as a means of physical therapy, both to promote relaxation and to relieve minor aches and pains. However, there is no evidence that any form of hydrotherapy is effective in preventing or treating cancer.

How is it promoted for use?

There are many medically accepted uses of hydrotherapy. Each involves water in the form of ice, liquid, or steam. Some of the more common examples of hydrotherapy include using water to clean wounds, use of warm moist compresses, ice packs, whirlpool or steam baths, and drinking water in order to prevent or reduce dehydration.

Warm compresses expand blood vessels, which can temporarily increase circulation, help to relax muscles, and reduce pain. Warm water in the form of a bath, Jacuzzi, or hot tub also provides relaxation and stress relief. The water vapor produced by a humidifier can reduce the discomfort of minor sore throats and colds. Warm water vapor from a sauna, hot shower, or "sweat lodge" can warm and moisten the nose and breathing passages. Hydrotherapy in the form of ice packs is used to reduce inflammation and swelling. The coldness constricts blood vessels and reduces circulation to the area, thereby decreasing fluid and swelling. The use of water for heating and cooling the body is also called hydrothermal therapy. Dehydration, which can be a serious medical problem, is treated by giving water or liquids, either by mouth or intravenously.

Hydrotherapy is also used in physical rehabilitation and exercise. When performed in water, exercises can cause less strain on the bones and joints. The water also offers resistance to movement, which helps build muscle strength.

Some claim that warm water baths or cleansing baths boost the immune system, invigorate the digestion, calm the lungs, and stimulate the mind. Streams of warm water directed at different parts of the body are claimed to help headaches, nervous disorders, paralysis, and multiple sclerosis, as well as liver, lung, and gallbladder disease.

Some proponents claim one form of hydrotherapy, which involves frequent enemas, cleanses the bowels and helps cure cancer (see "Colon Therapy," page 184).

What does it involve?

In most types of hydrotherapy, water is either directly applied to the desired area (an ice pack or a warm compress) or the body is immersed in water (a hot tub or bath). Internal means of hydrotherapy can include drinking the recommended amount of water daily, receiving an intravenous (IV) infusion, and getting a large amount of water in an enema.

In some alternative remedies, a stream of warm water is directed over a part of the body, such as the foot, back toward the heart. Or a person may be wrapped in a cold wet sheet and covered with blankets while the sheet dries. Other types of hydrotherapy may involve bathing or soaking in water that contains mud, herbs, aromatherapy oils, Epsom salts, Dead Sea salts, or other materials. Colon therapy involves introducing fluid into the colon and pulling it out again.

What is the history behind it?

Hydrotherapy has been used throughout history by many diverse cultures. Even the Old Testament mentions the healing powers of mineral waters. By the time of the ancient Greeks, the use of water as a healing agent was well established. The early Roman and Turkish baths are still popular tourist attractions today.

The modern use of hydrotherapy is linked to Vincent Preissnitz, who established the "Graefenberg cure" in the 1800s for treating almost every ailment. This treatment involved the use of water in every conceivable way, often alternating between hot and cold water.

Today, Native Americans use sweat lodges as a remedy. They believe sweating is a form of cleansing and purges poisons from the body. This belief is similar to the Scandinavians' use of saunas. Several of the springs first used by Native Americans have been converted into resorts and remain popular today. President Franklin D. Roosevelt's use of one such spring brought worldwide attention to the use of hydrotherapy.

What is the evidence?

Hydrotherapy has not been proven effective in slowing the growth or spread of cancer. Available scientific evidence does not support claims that alternative uses of hydrotherapy, such as cold body wraps or colon therapy, can cure cancer or any other disease.

Hydrotherapy is an accepted form of symptom treatment for many conditions, although many forms of it have not been studied carefully. It is often reported that hydrotherapy in many forms can promote relaxation. Some types of hydrotherapy are actually well-proven conventional therapies, such as ice packs for slight sprains and hot compresses for sore muscles. Hydrotherapy can be useful for patients with severe burns, rheumatoid arthritis, spinal cord injuries, and bone injuries. An analysis of studies done on hydrotherapy for lower back pain suggested that it might be helpful, although further studies are needed. Physical therapy is sometimes given in a pool, where the water can help to support the person's body weight and reduce impact on joints. Warm compresses or warm water soaks may be used in mainstream medicine to help treat local skin conditions, such as infection (see "Heat Therapy," page 199).

Are there any possible problems or complications?

Most forms of hydrotherapy are considered safe. However, colon therapy can cause perforation of the colon, which can lead to death. People who are frail, elderly, or very young may become dehydrated or develop blood chemistry imbalances in very warm water or saunas. People with diabetes, numbness, or poor sensation may be at higher risk for scalding or burns from hot soaks or compresses.

Those with poor circulation or problems such as Reynaud's disease or frostbite may find them worsened by cold water and cold wraps. Bacterial infection due to improperly cleaned whirlpools and hot tubs has also been reported. Fungal skin infection has resulted from mud baths. Excessively hot or cold water applied directly to the skin for long periods of time may cause pain and tissue damage.

Relying on this type of treatment alone and avoiding or delaying conventional medical care for cancer may have serious health consequences.

References

Burns SB, Burns JL. Hydrotherapy. *J Altern Complement Med.* 1997;3:105-107.

Cassileth B. *The Alternative Medicine Handbook: The Complete Reference Guide to Alternative and Complementary Therapies.* New York: W.W. Norton; 1998.

Hydrotherapy, balneotherapy. Aetna InteliHealth Web site. http://www.intelihealth.com/IH/ihtIH/WSIHW000/8513/34968/362192.html. Accessed June 2, 2008.

Pittler MH, Karagülle MZ, Karagülle M, Ernst E. Spa therapy and balneotherapy for treating low back pain: meta-analysis of randomized trials. *Rheumatology (Oxford).* 2006;45:880-884.

Ruiz de Casas A, Herrera A, Suárez AI, Camacho FM. Skin infection with Fusarium in an immunocompetent patient [in Spanish]. *Actas Dermosifiliogr.* 2006;97:278-280.

Tejirian T, Abbas MA. Sitz bath: where is the evidence? Scientific basis of a common practice. *Dis Colon Rectum.* 2005;48:2336-2340.

HYPERBARIC OXYGEN THERAPY

Other common name(s): hyperbaric medicine, hyperbarics, HBOT, HBO2
Scientific/medical name(s): none

Description

Hyperbaric oxygen therapy (HBOT) involves the breathing of pure oxygen while in a sealed chamber that has been pressurized at one and a half to three times the normal atmospheric pressure.

Overview

Research has shown HBOT is effective when used in addition to conventional treatment for the prevention and treatment of osteoradionecrosis, a term for delayed bone damage caused by radiation therapy. There is also some evidence suggesting HBOT may be helpful as an additional treatment for soft-tissue injury caused by radiation. There is no evidence that HBOT cures cancer. The U.S. Food and Drug Administration (FDA) has approved HBOT to treat decompression sickness, gangrene, brain abscess, and injuries in which tissues are not getting enough oxygen.

How is it promoted for use?

Hyperbaric oxygen therapy is used in conventional treatment for decompression sickness and severe carbon monoxide poisoning. Decompression sickness, commonly known as "the bends," is an extremely painful and potentially dangerous condition that strikes scuba divers who surface too quickly and, occasionally, miners and tunnel builders who come up too rapidly. It can also affect fighter pilots who climb very quickly.

Claims about alternative uses of HBOT include that it destroys disease-causing microorganisms, cures cancer, alleviates chronic fatigue syndrome, and decreases allergy symptoms. A few supporters also claim that HBOT helps patients with AIDS, arthritis, sports injuries, multiple sclerosis, autism, stroke, cerebral palsy, senility, cirrhosis, Lyme disease, and gastrointestinal ulcers. Available scientific evidence does not support these claims. Because of that lack of evidence, the FDA has sent a warning letter to at least one manufacturer about promoting HBOT for unproven uses. The FDA considers oxygen to be a drug, meaning it must be prescribed by a physician or licensed health care provider to treat illnesses or health conditions.

What does it involve?

HBOT can be done in single-person chambers or chambers that can hold more than a dozen people at a time. A single-person chamber, or monoplace, consists of a clear plastic tube about seven feet long. The patient lies on a padded table that slides into the tube. The chamber is gradually pressurized with pure oxygen. Patients are asked to relax and breathe normally during treatment. Chamber pressures typically rise to 2.5 times the normal atmospheric pressure. Patients may experience ear popping or mild discomfort, which usually disappears if the pressure is lowered a bit. At the end of the session, which can last from thirty minutes to two hours, technicians slowly depressurize the chamber.

After an HBOT session, patients often feel lightheaded and tired. Monoplace chambers cost less to operate than multiplace chambers and are relatively portable. Most health insurance policies cover medically approved uses of HBOT. Recently, Medicare and Medicaid have begun to cover them as well.

What is the history behind it?

In the early 1900s, Orville Cunningham noticed that people with some heart diseases did better if they lived closer to sea level than at high altitudes. He successfully treated a colleague with influenza who was near death because of lung restriction, and he later developed a hyperbaric chamber. After his attempts to use HBOT to treat a host of other conditions failed, the method was abandoned and his chamber was scrapped.

HBOT chambers were developed by the military in the 1940s to treat deep-sea divers who suffered from decompression sickness. In the 1950s, HBOT was first used during heart and lung surgery. In the 1960s, HBOT was used for carbon monoxide poisoning, and it has since been studied and used for a number of health-related applications. It has been the subject of a great deal of controversy because of the lack of scientific proof to support many of the other uses for which it is suggested.

What is the evidence?

There is strong scientific evidence showing HBOT is an effective treatment for decompression sickness, arterial gas embolism (bubbles of air in the blood vessels), and severe carbon monoxide poisoning. It may also be useful as an additional method for the prevention and treatment of osteoradionecrosis (bone damage caused by radiation therapy) and clostridial myonecrosis (a life-threatening bacterial infection that invades the muscle) and for helping skin graft and flap healing. Other evidence suggests HBOT may be helpful for less severe carbon monoxide poisoning, radiation-induced soft-tissue injury, anemia due to severe blood loss (when transfusions are not an option), crushing injuries, poor wound healing, and osteomyelitis (chronic bone inflammation) that does not respond to standard treatment. There is conflicting evidence about whether HBOT is helpful in treating burns and fast-spreading infections of the skin and underlying tissues.

The lack of randomized clinical studies makes it hard to judge the value of HBOT for many of its claims. Available scientific evidence does not support claims that HBOT stops the growth of cancer cells, destroys germs, improves allergy symptoms, or helps patients who have chronic fatigue syndrome, arthritis, multiple sclerosis, autism, stroke, cerebral palsy, senility, cirrhosis, or gastrointestinal ulcers.

Carefully controlled scientific studies are under way to find out whether HBOT may be helpful for lymphedema (swelling in arms or legs after surgery, which can happen after modified radical mastectomy or other treatments in which lymph nodes are removed or irradiated), diabetic ulcers, cluster headaches, heart attacks, and other conditions.

Are there any possible problems or complications?

HBOT is a relatively safe method for approved medical treatments. Complications can be reduced if pressures within the hyperbaric chamber remain below three times the normal atmospheric pressure and sessions last no longer than two hours.

Milder problems associated with HBOT include claustrophobia, fatigue, and headache. More serious complications include myopia (short-sightedness) that can last for weeks or months, sinus damage, ruptured middle ear, and lung damage. A complication called oxygen toxicity can result in seizures, fluid in the lungs, and even respiratory failure. Patients at high risk for oxygen toxicity may be given "air breaks" during which they breathe ordinary air rather than pure oxygen for short periods during treatment. People with severe congestive heart failure may have their symptoms worsened by HBOT. Patients with certain types of lung disease may be at higher risk for collapsed lung during HBOT. Pregnant women should be treated with HBOT only in serious situations where there are no other options. Hyperbaric oxygen chambers can also be a fire hazard: fires or explosions in hyperbaric chambers have caused about eighty deaths worldwide. Relying on this treatment alone and delaying or avoiding conventional medical care for cancer may have serious health consequences.

References

Al-Waili NS, Butler GJ, Beale J, Hamilton RW, Lee BY, Lucas P. Hyperbaric oxygen and malignancies: a potential role in radiotherapy, chemotherapy, tumor surgery and phototherapy. *Med Sci Monit.* 2005;11:RA279-RA289. Epub 2005 Aug 26.

Bennett MH, Feldmeier J, Hampson N, Smee R, Milross C. Hyperbaric oxygen therapy for late radiation tissue injury. *Cochrane Database Syst Rev.* 2005;(3):CD005005.

Bennett M, Feldmeier J, Smee R, Milross C. Hyperbaric oxygenation for tumour sensitisation to radiotherapy. *Cochrane Database Syst Rev.* 2005;(4):CD005007.

Brizel DM, Hage WD, Dodge RK, Munley MT, Piantadosi CA, Dewhirst MW. Hyperbaric oxygen improves tumor radiation response significantly more than carbogen/nicotinamide. *Radiat Res.* 1997;147:715-720.

Carl UM, Hartmann KA. Hyperbaric oxygen treatment for symptomatic breast edema after radiation therapy. *Undersea Hyperb Med.* 1998;25:233-234.

Coles C, Williams M, Burnet N. Hyperbaric oxygen therapy. Combination with radiotherapy in cancer is of proved benefit but rarely used. *BMJ.* 1999;318:1076-1077.

Heys SD, Smith IC, Ross JA, Gilbert FJ, Brooks J, Semple S, Miller ID, Hutcheon A, Sarkar T, Eremin O. A pilot study with long term follow up of hyperbaric oxygen pretreatment in patients with locally advanced breast cancer undergoing neo-adjuvant chemotherapy. *Undersea Hyperb Med.* 2006;33:33-43.

Indications for hyperbaric oxygen therapy. Undersea and Hyperbaric Medical Society Web site. http://www.uhms.org/Default.aspx?tabid=270. Accessed June 2, 2008.

Kalns J, Krock L, Piepmeier E Jr. The effect of hyperbaric oxygen on growth and chemosensitivity of metastatic prostate cancer. *Anticancer Res.* 1998;18:363-367.

Kohshi K, Kinoshita Y, Imada H, Kunugita N, Abe H, Terashima H, Tokui N, Uemura S. Effects of radiotherapy after hyperbaric oxygenation on malignant gliomas. *Br J Cancer.* 1999;80:236-241.

Landesberg R, Wilson T, Grbic JT. Bisphosphonate-associated osteonecrosis of the jaw: conclusions based on an analysis of case series. *Dent Today.* 2006;25:52, 54-57.

Leach RM, Rees PJ, Wilmshurst P. Hyperbaric oxygen therapy. *BMJ.* 1998;317:1140-1143.

London SD, Park SS, Gampper TJ, Hoard MA. Hyperbaric oxygen for the management of radionecrosis of bone and cartilage. *Laryngoscope.* 1998;108:1291-1296.

Morrison DS, Kirkby RD. Hyperbaric medicine: what works and what does not? Quackwatch Web site. http://www.quackwatch.org/01QuackeryRelatedTopics/HBOT/hmindex.html. Updated July 5, 2001. Accessed May 30, 2008.

Neheman A, Nativ O, Moskovitz B, Melamed Y, Stein A. Hyperbaric oxygen therapy for radiation-induced haemorrhagic cystitis. *BJU Int.* 2005;96:107-109.

Neumeister M. Hyperbaric oxygen therapy. E-Medicine Web site. http://www.emedicine.com/plastic/topic526.htm. Updated July 21, 2005. Accessed May 30, 2008.

Niezgoda JA, Cianci P, Folden BW, Ortega RL, Slade JB, Storrow AB. The effect of hyperbaric oxygen therapy on a burn wound model in human volunteers. *Plast Reconstr Surg.* 1997;99:1620-1625.

Tibbles PM, Edelsberg JS. Hyperbaric-oxygen therapy. *N Engl J Med.* 1996;334:1642-1648.

Warning letter. US Food and Drug Administration Web site. http://www.fda.gov/foi/warning_letters/m5272n.pdf. Accessed May 17, 2005. Content no longer available.

Woo TC, Joseph D, Oxer H. Hyperbaric oxygen treatment for radiation proctitis. *Int J Radiat Oncol Biol Phys.* 1997;38:619-622.

LIGHT THERAPY

Other common name(s):

light boxes, bright light treatment, ultraviolet light therapy, UV, ultraviolet blood irradiation, colored light therapy, chromatotherapy

Scientific/medical name(s):

phototherapy, ultraviolet phototherapy, photopheresis, extracorporeal photochemotherapy, photodynamic therapy

Description

Light therapy involves the use of visible light or nonvisible ultraviolet light to treat a variety of conditions.

Overview

Some forms of light therapy, such as light boxes, ultraviolet (UV) light therapy, and photodynamic therapy, are used in conventional medicine. However, available scientific evidence does not support claims that alternative uses of light or color therapy are effective in treating cancer or curing other illnesses.

How is it promoted for use?

Conventional medicine professionals may prescribe the use of light boxes, photopheresis, photodynamic therapy, or UV light therapy for the treatment of conditions for which studies have shown the methods to be safe and effective. For example, the use of light boxes to mimic sunlight is a proven medical treatment for seasonal affective disorder (SAD). Ultraviolet light therapy is used to treat psoriasis and cutaneous T-cell lymphoma (a type of cancer that first appears on the skin). Photodynamic therapy is helpful in treating certain cancers or precancers of the skin, esophagus, and lungs and is now being tested against other types of cancer. A special form of UV blood irradiation, called photopheresis or extracorporeal photochemotherapy, also inhibits T-cell lymphoma and may be helpful for other conditions.

However, several types of light therapy are also promoted for alternative uses. These include light boxes (or special bright lamps and visors), UV light or sun lamp therapy, most types of colored light therapy (chromatotherapy), and UV blood irradiation.

Colored light therapy: Supporters of colored light therapy (also called chromatotherapy) claim that colored light relieves a number of conditions, including sleep disorders, shoulder pain, diabetes, impotence, and allergies. Practitioners of one system of chromatotherapy believe that shining colored lights on the body harms cancer cells.

Light box therapy: Light box therapy is also sometimes called bright light therapy and can employ light boxes, bright lamps, or light visors. Proponents claim it relieves high blood pressure, insomnia, premenstrual syndrome, migraine headaches, carbohydrate cravings, and hyperactivity in children and that it improves sexual functioning.

Ultraviolet light: Proponents of UV light therapy, which is sometimes marketed as sun lamps, claim that it neutralizes toxins in the body and cures or helps immune system disorders, bacterial infections, AIDS, colds, bug bites, and cancer.

Ultraviolet blood irradiation: Proponents of UV blood irradiation claim that UV light exposure kills germs such as viruses, bacteria, and fungi inside the body and that it neutralizes toxins in the blood. Some claim that even a small amount of UV-treated blood can reenter the circulatory system of the patient and stimulate the immune system to increase attacks against invaders, including cancer cells.

What does it involve?

Colored light therapy involves the use of colored lights, such as blue, red, and violet lights, that the practitioner shines directly on the patient. In some cases, the patient purchases the device and uses it at home. Sometimes the lights flash in patterns.

One type of colored light therapy is used in conventional medicine for newborns who have a buildup of a waste product called bilirubin in the blood. The infant's skin is exposed to a special blue light, usually for several days. The blue light helps the bilirubin to break down into a substance that is easier for the baby to excrete.

Light boxes contain lights that simulate the wavelengths of sunlight. Patients undergoing this kind of therapy sit in front of the light box or special bright lamp for a prescribed amount of time each day. The person may read or do other tasks during the light exposure, but must sit close enough to the light to receive its full effect. The amount of time required will vary according to the person and the strength of light being used. For most people with SAD, light treatment is used early in the morning for a period of thirty minutes to two hours each day. A brighter light may require less time exposure.

In **ultraviolet light therapy**, the eyes and unaffected skin are protected while the patient is exposed to UV light for a prescribed length of time. Conventional treatment for psoriasis may involve the use of UV light and drugs that make one's skin sensitive to the light. A new type of UV light, called narrow-band UV light, is also being used now and may be more effective.

Ultraviolet blood irradiation is called photopheresis or extracorporeal photochemotherapy in conventional medicine and is mainly used to inhibit T-cell lymphoma. It may also be helpful for other conditions. During this procedure, blood is removed from the patient and separated into different types of cells. About a pint of blood, mostly white blood cells, is treated with a special drug to make it make it more sensitive to light. It is then treated with UV light, and the blood is infused back into the patient. This procedure is considered a form of immunotherapy and takes from three to five hours. In the alternative treatment setting, a small tube of blood is removed, treated with UV rays, and infused back into the patient.

Photodynamic therapy is used in conventional medicine for certain types of cancer. The patient is given a drug to make cancer cells more sensitive to light. The tumor area is then exposed to laser or another type of light.

What is the history behind it?

Interest in the relationship between light and health dates back centuries. All forms of light therapy now in use started during the twentieth century. The first reports of ultraviolet blood irradiation date back to the 1930s.

What is the evidence?

Available scientific evidence does not support claims that light box therapy can cure cancer; however, it does have some medically accepted uses. Light box therapy has been shown to be effective in treating SAD, a type of depression caused by insufficient exposure to bright light. Some researchers are testing light therapy to see whether it helps other types of depression. Early findings suggest it may be helpful given alone or with medicines. It may also be helpful for shift workers and those traveling to different time zones in helping to reset their internal clocks.

Ultraviolet light therapy (phototherapy) is commonly used to treat psoriasis. There is also evidence that UV light therapy inhibits the growth of cutaneous T-cell lymphoma. Researchers have found that it has resulted in long-term remission and cure among many patients in the early stage of the disease and prolonged survival even in patients treated in the later stages of disease. Early studies suggest that it may also be helpful for people with atopic dermatitis (an allergic skin condition) and vitiligo (uneven pigment in the skin). However, available scientific evidence does not support other health claims for UV light therapy.

Colored light therapy has been advocated since the early twentieth century for nearly every imaginable purpose. At least one maker of spectro-chrome (color) therapy devices has been prosecuted for making false claims. However, blue light has been used for years to treat newborns with high bilirubin levels and has proven to be very effective. The light helps to break down the bilirubin into a form that is easier to excrete from the body. At this time, available scientific evidence does not support claims that any other type of colored light therapy is effective in treating cancer or other illnesses.

Ultraviolet blood irradiation treatment is approved by the U.S. Food and Drug Administration (FDA) for treating T-cell lymphoma involving the skin. Photopheresis is sometimes used conventionally when organ transplant rejection or graft-versus-host disease (a complication related to bone marrow or stem cell transplants) does not respond to usual medical treatments. Some clinical trial results look promising for the treatment of immune system diseases such as multiple sclerosis, systemic sclerosis, rheumatoid arthritis, lupus, and type 1 diabetes. Available scientific evidence does not support claims for alternative uses of UV blood irradiation.

Are there any possible problems or complications?

Light therapy that involves only visible light (light boxes and colored light therapy) is generally considered safe. Light therapy for depressive disorders can push a few people into a hyperactive state called mania, which may pose some risk. Light or light box therapy should not be confused with a tanning bed or sun lamp, which is not a medical therapy and is dangerous because of high levels of ultraviolet radiation. Any treatment that exposes the patient to ultraviolet radiation presents some danger, including premature aging of the skin and an increased risk for skin cancer later in life.

Patients may be at higher risk for sunburn the day of UV treatment and are advised to avoid natural sunlight. Those having long-term UV light treatment for psoriasis or other conditions may have a greater-than-average number of cataracts and skin-related problems, including cancer.

Relying on unproven uses of light therapy while delaying or avoiding conventional therapy for cancer can have serious health consequences.

References

American Cancer Society. Questionable methods of cancer management: electronic devices. *CA Cancer J Clin.* 1994;44:115-127.

Boivin DB, James FO. Light treatment and circadian adaptation to shift work. *Ind Health.* 2005;43:34-48.

Cassileth B. *The Alternative Medicine Handbook: The Complete Reference Guide to Alternative and Complementary Therapies.* New York: W.W. Norton; 1998.

Gambichler T, Breuckmann F, Boms S, Altmeyer P, Kreuter A. Narrowband UVB phototherapy in skin conditions beyond psoriasis. *J Am Acad Dermatol.* 2005;52:660-670.

Golden RN, Gaynes BN, Ekstrom RD, Hamer RM, Jacobsen FM, Suppes T, Wisner KL, Nemeroff CB. The efficacy of light therapy in the treatment of mood disorders: a review and meta-analysis of the evidence. *Am J Psychiatry.* 2005;162:656-662.

Herrmann JJ, Roenigk HH Jr, Hönigsmann H. Ultraviolet radiation for treatment of cutaneous T-cell lymphoma. *Hematol Oncol Clin North Am.* 1995;9:1077-1088.

Ilhan O, Arat M, Arslan O, Ayyildiz E, Sanli H, Beksac M, Ozcan M, Gürman G, Akan H. Extracorporeal photoimmunotherapy for the treatment of steroid refractory progressive chronic graft-versus-host disease. *Transfus Apher Sci.* 2004;30:185-187.

Knobler R, Girardi M. Extracorporeal photochemoimmunotherapy in cutaneous T cell lymphomas. *Ann N Y Acad Sci.* 2001;941:123-138.

Lurie SJ, Gawinski B, Pierce D, Rousseau SJ. Seasonal affective disorder. *Am Fam Physician.* 2006;74:1521-1524.

Marques MB, Tuncer HH. Photopheresis in solid organ transplant rejection. *J Clin Apher.* 2006; 21:72-77.

McGinnis KS, Shapiro M, Vittorio CC, Rook AH, Junkins-Hopkins JM. Psoralen plus long-wave UV-A (PUVA) and bexarotene therapy: an effective and synergistic combined adjunct to therapy for patients with advanced cutaneous T-cell lymphoma. *Arch Dermatol.* 2003;139:771-775.

Photodynamic therapy for cancer: questions and answers. National Cancer Institute Web site. http://www.cancer.gov/cancertopics/factsheet/Therapy/photodynamic. Updated May 12, 2004. Accessed May 30, 2008.

PUVA. National Psoriasis Foundation Web site. http://www.psoriasis.org/treatment/psoriasis/phototherapy/puva.php. Accessed June 2, 2008.

Schwarcz J. Colorful nonsense: Dinshah Ghadiali and his spectro-chrome device. Quackwatch Web site. http://www.quackwatch.org/01QuackeryRelatedTopics/spectro.html. Updated July 10, 2003. Accessed May 30, 2008.

Triesscheijn M, Baas PM, Schellens JH, Stewart FA. Photodynamic therapy in oncology. *Oncologist.* 2006;11:1034-1044.

UVB phototherapy. National Psoriasis Foundation Web site. http://www.psoriasis.org/treatment/psoriasis/phototherapy/uvb.php. Accessed May 30, 2008.

Woltz P, Castro K, Park BJ. Care for patients undergoing extracorporeal photopheresis to treat chronic graft-versus-host disease: review of the evidence. *Clin J Oncol Nurs.* 2006;10:795-802.

MAGNETIC THERAPY

Other common name(s): magnetic field therapy, magnet therapy, bioenergy therapy
Scientific/medical name(s): none

Description

Magnetic therapy involves the use of magnets of varying sizes and strengths that are placed on the body to relieve pain and treat disease.

Overview

Although there are anecdotal reports of healing with magnetic therapy, available scientific evidence does not support these claims. The U.S. Food and Drug Administration (FDA) considers magnets harmless and of no use for medical purposes.

How is it promoted for use?

Many claims about magnetic therapy are based on the fact that some cells and tissues in the human body give off electromagnetic impulses. Some practitioners think the presence of illness or injury disrupts these fields. Magnets produce energy fields of different strengths, which proponents believe can penetrate the human body, correcting disturbances and restoring health to the afflicted systems, organs, and cells. Most magnets marketed to consumers are static magnets, also called constant magnets, because the magnetic field doesn't change. They are usually made of magnetized metal or lodestone. Static magnets are different from electromagnets, which have an energy field only while electricity is passing through them (see "Electromagnetic Therapy," page 194).

Proponents claim magnetic therapy can relieve pain caused by arthritis, headaches, migraines, and stress and can also heal broken bones, improve circulation, reverse degenerative diseases, and cure cancer. They also claim that placing magnets over areas of pain or disease strengthens the body's healing ability. Some believe that magnetic fields increase blood flow, alter nerve impulses, increase the flow of oxygen to cells, decrease fatty deposits on artery walls, and realign thought patterns to improve emotional well-being.

Proponents of magnetic therapy assert that magnetic fields produced from the negative pole of the magnet have healing powers. Negative magnetic fields are thought to stimulate metabolism, increase the amount of oxygen available to cells, and create a less acidic environment within the body. Because many people who use magnets believe cancer cells cannot thrive when acid is low, they claim that the effects of negative magnetic fields can halt or reverse the spread of tumors. For the same reasons, they believe that negative magnetic fields speed the healing of cuts, broken bones, and infections and that they counter the effects of toxic chemicals, addictive drugs, and other harmful substances.

What does it involve?

Magnetic therapy involves the use of thin metal magnets attached to the body alone or in groups. They are sometimes mounted on bracelets and necklaces or attached to adhesive patches that hold them in place. Some magnets are placed in bands or belts that can be wrapped around the wrist, elbow, knee, ankle, foot, waist, or lower back. There are even magnetic insoles, blankets, and slumber pads. These magnets may be worn for just a few minutes or for weeks, depending on the condition being treated and the practitioner.

What is the history behind it?

Interest in magnets as a source of healing dates back many centuries. A sixteenth century physician, Paracelsus, thought that because magnets attract iron, they might attract and eliminate diseases from the body. In the Middle Ages, doctors used magnets to treat gout, arthritis, poisoning, and baldness. The modern version of magnet therapy reportedly began in the 1970s, when researcher Albert Roy Davis, PhD, noticed that positive and negative magnetic charges had different effects on human biological systems. He claimed that magnets could kill cancer cells in animals and could also cure arthritis pain, glaucoma, infertility, and other conditions. Magnetic therapy has recently become a large industry in the United States and Europe and has been used widely in Japan and China for many years.

What is the evidence?

Magnetic therapy has undergone some scientific study. Most of the success stories have come from a few isolated sources who have not provided proof that the treatment actually works. One small but well-publicized randomized clinical trial conducted at the Baylor College of Medicine concluded that the permanent placement of small magnets reduced pain in people who had recovered from polio. However, several aspects of the study's methods have been criticized (for example, characteristics of patients in the two groups differed in ways that might have influenced their susceptibility to placebo effects). In addition, the study looked only at short-term results and was intended to be a pilot study. Pilot studies are done only to decide whether it is worthwhile to do larger studies. To date, larger studies have not been done.

To test the claim of improved blood flow, one study compared magnets and otherwise identical nonmagnetic disks on the arms of healthy volunteers. The researchers measured blood flow and found no difference between the real and fake magnets.

Clinical trials of static magnets for pain relief have generally had mixed results. One review noted that about half the studies found that magnets improved pain, and the other half did not. However, it has been difficult to conduct studies that exclude placebo effects because patients are generally able to tell whether their bracelet or patch is magnetic (as it attracts metallic objects like paperclips). Studies of electromagnets appear to be more promising (see "Electromagnetic Therapy," page 194).

We are not aware of any published clinical studies involving magnets as an anticancer treatment and know of only one study specifically involving cancer survivors. Researchers from the Vanderbilt University School of Nursing placed either magnets or nonmagnetic (placebo) objects at six acupressure points in breast cancer survivors suffering from hot flashes. The magnets were no more effective in reducing hot flash severity and turned out to be less effective in decreasing hot flash frequency, bother, interference with daily activities, and overall quality of life.

The FDA has not approved the marketing of magnets with claims of health benefits. In fact, the FDA and the Federal Trade Commission have taken action against several makers and sellers of magnets because they were making health claims that had not been proven.

Are there any possible problems or complications?

According to the FDA, magnets used for magnetic therapy are generally considered safe. However, implantable medical devices such as pacemakers, defibrillators, or infusion pumps may be adversely affected by magnets.

Relying on this type of treatment alone and avoiding or delaying conventional medical care for cancer may have serious health consequences.

References

Barrett S. Magnet therapy: a skeptical view. Quackwatch Web site. http://www.quackwatch.org/04ConsumerEducation/QA/magnet.html. Accessed May 30, 2008.

Cepeda MS, Carr DB, Sarquis T, Miranda N, Garcia RJ, Zarate C. Static magnetic therapy does not decrease pain or opioid requirements: a randomized double-blind trial. *Anesth Analg.* 2007;104:290-294.

Finegold L, Flamm BL. Magnet therapy. *BMJ.* 2006;332:4.

Questions and answers about using magnets to treat pain. National Center for Complementary and Alternative Medicine Web site. http://nccam.nih.gov/health/magnet/magnet.htm. Accessed June 20, 2008.

Ratterman R, Secrest J, Norwood B, Ch'ien AP. Magnet therapy: what's the attraction? *J Am Acad Nurse Pract.* 2002;14:347-353.

MASSAGE

Other common name(s):
Swedish massage, sports massage, deep tissue massage, myotherapy, massage therapy, therapeutic massage, neuromuscular therapy, trigger point massage, trigger point therapy
Scientific/medical name(s): none

Description

Massage involves manipulation, rubbing, and kneading of the muscles and soft tissue to enhance function of those tissues and promote relaxation.

Overview

Studies of massage for cancer patients suggest massage can decrease stress, anxiety, depression, pain, and fatigue. Many health care professionals recognize massage as a useful, noninvasive addition to standard medical treatment. Therapeutic massage is most often given by trained massage therapists. Caregivers can also be trained in safe massage techniques.

How is it promoted for use?

Massage is recommended by some health care professionals as a complementary therapy. Supporters believe massage can help reduce stress, anxiety, and pain in people who have serious illnesses such as cancer. It is also known to help relax muscles. Many people find that massage brings a temporary feeling of well-being and relaxation. Massage is also used to relieve pain and stiffness, increase mobility, rehabilitate injured muscles, and reduce the pain of headaches and backaches.

Some practitioners claim massage raises the body's production of endorphins (chemicals believed to improve overall mood) and flushes the waste product lactic acid out of muscles. Proponents also claim massage promotes recovery from fatigue produced by excessive exercise, breaks up scar tissue, loosens mucus in the lungs, promotes sinus drainage, and helps arthritis, colds, and constipation.

Proponents claim a type of massage called myotherapy can reduce 95 percent of all muscle-related pain and, in some cases, can take the place of pain-relieving drugs. They say the techniques used in myotherapy relax muscles and improve muscle strength, flexibility, and coordination; relieve pain; reduce the need for pain medications; increase blood circulation; improve stamina and sleep patterns; and correct posture imbalances.

What does it involve?

There are many types of massage, including Swedish massage, sports massage, neuromuscular therapy, myotherapy, and others (see also "Acupressure, Shiatsu, and Other Asian Bodywork," page 151, and "Myofascial Release," page 226). Swedish massage is one of the most common types of massage used in the United States today, although most massage therapists combine a number of different styles and techniques.

In all forms of massage, therapists use their hands (and sometimes forearms, elbows, and massage tools) to manipulate the body's soft tissue. Massage strokes can vary from light and shallow to firm and deep and from slow steady pressure to quick tapping. The type of massage stroke will depend on the health and needs of the individual and the training and style of the massage therapist. During active treatment for cancer, special considerations may apply (see page 221).

Swedish massage uses several techniques to apply pressure to muscles in order to relax them and encourage circulation. Deep tissue massage focuses on deep layers of muscle tissue and connective tissue with the goal of releasing chronic tension or tightness. Sports massage is used in different ways depending on the sport, but the overall goals are to reduce fatigue and improve mobility.

Myotherapy and neuromuscular therapy focus on finding "trigger points" and use techniques such as deep pressure to reduce them. Trigger points are abnormally sensitive, highly irritable knots of tight muscle tissue that may cause pain or limit range of motion. These types of massage are also called trigger point therapies.

Massage usually takes place on a massage table. The client may wear minimal clothing and be covered by a sheet, light blanket, or towel. Oils or lotions are often used to keep friction from irritating the skin. Typical massage therapy sessions last from thirty minutes to one hour. Massage therapists often play soothing music and use dim lighting to increase relaxation and comfort.

Some massages take place with the client fully clothed and seated on a massage chair. Chair massage focuses on the head, neck, shoulders, back, arms, and hands. These massages tend to last fifteen to thirty minutes.

Many hospitals and cancer centers now offer massage to cancer patients. When provided to patients undergoing inpatient procedures, these massages generally last a shorter time.

What is the history behind it?

Massage has been used in many ancient cultures, including those of China, India, Persia, Arabia, Greece, and Egypt. Chinese texts dating back to 2700 BC recommended massage and other types of body movements as treatments for paralysis, chills, and fever. Hippocrates, known as the father of western medicine, recommended massage for sports and war injuries.

Swedish massage, one of the most common forms of massage used today in the United States, is usually attributed to the nineteenth century Swedish physician Per Henrik Ling. A number of writings from the late 1800s discuss techniques that have been incorporated into what we call Swedish massage.

Trigger point therapy was developed as a result of the work of Janet Travell, MD, and colleagues in the 1940s. Travell developed a technique called trigger point injections, in which pain-relieving drugs are injected directly into the tender area of painful muscles. Later therapists noted that external pressure could help relieve trigger point pain without injections. Neuromuscular techniques emerged during the last half-century in Europe and North America.

In 1992, massage therapists set up the National Certification Board for Therapeutic Massage and Bodywork so that their qualifications could be standardized and officially recognized. A person who completes required training and passes the Board's exam can say that he or she is Nationally Certified in Therapeutic Massage and Bodywork (NCTMB). In 2005, the board created a new level of certification, which allows a person to call himself or herself Nationally Certified in Therapeutic Massage (NCTM). The newer title requires the same basic knowledge as the NCTMB certification, but the person is tested on fewer types of massage. Both credentials must be renewed every four years through continuing education and practice. The massage therapists' certifying board is recognized by the National Commission for Certifying Agencies.

In addition, massage therapists have asked state legislatures to require licensing so that untrained people cannot call themselves massage therapists. According to the U.S. Department of Labor, thirty-eight states and the District of Columbia now regulate massage therapists. Certification and licensure make it easier to find a professional massage therapist.

What is the evidence?

While massage appears promising for symptom management and improving quality of life, available scientific evidence does not support claims that massage slows or reverses the growth or spread of cancer. A growing number of health care professionals recognize massage as a useful addition to conventional medical treatment. In a 1999 publication, the National Cancer Institute found that about half of their cancer centers offered massage as an adjunctive therapy to cancer treatment. Some studies of massage for cancer patients suggest that it can decrease stress, anxiety, depression, pain, and fatigue. These potential benefits hold great promise for people who have cancer, who often must deal with the stresses of a serious illness in addition to unpleasant side effects of conventional medical treatment. While some evidence from research studies with cancer patients supports the use of massage for short-term symptom relief, additional research is needed to find out whether there are measurable, long-term physical or psychological benefits.

Meanwhile, most patients do indeed seem to feel better after massage, which may result in substantial relief. A 2005 review of research reported that massage therapy has been shown to reduce pain and anxiety in randomized controlled trials. Large, well-controlled studies are still needed to determine the long-term health benefits of massage.

Are there any possible problems or complications?

People with rheumatoid arthritis, cancer that has spread to the bone, spine injuries, osteoporosis, or other bone diseases that could be worsened by physical manipulation should avoid physical manipulation or deep pressure. Manipulation of a bone in an area of cancer metastasis could result in a bone fracture. Also, people who have had radiation may find even light touch on the treatment area to be uncomfortable. A few people have allergic reactions to lotions or oils used during massage, and this may be more common among patients receiving radiation treatment. People with cancer and chronic conditions such as arthritis and heart disease should consult their physicians before undergoing any type of therapy that involves manipulation of joints and muscles. It is important that massage be given by trained massage therapists and that the massage therapist know about your cancer and its treatment. Generally, gentle massage and bodywork can be adapted to meet the needs of cancer patients.

Another concern for people who have cancer is that tissue manipulation in the area of a tumor might increase the risk that cancer cells will travel to other parts of the body. It may be prudent for cancer patients to avoid massage near tumors and lumps that could be cancerous until this question is clearly answered.

Patients with low blood platelet counts (a common side effect of chemotherapy) or who are taking blood-thinning medication such as warfarin (Coumadin) may be susceptible to easy bruising and should ask their doctor whether massage is safe for them.

It is important for people who have cancer to let their health care providers know they are receiving massage. Massage should be provided by a trained professional with expertise in working safely with people with cancer and with cancer survivors. Family members and other caregivers can be instructed in certain massage techniques as well. Relying on this treatment alone and delaying or avoiding conventional medical care for cancer may have serious health consequences.

References

Ahles TA, Tope DM, Pinkson B, Walch S, Hann D, Whedon M, Dain B, Weiss JE, Mills L, Silberfarb PM. Massage therapy for patients undergoing autologous bone marrow transplantation. *J Pain Symptom Manage.* 1999;18:157-163.

Bass SS, Cox CE, Salud CJ, Lyman GH, McCann C, Dupont E, Berman C, Reintgen DS. The effects of postinjection massage on the sensitivity of lymphatic mapping in breast cancer. *J Am Coll Surg.* 2001;192:9-16.

Calvert RN. Pages from history: Swedish massage. Massage Magazine Web site. http://www.massagemag.com/Magazine/2002/issue100/history100.php. Accessed June 2, 2008.

Cassileth B, Vickers AJ. Massage therapy for symptom control: outcome study at a major cancer center. *J Pain Symptom Manage.* 2004; 28:244-249.

Corley MC, Ferriter J, Zeh J, Gifford C. Physiological and psychological effects of back rubs. *Appl Nurs Res.* 1995;8:39-42.

Deng G, Cassileth BR. Integrative oncology: complementary therapies for pain, anxiety, and mood disturbance. *CA Cancer J Clin.* 2005;55:109-116.

Fellowes D, Barnes K, Wilkinson S. Aromatherapy and massage for symptom relief in patients with cancer. *Cochrane Database Syst Rev.* 2004;(2):CD002287.

Hernandez-Reif M, Ironson G, Field T, Hurley J, Katz G, Diego M, Weiss S, Fletcher MA, Schanberg S, Kuhn C, Burman I. Breast cancer patients have improved immune and neuroendocrine functions following massage therapy. *J Psychosom Res.* 2004;57:45-52.

Manipulation & body-based methods: massage & related bodywork. Complementary/Integrative Medicine Education Resources, The University of Texas M. D. Anderson Cancer Center Web site. http://www.mdanderson.org/departments/CIMER/display.cfm?id=254B81AA-6D52-42D3-94DDF74AC23EFEC4&method=displayFull. Accessed June 20, 2008.

Manipulative and body-based practices: an overview. National Center for Complementary and Alternative Medicine Web site. http://nccam.nih.gov/health/backgrounds/manipulative.htm. Accessed June 13, 2007.

Massage therapy as CAM. National Center for Complementary and Alternative Medicine Web site. http://nccam.nih.gov/health/massage/. Accessed December 9, 2006.

Occupational Outlook Handbook, 2006–07 Edition. Massage therapists. US Department of Labor, Bureau of Labor Statistics Web site. http://www.bls.gov/oco/ocos295.htm. Accessed April 2, 2007.

Post-White J, Kinney ME, Savik KS, Gau JB, Wilcox C, Lerner I. Therapeutic massage and healing touch improve symptoms in cancer. *Integr Cancer Ther.* 2003;2:332-344.

Rosser RJ. Sentinel lymph nodes and postinjection massage: it is premature to reject caution. *J Am Coll Surg.* 2001;193:338-339.

Smith MC, Kemp J, Hemphill L, Vojir CP. Outcomes of therapeutic massage for hospitalized cancer patients. *J Nurs Scholarsh.* 2002;34:257-262.

Weinrich SP, Weinrich MC. The effect of massage on pain in cancer patients. *Appl Nurs Res.* 1990;3:140-145.

MOXIBUSTION

Other common name(s): acumoxa, auricular mo, moxabustion
Scientific/medical name(s): none

Description

Moxibustion is the application of heat resulting from the burning of a small bundle of tightly bound herbs, or moxa, to targeted acupoints. It is used along with acupuncture (see "Acupuncture," page 156).

Overview

Available scientific evidence does not support claims that moxibustion is effective in preventing or treating cancer or any other disease. Oils from the herbs used in moxibustion are dangerous if consumed.

How is it promoted for use?

Moxibustion is a practice of both traditional Chinese and Tibetan medicine that stimulates acupoints in order to promote the body's ability to heal itself. Practitioners claim the radiant heat produced by moxibustion penetrates deeply into the body, restoring the balance and flow of vital energy or life force called qi or chi. Moxibustion is promoted for improving general health and treating cancer and chronic conditions such as arthritis, digestive disorders, and ulcers.

What does it involve?

Moxibustion involves the burning of moxa, which is created by gathering dried leaves from mugwort or wormwood plants and forming them into a small cone or cigar-like shape (see "Mugwort," page 432, and "Wormwood," page 571). The two main types of moxibustion are direct and indirect.

In its earliest uses, direct moxibustion was most often applied over the acupuncture point, with the moxa cone placed directly on the skin. However, this often produced pain and scarring. Some Chinese traditions still deliberately induce scarring, although that technique is not usually done in the United States.

Indirect moxibustion, the method most commonly used today, involves either burning the moxa on top of an acupuncture needle or applying heat to needle points from an electrical source. Other practitioners hold the burning moxa above the skin for a few minutes or place a layer of ginger, garlic, or salt on the person's skin, with the burning moxa on top of it. For people who have asthma or respiratory problems, smokeless moxa can be used.

Other kinds of moxibustion include burnt match moxibustion, in which the practitioner taps one or two acupoints on the ear rapidly with the head of a burnt match; thread incense moxibustion, in which the practitioner burns thin strips of moxa; and warm needle moxibustion, which involves the use of acupuncture needles that have been heated with a match or lighter.

What is the history behind it?

Moxibustion evolved thousands of years ago in early northern China. It is part of traditional Chinese medical practices and came about at the same time as acupuncture. In such a cold, mountainous region, heating the body on energetically active points was thought to be effective for preventing illness and promoting healing. Chinese medicine practitioners currently use moxibustion in some parts of the United States.

What is the evidence?

In general, most studies that have looked at moxibustion have not followed rigorous scientific guidelines to be sure that the outcomes were due to the moxibustion treatment. It is also difficult to find studies where moxibustion is used without acupuncture so that its effect can be evaluated alone.

A Chinese study of 230 women in the 1990s suggested that moxibustion may have helped some fetuses in breech (bottom-first) position return to a normal, head-first position before birth. In the study, 75 percent of the babies in the moxibustion group were born in the normal position, as opposed to 62 percent of those in the control group. Other studies have had similar findings. Further research is needed to be sure of the procedure's safety and its effects.

In general, most studies that have looked at moxibustion have not followed rigorous scientific guidelines to be sure that the outcomes were due to the moxibustion treatment. For example, a 2005 review concluded that only three of eleven published studies of moxibustion and breech delivery provided useful clinical evidence and that although these studies suggested moxibustion might be useful, there was "… insufficient evidence to support the use of moxibustion to correct a breech presentation" (*Cochrane Database Syst Rev*. 2005;2:D003928).

Other research in China has examined the use of moxibustion in asthma and ulcerative colitis (chronic inflammation of the colon). A small study of moxibustion and acupuncture found that this approach was not helpful in treating obesity.

There have been no human studies on the effects of moxibustion and cancer; however, a study in Taiwan found that mice with tumors that had been treated with moxibustion lived longer than mice with tumors that had not. Further studies are needed to determine whether the results apply to humans.

Are there any possible problems or complications?

Direct moxibustion can burn the skin. Oils from mugwort and wormwood can cause toxic reactions if taken internally, although their toxicity is much lower when applied externally. Mugwort is on the Commission E (Germany's regulatory agency for herbs) list of unapproved herbs. This means that it is not recommended for internal use because it has not been proven to be safe or effective and because of the possibility that it may cause miscarriage in pregnant women. Moxibustion can result in burns and may be dangerous for diabetic patients because of reduced sensation and problems with infection.

Relying on this type of treatment alone and avoiding or delaying conventional medical care for cancer may have serious health consequences.

References

Cardini F, Weixin H. Moxibustion for correction of breech presentation: a randomized controlled trial. *JAMA.* 1998;280:1580-1584.

Cassileth B. *The Alternative Medicine Handbook: The Complete Reference Guide to Alternative and Complementary Therapies.* New York: W. W. Norton; 1998.

Coyle ME, Smith CA, Peat B. Cephalic version by moxibustion for breech presentation. *Cochrane Database Syst Rev.* 2005;(2):CD003928.

Gruenwald J. *PDR for Herbal Medicines.* 3rd ed. Montvale, NJ: Thomson PDR; 2004.

Hau DM, Lin IH, Lin JG, Chang YH, Lin CH. Therapeutic effects of moxibustion on experimental tumor. *Am J Chin Med.* 1999;27:157-166.

Jarvis WT. How quackery harms cancer patients. Quackwatch Web site. http://www.quackwatch.org/01QuackeryRelatedTopics/harmquack.html. Accessed June 2, 2008.

Mazzoni R, Mannucci E, Rizzello SM, Ricca V, Rotella CM. Failure of acupuncture in the treatment of obesity: a pilot study. *Eat Weight Disord.* 1999;4:198-202.

Moxibustion. Acupuncture Today Web site. http://www.acupuncturetoday.com/abc/moxibustion.php. Accessed May 30, 2008.

National Institutes of Health. *Alternative Medicine: Expanding Medical Horizons: A Report to the National Institutes of Health on Alternative Medical Systems and Practices in the United States.* Washington, DC: US Government Printing Office; 1994. NIH publication 94-066.

Wu H, Chen H, Hua X, Shi Z, Zhang L, Chen J. Clinical therapeutic effect of drug-separated moxibustion on chronic diarrhea and its immunologic mechanisms. *J Tradit Chin Med.* 1997;17:253-258.

MYOFASCIAL RELEASE

Other common name(s): none
Scientific/medical name(s): none

Description

Myofascial release is a bodywork technique that focuses on the body's fascia, a connective tissue system that weaves through the entire body. Practitioners use manual massage techniques with the goal of relieving pain and increasing range of motion.

Overview

There is little scientific evidence available to support proponents' claims that myofascial release relieves pain or restores flexibility. A small preliminary study found that it seemed to help chronic pain related to prostatitis, but additional research is needed.

How is it promoted for use?

Myofascial release is promoted to restore flexibility and relieve pain. According to practitioners of myofascial release, poor posture, injury, illness, or stress can negatively affect the body's alignment and cause fascia to become restricted. They believe that these effects can cause pain and impair movement. A gentle form of stretching and manual compression is said to restore flexibility to this connective tissue and provide relief from fascial restrictions and pain.

What does it involve?

Fascia is a connective tissue system that weaves through the entire body. Sheets of this fibrous material surround muscles, joints, nerves, blood vessels, and organs. Fascia is flexible but has limited stretch, and it provides support and protection for softer tissues. There are two main schools of myofascial release: the direct and indirect method, depending on whether the fascia is manipulated directly or indirectly. Generally speaking, myofascial release consists of a gentle form of stretching and manual compression. It is said to restore flexibility to this connective tissue and provide relief from fascial restrictions and pain. Myofascial release is often practiced by physical therapists but may also be offered by osteopathic physicians, chiropractors, massage therapists, and others who are trained in this method (see also "Massage," page 218, "Bodywork," page 167).

What is the history behind it?

Massage has been used in many ancient cultures, including those of China, India, Persia, Arabia, Greece, and Egypt. Chinese texts dating back to 2700 BC recommended massage and other types of body movements as treatments for paralysis, chills, and fever. Hippocrates, known as the father of western medicine, recommended massage for sports and war injuries.

The term myofascial was used by Janet Travell, MD, in the 1940s, and the term was used throughout the 1970s and 1980s as part of her trigger point therapy, a massage technique focusing on trigger points, or points of extreme tension in the body. There are now two main schools of myofascial release: the direct and indirect method.

What is the evidence?

There is little scientific evidence available to support proponents' claims that myofascial release relieves pain or restores flexibility. One study has found that myofascial release, when combined with electrical current, improved pain and neck flexibility in people with neck and shoulder pain. A small preliminary study that looked at the use of myofascial release with relaxation therapy found that it seemed to help men with chronic pelvic pain related to prostatitis, but additional research is needed to confirm its effect.

Are there any possible problems or complications?

People with rheumatoid arthritis, cancer that has spread to the bone, spine injuries, osteoporosis, or other bone diseases that could be worsened by physical manipulation should avoid physical manipulation or deep pressure. Manipulation of a bone in an area of cancer metastasis could result in a bone fracture. Also, people who have had radiation may find even light touch on the treatment area to be uncomfortable. A few people have allergic reactions to lotions or oils used during massage, and this may be more common among patients receiving radiation treatment. People with cancer and chronic conditions such as arthritis and heart disease should consult their physicians before undergoing any type of therapy that involves manipulation of joints and muscles. It is important that massage be given by trained massage therapists and that the massage therapist know about your cancer and its treatment. Generally, gentle massage and bodywork can be adapted to meet the needs of cancer patients.

Another concern for people who have cancer is that tissue manipulation in the area of a tumor might increase the risk that cancer cells will travel to other parts of the body. It may be prudent for cancer patients to avoid massage near tumors and lumps that could be cancerous until this question is clearly answered.

Patients with low blood platelet counts (a common side effect of chemotherapy) or who are taking blood-thinning medication such as warfarin (Coumadin) may be susceptible to easy bruising and should ask their doctors whether massage is safe for them.

It is important for people who have cancer to let their medical care providers know they are receiving any type of massage or bodywork. Massage should be provided by a trained professional with expertise in working safely with people with cancer and with cancer survivors.

Relying on this treatment alone and delaying or avoiding conventional medical care for cancer may have serious health consequences.

References

Anderson RU, Wise D, Sawyer T, Chan C. Integration of myofascial trigger point release and paradoxical relaxation training treatment of chronic pelvic pain in men. *J Urol.* 2005;174:155-160.

Hou CR, Tsai LC, Cheng KF, Chung KC, Hong CZ. Immediate effects of various physical therapeutic modalities on cervical myofascial pain and trigger-point sensitivity. *Arch Phys Med Rehabil.* 2002;83:1406-1414.

Manheim C. What is myofascial release? Myofascial Release Web site. http://www.myofascial-release.com/. Accessed June 2, 2008.

Manipulation & body-based methods: massage & related bodywork. Complementary/Integrative MedicineEducation Resources, The University of Texas M. D. Anderson Cancer Center Web site. http://www.mdanderson.org/departments/CIMER/display.cfm?id=254B81AA-6D52-42D3-94DDF74AC23EFEC4&method=displayFull. Accessed June 20, 2008.

NEURAL THERAPY

Other common name(s): none
Scientific/medical name(s): none

Description

Neural therapy involves the injection of anesthetics (drugs that normally cause numbness or reduce pain) into various places in the body to eliminate pain and cure illness.

Overview

Research into neural therapy has been done mainly in Germany, where the therapy is widely used. No reports of clinical research on the effectiveness of neural therapy for pain management or any other health problems could be found in the available U.S. scientific journals.

How is it promoted for use?

The practice of neural therapy is based on the belief that energy flows freely through the body of a healthy person. Proponents claim injury, disease, malnutrition, stress, and even scar tissue disrupt this flow, creating energy imbalances called "interference fields." Some proponents of this theory in Germany have stated that 40 percent of all illness and chronic pain may be caused by interference fields in the body.

There are other explanations for how neural therapy works, including the electrical disturbance theory, the restricted lymphatic system theory, and the idea that illness is caused by distortion in the connective tissue of the body. All of these theories assume that any interference in structure, lymphatic flow, or electrical conduction can cause illness. The goal of neural therapy is to correct the interference and heal the illness or symptom. However, even those who practice neural therapy acknowledge that the process is not well understood.

Neural therapy is promoted mainly to relieve chronic pain. It is also thought to be helpful for people with allergies; hay fever; headaches; arthritis; asthma; hormone imbalances; sports or muscle injuries; gallbladder, heart, or liver disease; dizziness; depression; menstrual cramps; and skin and circulation problems.

There are conflicting beliefs about the usefulness of neural therapy for easing cancer-related pain. Proponents of the therapy for other uses generally suggest that people who have cancer should not use neural therapy. They say that it is unlikely to help and may even cause the cancer to spread. Finally, they maintain that neural therapy is not helpful in genetic diseases, nutritional deficiencies, end-stage chronic diseases, and mental health disorders other than depression.

This method is not to be confused with the nerve blocks and local anesthesia used in conventional medicine. Nerve blocks involve injections of medication to relieve pain caused by stimulation of a peripheral nerve. Local anesthesia is medication given at a local site to relieve localized pain. For example, a local anesthetic may be given before a tooth is removed, before removing a small skin lesion, or to help chronic pain in cancer. This type of anesthetic use has been proven to be effective.

What does it involve?

Practitioners begin by asking questions about the current problem and any past illnesses and injuries. They decide what is most likely to be the cause of the energy flow disturbance in the body and then inject anesthetics such as lidocaine and procaine at key points, which may be far from the pain source. These injections are meant to eliminate the interference and restore the body's natural energy flow. The injections may be given into nerves, acupuncture points, glands, scars, and trigger points (abnormally sensitive knots of tight muscle tissue that may cause pain or limit range of motion). A course of treatment may involve one or more injections spread over several weeks. A few practitioners use electrical current and lasers instead of injected drugs. The patient may be asked to keep a log of changes in the body for a day or two after injections are done. This record may be used to guide future treatments.

Some practitioners combine neural therapy with other types of treatment, such as homeopathy, applied kinesiology, and biological dentistry. In fact, some practitioners believe that root canals, metal tooth fillings, and even jewelry can cause interference fields.

What is the history behind it?

The idea behind neural therapy—that the nervous system influences all bodily functions—originated in Germany in the late 1800s with a Russian physiologist named Ivan Petrov. In the 1940s, Ferdinand and Walter Huneke, both physicians, carried this idea further. They believed that injecting local anesthetics could affect distant parts of the body, a theory based on a clinical experience with a patient who complained of shoulder pain. When Ferdinand Huneke injected an anesthetic drug directly into an existing scar on the patient's leg, the patient's shoulder pain reportedly disappeared in minutes. From this experience arose the notion of interference fields and the development of neural therapy.

Today, neural therapy is practiced at only a few clinics in the United States. However, it is widely used in Europe and South America.

What is the evidence?

Most articles on neural therapy have been published in Germany, where neural therapy is popular, and most of the literature focuses on pain relief. Many of the promoters have claimed positive results, but no clinical studies have been done in the United States. A study done in Scotland in 1999 seemed to suggest that neural therapy might be helpful for people with multiple sclerosis. However, it was an uncontrolled study, so no reliable conclusions can be drawn. Available scientific evidence does not support claims that neural therapy is effective in treating cancer or any other disease.

Are there any possible problems or complications?

Since there are few studies done on the use of neural therapy, information about side effects is limited. At least one person had bleeding of the brain while undergoing neural therapy, which was reported in German medical literature. Neural therapy practitioners suggest that people who have cancer, kidney failure, blood-clotting disorders, or myasthenia gravis (a condition in which muscles are very weak) should not use neural therapy. Patients taking blood-thinning medications may have problems with this treatment, as might those taking morphine or heart rhythm drugs that may be somewhat similar to the anesthetic drugs used in neural therapy. People with allergies to the anesthetic drugs are not candidates for the therapy. Relying on this treatment alone and delaying or avoiding conventional medical care for cancer may have serious health consequences.

References

Cassileth B. *The Alternative Medicine Handbook: The Complete Reference Guide to Alternative and Complementary Therapies.* New York: W.W. Norton; 1998.

Gibson RG, Gibson SL. Neural therapy in the treatment of multiple sclerosis. *J Altern Complement Med.* 1999;5:543-552.

Heyll U, Ziegenhagen DJ. Subarachnoid hemorrhage as life-threatening complication of neural therapy. Case report [in German]. *Versicherungsmedizin.* 2000;52:33-36.

Kaslow JE. Neural therapy. Dr. Kaslow Web site. http://www.drkaslow.com/html/neural_therapy.html. Accessed June 2, 2008.

Kennedy R. Neural therapy. The Doctors' Medical Library Web site. http://www.medical library.net/content/view/63/45/. Accessed June 2, 2008.

Klinghardt D. Neural therapy and the brain. Neural Therapy Web site. http://www.neuraltherapy.com/a_neural_therapy_brain.asp. Accessed May 30, 2008.

NCCN clinical practice guidelines in oncology: adult cancer pain, v 1.2006. National Comprehensive Cancer Network Web site. http://www.nccn.org/professionals/physician_gls/PDF/pain.pdf. Accessed March 30, 2007.

Neural therapy. American Association of Orthopedic Medicine Web site. http://www.aaomed.org/page.asp?id=93&name=Neural+Therapy. Accessed June 2, 2008.

Raso J. The expanded dictionary of metaphysical healthcare, alternative medicine, paranormal healing, and related methods. Quackwatch Web site. http://www.quackwatch.org/01QuackeryRelatedTopics/dictionary/md00.html. Accessed May 30, 2008.

OSTEOPATHY

Other common name(s): osteopathic medicine
Scientific/medical name(s): none

Description

Osteopathy is a form of physical manipulation (moving the joints and muscles) used to restore the structural balance of the body's system of bones and muscles. The word osteopathy comes from two Greek words meaning "bone" and "disease." Osteopathic physicians may combine this physical treatment with standard medical care.

Overview

There is little scientific evidence that osteopathic medicine is effective in treating cancer or any condition other than musculoskeletal problems. Doctors of osteopathy (called DOs) are educated in standard medical practices, and most of the methods that they use are based on the same scientific studies that medical doctors (MDs) use. In addition to bone and muscle movement, DOs prescribe drugs and generally do everything that MDs do.

How is it promoted for use?

Osteopathy is based on the belief that all systems in the human body work together. Doctors of osteopathy observe the patient, ask questions about medical history, and use their hands to diagnose and correct muscle, tendon, and joint abnormalities, which they claim are the cause of many diseases. Some osteopaths claim that if bones and muscles are in balance and functioning properly, the body can heal itself. Practitioners most often recommend osteopathy for head, neck, and back pain; headaches; joint pain; muscle strain; repetitive strain injuries; and sports-related problems.

Osteopathy is sometimes promoted as an alternative method to ease pain, improve quality of life, minimize the side effects of treatment, enhance other types of treatments, and extend the life of some cancer patients. Some proponents claim that people with cancer, heart disorders, high blood pressure, stomach disorders, and a variety of other conditions can benefit from osteopathy. Some supporters claim that osteopathy, when used with conventional medicine, can reduce the pain from arthritis, chronic fatigue, and some gynecological problems.

What does it involve?

In treating people with various conditions, DOs use several different forms of physical manipulation:

- Articulation involves moving the patient's joints through the normal range of motion.
- Counterstrain techniques involve placing a joint or muscle in a relaxed position and then pulling to stretch and loosen it.
- Cranial techniques involve the moving of bones in the skull, especially in the jaw, to relieve pain and treat other conditions.
- Functional techniques involve gently moving the patient's joints until the practitioner finds restrictions to movement.
- Muscle energy techniques involve stretching the patient's muscles and then forcing the muscles to move against resistance.
- Hands-on massage may also be used in osteopathy.

These techniques are sometimes used alongside standard medical treatment or after conventional treatment has failed. For example, an osteopath who treats cancer patients may use the same chemotherapy, radiation therapy, or surgical treatments as would a physician but may also look at how the disease has affected the patient's body structure and provide osteopathy to correct other physical abnormalities.

Some DOs limit their practice to conventional medicine only, while others may practice manipulative therapy almost exclusively. In recent years, there are fewer differences between the practices of osteopaths and conventional medical doctors.

What is the history behind it?

Originally started in the 1800s as a reaction to conventional medicine's reliance on drug therapy, osteopathy today is quite similar to conventional medicine, except for its use of osteopathic manipulative therapy. Andrew Taylor Still, MD, first expressed the philosophy and principles of osteopathy in 1874. Dr. Still rejected reliance on drug treatment and considered surgery a last resort in treating diseases. He believed that diseases could be cured through the manipulation of misplaced bones, nerves, and muscles, which cleared "obstructions."

In 1892 he founded the first osteopathic medical school in Kirksville, Missouri, to promote his philosophy of medicine. Today, there are twenty osteopathic medical colleges in the United States, and osteopathy has evolved to incorporate the theories and practices of conventional medicine as well. There are nearly sixty thousand DOs practicing in the United States, about half in general practice or one of the primary-care specialties—family practice, internal medicine, pediatrics, and obstetrics and gynecology. Osteopaths make up about 5 percent of the doctors practicing in the United States but represent almost 10 percent of primary-care providers.

Doctors of osteopathy are allowed to do more in the United States than in any other country. Laws in every state and in the military permit DOs unlimited medical practice once they are licensed by the state, following training in an accredited osteopathic medical school and a one-year internship in an approved hospital. Osteopaths may also undertake residency training in any medical specialty and become board certified by passing a certification exam.

Once barred from conventional hospitals and restricted to their own hospitals, most osteopaths now receive at least some of their training in conventional hospitals and may practice in conventional medical settings. Osteopathic medical schools have education programs that are similar to conventional medical schools, with the exception that they include up to three hundred hours of training in manipulation therapy.

What is the evidence?

Although most osteopaths use standard medical treatments that are proven in scientific studies, a few osteopaths use unproven methods, such as craniosacral therapy and chelation therapy. Available scientific evidence does not support claims that osteopathic manipulation alone is helpful in most diseases, although studies have indicated that the therapy may help relieve some musculoskeletal problems and related pain. A review of research studies that looked at lower back pain suggested that osteopathic manipulation was no better or worse than the usual medical management.

Are there any possible problems or complications?

As with any medical treatment, osteopathic manipulation may carry risks of failure or may have serious effects. There may be some risk for injury or fracture to anyone with bone cancer or severe osteoporosis. People who have cancer and chronic conditions such as arthritis and heart disease should consult their physicians before undergoing any type of therapy that involves manipulation of joints and muscles.

Relying on osteopathic manipulation alone and avoiding or delaying conventional medical treatment for cancer can result in serious consequences.

References

Assendelft WJ, Morton SC, Yu EI, et al. Spinal manipulative therapy for low back pain. *Cochrane Database Syst Rev.* 2004;(1):CD000447.

Barrett S. Dubious aspects of osteopathy. Quackwatch Web site. http://www.quackwatch.org/04ConsumerEducation/QA/osteo.html. Updated August 18, 2003. Accessed May 30, 2008.

Lesho EP. An overview of osteopathic medicine. *Arch Fam Med.* 1999;8:477-484.

Magee M. Rethinking physician supply [transcript]. *Health Politics with Dr. Mike Magee.* Health Politics Web site. http://www.healthpolitics.org/program_transcript.asp?p=prog_52. Accessed June 3, 2008.

Osteopathic fact sheet. Oklahoma State University Center for Health Sciences Web site. http://www.healthsciences.okstate.edu/student/factsheet.cfm. Accessed June 2, 2008.

Still AT. Autobiography with a history of the discovery and development of the science of osteopathy. Reprinted, New York: Arno Press and the New York Times; 1972.

Wood DL. Research lacking in osteopathic medical profession. *J Am Osteopath Assoc.* 1997;97:23.

POLARITY THERAPY

Other common name(s): polarity balancing, polarity energy balancing
Scientific/medical name(s): none

Description

Polarity therapy is based on the idea that a person's health and well-being are determined by the natural flow of energy through the body. Polarity refers to the positive and negative charges of the body's electromagnetic energy field. Practitioners use touch, movement, and other methods to help this energy flow.

Overview

Available scientific evidence does not support claims that polarity therapy is effective in treating cancer or any other disease. However, it is sometimes recommended by physicians as a tool for relaxation when conducted by a trained professional.

How is it promoted for use?

Polarity therapy is based on the theory that a smooth flow of energy maintains health, while disruptions in the flow caused by trauma, stress, poor nutrition, and other factors lead to energy imbalances, fatigue, and illness. There are believed to be three types of energy fields in the human body: long-line currents that run north to south on the body, transverse currents that run east-west in the body, and spiral currents that start at the navel and expand outward.

Practitioners of polarity therapy claim they can identify the sources of energy blockages and disruptions by observing symptoms such as headaches, tight shoulders and back muscles, muscle spasms, pain, abdominal discomfort, and even tumors. They also claim polarity therapy can be used to promote relaxation and range of motion, relieve tension, increase energy, and reduce pain, inflammation, and swelling. They further state that polarity therapy enhances the body's ability to fight off serious illness, including cancer.

What does it involve?

The first polarity therapy session includes detailed questions about physical and mental health, diet and exercise, health concerns, work, and more. The patient lies on a massage table while the therapist scans for imbalances and checks energy flow in the body. The polarity therapist may use a variety of techniques to balance and clear energy field paths. Some of these include twisting the torso, spinal realignment, curling toes, rocking motions, and moving the hands or crystals along the body's natural energy pathways. Some techniques are similar to those used by chiropractors (see page 177). Other aspects of polarity therapy may include supportive counseling, deep-breathing exercises, dietary changes, hydrotherapy (see page 203), stretching, and yoga (see page 145).

Because polarity therapy is based on the unique needs of the patient at the time, no two sessions are exactly alike. Most often, weekly sessions are suggested for six to eight weeks, although this may vary depending on the person and his or her needs. During a successful session of polarity therapy, the patient is said to reach a state of deep relaxation. A polarity therapy session lasts about an hour or more. Generally, polarity therapy is recommended for use in addition to standard medical care.

What is the history behind it?

Polarity therapy was developed in the late 1940s by Randolph Stone, a chiropractor, osteopath, and naturopath. Dr. Stone studied several forms of traditional medicine practices from India and China. He taught that each person is responsible for his or her own health and that simple steps such as those involved in polarity therapy improve physical and spiritual well-being. According to the American Polarity Therapy Association, about one thousand polarity therapists are registered in the United States. Various schools and people from around the world teach polarity therapy. Some organizations have training programs to certify polarity therapists. However, these organizations are not regulated by any government agency.

What is the evidence?

Claims that polarity therapy is an effective treatment for cancer and other serious diseases have not been proven. The existence of energy field paths in the human body has also not been proven. Little clinical research has been published in peer-reviewed medical journals on polarity therapy. A very small pilot study looked at fatigue in women undergoing radiation therapy for breast cancer and found that the women who received polarity treatments reported better quality of life a few days afterward. However, no treatment was used in the comparison group, and the patients' expectation of improvement may have affected the results. A 2007 review study that looked at research on complementary methods to help cancer-related fatigue did not find enough evidence to recommend polarity therapy for this problem.

Patients often report feeling relaxed and less tense after a polarity therapy session. Some physicians encourage patients to undergo bodywork therapies (such as polarity therapy and massage) because some of these therapies make people feel better, if only for a short time. Others believe the prolonged physical contact involved in hands-on techniques is relaxing and therefore helpful to some people.

Are there any possible problems or complications?

Polarity therapy, when done by a trained professional, is considered safe for relaxation purposes. Improperly applied techniques may cause injury. People with cancer and chronic conditions such as arthritis and heart disease should talk to their doctors before having any type of treatment that involves manipulation of joints and muscles. Relying on this treatment alone and delaying or avoiding conventional medical care for cancer may have serious health consequences.

References

Cassileth B. *The Alternative Medicine Handbook: The Complete Reference Guide to Alternative and Complementary Therapies.* New York: W.W. Norton; 1998.

National Institutes of Health. *Alternative Medicine: Expanding Medical Horizons: A Report to the National Institutes of Health on Alternative Medical Systems and Practices in the United States.* Washington, DC: US Government Printing Office; 1994. NIH publication 94-066.

Polarity. Aetna InteliHealth Web site. http://www.intelihealth.com/IH/ihtIH?d=dmtContent&c=358862. Accessed June 2, 2008.

Roscoe JA, Matteson SE, Mustian KM, Padmanaban D, Morrow GR. Treatment of radiotherapy-induced fatigue through a nonpharmacological approach. *Integr Cancer Ther.* 2005;4:8-13.

Sood A, Barton DL, Bauer BA, Loprinzi CL. A critical review of complementary therapies for cancer-related fatigue. *Integr Cancer Ther.* 2007;6:8-13.

Wilson W. Polarity therapy: in introduction. American Polarity Therapy Association Web site. http://www.polarity therapy.org/page.asp?PageID=24. Accessed June 2, 2008.

PSYCHIC SURGERY

Other common name(s): none

Scientific/medical name(s): none

Description

Psychic surgery is used to remove spirits or physical manifestations of spiritual problems from a patient by the use of bare fingers and hands without any actual surgery.

Overview

Psychic surgeons create the illusion that they can remove tumors, unhealthy tissue, and organs by making an invisible incision using only their fingers and hands. Available scientific evidence does not support claims that psychic surgery offers any value to people with cancer or any other disease.

How is it promoted for use?

Some psychic surgeons claim they can cure cancer and other serious illnesses by removing tumors or other unhealthy tissue from a patient's body without leaving an incision or wound.

What does it involve?

No anesthesia or surgical instruments are used in psychic surgery. During the procedure, practitioners appear to press their fingers and hands into the patient's body (usually the abdomen) in order to remove tissue, tumors, or other material that is believed to be making the patient sick. The practitioners often show their bloodied hands or objects supposedly removed from the body to patients as proof of their ability to enter the body without surgical instruments. Close observers have noted that the removed material is often cotton or another object soaked in animal blood. They have reported seeing the psychic surgeon remove the materials from a plastic bag or other container hidden so as not to be seen by the patient and others.

Some psychic surgeons hold up objects such as animal organs, fatty tumors, and other materials that are presented as human organs. In Filipino cultures, where people believe in evil spirits that can put foreign objects into a person's body, the psychic surgeon may display palm leaves, glass, or corncobs they supposedly removed from the patient. Practitioners will then "close" the wound using their fingers and hands and wipe the blood away. During the procedure, patients feel no pain. The patient is asked to stand and walk immediately after the procedure has ended. The skin shows no scars or wounds where the "incision" has been made.

Although some psychic surgeons publicly claim that they charge no fees, they may ask for large donations from patients who have money.

What is the history behind it?

Psychic surgery began in rural parts of the Philippines during the twentieth century. In the 1940s, Philippines native Eleuterio Terte was reportedly the first person to perform psychic surgery. Medical anthropologists have described the development of psychic surgery as a transition from traditional shamanism. Some shamans learned to use animal parts and blood as part of a dramatic ritual to remove the effects of evil spirits.

Legal authorities have convicted some psychic surgeons for practicing medicine without a license and others for fraud. Psychic surgery is mainly practiced in the Philippines and Brazil, although it sometimes is done in the United States. In the United States, practitioners may claim that psychic surgery is part of their religious practice in an attempt to avoid prosecution. To receive psychic surgery, some Americans travel abroad, where it is practiced in the original surroundings of religious and traditional healing.

What is the evidence?

Available scientific evidence does not support claims that psychic surgery has any medical value. It has never been known to remove tumors or cure cancer or any other disease. In fact, following up on people who had cancerous tumors "removed" in this way revealed that the tumors were still present. Some patients also report being told that the psychic surgeon had removed their cancer, when in fact the patient never had cancer at all.

Are there any possible problems or complications?

People should be aware that claims made by practitioners of psychic surgery have not been proven. There has been at least one report of a psychic surgeon in the Philippines who uses human blood for this procedure. There is a very slight chance of infection with human immunodeficiency virus or hepatitis if human blood (instead of animal blood) is used by a psychic surgeon.

Relying on this type of treatment alone and avoiding or delaying traditional medical care for cancer may have serious health consequences.

References

Barrett S, Herbert V. Questionable cancer therapies. Quackwatch Web site. http://www.quackwatch.org/01QuackeryRelatedTopics/cancer.html. Updated July 6, 2001. Accessed May 30, 2008.

Cassileth B. *The Alternative Medicine Handbook: The Complete Reference Guide to Alternative and Complementary Therapies*. New York: W.W. Norton; 1998.

Psychic surgery. BC Cancer Agency Web site. http://www.bccancer.bc.ca/HPI/UnconventionalTherapies/PsychicSurgery.htm. Accessed June 2, 2008.

True GN II. The facts about faith healing and psychic surgery. True Health Web site. http://georgenavatrue.spaces.live.com/Blog/cns!2C2DFB94368AB40F!113.entry. Accessed June 3, 2008.

US Congress, Office of Technology Assessment. *Unconventional Cancer Treatments: OTA-H-405*. Washington, DC: US Government Printing Office; 1990.

REFLEXOLOGY

Other common name(s): zone therapy, reflex therapy, foot reflexology, hand reflexology
Scientific/medical name(s): none

Description

Reflexology is a treatment that uses pressure on specific areas of the feet (or the hands) with the goal of relieving a variety of problems and balancing the flow of vital energy throughout the body.

Overview

There is early scientific evidence that reflexology may be useful for relaxation and reducing some types of pain and anxiety in some patients. Available scientific evidence does not support reflexology as a treatment for cancer or any other disease.

How is it promoted for use?

Reflexology is based on the theory that reflex points, located in the feet or hands, are linked to various organs and parts of the body. According to this theory, stimulation of these points is thought to affect the connected organ or body part. By stimulating the reflex points, reflexologists claim that they can relieve a wide variety of health problems and promote well-being and relaxation.

Some proponents claim that reflexology can help conditions such as respiratory infections, headaches, asthma, diabetes, back pain, premenstrual syndrome, and problems with the skin and gastrointestinal tract. They also say reflexology can stimulate internal organs, boost circulation, and restore bodily functions to normal. According to their beliefs, energy travels from the foot to the spine, where it is released to the rest of the body. They believe that reflexology releases endorphins (the body's own natural painkillers) and detoxifies the body by dissolving uric acid crystals in the feet. Some reflexologists say that a tender or gritty area of the foot or hand reflects a current or past disease in the organ linked to that area.

What does it involve?

The reflexologist may start by asking health-related questions before examining the feet. He or she will gently examine a person's feet while the client sits in a special chair or lies on a massage table, then apply pressure to selected reflex points on the feet. Sometimes the client will notice tender areas on the feet as they are touched. Some people report tingling sensations in other areas of the body while the reflex points are being touched. Most sessions take from thirty minutes to an hour. Some people learn to apply reflex pressure to their own or a family member's feet. A few reflexologists work on the hands, and some work on both the hands and the feet.

Since reflexology is not legally regulated at this time, no formal training is required before a person can call himself or herself a reflexologist. The practitioner may have taken courses from a massage school or other source, studied reflexology books, apprenticed with another practitioner, or be self-taught. Some massage therapists, nurses, and others incorporate reflexology techniques into their practices.

What is the history behind it?

Reflexology traces its roots to ancient Egypt and China. In the early twentieth century, an American physician, William Fitzgerald, MD, decided the foot was the best place to "map" parts of the body for diagnosis and treatment. He divided the body into ten zones and decided which section of the foot controlled each zone. Dr. Fitzgerald believed gentle pressure on a particular area of the foot would generate relief in the targeted zone. This process was originally named zone therapy. A few years later, another doctor named Joe Shelby Riley published drawings of zones on both the feet and the hands to promote what he called Zone Reflex. He also mapped zones on the outer ear.

In the 1930s, Eunice Ingham, a nurse and physiotherapist, further developed Dr. Fitzgerald's maps to include reflex points, which were much more specific than the zones used in Fitzgerald's maps. It was Ingham who changed the name of zone therapy to reflexology.

What is the evidence?

Available scientific evidence does not support claims that reflexology cures cancer or any other disease. However, it has been shown to help promote relaxation and reduce pain in some people. Most evidence regarding reflexology is based on anecdotal reports or small studies.

A 2003 study looked at patients with cancer pain and found that reflexology seemed to help symptoms for a short time. However, the effects were gone three hours after the treatment. A recheck at twenty-four hours showed no difference between the groups. A 2007 study of eighty-six people with metastatic cancer compared reflexology administered by patients' partners with reading to patients by their partners. The reflexology group reported less anxiety and less pain.

A study done in 2002 looked at symptoms in menopausal women. All the women received either a reflexology treatment or a placebo foot massage. They reported improved menopausal symptoms, with no difference between the foot massage and reflexology groups.

In a Danish study in the early 1990s, 220 people suffering from migraine headaches or tension headaches were evaluated. Of those, 81 percent said they were helped or cured by reflexology, and 19 percent of those who had been taking medication were able to stop after six months of reflexology treatments. However, since there was no control group, scientists who conducted the study cautioned that the patients' improved well-being could have been due to other factors. They concluded that further study would be needed to determine the benefits, if any, of reflexology.

Are there any possible problems or complications?

As with massage and other forms of bodywork, reflexology can generally be adapted to meet the needs of cancer patients. Deep pressure and vigorous manipulation of the foot should be avoided during times of active treatment for cancer, or if there is edema in the foot or lower leg. It is recommended that cancer patients not have pressure applied directly to known tumor sites or to lumps that may be cancerous. People with cancer that has spread to the bone or who have fragile bones should avoid physical manipulation or deep pressure because of the risk for fracture. Bodywork should be provided by a trained professional with expertise in working safely with people who have cancer and with cancer survivors.

People with cancer and chronic conditions such as arthritis and heart disease should talk to their doctors before having any type of therapy that involves moving joints and muscles. Relying on this type of treatment alone and avoiding or delaying conventional medical care for cancer may have serious health consequences.

References

Barrett S. Reflexology: a close look. Quackwatch Web site. http://www.quackwatch.org/01QuackeryRelatedTopics/reflex.html. Updated September 25, 2004. Accessed May 30, 2008.

Botting D. Review of literature on the effectiveness of reflexology. *Complement Ther Nurs Midwifery.* 1997;3:123-130.

Cassileth B. *The Alternative Medicine Handbook: The Complete Reference Guide to Alternative and Complementary Therapies.* New York: W.W. Norton; 1998.

History of reflexology. American Academy of Reflexology Web site. http://www.americanacademyofreflexology.com/HistoryOf.shtml. Accessed June 2, 2008.

Hodgson H. Does reflexology impact on cancer patients' quality of life? *Nurs Stand.* 2000;14:33-38.

Launsø L, Brendstrup E, Arnberg S. An exploratory study of reflexological treatment for headache. *Altern Ther Health Med.* 1999;5:57-65.

Oleson T, Flocco W. Randomized controlled study of premenstrual symptoms treated with ear, hand, and foot reflexology. *Obstet Gynecol.* 1993;82:906-911.

Quattrin R, Zanini A, Buchini S, Turello D, Annunziata MA, Vidotti C, Colombatti A, Brusaferro S. Use of reflexology foot massage to reduce anxiety in hospitalized cancer patients in chemotherapy treatment: methodology and outcomes. *J Nurs Manag.* 2006;14:96-105.

Reflexology. Aetna InteliHealth Web site. http://www.intelihealth.com/IH/ihtIH/WSIHW000/8513/34968/360060.html. Accessed June 2, 2008.

Ross CS, Hamilton J, Macrae G, Docherty C, Gould A, Cornbleet MA. A pilot study to evaluate the effect of reflexology on mood and symptom rating of advanced cancer patients. *Palliat Med.* 2002;16:544-545.

Stephenson N, Dalton JA, Carlson J. The effect of foot reflexology on pain in patients with metastatic cancer. *Appl Nurs Res.* 2003;16:284-286.

Williamson J, White A, Hart A, Ernst E. Randomised controlled trial of reflexology for menopausal symptoms. *BJOG.* 2002;109:1050-1055.

REIKI

Other common name(s): Reiki healing, Usui system of Reiki, distant Reiki
Scientific/medical name(s): none

Description

Reiki is based on the belief that spiritual energy can be channeled through a Reiki practitioner to heal the patient's spirit. This is thought to help liberate the body's natural healing powers. Reiki is most often given as a hands-on treatment, but it may also be sent from a distance. Reiki is a Japanese term meaning "universal life energy."

Overview

There are anecdotal reports that Reiki increases relaxation and the sense of well-being. There is early scientific evidence that Reiki may be useful for reducing pain in some patients with advanced cancer. Available scientific evidence does not support claims that Reiki can treat cancer.

How is it promoted for use?

Many practitioners explain that Reiki is not used to diagnose or treat specific illnesses. Rather, Reiki is said to promote relaxation, decrease stress and anxiety, and increase a person's general sense of well-being. The Reiki practitioner delivers the therapy through his or her hands, with the goal of raising the amount of universal life energy (called qi or chi) in and around the client. Proponents claim that when the energy paths of the body are blocked or disturbed, the result can be illness, weakness, and pain. Reiki practitioners intend to realign and strengthen the flow of energy, thereby decreasing pain, easing muscle tension, speeding healing, improving sleep, and generally enhancing the body's natural ability to heal itself.

What does it involve?

During a Reiki session, the practitioner places his or her hands in twelve to fifteen positions on or above parts of the patient's clothed body. The hands are intended to be a conduit for universal life energy, balancing energy within and around the body. The hands are held in place for approximately two to five minutes in each position. A Reiki session usually lasts about one hour. Some practitioners say that they achieve the best results when patients have three Reiki sessions within a relatively short time, take a break, and then repeat the process. There are three levels of Reiki practice: a Reiki I practitioner can offer hands-on sessions, a Reiki II practitioner can offer hands-on or distant Reiki, and a Reiki master can offer hands-on Reiki, distant Reiki, and Reiki instruction. Second-degree Reiki practitioners and Reiki masters believe that they can send healing universal life energy over a distance, similar to claims by qigong masters who practice traditional Chinese healing concepts (see "Qigong," page 128).

What is the history behind it?

The basis for modern-day Reiki practice may have originated in Tibet more than twenty-five hundred years ago. Reiki was rediscovered in the early 1900s by a Japanese doctor named Mikao Usui. During a lengthy period of travel and research, Dr. Usui found ancient texts that described Reiki and its power to heal by using the energy that flows through all living things. From his studies and meditations, he developed what came to be known as the Usui system of Reiki. Other systems of Reiki have been developed as well.

Training programs and certification are available from Reiki organizations. However, these organizations are not regulated by any government agency.

What is the evidence?

There are many individual reports about Reiki's power to increase feelings of well-being and refresh the spirit. Some cancer patients undergoing active treatment have reported an increased sense of well-being, reduced pain, and reduced nausea and vomiting after Reiki sessions. One small controlled pilot study found that Reiki was linked with reduced self-reports of pain in patients with advanced cancer, but it had no effect on the amount of pain medicine used by the patients to control their pain.

A nonrandomized study reported that Reiki improved anxiety among women after hysterectomy, whereas a randomized study reported no effect on anxiety of women undergoing breast biopsies.

Available scientific evidence does not support claims that Reiki can help treat cancer or any other illness. More study may help determine to what extent, if at all, it can improve a patient's sense of well-being.

Are there any possible problems or complications?

Reiki involves very light touch or no touch and is considered safe. However, relying on this type of treatment alone and avoiding or delaying standard medical care for cancer may have serious health consequences.

References

Energy medicine: an overview. National Center for Complementary and Alternative Medicine Web site. http://nccam.nih.gov/health/backgrounds/energymed.htm. Accessed April 2, 2007.

Federal News Service. Prepared testimony of Susan Silver, the Center for Integrative Medicine, George Washington University, before the House Government Reform Committee: The role of early detection and complementary and alternative medicine in women's cancers. June 10, 1999. http://www.fnsg.com/. Accessed June 20, 2008.

An introduction to Reiki. National Center for Complementary and Alternative Medicine Web site. http://nccam.nih.gov/health/reiki/. Accessed December 9, 2006.

Mansour AA, Beuche M, Laing G, Leis A, Nurse J. A study to test the effectiveness of placebo Reiki standardization procedures developed for a planned Reiki efficacy study. *J Altern Complement Med.* 1999;5:153-164.

Miles P, True G. Reiki—review of a biofield therapy: history, theory, practice, and research. *Altern Ther Health Med.* 2003;9:62-72.

Olson K, Hanson J, Michaud M. A phase II trial of Reiki for the management of pain in advanced cancer patients. *J Pain Symptom Manage.* 2003;26:990-997.

Olson K, Hanson J. Using Reiki to manage pain: a preliminary report. *Cancer Prev Control.* 1997;1:108-113.

Reiki. Aetna InteliHealth Web site. http://www.intelihealth.com/IH/ihtIH/WSIHW000/8513/34968/360056.html. Accessed June 2, 2008.

Shiflett SC, Nayak S, Bid C, Miles P, Agostinelli S. Effect of Reiki treatments on functional recovery in patients in poststroke rehabilitation: a pilot study. *J Altern Complement Med.* 2002;8:755-763.

ROSEN METHOD

Other common name(s): Rosen Method bodywork, Rosen Method psychospiritual bodywork

Scientific/medical name(s): none

Description

The Rosen Method combines bodywork with talk therapy. The purpose is to reach the unconscious mind through touch, making the patient aware of subconscious thoughts and painful emotions that are thought to be stored in the body as muscle tension or tightness.

Overview

People who subscribe to the Rosen philosophy believe that people protect themselves by tightening muscles to help shut down the emotional pain of difficult situations. This muscle tension can become persistent and can lead to limited movement or chronic muscle pain. It can also serve to keep the conscious mind from being aware of emotional pain. Proponents of this therapy claim that these feelings and memories may be reclaimed and let go through touch, awareness, and breathwork.

How is it promoted for use?

The Rosen method is promoted as a complementary therapy to be used along with talk therapy or traditional psychotherapy and as a measure to enhance health and wellness. It is promoted for diverse groups, including people with physical pain, poor posture, or restricted breathing, as well as for people wanting to know more about themselves, artists, dancers, musicians, singers, actors who use their bodies for creative expression, people who want to explore body-mind connections, and people in psychotherapy or counseling who may feel "stuck."

It is not recommended for people with severe emotional disturbance or acute physical pain.

What does it involve?

The patient lies down on a massage table, and the therapist sits or stands nearby to touch the muscles and watch for changes in the patient's breathing and other responses. These changes guide the therapist's touch and words, which are said to help the client recognize repressed memories and feelings. A period of quiet reflection is often recommended after the session, which typically lasts about one hour.

What is the history behind it?

A physical therapist named Marion Rosen developed this treatment method in the 1970s based on the belief that repressed emotions cause muscular tension.

What is the evidence?

No research results relevant to the Rosen method as a treatment for cancer or its symptoms have been published in medical or scientific journals. Available scientific evidence does not support the idea that discovery of repressed feelings can influence the course of diseases such as cancer.

Are there any possible problems or complications?

The Rosen method involves light touch and is considered safe. However, relying on this type of treatment alone and avoiding or delaying standard medical care for cancer may have serious health consequences.

References

Alternative medicine encyclopedia: Rosen method. Answers Web site. http://www.answers.com/topic/rosen-method. Accessed June 12, 2008.

Murphy J. Rosen method releases pain and emotion. Rosen Method Bodywork Australia Web site. http://www.rosenmethod.com.au/Artcl3.html. Accessed June 2, 2008.

Wooten S. Rosen method bodywork. Two Rivers Center Web site. http://www.rosensouthwest.com/rmbodywork.html. Accessed June 2, 2008.

RUBENFELD SYNERGY METHOD

Other common name(s): the listening hand
Scientific/medical name(s): none

Description

Practitioners of the Rubenfeld Synergy Method identify and touch tense muscles to help the patient become aware of painful feelings and beliefs that are suppressed and kept in the body. This method includes talk, imagery, hypnosis, movement, and work with dreams.

Overview

The Rubenfeld Synergy Method uses light touch to help clients identify repressed feelings and memories. It combines elements of the Alexander Technique, the Feldenkrais Method, Gestalt therapy, and hypnotherapy practices (see “Bodywork,” page 167, “Psychotherapy,” page 123, “Hypnosis,” page 94).

How is it promoted for use?

The Rubenfeld Synergy Method is typically not promoted as a treatment for physical illnesses. Rather, it is intended to provide benefits such as resolution of painful issues and experiences, increased inner peace and calm, recovery from physical and/or emotional trauma, and maintenance of physical/emotional health and well-being.

What does it involve?

The patient usually lies on a table but may sit, stand, or move about in some of the sessions, which typically last forty-five to fifty minutes. The therapist uses light touch to help patients recall and discuss repressed memories and experiences.

What is the history behind it?

Developed in the 1960s by Ilana Rubenfeld, the Rubenfeld Method has the aim of personal growth and awareness, allowing memories, emotions, and habitual patterns to surface and be dealt with.

What is the evidence?

No research results relevant to the Rubenfeld Method have been published in medical or scientific journals.

Are there any possible problems or complications?

The Rubenfeld Method involves light touch and is considered safe. However, relying on this type of treatment alone and avoiding or delaying standard medical care for cancer may have serious health consequences.

References

Granstrom K. What is Rubenfeld synergy? Karin Granstrom Web site. http://www.karingranstrom.net/method.htm. Accessed June 2, 2008.

The listening hand. Ilana Rubenfeld Web site. http://www.thelisteninghand.com. Accessed April 2, 2007.

Nadler DL. The Rubenfeld synergy method: when words are not enough. *Counselor, The Magazine for Addiction Professionals.* February 2004;5:46-48. http://www.counselormagazine.com/content/view/380/55/. Accessed June 20, 2008.

THERAPEUTIC TOUCH

Other common name(s): energy field therapy, biofield therapy, TT

Scientific/medical name(s): none

Description

Therapeutic Touch (TT) is a technique in which the hands are used to direct human energy for healing purposes. There is usually no actual physical contact.

Overview

Available scientific evidence does not support many of the claims made for TT or the claim that energy is balanced or transferred by the use of TT. However, it may be useful in reducing anxiety and increasing the sense of well-being in some people.

How is it promoted for use?

The practice of Therapeutic Touch is based on the belief that problems in the patient's energy field that cause illness and pain can be identified and rebalanced by a healer. Harmful energy is believed to cause blockages and other problems in the patient's normal energy flow, and proponents of TT claim the treatment removes those blockages. TT is promoted by some to improve conditions such as pain, fever, swelling, infections, wounds, ulcers, thyroid problems, colic, burns, nausea, premenstrual syndrome, diarrhea, and headaches. They also say that TT is useful in treating diseases such as measles, Alzheimer's disease, AIDS, asthma, autism, multiple sclerosis, stroke, comas, and cancer. In practice, TT is generally promoted as a complementary therapy, to be used with standard medical care.

What does it involve?

The clothed patient is normally lying down, but may also be sitting or standing. There are four steps involved in a TT session, which takes between ten and thirty minutes to complete. The first step is called centering. During centering, the therapist makes an effort to clear his or her mind in order to communicate with the patient's energy field and locate areas of energy blockage that are believed to cause pain or illness.

The second part of TT involves an assessment in which the therapist's hands are held about two to six inches above the patient's body. The therapist then passes both hands, palms facing downward, head to toe along the patient's body. This process is used to locate irregularities or blockages in the patient's energy field that signal a health problem.

In the third step, the therapist conducts several passes over the body with his or her hands. At the end of each pass, the therapist releases the harmful energy by flicking his or her hands into the air past the toes of the patient. Finally, in the final step, the therapist transfers his or her own excess healthy energy to the patient.

What is the history behind it?

Therapeutic Touch is similar to the "laying on of hands" practiced by some religious sects as a means of transferring healing energy to the believer. The idea of an energy field can be traced back to the eighteenth century work of Franz Anton Mesmer, a German doctor who believed that illness was caused by imbalances in the body's magnetic forces. He believed he could restore magnetic balance through the use of soothing words and quieting gestures, a technique he called Mesmerism.

Dora Kunz, a natural healer, theosophy promoter, and one-time president of the Theosophical Society of America, and Dolores Krieger, PhD, RN, nursing educator at New York University, developed Therapeutic Touch in the 1970s.

More than a hundred colleges and universities in seventy-five countries teach TT. It is promoted by many professional nursing organizations and practiced by nurses in at least eighty hospitals in the United States and Canada. There are more than fifty thousand health care professionals, mostly nurses, who have learned TT worldwide. Many nonprofessionals have also learned the technique.

What is the evidence?

A good deal of the information about TT is based on individual reports and small studies. There have been few well-designed studies. An article published in the *Journal of the American Medical Association* (*JAMA*) reported that only one study out of eighty-three confirmed positive results for TT. The authors stated that some of the clinical studies found positive effects, such as help with wound healing and headaches; however, they reported that most of those studies had questionable study designs. The authors of the *JAMA* article conducted their own small study, which did not test any effect of TT but looked at the ability of twenty one practitioners to detect the relative closeness of human energy fields under experimental conditions. The authors found that when the practitioners' views were blocked, they were not able to sense the investigator's location.

In one scientific review of available published studies, it was concluded that TT may help reduce anxiety and some types of pain, but more study is needed. Another review of studies showed mixed results on whether TT helped wound healing, with some outcomes favoring the TT groups and others the control groups.

A recent controlled clinical trial on the effects of dialogue and TT on patients having breast cancer surgery found that ten minutes of TT and twenty minutes of talking lowered anxiety before surgery. No effects were found after surgery. A more recent controlled study on women with early-stage breast cancer found that those who spent quiet time talking with a nurse noticed feeling just as calm, comfortable, and relaxed as those who had TT. On the other hand, another study of nursing home residents with dementia found that TT reduced symptoms of restlessness, pacing, and wandering when compared with a placebo group. Further study is needed to prove the helpfulness of Therapeutic Touch in people with dementia.

Research funded by the U.S. Department of Defense to study the effect of TT on burn patients produced mixed results. Patients reported a reduction in pain and anxiety, but there was no difference in the amount of pain medicine requested.

Many researchers believe the positive results claimed for TT are due to the placebo effect. Researchers also believe the simple presence of a person who is interested in helping can promote relaxation and increase one's sense of well-being. Available scientific evidence does not support any claims that TT can cure cancer or other diseases.

Are there any possible problems or complications?

Therapeutic Touch is generally considered safe when given by trained professionals. Some of the reported side effects include nausea, dizziness, restlessness, and irritability. Relying on this treatment alone and delaying or avoiding conventional medical care for cancer may have serious health consequences.

References

Cassileth B. *The Alternative Medicine Handbook: The Complete Reference Guide to Alternative and Complementary Therapies.* New York: W.W. Norton; 1998.

Energy therapies: therapeutic touch detailed scientific review. Complementary/ Integrative Medicine Education Resources, The University of Texas M. D. Anderson Cancer Center Web site. http://www.mdanderson.org/departments/cimer/display.cfm?id=6ef12958-d712-4533-8ccef3307e8137dc&method=displayfull. Accessed June 2, 2008.

Hutchison CP, D'Alessio B, Forward JB, Newshan G. Body-mind-spirit: healing touch: an energetic approach. *Am J Nurs.* 1999;99:43-48.

Kelly AE, Sullivan P, Fawcett J, Samarel N. Therapeutic touch, quiet time, and dialogue: perceptions of women with breast cancer. *Oncol Nurs Forum.* 2004;31:625-631.

O'Mathuna DP. TT: what could be the harm? *Sci Rev Altern Med.* Spring, 1998.

O'Mathuna DP, Ashford RL. Therapeutic touch for healing acute wounds. *Cochrane Database Syst Rev.* 2003;(4):CD002766.

Rosa L, Rosa E, Sarner L, Barrett S. A close look at therapeutic touch. *JAMA.* 1998;279:1005-1010.

Samarel N, Fawcett J, Davis MM, Ryan FM. Effects of dialogue and therapeutic touch on preoperative and postoperative experiences of breast cancer surgery: an exploratory study. *Oncol Nurs Forum.* 1998;25:1369-1376.

Woods DL, Craven RF, Whitney J. The effect of therapeutic touch on behavioral symptoms of persons with dementia. *Altern Ther Health Med.* 2005;11:66-74.

TRANSCUTANEOUS ELECTRICAL NERVE STIMULATION

Other common name(s): TENS
Scientific/medical name(s): none

Description

Transcutaneous electrical nerve stimulation (TENS) is a method of pain relief in which a special device transmits low-voltage electrical impulses through electrodes on the skin to an area of the body that is in pain.

Overview

There is some evidence that TENS may help reduce certain types of pain, especially mild pain, for a short period of time. However, it does not appear to reduce chronic pain.

How is it promoted for use?

Supporters claim that transcutaneous electrical nerve stimulation is an effective method for relieving acute and chronic pain caused by surgery, childbirth, migraine headaches, tension headaches, injuries, arthritis, tendonitis, bursitis, chronic wounds, cancer, and other problems. Some practitioners claim that TENS stimulates the production of endorphins, the body's natural painkillers. Most TENS practitioners do not claim the therapy cures the underlying causes of pain.

What does it involve?

A TENS system consists of an electrical power unit connected by wires to a pair of electrodes. The electrodes are attached to the patient's skin near the source of pain. When the unit is switched on, a mild electrical current travels through the electrodes into the body. Patients may feel tingling or warmth during treatment. A session typically lasts from five to fifteen minutes, and treatments may be applied as often as necessary, depending on the severity of pain. Some practitioners refer to TENS as a sort of "electrical massage."

TENS is used widely by physical therapists and other medical practitioners but can also be performed at home by patients using a portable TENS system. There are more than a hundred types of TENS units approved for use by the U.S. Food and Drug Administration. A prescription is needed to obtain a system. In a variation of TENS called percutaneous electrical nerve stimulation, the electrical impulses are sent through acupuncture needles (see "Acupuncture," page 156).

What is the history behind it?

Dr. Ronald Melzac and Dr. Patrick Wall developed the Gate Control Theory in 1965, which claims that when nerves are electrically stimulated, a gate mechanism is closed in the spinal cord, thereby preventing the awareness of pain. After the introduction of their theory, TENS was widely used to treat pain. TENS became a relatively common therapy in the early 1970s. It is still widely used by physical therapists and physiotherapists.

What is the evidence?

Research on the effectiveness of TENS therapy for cancer pain is somewhat conflicting and is limited to small clinical studies and case reports. Some cancer patients, particularly those with mild neuropathic pain (pain related to nerve tissue damage), may benefit from TENS for brief periods of time. TENS may also work better when used with pain medicines.

One review of TENS reported that many studies have found it useful in easing pain related to acute injuries of the muscles and bones, pain after surgery, and some other types of pain. A second review of fifteen years of TENS research found some evidence to suggest that it is a useful addition to pain relief, although a number of the studies under review failed to show TENS was helpful in pain control. One study found that TENS was not effective for relieving pain after surgery or during labor. Another study found that percutaneous electrical nerve stimulation—in which electrical current is transmitted through acupuncture needles instead of surface electrodes—was more effective than TENS for relieving lower back pain.

A 2005 review of studies that looked at the effectiveness of TENS in relieving lower back pain found very few high-quality studies. Of the two studies that met all criteria for scientifically sound research, one showed significant relief of lower back pain in the TENS group, while the other study showed no difference in pain relief between the TENS group and the control group.

Overall, there is limited evidence to show TENS effectively decreases chronic pain. More clinical studies are needed to determine what benefit TENS may have for people with cancer in managing cancer-related pain. At present, it is usually prescribed to be used with pain medicines.

Are there any possible problems or complications?

TENS is generally considered safe. However, electrical current that is too intense or that is used incorrectly can burn or irritate the skin. The electrodes should not be placed over the eyes, heart, brain, or front of the throat. People with heart problems should not use TENS. The effects of long-term use of TENS on fetuses is unknown, and pregnant women should not undergo the therapy. People with allergies to adhesives may react to the electrode pads. Those with implanted pacemakers, defibrillators, infusion pumps, and other such devices should avoid exposure to electric current. Relying on this treatment alone and delaying or avoiding conventional medical care for cancer may have serious health consequences.

References

Barrett D. Ten tips on living with fibromyalgia syndrome. Quackwatch Web site. http://www.quackwatch.org/03HealthPromotion/fibromyalgia/fms02.html. Updated February 15, 2000. Accessed May 30, 2008.

Ghoname EA, Craig WF, White PF, Ahmed HE, Hamza MA, Henderson BN, Gajraj NM, Huber PJ, Gatchel RJ. Percutaneous electrical nerve stimulation for low back pain: a randomized crossover study. *JAMA.* 1999;281:818-823.

Khadilkar A, Milne S, Brosseau L, Robinson V, Saginur M, Shea B, Tugwell P, Wells G. Transcutaneous electrical nerve stimulation (TENS) for chronic low-back pain. *Cochrane Database Syst Rev.* 2005;(3):CD003008.

Long DM. Fifteen years of transcutaneous electrical stimulation for pain control. *Stereotact Funct Neurosurg.* 1991;56:2-19.

McQuay HJ, Moore RA, Eccleston C, Morley S, Williams AC. Systematic review of outpatient services for chronic pain control. *Health Technol Assess.* 1997;1:i-iv, 1-135.

Spencer JW, Jacobs JJ. *Complementary/Alternative Medicine: An Evidence-Based Approach.* St. Louis, MO: Mosby; 1999.

Sykes J, Johnson R, Hanks GW. ABC of palliative care. Difficult pain problems. *BMJ.* 1997;315:867-869.

Transcutaneous electrical nerve stimulation. Aetna InteliHealth Web site. http://www.intelihealth.com/IH/ihtIH/WSIHW000/8513/34968/363973.html. Accessed June 2, 2008.

Chapter Seven

Herb, Vitamin, and Mineral Therapies

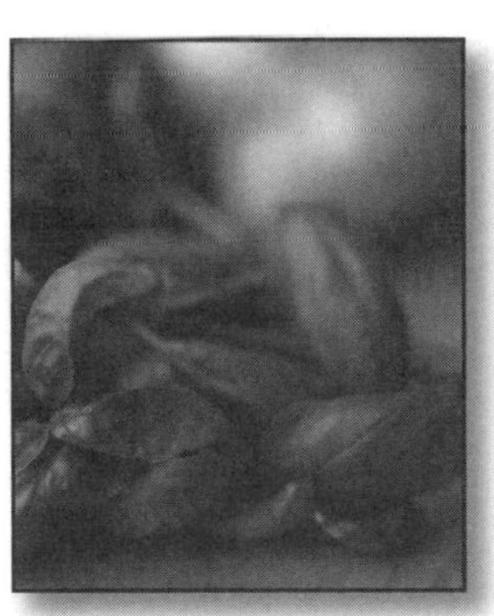

ACONITE

Other common name(s): monkshood, wolfsbane, fu-tzu
Scientific/medical name(s): *Aconitum napellus*

Description

Aconite is an herb related to the buttercup family *(Ranunculaceae)*, native to Asia and common to the Alps and other areas of Europe. Some varieties grow in the United States, although they are rare.

Overview

Available scientific evidence does not support the use of aconite to prevent or treat cancer or other health problems. It is extremely toxic and can cause irregular heartbeat, heart failure, and death. For this reason, few sources promote the use of this herb for medicinal purposes.

How is it promoted for use?

When used in traditional Chinese and Ayurvedic (Indian) medicine, aconite is first processed to reduce its toxicity, and small doses are used to treat pain related to arthritis, cancer, gout, inflammation, migraine headaches, neuralgia, rheumatism, and sciatica.

What does it involve?

Certain ingredients are extracted from the leaves, flowers, and roots of the plant. It is available as a tincture, tea, ointment, or highly diluted into a homeopathic remedy (see "Homeopathy," page 753). Although it can be purchased online, it is not commercially prepared in the United States.

What is the history behind it?

Aconite has been used since ancient times in traditional Asian (Chinese, Japanese, and Indian/Ayurvedic) medicine, as well as in ancient Greek and Roman medicine. Aconite was also used in Western medicine until it was replaced by safer and more effective treatments in the mid-1900s. In addition to its medical uses, aconite has been used to poison arrows in hunting. Also known as wolfsbane, aconite has been considered variably in folklore as a causative agent in transforming a person into a werewolf or as a treatment for werewolves. References in mythology and literature extend from the ancient Greeks (in an attempt to poison Theseus) to modern literature (as treatment for a werewolf in J. K. Rowling's *Harry Potter* series).

What is the evidence?

Although there have been some modern laboratory and animal studies, as well as a few clinical trials, of various chemical compounds from aconite for use as anesthetics and as treatments for circulatory and neurologic conditions, none of these uses are recommended in conventional medical practice. A few preclinical studies have tested chemicals from aconite as anticancer drugs, but none of the chemicals has been evaluated in clinical trials.

Are there any possible problems or complications?

Because aconite is extremely toxic and can cause irregular heartbeat, heart failure, and death, few sources promote the use of this herb for medicinal purposes. It is dangerous even when used as an ointment because it can be absorbed through the skin. Handling the plant can cause allergic reactions and rashes.

Aconite is on the German Commission E's list of unapproved herbs. This means that it is not recommended for use because it has not been proven to be safe or effective. This herb should be avoided, especially by women who are pregnant or breastfeeding.

References

Aconitum. Wikipedia Web site. http://en.wikipedia.org/wiki/Aconitum. Accessed June 6, 2008.

Blumenthal M, ed. *The Complete German Commission E Monographs: Therapeutic Guide to Herbal Medicines.* Austin, TX: American Botanical Council; 1998.

Cantrell FL. Look what I found! Poison hunting on eBay. *Clin Toxicol (Phila).* 2005;43:375-379.

Dasyukevich OI, Solyanik GI. Comparative study of anticancer efficacy of acnitine-containing agent BC1 against ascite and solid forms of Ehrlich's carcinoma. *Exp Oncol.* 2007;29:317-319.

Gruenwald J. *PDR for Herbal Medicines.* 3rd ed. Montvale, NJ: Thomson PDR; 2004.

Kadyrova MM, Sobol' IuS, Sokolov SF, Ageev FT, Smetnev AS. Effect of a new anti-arrhythmia drug allapinin on hemodynamics in patients with a persistent form of atrial fibrillation before and after restoration of sinus rhythm [in Russian]. *Kardiologiia.* 1990;30:87-91.

Lowe L, Matteucci MJ, Schneir AB. Herbal aconite tea and refractory ventricular tachycardia. *N Engl J Med.* 2005;353:1532.

Poon WT, Lai CK, Ching CK, Tse KY, So YC, Chan YC, Hau LM, Mak TW, Chan AY. Aconite poisoning in camouflage. *Hong Kong Med J.* 2006;12:456-459.

Sun K, Yang J, Shen DK. Clinical observation on treatment of primary knee osteoarthritis of liver and kidney deficiency type with Aconite cake-separated moxibustion [in Chinese]. *Zhongguo Zhen Jiu.* 2008;28:87-90.

Wang CF, Gerner P, Wang SY, Wang GK. Bulleyaconitine A isolated from aconitum plant displays long-acting local anesthetic properties in vitro and in vivo. *Anesthesiology.* 2007;107:82-90.

ALOE

Other common name(s): aloe vera, aloe vera gel, T-UP
Scientific/medical name(s): *Aloe barbadensis, Aloe capensis*

Description

The aloe plant, a member of the lily family, is a common household plant originally from Africa. The most common and widely known species of aloe plant is aloe vera. Aloe vera plants have dark green leaves that look like small cacti but are soft and supple. Aloe vera gel is the thin, clear, jelly-like substance that oozes from the inside of the aloe leaves. The extract taken from inside the outer lining of the leaves is called aloe juice or aloe latex and is often dried into brownish granules. Unprocessed aloe gel often contains some aloe latex.

Overview

Available scientific evidence does not support claims that aloe can treat any type of cancer. In fact, used as a cancer treatment, aloe is dangerous and may even be deadly. The gel inside aloe leaves may be effective in treating minor burns and skin irritations. There are mixed reports about its use as a laxative.

How is it promoted for use?

Aloe juice or latex is used mostly for constipation, whereas aloe gel is used for skin conditions. However, proponents of alternative treatments claim aloe also boosts the immune system and acts directly on abnormal cells, thus preventing or treating cancer.

The main aloe product promoted as a cancer cure is an unapproved drug called T-UP, which comes in an oral form or can be injected. Aloe proponents claim it is effective against all types of cancer.

What does it involve?

Aloe vera gel is a common ingredient in many skin creams and lotions, cosmetics, and burn and wound ointments. When used on skin for minor burns or irritations, aloe gel is usually applied to the affected area three to five times a day. The aloe gel may be purchased as a commercial gel or cream or applied directly from a cut aloe leaf. Since some compounds in aloe gel break down quickly, some supporters recommend fresh aloe gel taken directly from the leaf as the best source.

Commission E (Germany's regulatory agency for herbs) has approved aloe for treating constipation. A common dosage is 50 to 200 milligrams of aloe latex (the bitter substance from inside the outer lining of the leaf), taken in liquid or capsule form once a day for up to ten days. The U.S. Food and Drug Administration (FDA) has ruled that aloe products cannot be sold as nonprescription drugs for treatment of constipation because of insufficient information on safety and effectiveness. Aloe products can be sold as dietary supplements in the United States.

T-UP, a concentrated liquid form of aloe, has been promoted to be taken orally or injected directly into the tumor or bloodstream. Practitioners give T-UP injections to people with advanced cancer. Aloe injections are illegal in the United States but are available at clinics in other countries.

What is the history behind it?

The earliest known references to the medicinal use of aloe come from the ancient Egyptians, who used it as a treatment for cuts, burns, and skin irritations. Many other cultures have also used aloe for similar purposes. Since the 1930s, aloe has been used frequently for the treatment of minor skin ailments and skin reactions to radiation burns.

In 1996, a company based in Maryland began producing and selling a concentrated form of aloe called T-UP to be used orally and by injection for the treatment of cancer, AIDS, herpes, and other autoimmune disorders. In the summer of 1999, the U.S. Attorney's Office and the FDA indicted the makers of T-UP on twenty different charges including fraud, promoting and selling an unapproved drug, and conspiracy. The makers of T-UP were charged with misleading cancer patients by making false claims, including claiming FDA approval for their drug when approval was never granted.

What is the evidence?

Aloe contains many chemicals. A group of chemicals called anthraquinones give aloe its stimulant laxative properties. Preliminary studies of cell cultures grown in laboratory dishes and laboratory animals suggest that some of the chemicals found in aloe may have helpful effects on the immune system. However, the safety and effectiveness of most of these chemicals have not been tested in humans. The aloe products being promoted for internal use contain a wide variety of chemicals, some of which can cause very serious side effects.

Available scientific evidence does not support the claim that aloe is effective in treating people with cancer. Several cancer patients have died as a direct result of receiving aloe injections. Animal and laboratory studies have found mixed results. One study reported that aloe reduced the growth of liver cancer cells in rats, but another found that it promoted the growth of human liver cancer cells in tissue culture. Another rat study reported aloe reduced precancerous liver changes in rats treated with cancer-causing chemicals. Another recent laboratory study reported that aloe promotes the growth of endothelial (blood vessel) cells, raising the concern that it might promote angiogenesis, the growth of blood vessels that help "feed" a cancer.

Although aloe has been used since the 1930s in the treatment of skin reactions resulting from radiation therapy, recent clinical trials found that an aloe vera gel did not protect against skin inflammation caused by radiation therapy. Some studies suggest that aloe gel may be effective for minor cuts and burns, but other studies report that aloe can delay healing of infected surgical wounds. People with severe skin trauma or deep injuries may need other treatments.

Aloe gel and juice contain chemicals with laxative properties. These substances are classified as stimulant laxatives and can be irritating to the intestines. There are a number of dietary and medical approaches to treating constipation that are safer and more effective than aloe products.

Are there any possible problems or complications?

The use of aloe on the skin for the relief of minor cuts and burns appears to be safe. There are mixed reports about the safety of taking aloe internally. One report suggested that aloe taken by mouth might increase cancer risk to humans. Side effects of the internal use of aloe may include abdominal pain, nausea and vomiting, diarrhea, and electrolyte (chemical) imbalance in the blood, especially at high doses. It should not be used as a laxative for more than two weeks. Women who are pregnant or breastfeeding should not use aloe internally.

Taking aloe internally may cause dangerous interactions with prescription drugs and with other herbal supplements. Aloe injections are dangerous, are illegal in the United States, and have caused the deaths of several people.

Some people who have used aloe gel for long periods of time have had allergic reactions such as hives and rashes. Those who are allergic to garlic, onions, tulips, and similar plants may be more likely to have an allergic reaction to aloe. Relying on this type of treatment alone and avoiding or delaying conventional medical care for cancer may have serious health consequences.

This product is sold as a dietary supplement in the United States. Unlike companies that produce drugs (which must provide the FDA with results of detailed testing showing their product is safe and effective before the drug is approved for sale), the companies that make supplements do not have to show evidence of safety or health benefits to the FDA before selling their products. Supplement products without any reliable scientific evidence of health benefits may still be sold as long as the companies selling them do not claim the supplements can prevent, treat, or cure any specific disease. Some such products may not contain the amount of the herb or substance that is written on the label, and some may include other substances (contaminants). Though the FDA has written new rules to improve the quality of manufacturing processes for dietary supplements and the accurate listing of supplement ingredients, these rules do not take full effect until 2010. The new rules also do not address the safety

of supplement ingredients or their effects on health when proper manufacturing techniques are used.

Most such supplements have not been tested to find out if they interact with medicines, foods, or other herbs and supplements. Even though some reports of interactions and harmful effects may be published, full studies of interactions and effects are not often available. Because of these limitations, any information on ill effects and interactions should be considered incomplete.

References

Aloe vera. Memorial Sloan-Kettering Cancer Center Web site. http://www.mskcc.org/mskcc/html/69116.cfm. Accessed June 4, 2008.

Blumenthal M, ed. *The Complete German Commission E Monographs: Therapeutic Guide to Herbal Medicines.* Austin, TX: American Botanical Council; 1998.

Department of Health and Human Services. Status of certain additional over-the-counter drug category II and II active ingredients. May 9, 2002. 21 CFR Part 310. [Docket No. 78N-036L]. RIN 0910-AA01. US Food and Drug Administration Web site. http://www.fda.gov/OHRMS/DOCKETS/98fr/78n-036L-nfr0004-vol107.pdf. Accessed June 4, 2008.

Gruenwald J. *PDR for Herbal Medicines.* 3rd ed. Montvale, NJ: Thomson PDR; 2004.

Heggie S, Bryant GP, Tripcony L, Keller J, Rose P, Glendenning M, Heath J. A phase III study on the efficacy of topical aloe vera gel on irradiated breast tissue. *Cancer Nurs.* 2002;25:442-451.

Meadows M. Investigators' reports: Maryland man, Virginia physician sentenced for illegally marketing aloe vera 'treatments.' *FDA Consumer: The Magazine of the US Food and Drug Administration.* May-June 2002. http://www.fda.gov/fdac/departs/2002/302_irs.html. Accessed June 4, 2008.

Natural Standard. Herbal/plant therapies: aloe (aloe vera). Complementary/Integrative Medicine Education Resources, The University of Texas M. D. Anderson Cancer Center Web site. http://www.mdanderson.org/departments/cimer/display.cfm?id=ee033c9d-ec7b-11d4-810100508b603a14&method=displayfull. Accessed June 4, 2008.

Olsen DL, Raub W Jr, Bradley C, Johnson M, Macias JL, Love V, Markoe A. The effect of aloe vera gel/mild soap versus mild soap in preventing skin reactions in patients undergoing radiation therapy. *Oncol Nurs Forum.* 2001;28:543-547.

ARNICA

Other common name(s): arnica root, common arnica, arnica flowers, mountain arnica, mountain tobacco, leopardsbane, wolfsbane

Scientific/medical name(s): *Arnica montana*

Description

Arnica is a perennial herb that grows in Europe, the northern United States, Canada, and eastern Asia. Its daisy-like flower and root, or rhizome, are often used in herbal medicines.

Overview

This herbal remedy is used on the skin for wounds, infections, and inflammation. It also is used to prepare a homeopathic medicine (see "Homeopathy," page 753). Available scientific evidence does not support most of the claims about arnica's effectiveness. If the herb is taken by mouth, it can be poisonous. It has caused a number of serious reactions, including allergies and at least one death.

How is it promoted for use?

Arnica is promoted for use on the skin to help soothe and heal wounds, sunburn, bruises, sprains, sore muscles, arthritis, ulcers, acne, eczema, chapped lips, and irritated nostrils. Arnica contains organic chemicals such as sesquiterpene lactones and flavonoid glycosides that are claimed to reduce the swelling, redness, and pain associated with inflammation and help heal bacterial infections.

The herb is not usually recommended for internal use because it can irritate the stomach and may result in vomiting, diarrhea, and nosebleeds. However, some homeopathic practitioners claim that a very diluted solution can be taken by mouth to treat low-grade fevers, colds, bronchitis, seasickness, inflammation of the mouth and throat, and epilepsy.

Germany's Commission E has approved arnica only for external use in treating injury and effects of accidents, inflammation of the mouth and throat area, and insect bites. It is considered unsafe for internal use.

Arnica is an ingredient in some herbal skin care products and shampoos.

What does it involve?

Arnica is used as a whole or cut herb, powder, tea, liquid, gel, cream, ointment, oil, tincture, spray, or salve. The herb can be soaked with water and made into a poultice (a soft, moist mass of herbs) that is applied directly to the skin. Arnica ointments usually contain up to 15 percent of arnica oil or 25 percent of a tincture of arnica (the herb mixed with alcohol). Blistering and inflammation may be more likely to occur if very strong solutions are used on the skin. Homeopathic liquids reportedly contain little or no actual arnica and are usually placed under the tongue. Homeopathic tablets are also reported to contain extremely small or undetectable amounts of arnica, but the dose may vary.

What is the history behind it?

Herbal medicines made from arnica flowers and roots have been popular for hundreds of years. It has been said that Goethe drank arnica tea to relieve chest pains. The leaves were reportedly smoked, like tobacco. More recently, arnica has been used mainly in homeopathic and topical forms due to the possible harm in taking the herb by mouth.

What is the evidence?

Available scientific evidence does not support most of the claims about arnica's effectiveness. In 1998, a review in the *Archives of Surgery* of eight controlled human trials studying the effectiveness of arnica found that arnica was no more effective in treating injuries than the placebo with which it was compared. The authors found that the studies had serious flaws in the methods used to evaluate the effectiveness of arnica. They concluded that the human trials did not indicate that arnica was helpful or beneficial. One randomized clinical trial actually found that arnica appeared to increase pain and cause more swelling than the placebo in patients who had their wisdom teeth removed.

A 2003 study of sixty-two patients tested homeopathic arnica to determine whether it reduced pain and bruising in patients having surgery for carpal tunnel syndrome. There were no differences in pain or bruising between the arnica and placebo groups.

A double-blind, randomized British study of thirty-seven patients looked at homeopathic arnica in tablet and ointment form to determine whether it helped people having surgery for carpal tunnel syndrome. A week after surgery, there were no differences in grip strength, wrist swelling, or pain between the group that was given arnica and the placebo group. Two weeks after surgery, the group that had arnica reported somewhat less pain than the other group, although there were still no differences in grip strength or swelling. Further studies are needed to find out whether this one difference is due to chance or to the effects of the arnica.

In 2002, a small Miami study looked at arnica gel to see whether it would reduce bruising after laser surgery to the face. No difference in bruising was noted between the patients who used plain gel and those who used the arnica gel.

In 2006, German researchers analyzed three studies on the use of arnica after knee surgery. Homeopathic arnica was given before and after surgery in all three studies. There were no significant differences in swelling after surgery between the arnica groups and the placebo groups in two out of three of the studies.

A 2007 controlled study looked at homeopathic arnica in patients who had their tonsils removed. One group received arnica and the other a placebo. Patients were surveyed afterward, with 111 out of 190 patients returning their questionnaires. The arnica group reported slightly lower pain levels than the placebo group, although there was no difference in how much pain medicine they needed, the period of time before they went back to work, and the number of visits they made to the doctor afterward. There was also no difference between the groups in bleeding and infection after surgery.

A toxicology assessment completed in 2001 concluded that there was not enough safety information on arnica to support allowing its use in cosmetics.

One 1994 study found that some of the chemicals extracted from arnica can kill colon and lung cancer cells growing in laboratory dishes. No follow-up studies in animals or humans have been published since that time.

Are there any possible problems or complications?

Small, single doses of the herb are considered safe if applied externally. However, repeated use can cause skin reactions, severe inflammation, itching, blisters, skin ulcers, and other allergy-related skin problems. Use of very concentrated herb on the skin can increase the risk for irritation. Use of the herb on broken skin or mucous membranes can cause irritation and increase the risk for more serious reactions.

Internal use is not recommended because arnica may cause vomiting, diarrhea, internal bleeding, rapid heartbeat, muscle weakness, nervousness, nosebleeds, and coma. At least one death has been reported. Arnica may reduce the effectiveness of medications for high blood pressure and increase the risk for bleeding in people who take blood-thinning medications. People taking medicines that affect the heart's rhythm or function may have worse effects if they take arnica.

People who are allergic to arnica may suffer runny nose, itching, hives, shortness of breath, and shock. Those with allergies to sunflowers, marigolds, or chamomile may be more likely to be allergic to arnica.

Effects on pregnant women and children are not well known. Women who are pregnant or breastfeeding should not use this herb. Relying on this type of treatment alone and avoiding or delaying conventional medical care for cancer may have serious health consequences.

References

Alonso D, Lazarus MC, Baumann L. Effects of topical arnica gel on post-laser treatment bruises. *Dermatol Surg.* 2002;28:686-688.

Arnica. Drug Digest Web site. http://www.drugdigest.org/DD/DVH/HerbsWho/0,3923,4075|Arnica,00.html. Accessed June 4, 2008.

Arnica. PDRhealth Web site. http://www.pdrhealth.com/drugs/altmed/altmed-mono.aspx?contentFileName=ame0009.xml&contentName=Arnica. Accessed June 4, 2008.

Blumenthal M, ed. *The Complete German Commission E Monographs: Therapeutic Guide to Herbal Medicines.* Austin, TX: American Botanical Council; 1998.

Bown D. *New Encyclopedia of Herbs & Their Uses.* New York: DK Publishing Inc; 2001.

Brinkhaus B, Wilkens JM, Lüdtke R, Hunger J, Witt CM, Willich SN. Homeopathic arnica therapy in patients receiving knee surgery: results of three randomised double-blind trials. *Complement Ther Med.* 2006;14:237-246. Epub 2006 Oct 13.

Cosmetic Ingredient Review. Final report on the safety assessment of *Arnica montana* extract and *Arnica montana*. *Int J Toxicol.* 2001;20 (suppl 2):1-11.

Ernst E, Pittler MH. Efficacy of homeopathic arnica: a systematic review of placebo-controlled clinical trials. *Arch Surg.* 1998;133:1187-1190.

Fetrow CW, Avila JR. *Professional's Handbook of Complementary & Alternative Medicines.* Philadelphia, PA: Lippincott Williams & Wilkins; 2004.

Gibson J, Haslam Y, Laurneson L, Newman P, Pitt R, Robins M. Double-blind trial of arnica in acute trauma patients. *Homeopathy.* 1991;41:54-55.

Jeffrey SL, Belcher HJ. Use of arnica to relieve pain after carpal-tunnel release surgery. *Altern Ther Health Med.* 2002;8:66-68.

Kaziro GS. Metronidazole (Flagyl) and Arnica Montana in the prevention of post-surgical complications, a comparative placebo controlled clinical trial. *Br J Oral Maxillofac Surg.* 1984;22:42-49.

Medical Economics. *PDR for Herbal Medicines.* Montvale, NJ: Medical Economics Co; 1998.

Paulsen E, Chistensen LP, Andersen KE. Cosmetics and herbal remedies with Compositae plant extracts - are they tolerated by Compositae-allergic patients? *Contact Dermatitis.* 2008;58:15-23.

Reider N, Komericki P, Hausen BM, Fritsch P, Aberer W. The seamy side of natural medicines: contact sensitization to arnica (*Arnica montana* L.) and marigold (*Calendula officinalis* L.). *Contact Dermatitis.* 2001;45:269-272.

Robertson A, Suryanarayanan R, Banerjee A. Homeopathic *Arnica montana* for post-tonsillectomy analgesia: a randomised placebo control trial. *Homeopathy.* 2007;96:17-21.

Stevinson C, Devaraj VS, Fountain-Barber A, Hawkins S, Ernest E. Homeopathic arnica for prevention of pain and bruising: randomized placebo-controlled trial in hand surgery. *J R Soc Med.* 2003;96:60-65.

Woerdenbag HJ, Merfort I, Passreiter CM, Schmidt TJ, Willuhn G, van Uden W, Pras N, Kampinga HH, Konings AW. Cytotoxicity of flavonoids and sesquiterpene lactones from *Arnica* species against the GLC4 and the COLO 320 cell lines. *Planta Med.* 1994;60:434-437.

ASTRAGALUS

Other common name(s): milk vetch, huang qi, huang chi, radix astragali, goat's horn, green dragon, locoweed
Scientific/medical name(s): *Astragalus membranaceus*

Description

Astragalus is a traditional Chinese herbal medicine taken from a plant known as *Astragalus membranaceus*, which is a type of bean or legume. The root is used in herbal remedies.

Overview

Animal studies and preliminary human clinical studies suggest that astragalus may improve functioning of the immune system and might enhance the effects of conventional immune therapy for some cancers. However, available scientific evidence does not support claims that astragalus can prevent cancer, cure cancer, or reduce side effects of conventional cancer treatment in humans. There is some suggestion that it may enhance the effects of certain chemotherapy drugs, but more testing is needed.

How is it promoted for use?

The herb is promoted to kill cancer cells, reduce the toxic effects of chemotherapy, help heal burns, protect against heart disease, fight the common cold, and help improve overall weakness. Proponents also claim astragalus can stimulate the spleen, liver, lungs, circulatory system, and urinary system and help treat arthritis, asthma, and nervous conditions. They further claim it can lower blood sugar levels and blood pressure.

What does it involve?

When dried, the root of the astragalus plant is used in teas, tinctures, and capsules. It is also available as dried slices of the root and as a powder. In China, healers sometimes use the dried root in soups or roast the root in honey for use as a medicinal tonic. Astragalus is usually combined with other Chinese herbal remedies to enhance the herbs' effects.

What is the history behind it?

For more than two thousand years, Chinese herbalists have recommended astragalus for helping the human body build up energy and resist diverse diseases including cancer, heart disease, liver and kidney problems, and infections. It is the most commonly used herb in Chinese medicine.

Conventional medical practitioners have recently become interested in the possibility that astragalus might lessen the side effects of chemotherapy.

What is the evidence?

The scientific evidence for the ability of astragalus to enhance the immune system and fight diseases, including cancer and heart disease, comes mostly from laboratory and animal studies. Researchers at The University of Texas M. D. Anderson Cancer Center found that astragalus extract enhanced the cell-destroying ability, or cytotoxicity, of the conventional immunotherapy treatment interleukin-2 by improving the immune system's response. It also partly restored the immune function of cells in test tubes. Astragalus has also been found to reduce the length of colds and stimulate the production of interferons, a group of substances produced by the body as part of the normal defense mechanism against viral infections.

Though animal and laboratory studies show promise, more studies are needed to find out whether the results apply to humans. A few studies of humans have been done, mostly in China, and some suggest that this herb might have some benefit for immune system cells in people who have cancer. However, most experts who have reviewed these studies said that flaws in the way the research was designed, conducted, or analyzed make it difficult to say whether the results are valid. A 2006 review of the most reliable studies of astragalus and lung cancer found some evidence that this herb might enhance the effects of some chemotherapy drugs and recommended that more rigorously designed studies be conducted.

The consensus of available scientific evidence does not support claims that astragalus can prevent or cure cancer in humans or decrease the toxic effects of chemotherapy or other conventional cancer treatments. Large-scale human trials are needed to verify the benefits, if any, of astragalus in people with cancer.

Are there any possible problems or complications?

Astragalus is generally considered safe. Reported side effects include abdominal bloating, loose stools, low blood pressure, and dehydration. People with autoimmune diseases (such as rheumatoid arthritis or lupus) or people taking immune-suppressing medicines (such as corticosteroids or cyclosporin) should talk to their doctors before taking this herb. There is some concern that astragalus might interfere with blood clotting, so some doctors recommend it not be taken before surgery or in people taking aspirin-like drugs or blood-thinning medications. It may also affect blood pressure in some, so those taking blood pressure medicines may need to be monitored by their doctors. There have also been reports of lowered blood sugar, which could be dangerous for those with diabetes or hypoglycemia. Other potential interactions between herbs and medicines are possible, some of which may be dangerous. Always tell your doctor and pharmacist about the herbs you are taking.

Allergic reactions are rare. People who are allergic to other legumes may be more likely to be allergic to astragalus. Relying on this type of treatment alone and avoiding or delaying conventional medical care for cancer may have serious health consequences.

This product is sold as a dietary supplement in the United States. Unlike companies that produce drugs (which must provide the FDA with results of detailed testing showing their product is safe and effective before the drug is approved for sale), the companies that make supplements do not have to show evidence of safety or health benefits to the FDA before selling their products. Supplement products without any reliable scientific evidence of health benefits may still be sold as long as the companies selling them do not claim the supplements can prevent, treat, or cure any specific disease. Some such products may not contain the amount of the herb or substance that is written on the label, and some may include other substances (contaminants). Though the FDA has written new rules to improve the quality of manufacturing processes for dietary supplements and the accurate listing of supplement ingredients, these rules do not take full effect until 2010. The new rules also do not address the safety of supplement ingredients or their effects on health when proper manufacturing techniques are used.

Most such supplements have not been tested to find out if they interact with medicines, foods, or other herbs and supplements. Even though some reports of interactions and harmful effects may be published, full studies of interactions and effects are not often available. Because of these limitations, any information on ill effects and interactions should be considered incomplete.

References

Astralagus. Memorial Sloan-Kettering Cancer Center Web site. http://www.mskcc.org/mskcc/html/69128.cfm. Updated September 20, 2007. Accessed June 4, 2008.

Chu DT, Lepe-Zuniga J, Wong WL, LaPushin R, Mavligit GM. Fractionated extract of Astragalus membranaceus, a Chinese medicinal herb, potentiates LAK cell cytotoxicity generated by a low dose of recombinant interleukin-2. *J Clin Lab Immunol.* 1988;26:183-187.

Cui R, He J, Wang B, Zhang F, Chen G, Yin S, Shen H. Suppressive effect of *Astragalus membranaceus* Bunge on chemical hepatocarcinogenesis in rats. *Cancer Chemother Pharmacol.* 2003;51:75-80. Epub 2002 Nov 26.

Khoo KS, Ang PT. Extract of *Astragalus membranaceus* and *Ligustrum lucidum* does not prevent cyclophosphamide-induced myelosuppression. *Singapore Med J.* 1995;36:387-390.

Lau BH, Ruckle HC, Botolazzo T, Lui PD. Chinese medicinal herbs inhibit growth of murine renal cell carcinoma. *Cancer Biother.* 1994;9:153-161.

McCulloch M, See C, Shu XJ, Broffman M, Kramer A, Fan WY, Gao J, Leib W, Shieh K, Colfrod JM Jr.

Astragalus-based Chinese herbs and platinum-based chemotherapy for advanced non-small-cell lung cancer: meta-analysis of randomized trials. *J Clin Oncol.* 2006:24:419-430.

Miller AL. Botanical influences on cardiovascular disease. *Altern Med Rev.* 1998;3:422-431.

Natural Standard. Herbal/plant therapies: Astragalus (*Astragalus membranaceus*). Complementary/Integrative Medicine Education Resources, The University of Texas M. D. Anderson Cancer Center Web site. http://www.mdanderson.org/depart nts/cimer/display.cfm?id=1513AA63-4EC5-42EE-96425F81F9D3FAD6&method=displayFull. Accessed June 4, 2008.

Rittenhouse JR, Lui PD, Lau BH. Chinese medicinal herbs reverse macrophage suppression induced by urological tumors. *J Urol.* 1991;146:486-490.

Taixiang W, Munro AJ, Guanjian L. Chinese medical herbs for chemotherapy side effects in colorectal cancer patients. *Cochrane Database Syst Rev.* 2005;(1):CD004540.

Zhao KS, Mancini C, Doria G. Enhancement of the immune response in mice by *Astragalus membranaceus* extracts. *Immunopharmacology.* 1990;20:225-233.

AVELOZ

Other common name(s): pencil cactus, pencil tree, milkbush, petroleum plant
Scientific/medical name(s): *Euphorbia tirucalli, Euphorbia viminalis, Euphorbia insulana*

Description

Aveloz is the Spanish name for a succulent shrub that grows in tropical areas of Africa, Brazil, and Madagascar. This relative of the poinsettia is sometimes grown as a houseplant. The sap, leaves, and root of various species of the shrub have been used in folk medicine for centuries.

Overview

Aveloz sap is promoted for use as an anticancer agent. However, laboratory and animal studies do not support this claim and have shown that aveloz sap may actually suppress the immune system, promote tumor growth, and lead to the development of certain types of cancer. The sap can burn the skin and damage the eyes. If taken internally, it can cause burning of the mouth and throat, vomiting, diarrhea, and other serious problems.

How is it promoted for use?

The sap of the aveloz shrub has been promoted as a tumor-killing agent for people with cancer.

It is promoted for use on the skin or to be taken by mouth. It is said to burn off warts, cysts, and skin cancers, especially on the face. In various parts of the world, the plant is also used to treat leprosy, earaches, abscesses, toothaches, asthma, colic, cough, rheumatism, and fractures.

What does it involve?

In the United States, aveloz is sold in liquid form by some health food stores and herbal practitioners. To treat cancer, benign tumors, warts, and cysts, practitioners recommend drinking five drops of the liquid dissolved in half a glass of water or tea. Aveloz is also sold as an ointment to be applied directly to warts, skin growths, and tumors.

What is the history behind it?

Thousands of years ago, Amazon Indians in Brazil began applying the sap of the aveloz plant to warts and tumors on the skin. In some tropical areas of Africa, *Euphorbia tirucalli* has long been recognized as a fish poison. The plants are crushed and placed into rivers so that fish can be easily caught when they float to the surface. By the 1770s, it was used against cancerous tumors in African folk medicine. In the 1880s, a Brazilian physician introduced the plant to conventional medicine.

In the 1970s, some U.S. tabloids began proclaiming aveloz as a cure for cancer when taken internally, saying, "One drop of sap, diluted in a glass of distilled water and taken by the tablespoon every hour, eliminates cancerous growths in one week." The craze over aveloz as a cure for cancer peaked in the 1980s, but it is still sold on the Internet as an alternative treatment for cancer.

What is the evidence?

The effects of aveloz have only been studied in the laboratory and in animals, but the results suggest that aveloz may actually promote tumor growth. These early studies have suggested that the sap and the plant itself may suppress the body's immune system, making it less resistant to infections and some types of cancer. This effect may lead to an activation of the Epstein-Barr virus (the same virus that causes mononucleosis) and the development of a type of cancer known as Burkitt's lymphoma. In light of this information, no recent cancer studies in humans have been completed on this particular plant.

Plants in the *Euphorbia* genus are being tested for use against leukemia, and some of their extracts look promising in laboratory experiments. One study suggests that chemicals from *Euphorbia tirucalli* may enhance the immune system of mice with cancer. However, no human studies have been published. Extensive testing will be necessary to determine whether any of these extracts might be suitable for human use.

Are there any possible problems or complications?

Aveloz sap can cause chemical burns, making blisters or ulcers on skin and mucous membranes (the moist pink layer of cells that lines the eyes, nose, mouth, and other cavities in the body). Sap from the plant can irritate skin and damage the eyes. Blindness has even been reported after untreated eye exposure.

If taken internally, the plant or its sap can cause burning of the mouth and throat, nausea, vomiting, diarrhea, and stomach cramps. It has been reported to have caused some deaths in eastern Africa. Children and pets may be harmed if they eat the plants or sap. Relying on this type of treatment alone and avoiding or delaying conventional medical care for cancer may have serious health consequences.

This product is sold as a dietary supplement in the United States. Unlike companies that produce drugs (which must provide the FDA with results of detailed testing showing their product is safe and effective before the drug is approved for sale), the companies that make supplements do not have to show evidence of safety or health benefits to the FDA before selling their products. Supplement products without any reliable scientific evidence of health benefits may still be sold as long as the companies selling them do not claim the supplements can prevent, treat, or cure any specific disease. Some such products may not contain the amount of the herb or substance that is written on the label, and some may include other substances (contaminants). Though the FDA has written new rules to improve the quality of manufacturing processes for dietary supplements and the accurate listing of supplement ingredients, these rules do not take full effect until 2010. The new rules also do not address the safety of supplement ingredients or their effects on health when proper manufacturing techniques are used.

Most such supplements have not been tested to find out if they interact with medicines, foods, or other herbs and supplements. Even though some reports of interactions and harmful effects may be published, full studies of interactions and effects are not often available. Because of these limitations, any information on ill effects and interactions should be considered incomplete.

References

Eke T. Euphorbia sap keratouveitis. *Br J Ophthalmol.* 1997;81:518.

Euphorbiaceae -10 Euphorbia ramosissima- Euphorbia virosa (Spurge family). Botanical Dermatology Data Base Web site. http://bodd.cf.ac.uk/BotDermFolder/BotDermE/EUPH-10.html. Accessed June 4, 2008.

Fürstenburger G, Hecker E. On the active principles of the Euphorbiaceae, XII. Highly unsaturated irritant diterpene esters from *Euphorbia tirucalli* originating from Madagascar. *J Nat Prod.* 1986;49:386-397.

Hsueh KF, Lin PY, Lee SM, Hsieh CF. Ocular injuries from plant sap of genera Euphorbia and Dieffenbachia. *J Chin Med Assoc.* 2004;67:93-98.

Imai S, Sugiura M, Mizuno F, Ohigashi H, Koshimizu K, Chiba S, Osato T. African Burkitt's lymphoma: a plant, *Euphorbia tirucalli*, reduces Epstein-Barr virus-specific cellular immunity. *Anticancer Res.* 1994;14:933-936.

MacNeil A, Sumba OP, Lutzke ML, Moormann A, Rochford R. Activation of the Epstein-Barr virus lytic cycle by the latex of the plant *Euphorbia tirucalli*. *Br J Cancer.* 2003;88:1566-1569.

Neuwinger HD. Plants used for poison fishing in tropical Africa. *Toxicon.* 2004;44:417-430.

Osato T, Mizuno F, Imai S, Aya T, Koizumi S, Kinoshita T, Tokuda H, Ito Y, Hirai N, Hirota M, et al. African Burkitt's lymphoma and an Epstein-Barr virus-enhancing plant *Euphorbia tirucalli*. *Lancet.* 1987;1:1257-1258.

Tyler VA. Aveloz. Quackwatch Web site. http://www.quackwatch.org/01QuackeryRelatedTopics/DSH/aveloz.html. Accessed June 4, 2008.

Valadares MC, Carrucha SG, Accorsi W, Queiroz ML. *Euphorbia tirucalli* L. modulates myelopoiesis and enhances the resistance of tumour-bearing mice. *Int Immunopharmacol.* 2006;6:294-299.

van den Bosch CA. Is endemic Burkitt's lymphoma an alliance between three infections and a tumour promoter? *Lancet Oncol.* 2004;5:738-748.

BLACK COHOSH

Other common name(s): black snakeroot, bugbane, bugwort, Remifemin
Scientific/medical name(s): *Cimicifuga racemosa*

Description

Black cohosh is a perennial woodland plant of the eastern United States and Canada that grows from four to eight feet tall and has feathery white flowers. The root is used in herbal remedies.

Overview

Available scientific evidence does not support claims that black cohosh is effective in treating cancer. Some studies suggest it might interfere with some drugs used in chemotherapy. The safety of long-term use is not known. Serious side effects are rare but have been reported. There is inconsistent evidence regarding whether black cohosh is effective in relieving menopausal symptoms for women in general. Its safety and effectiveness for women with menopausal symptoms caused by treatment of breast cancer is also not clear.

How is it promoted for use?

Black cohosh is often referred to as a "woman's remedy" because it is used mainly to relieve premenstrual problems, menstrual cramps, and symptoms of menopause such as hot flashes. Commission E (Germany's regulatory agency for herbs) has approved black cohosh for these symptoms. Black cohosh is also a source of vitamin A and pantothenic acid.

In the past, the helpful effects of black cohosh were thought to be due to chemicals in the plant that resemble and mimic the effects of the female hormone estrogen. However, the strength of the plant's estrogen-like effects has been disputed, and the exact way black cohosh works in the body is not well understood.

Because some types of cancer, such as breast and endometrial cancer, are stimulated by estrogen, some herbalists state that black cohosh may be dangerous for people who have cancer. But another view holds that since the herb does not actually contain estrogen, it is safe for cancer patients. Some promoters of black cohosh state that the herb reduces the risk for breast and prostate cancer.

Black cohosh has also been used to treat pain before, during, and after childbirth; breast pain; ovarian pain; and uterine pain. Other reported uses of black cohosh include arthritis pain relief, lowering blood pressure, sedation, treatment of bronchial infections, treatment for spasms associated with whooping cough, and treatment of diarrhea.

What does it involve?

Black cohosh is the main ingredient in an over-the-counter German menopausal remedy called Remifemin. In addition, black cohosh can be found in several different forms including capsules, solutions, tablets, tinctures, and powders. There is no standardized treatment plan for the use of the herb. The typical dose suggested is 20 to 40 milligrams of Remifemin twice daily or 40 to 200 milligrams of dried root powder.

What is the history behind it?

Cohosh is a Native American word that means "knobby rough roots," which describes the appearance of the plant's roots. Native Americans used black cohosh to treat uterine disorders, such as menstrual and menopausal symptoms, as well as other ailments, such as diarrhea, sore throat, arthritis, and general weakness. The herb has been approved in Germany for the same purposes for more than fifty years and is commonly prescribed in other European countries.

What is the evidence?

There is inconsistent evidence of effectiveness from clinical trials. Some studies report that black cohosh relieves menopausal symptoms while others do not. Some of the disagreement may be because of differences in the herbal products tested. A 2005 study of 304 women found that, compared with a placebo, black cohosh helped relieve symptoms of menopause. It seemed more effective for women whose symptoms had begun recently than for those who had been postmenopausal for a longer time. On the other hand, a 2006 study of 351 women found that menopausal symptoms were helped by hormone therapy but not by black cohosh (either alone or with other herbs). Clinical trial results published in 2008 reported no difference between black cohosh and placebo with regard to vaginal dryness, menstrual irregularity, female hormones, or the structure of vaginal cells in Pap test samples. The North American Menopause Society recommends considering black cohosh as one of the nonprescription remedies for mild menopausal symptoms, but it points out that the safety of this herb for women with breast cancer remains uncertain.

In a smaller study of twenty-one women, thirteen of whom had breast cancer, participants also reported less trouble with sleeping, less fatigue, and less abnormal sweating after they started taking black cohosh, although this study did not use a placebo control group. Therefore, it was impossible to conclude whether the results were due to black cohosh and not a placebo effect.

A 2001 study of black cohosh and an inactive placebo for breast cancer survivors found no difference in severity or number of hot flashes, although there was a slight reduction in sweating. About two-thirds of these patients were also taking tamoxifen, an anti-estrogen drug that is commonly used in the treatment of breast cancer. Two years later, another study of women with breast cancer being treated with tamoxifen found that hot flashes were less severe and occurred less often in women taking black cohosh. However, a 2006 study of 132 cancer survivors found no effect on hot flashes.

Are there any possible problems or complications?

Serious reactions to moderate doses of black cohosh are very uncommon. Common side effects include upset stomach, nausea, and vomiting. A very high dose may cause slow heart rate, uterine cramps, headache, dizziness, tremors, joint pain, and lightheadedness. There have been a few reports of serious liver disease among women who had recently started using black cohosh. For this reason, some doctors suggest that people who already have liver problems should not use this supplement.

Some doctors are concerned that taking black cohosh might affect how conventional cancer treatments work. There are conflicting results among studies of cancer cells grown in laboratory dishes. Black cohosh does not seem to have an impact on the effectiveness of radiation therapy in these cells, while the herb seems to make some chemotherapy drugs less effective and others more effective. Some studies found black cohosh may reduce the growth of breast cancer cells in laboratory dishes, but another study suggested that it can increase the spread of breast cancer in mice. Because of these conflicting reports, until more is known about this issue, many oncologists recommend a cautious approach and suggest delaying use of black cohosh until treatment is over.

Allergic reactions are possible but rarely reported. Those who are allergic to other members of the buttercup family may be more likely to react to black cohosh. The herb also contains small amounts of salicylic acid and should be used with caution by those allergic to aspirin.

Commission E (Germany's regulatory agency for herbs) recommends that the herb not be taken for more than six months in a row. It should be used with caution in people with high blood pressure and those taking medication for high blood pressure. Women who are thinking about any form of hormone replacement therapy should consult their doctors before taking black cohosh. Women who are pregnant or breastfeeding should not use this herb. Relying on this type of treatment alone and avoiding or delaying conventional medical care for cancer may have serious health consequences.

This product is sold as a dietary supplement in the United States. Unlike companies that produce drugs (which must provide the FDA with results of detailed testing showing their product is safe and effective before the drug is approved for sale), the companies that make supplements do not have to show evidence of safety or health benefits to the FDA before selling their products. Supplement products without any reliable scientific evidence of health benefits may still be sold as long as the companies selling them do not claim the supplements can prevent, treat, or cure any specific disease. Some such products may not contain the amount of the herb or substance that is written on the label, and some may include other substances (contaminants). Though the FDA has written new rules to improve the quality of manufacturing processes for dietary supplements and the accurate listing of supplement ingredients, these rules do not take full effect until 2010. The new rules also do not address the safety of supplement ingredients or their effects on health when proper manufacturing techniques are used.

Most such supplements have not been tested to find out if they interact with medicines, foods, or other herbs and supplements. Even though some reports of interactions and harmful effects may be published, full studies of interactions and effects are not often available. Because of these limitations, any information on ill effects and interactions should be considered incomplete.

References

Black cohosh. Memorial Sloan-Kettering Cancer Center Web site. http://www.mskcc.org/mskcc/html/69140.cfm. Accessed April 6, 2007.

Blumenthal M, ed. *The Complete German Commission E Monographs: Therapeutic Guide to Herbal Medicines.* Austin, TX: American Botanical Council; 1998.

Cohen SM, O'Connor AM, Hart J, Merel NH, Te HS. Autoimmune hepatitis associated with the use of black cohosh: a case study. *Menopause.* 2004;11:575-577.

Davis V, Jayo MJ, Hardy ML, et al. Effects of black cohosh on mammary tumor development and progression in MMTV-neu transgenic mice [abstract R910]. *Proc Am Assoc Cancer Res.* 2nd ed. 2003;44:R910.

Hernández Muñoz G, Pluchino S. *Cimicifuga racemosa* for the treatment of hot flushes in women surviving breast cancer. *Maturitas.* 2003;44 (suppl 1):S59-S65.

Jacobson JS, Troxel AB, Evans J, Klaus L, Vahdat L, Kinne D, Lo KM, Moore A, Rosenman PJ, Kaufman EL, Neugut AI, Grann VR. Randomized trial of black cohosh for the treatment of hot flashes among women with a history of breast cancer. *J Clin Oncol.* 2001;19:2739-2745.

Low Dog T, Powell KL, Weisman SM. Critical evaluation of the safety of *Cimicifuga racemosa* in menopause symptom relief. *Menopause.* 2003;10:299-313.

Lynch CR, Folkers ME, Hutson WR. Fulminant hepatic failure associated with the use of black cohosh: a case report. *Liver Transpl.* 2006;12:989-992.

Natural Standard. Herbal/plant therapies: black cohosh (*Cimicifuga racemosa* [l.] nutt.) Complementary/Integrative Medicine Education Resources, The University of Texas M.D. Anderson Cancer Center Web site. http://www.mdanderson.org/departments/cimer/display.cfm?id=454642F6-FA6F-4259-9CC981E93779D461&method=displayFull. Accessed June 4, 2008.

Neff MJ. NAMS releases position statement on the treatment of vasomotor symptoms associated with menopause. *Am Fam Physician.* 2004;70:393-394, 396, 399.

Newton KM, Reed SD, LaCroix AZ, Grothaus LC, Ehrlich K, Guiltinan J. Treatment of vasomotor symptoms of menopause with black cohosh, multibotanicals, soy, hormone therapy, or placebo: a randomized trial. *Ann Intern Med.* 2006;145:869-879.
Summary for patients in:
Ann Intern Med. 2006;145:I25.

North American Menopause Society. Treatment of menopause-associated vasomotor symptoms: position statement of The North American Menopause Society. *Menopause.* 2004;11:11-33.

Osmers R, Friede M, Liske E, Schnitker J, Freudenstein J, Henneicke-von Zepelin HH. Efficacy and safety of isopropanolic black cohosh extract for climacteric symptoms. *Obstet Gynecol.* 2005;105:1074-1083.

Pockaj BA, Gallagher JG, Loprinzi CL, Stella PJ, Barton DL, Sloan JA, Lavasseur BI, Rao RM, Fitch TR, Rowland KM, Novotny PJ, Flynn PJ, Richelson E, Fauq AH. Phase III double-blind, randomized, placebo-controlled crossover trial of black cohosh in the management of hot flashes: NCCTG Trial N01CC1. *J Clin Oncol.* 2006;24:2836-2841.

Pockaj BA, Loprinzi CL, Sloan JA, Novotny PJ, Barton DL, Hagenmaier A, Zhang H, Lambert GH, Reeser KA, Wisbey JA. Pilot evaluation of black cohosh for the treatment of hot flashes in women. *Cancer Invest.* 2004;22:515-521.

Reed SD, Newton KM, LaCroix AZ, Grothaus LC, Grieco VS, Ehrlich K. Vaginal, endometrial, and reproductive hormone findings: randomized, placebo-controlled trial of black cohosh, multibotanical herbs, and dietary soy for vasomotor symptoms: the Herbal Alternatives for Menopause (HALT) Study. *Menopause.* 2008;15:51-58.

Rockwell S, Liu Y, Higgins SA. Alteration of the effects of cancer therapy agents on breast cancer cells by the herbal medicine black cohosh. *Breast Cancer Res Treat.* 2005;90:233-239.

Stoll W. Phytopharmacon influences atrophic vaginal epithelium. Double-blind study of Cimicifuga vs. estrogenic substances [in German]. *Therapeutikon.* 1987;1:23-31.

Wuttke W, Seidlová-Wuttke D, Gorkow C. The Cimicifuga preparation BNO 1055 vs conjugated estrogens in a double-blind placebo-controlled study: effects on menopause symptoms and bone markers. *Maturitas.* 2003;44 (suppl 1):S67-S77.

BLACK WALNUT

Other common name(s): black walnut hulls, English walnut, butternut, oilnut
Scientific/medical name(s): *Juglans nigra*

Description

The black walnut is a hardwood tree that grows widely in the United States, Canada, and parts of Europe. It can reach a height of more than a hundred feet. The nut hulls, inner bark, leaves, and nut (also called the fruit) are used in herbal remedies.

Overview

Available scientific evidence does not support claims that hulls from black walnuts remove parasites from the intestinal tract or that they are effective in treating cancer or any other disease. Early evidence from laboratory research suggests that juglone, a compound in black walnut, may possibly reduce cancer risk. However, studies in humans have not been completed.

How is it promoted for use?

A small number of herbal medicine practitioners claim that cancer is caused by a parasite. Some of these practitioners claim that a tincture made from black walnut hulls, wormwood, and cloves will kill the cancer-causing parasites, preventing or curing the disease without causing significant side effects. Black walnut is claimed to effectively kill more than a hundred types of parasites.

Black walnut is also promoted as a natural remedy for such wide-ranging conditions as acne, thyroid disease, colitis, eczema, hemorrhoids, ringworm, sore throats, tonsillitis, skin irritations, and wounds. Supporters claim black walnut hulls can be used as a mild laxative that eases general digestive problems. Because of its claimed antiparasitic properties in the stomach and intestines, proponents recommend black walnut for people who travel to areas with contaminated water supplies.

What does it involve?

One part of the black walnut tree used as a remedy is the hull of the fruit (the outside of the nut), which is harvested when it is green. Black walnut hull is available in tablets, capsules, and tinctures. However, some claim that only a tincture, a preparation in which the substance is mixed with alcohol, is effective. Some companies include powdered bark from the tree along with the hulls in their black walnut supplements.

The leaves of the black walnut tree are sometimes used to make tea or placed directly on affected skin to treat ringworm or other skin conditions. Black walnut leaves are available in capsules and tea bags. The inner bark can be used to make infusions and is sometimes ground with the hulls.

What is the history behind it?

Ancient Greeks and Romans called black walnut fruit the "imperial nut" and reportedly used the hull to treat intestinal ailments. Black walnut has also played a part in Russian folk medicine since the seventeenth century. Throughout history, every part of the tree has been used in folk medicine to treat dozens of conditions, including the bite of a mad dog. According to traditional Chinese medicine, eating black walnuts builds physical strength. In Texas folk medicine, black walnut extract is considered an effective treatment for scorpion bites.

Today, craftspeople and artists prize the tree's fine-grained wood for making furniture and carvings, and the nuts are a safe and very popular food for people without nut allergies. Walnuts have been noted to contain omega-3 fatty acids as well as antioxidants such as folate and vitamin E.

What is the evidence?

Available scientific evidence does not support claims that black walnut hulls, bark, or leaves can cure or prevent any disease, including cancer. The notion that parasites cause cancer or that they can be killed with herbal remedies is also unsupported by the available scientific evidence.

Of interest, a few small laboratory studies have suggested that a compound called juglone, which is present in black walnut, may have some antitumor activity. However, studies have not been completed to find out if juglone can help prevent cancer in humans.

In addition, some studies in humans have suggested that eating walnuts (the nut itself, not the hull) can lower "bad" cholesterol and reduce the risk for heart disease. Most of these studies were done on the English walnut, a close relative of the black walnut. The study findings may not pertain to black walnuts.

Are there any possible problems or complications?

Because of the lack of research, little is known about the potential side effects of black walnut hulls or leaves. However, allergy to tree nuts is common, and severe allergic reactions to walnuts have taken place. People who are allergic to other nuts, especially pecans, may also react to walnuts or walnut products. Relying on this type of treatment alone and avoiding or delaying conventional medical care for cancer may have serious health consequences.

This product is sold as a dietary supplement in the United States. Unlike companies that produce drugs (which must provide the FDA with results of detailed testing showing their product is safe and effective before the drug is approved for sale), the companies that make supplements do not have to show evidence of safety or health benefits to the FDA before selling their products. Supplement products without any reliable scientific evidence of health benefits may still be sold as long as the companies selling them do not claim the supplements can prevent, treat, or cure any specific disease. Some such products may not contain the amount of the herb or substance that is written on the label, and some may include other substances (contaminants). Though the FDA has written new rules to improve the quality of manufacturing processes for dietary supplements and the accurate listing of supplement ingredients, these rules do not take full effect until 2010. The new rules also do not address the safety of supplement ingredients or their effects on health when proper manufacturing techniques are used.

Most such supplements have not been tested to find out if they interact with medicines, foods, or other herbs and supplements. Even though some reports of interactions and harmful effects may be published, full studies of interactions and effects are not often available. Because of these limitations, any information on ill effects and interactions should be considered incomplete.

References

Black walnut. Drug Digest Web site. http://www.drugdigest.org/DD/DVH/HerbsWho/0,3923,4080|Black+Walnut,00.html. Accessed June 4, 2008.

Black walnut. PDRhealth Web site. http://www.pdrhealth.com/drugs/altmed/altmed-mono.aspx?contentFileName=ame0211.xml&contentName=Black+Walnut. Accessed June 18, 2008.

Feldman EB. The scientific evidence for a beneficial health relationship between walnuts and coronary heart disease. *J Nutr.* 2002;132:1062S-1101S.

Kruger J, Savitsky K, Gilovich T. Superstition and the regression effect. *Skeptical Inquirer.* 1999;23:24.

McGuffin M, ed. *American Herbal Products Association's Botanical Safety Handbook.* Boca Raton, FL: CRC Press; 1997.

Munday R, Munday CM. Induction of quinone reductase and glutathione transferase in rat tissues by juglone and plumbagin. *Planta Med.* 2000;66:399-402.

Pong AH. Tree nut allergies. Calgary Allergy Network Web site. http://www.calgaryallergy.ca/Articles/English/treenuthp.htm. Accessed June 4, 2008.

Sugie S, Okamoto K, Rahman KM, Tanaka T, Kawai K, Yamahara J, Mori H. Inhibitory effects of plumbagin and juglone on azoxymethane-induced intestinal carcinogenesis in rats. *Cancer Lett.* 1998;127:177-183.

Walsh T. Debunking the detoxification theory. *Nutrition Forum.* 1999;16:1.

BROMELAIN

Other common name(s): bromelin, bromeline, pineapple enzyme, pineapple extract, Ananase, Traumanase, and others

Scientific/medical name(s): sulphydryl proteolytic enzyme, cysteine-proteinase, both made from the plant *Ananas comosus*

Description

Bromelain is a natural enzyme found in the stem and fruit of the pineapple, a tropical fruit native to Central and South America. Bromelain supplements are promoted as an alternative remedy for various health problems, including joint inflammation and cancer.

Overview

Some small studies have suggested bromelain may have some effect on immune function or that it may help reduce the ill effects of some types of chemotherapy. Early studies have also looked at the possible use of bromelain for tissues damaged by burns, as a digestive enzyme, and for the treatment of diarrhea. However, there are no available scientific studies that have looked at whether bromelain shrinks tumors, improves comfort, or extends the life of people with cancer.

How is it promoted for use?

Proponents claim bromelain reduces swelling and inflammation associated with soft-tissue injuries. Some people also believe that the enzyme is an effective treatment for a number of digestive problems because it stimulates the muscles of the intestines. Some practitioners claim bromelain relieves the pain and inflammation caused by joint disorders such as arthritis and carpal tunnel syndrome and that it inhibits cancer cell growth when combined with chemotherapy. There are some who claim that bromelain can "digest fat" and that people who take bromelain pills can lose weight without diet or exercise. Some supporters also state that bromelain fights bacterial and viral infections.

What does it involve?

Although bromelain can be obtained naturally by eating fresh pineapple, some people also use supplements. They are available as capsules, tablets, and ointments in most health food stores and on the Internet. Bromelain is also a common ingredient in supplements sold for joint health. Recommended doses vary by manufacturer.

What is the history behind it?

Bromelain has been used for hundreds of years in folk medicine as a digestive aid and to treat inflammation and other health problems. Christopher Columbus found pineapples growing on the island of Guadeloupe in 1493 and brought them back to Spain. By the 1600s, they were very popular in Europe. In the sixteenth and seventeenth centuries, the plants were distributed to the Pacific Islands, India, and Africa. Pineapple was first established as a commercial crop in Hawaii in 1885. Recently, bromelain has been investigated for medical uses, including possible anticancer activity.

What is the evidence?

There are some suggestions that bromelain may be beneficial for a number of conditions. However, further research is needed to learn more about bromelain's possible benefits for humans. A clinical study of sixteen breast cancer patients in Germany found that a bromelain drug taken by mouth may stimulate one aspect of immune function. However, this study did not measure actual benefit, such as improvement or survival, of the treated women. Other studies suggest that bromelain increases the quantities of immune system hormones, called cytokines, that are produced by white blood cells. There are newer studies suggesting that bromelain and other such enzymes may be used with standard cancer treatment to help reduce some side effects of therapy and possibly some symptoms of the cancer itself. No scientific data are available on bromelain's impact on survival or quality of life in people who have cancer. Additional well-controlled research is needed to understand its role, if any, in cancer treatment.

A number of laboratory and animal studies suggest that bromelain may help treat diarrhea related to *E. coli* infections. The health benefits to humans have not been proven. It also appears to help keep platelets in the blood from sticking together, which in turn may help prevent blood clots. Although animal and laboratory studies look promising for some of these uses, further studies are necessary to determine whether the results apply to humans.

The German Commission E approved bromelain to be used with other treatments for swelling or inflammation of the nose and sinuses caused by surgery. Some studies have suggested that bromelain may speed recovery time, although not all studies have found it helpful. A 2006 review of three studies suggested that bromelain may help relieve the symptoms of sinusitis. However, sinusitis caused by allergies or different forms of infection may vary in response to bromelain.

Studies on joint injuries and muscle pain have also shown mixed results. Bromelain may have an anti-inflammatory effect. Some clinical trials that compared bromelain to standard treatment found it less effective, while others reported it as a possible alternative. More research is needed.

Early studies suggest that bromelain may be helpful when used directly on burns to remove damaged tissue without surgery. A few clinical studies have used bromelain to clean dead or dying tissue from burns that were severe enough to injure or kill layers of skin. The results suggested that bromelain may speed healing and reduce the need for surgery to remove dead and injured tissues in some patients. More research is needed to confirm these findings.

Because bromelain is an enzyme that breaks down proteins, it is a possible alternative to help digestion in people who don't make enough digestive enzymes on their own. More research is needed to directly compare bromelain's effectiveness to that of the enzymes generally used for this purpose.

Are there any possible problems or complications?

Bromelain is generally considered safe, although it may speed up the heart rate. Some people may be allergic to bromelain and pineapple, especially those with allergies to kiwi fruit, papaya (including papain), or natural rubber latex, and serious reactions may occur. Those allergic to honeybee stings, birch or cypress pollen, grass pollen, carrots, celery, fennel, wheat flour, or rye flour may also have a higher risk for reacting to bromelain. People who are allergic to pineapple should not take bromelain.

Upset stomach with nausea, vomiting, and diarrhea have been noted. A few women have reported increased menstrual bleeding while taking bromelain. Some practitioners advise caution when giving bromelain to people with high blood pressure, liver disease, kidney disease, or bleeding disorders.

When bromelain is taken with blood-thinning medications or aspirin, it may raise the risk for bleeding. Some antibiotics may reach higher levels in the body when taken with bromelain. There may be other potential interactions between bromelain and medicines or herbs, and some may be dangerous. Always tell your doctor and pharmacist about any herbs you are taking. Relying on this treatment alone and avoiding or delaying conventional medical care for cancer may have serious health consequences.

This product is sold as a dietary supplement in the United States. Unlike companies that produce drugs (which must provide the FDA with results of detailed testing showing their product is safe and effective before the drug is approved for sale), the companies that make supplements do not have to show evidence of safety or health benefits to the FDA before selling their products. Supplement products without any reliable scientific evidence of health benefits may still be sold as long as the companies selling them do not claim the supplements can prevent, treat, or cure any specific disease. Some such products may not contain the amount of the herb or substance that is written on the label, and some may include other substances (contaminants). Though the FDA has written new rules to improve the quality of manufacturing processes for dietary supplements and the accurate listing of supplement ingredients, these rules do not take full effect until 2010. The new rules also do not address the safety of supplement ingredients or their effects on health when proper manufacturing techniques are used.

Most such supplements have not been tested to find out if they interact with medicines, foods, or other herbs and supplements. Even though some reports of interactions and harmful effects may be published, full studies of interactions and effects are not often available. Because of these limitations, any information on ill effects and interactions should be considered incomplete.

References

Akhtar NM, Naseer R, Farooqi AZ, Aziz W, Nazir M. Oral enzyme combination versus diclofenac in the treatment of osteoarthritis of the knee—a double-blind prospective randomized study. *Clin Rheumatol.* 2004;23:410-415. Epub 2004 Jul 24.

Barrett S. Bromeline "diet pills". Quackwatch Web site. http://www.quackwatch.org/04ConsumerEducation/QA/bromeline.html. Posted October 18, 1999. Accessed June 4, 2008.

Blumenthal M, ed. *The Complete German Commission E Monographs: Therapeutic Guide to Herbal Medicines.* Austin, TX: American Botanical Council; 1998.

Bromelain. Medline Plus Web site. http://www.nlm.nih.gov/medlineplus/druginfo/natural/patient-bromelain.html. Accessed June 4, 2008.

Bromelain. Memorial Sloan-Kettering Cancer Center Web site. http://www.mskcc.org/mskcc/html/69152.cfm. Accessed June 4, 2008.

Bromelain. PDRhealth Web site. http://www.pdrhealth.com/drugs/altmed/altmed-mono.aspx?contentFileName=ame0025.xml&contentName=Bromelain. Accessed June 4, 2008.

Cassileth B. *The Alternative Medicine Handbook: The Complete Reference Guide to Alternative and Complementary Therapies.* New York: W.W. Norton; 1998.

Chandler DS, Mynott TL. Bromelain protects piglets from diarrhea caused by oral challenge with K88 positive enterotoxigenic *Escherichia coli. Gut.* 1998;43:196-202.

Desser L, Holomanova D, Zavadova E, Pavelka K, Mohr T, Herbacek I. Oral therapy with proteolytic enzymes decreases excessive TGF-beta levels in human blood. *Cancer Chemother Pharmacol.* 2001;47(suppl):S10-S15.

Desser L, Rehberger A, Kokron E, Paukovits W. Cytokine synthesis in human peripheral blood mononuclear cells after oral administration of polyenzyme preparations. *Oncology.* 1993;50:403-407.

Eckert K, Grabowska E, Stange R, Schneider U, Eschmann K, Maurer HR. Effects of oral bromelain administration on the impaired immunocytotoxicity of mononuclear cells from mammary tumor patients. *Oncol Rep.* 1999;6:1191-1199.

Gruenwald J. *PDR for Herbal Medicines.* 3rd ed. Montvale, NJ: Thomson PDR; 2004.

Guo R, Canter PH, Ernst E. Herbal medicines for the treatment of rhinosinusitis: a systematic review. *Otolaryngol Head Neck Surg.* 2006;135:496-506.

Kerkhoffs GM, Struijs PA, de Wit C, Rahlfs VW, Zwipp H, van Dijk CN. A double blind, randomised, parallel group study on the efficacy and safety of treating acute lateral ankle sprain with oral hydrolytic enzymes. *Br J Sports Med.* 2004;38:431-435.

Metzig C, Grabowska E, Eckert K, Rehse K, Maurer HR. Bromelain proteases reduce human platelet aggregation in vitro, adhesion to bovine endothelial cells and thrombus formation in rat vessels in vivo. *In Vivo.* 1999;13:7-12.

Pineapple-*Ananas comosus.* University of Georgia Web site. www.uga.edu/fruit/pinapple.html. Accessed June 4, 2008

Sinusitis. University of Maryland Medical Center Web site. http://www.umm.edu/ency/article/000647.htm. Accessed June 4, 2008.

Stone MB, Merrick MA, Ingersoll CD, Edwards JE. Preliminary comparison of bromelain and ibuprofen for delayed onset muscle soreness management. *Clin J Sport Med.* 2002;12:373-378.

CALCIUM

Other common name(s): calcium carbonate, calcium gluconate, calcium citrate
Scientific/medical name(s): Ca, Ca++

Description

Calcium is a mineral that is vital for a number of bodily functions, such as contraction of muscles (including the heart), secretion of hormones, and sending messages through the nervous system. Most of the body's calcium is in the bones and teeth, but some of it circulates in the blood for these important tasks. Calcium is found naturally in many dairy products, leafy green vegetables, and fish. Because humans cannot make calcium, it must be obtained from foods or supplements.

Overview

Many people, especially women, can benefit from keeping up with their calcium intake to help prevent bone problems such as osteoporosis. Calcium supplements will not slow the growth of most cancers, although they appear to reduce the risk for precancerous polyps of the colon. Calcium supplements may be important for some people with cancer, depending on their specific cancer type and stage and the type of treatments received.

How is it promoted for use?

Calcium is best known for its role in growing and maintaining the bones and teeth. It also helps the heart and other muscles do their work. There is strong evidence that low calcium intake can lead to fragile bones, high blood pressure, and certain types of cancer. Recent studies have shown that calcium may reduce the risk for colon cancer and perhaps some other types of cancer. When combined with vitamin D, calcium may have the potential to help prevent cancers of the breast and pancreas. Calcium has also been found helpful in reducing certain symptoms of premenstrual syndrome. There is some early evidence that calcium may play a role in helping to prevent heart disease and reducing insulin resistance in diabetic patients.

Because calcium plays a crucial role in building and maintaining bone mass and strength, its greatest benefit to people with cancer may be to reduce the risk for osteopenia (reduced bone mass) and osteoporosis, a condition that results in fragile bones and a severe loss of bone mass and strength. Both conditions are linked mainly with aging, and osteoporosis is a common problem for women after menopause. Osteopenia and osteoporosis can also result from poor nutrition, prolonged drug therapy, disease, and poor mobility, all of which may apply to people who have cancer.

What does it involve?

The body's use of calcium is complex. It is affected by many hormones and factors other than how much calcium a person eats or takes in. There are many ways to treat bone problems and calcium imbalance in the body, depending on their causes.

The best source of calcium is a balanced diet, which helps to avoid bone problems and decreases the risk for some types of cancer. Foods and beverages high in calcium include milk and other dairy products (low-fat products are healthier), leafy green vegetables such as broccoli and greens, nuts, seeds, beans, tofu prepared with calcium, cheese, dried figs, kelp, oysters, and canned fish that can be eaten with the bones still in it, such as sardines and salmon. Certain brands of cereals, orange juices, and soy milks are fortified with calcium and are clearly marked as such on the label.

Although calcium intake from healthy foods is the best source, calcium supplements are also available in drug stores, grocery stores, and many health food stores. The Adequate Intake (AI) for calcium is 1,000 milligrams per day for men and women between the age of nineteen and fifty, and 1,200 milligrams per day for people over fifty. Some nutritionists and doctors recommend that calcium supplements be taken with supplements of vitamin D and other important minerals, such as magnesium and potassium.

What is the history behind it?

The importance of calcium for maintaining overall health and promoting bone strength has been known for decades. Some scientists believe that humans became accustomed to diets high in calcium as far back as thirty-five thousand years ago. Calcium's role in preventing or slowing the growth of cancer has only become a notable subject of research within the last fifteen to twenty years.

What is the evidence?

A number of important studies to measure calcium's impact on cancer have been published in peer-reviewed medical journals. Several studies have suggested that foods high in calcium might help reduce the risk for colorectal cancer. These studies also suggest that calcium supplements may somewhat reduce the risk for adenomas, a type of polyps in the colon and rectum that can progress to cancer. More recent studies have noted that women with higher dietary calcium intake seemed to have a lower risk for breast cancer. This risk was not affected by calcium supplements.

One researcher reviewed several dozen studies of the effects of calcium on various diseases and concluded that long-term deficiencies in calcium and vitamin D may lead not only to fragile bones but also to colorectal cancer and high blood pressure in some people. Adequate calcium intake may help to prevent these conditions in some people. A randomized clinical trial reported in 2007 found a lower risk for all cancers combined in women given calcium supplements than in women taking the placebo. Cancer risk was even lower among women taking both calcium and vitamin D.

While further research is needed to clarify the role of calcium in preventing or reversing cancer growth, there is little doubt that adequate calcium intake is required for preventing bone shrinkage and weakening. For people who have cancer, calcium and vitamin D intake may help keep bones strong.

Some chemotherapy medications can reduce appetite, create swallowing difficulties, cause nausea and vomiting, and result in osteopenia. The chemotherapy drugs methotrexate and doxorubicin may directly damage bones. Some hormonal therapies used in the treatment of breast or prostate cancer can also weaken bones. Radiation therapy can cause osteopenia within the area being treated, and the combination of radiation therapy and chemotherapy can cause even greater damage to bone structure. Some cancers also can harm bones. Although adequate calcium intake is important for bone health in the general public and in cancer survivors, and especially in those with osteoporosis, calcium intake is not the only factor that determines bone health. Physical activity is also important in keeping bones strong. In addition, there are several kinds of medications available for treatment of osteoporosis.

Are there any possible problems or complications?

The greatest risk with calcium comes from not getting enough of it. In rare cases, taking in very high levels of calcium (usually more than 2,400 milligrams a day) can lead to high levels of calcium in the blood, a condition called hypercalcemia. Hypercalcemia can cause kidney stones, muscle pain, and mental confusion and is considered a serious medical condition. It is also possible to get high calcium levels from taking in too much vitamin D, such as from supplement overuse. However, most cases of high calcium levels are caused by the cancer itself, especially in its later stages.

Calcium can keep other minerals such as iron, zinc, magnesium, and phosphorus from being absorbed. Calcium can also interfere with the absorption of several types of medicine, so it is helpful to talk with your doctor or pharmacist about all medicines and supplements that you are taking.

There is some evidence that a high calcium intake, mainly through supplements, is linked with increased risk for prostate cancer, especially for prostate cancer that is more aggressive. Both men and women should try to take in recommended levels of calcium, mainly through food sources. Dairy products are excellent sources of calcium, as are some leafy vegetables and greens. People who get much of their calcium from dairy products may want to select low-fat or fat-free choices to reduce their intake of saturated fat.

Some conditions can interfere with the absorption of calcium from the stomach. Poor vitamin D intake and inactivity decrease calcium absorption. Low stomach acid can cause calcium carbonate to be poorly absorbed, although it does not affect other forms of calcium the same way. For those who either have low stomach acid or take medicine to block stomach acid, calcium citrate is better absorbed.

Those who have kidney stones, kidney failure, or high parathyroid levels should talk with their doctors before taking calcium supplements. People who are having treatment for cancer should talk to their doctors or cancer team before taking vitamins, minerals, or other supplements that might interact with the cancer drugs prescribed. Relying on this type of treatment alone and avoiding or delaying conventional medical care for cancer may have serious health consequences.

This product is sold as a dietary supplement in the United States. Unlike companies that produce drugs (which must provide the FDA with results of detailed testing showing their product is safe and effective before the drug is approved for sale), the companies that make supplements do not have to show evidence of safety or health benefits to the FDA before selling their products. Supplement products

without any reliable scientific evidence of health benefits may still be sold as long as the companies selling them do not claim the supplements can prevent, treat, or cure any specific disease. Some such products may not contain the amount of the herb or substance that is written on the label, and some may include other substances (contaminants). Though the FDA has written new rules to improve the quality of manufacturing processes for dietary supplements and the accurate listing of supplement ingredients, these rules do not take full effect until 2010. The new rules also do not address the safety of supplement ingredients or their effects on health when proper manufacturing techniques are used.

Most such supplements have not been tested to find out if they interact with medicines, foods, or other herbs and supplements. Even though some reports of interactions and harmful effects may be published, full studies of interactions and effects are not often available. Because of these limitations, any information on ill effects and interactions should be considered incomplete.

References

Baron JA, Beach M, Mandel JS, van Stolk RU, Haile RW, Sandler RS, Rothstein R, Summers RW, Snover DC, Beck GJ, Bond JH, Greenberg ER. Calcium supplements for the prevention of colorectal adenomas. *N Engl J Med.* 1999;340:101-107.

Calcium. Memorial Sloan-Kettering Cancer Center Web site. http://www.mskcc.org/mskcc/html/69157.cfm. Accessed June 4, 2008.

Cassileth B. *The Alternative Medicine Handbook: The Complete Reference Guide to Alternative and Complementary Therapies.* New York: W.W. Norton; 1998.

Cats A, Kleibeuker JH, van der Meer R, Kuipers F, Sluiter WJ, Hardonk MJ, Oremus ET, Mulder NH, de Vries EG. Randomized, double-blinded, placebo-controlled intervention study with supplemental calcium in families with hereditary nonpolyposis colorectal cancer. *J Natl Cancer Inst.* 1995;87:598-603.

Dietary supplement fact sheet: calcium. Office of Dietary Supplements Web site. http://dietary-supplements.info.nih.gov/factsheets/calcium.asp. Accessed June 4, 2008.

Giovannucci E, Rimm EB, Wolk A, Ascherio A, Stampfer MJ, Colditz GA, Willett WC. Calcium and fructose intake in relation to risk of prostate cancer. *Cancer Res.* 1998;58:442-447.

Guise TA. Bone loss and fracture risk associated with cancer therapy. *Oncologist.* 2006;11:1121-1131.

Holt PR. Dairy foods and prevention of colon cancer: human studies. *J Am Coll Nutr.* 1999;18:379S-391S.

Hyman J, Baron JA, Dain BJ, Sandler RS, Haile RW, Mandel JS, Mott LA, Greenberg ER. Dietary and supplemental calcium and the recurrence of colorectal adenomas. *Cancer Epidemiol Biomarkers Prev.* 1998;7:291-295.

Kushi LH, Byers T, Doyle C, Bandera EV, McCullough M, McTiernan A, Gansler T, Andrews KS, Thun MJ; American Cancer Society 2006 Nutrition and Physical Activity Guidelines Advisory Committee. American Cancer Society guidelines on nutrition and physical activity for cancer prevention: reducing the risk of cancer with healthy food choices and physical activity. *CA Cancer J Clin.* 2006;56:254-281.

Lappe JM, Travers-Gustafson D, Davies KM, Recker RR, Heaney RP. Vitamin D and calcium supplementation reduces cancer risk: results of a randomized trial. *Am J Clin Nutr.* 2007;85:1586-1591.

Lipkin M, Newmark HL. Vitamin D, calcium and prevention of breast cancer: a review. *J Am Coll Nutr.* 1999;18:392S-397S.

Martinez ME, Jacobs ET. Calcium supplementation and prevention of colorectal neoplasia: lessons from clinical trials. *JNCI J Natl Cancer Inst.* 2007;99:99-100.

McCullough ML, Rodriguez C, Diver WR, Feigelson HS, Stevens VL, Thun MJ, Calle EE. Dairy, calcium, and vitamin D intake and postmenopausal breast cancer risk in the Cancer Prevention Study II Nutrition Cohort. *Cancer Epidemiol Biomarkers Prev.* 2005;14:2898-2904.

Neugut AI, Horvath K, Whelan RL, Terry MB, Garbowski GC, Bertram A, Forde KA, Treat MR, Waye J. The effect of calcium and vitamin supplements on the incidence and recurrence of colorectal adenomatous polyps. *Cancer.* 1996;78:723-728.

Thys-Jacobs S, Starkey P, Bernstein D, Tian J; Premenstrual Syndrome Study Group. Calcium carbonate and the premenstrual syndrome: effects on premenstrual and menstrual symptoms. *Am J Obstet Gynecol.* 1998;179:444-452.

CAPSICUM

Other common name(s): capsaicin, cayenne, chili pepper, hot pepper, red pepper, paprika, pimiento, long pepper, conoids

Scientific/medical name(s): *Capsicum annum, Capsicum frutescens*

Description

Capsicum is the name of a group of annual plants in the nightshade (*Solanaceae*) family. They are native to Mexico and Central America but are cultivated for food in many warmer regions of the world. Capsicum varieties include the cayenne pepper, jalapeño pepper, other hot peppers, and paprika. Capsaicin is the most-studied active ingredient in the plant and has been approved by the U.S. Food and Drug Administration (FDA) for use on the skin.

Overview

Although little research has been reported using the whole *Capsicum annum* or *Capsicum frutescens* plant for people with cancer, capsaicin (a major active ingredient) has been studied in oral and topical forms. Several studies have shown that capsaicin may be somewhat useful for managing pain related to surgery and mouth sores due to chemotherapy and radiation therapy.

However, more research is needed on other uses of capsaicin and to find out whether the whole herb is helpful for treating or preventing illness.

How is it promoted for use?

Capsaicin in topical form is promoted mainly for pain caused by conditions such as arthritis and general muscle soreness. The FDA approved a topical form of capsaicin for treating pain more than twenty years ago that is still sold without a prescription. There is some evidence that capsaicin may be useful in managing postsurgical pain from mastectomy, thoracotomy (chest surgery), amputation, and other surgery related to mainstream cancer treatment. Researchers have found that capsaicin may provide temporary relief for pain from mouth sores caused by chemotherapy and radiation therapy.

Some proponents claim that capsaicin has antioxidant properties that help to fight nitrosamine, a cancer-causing agent. An antioxidant is a compound that blocks the action of free radicals, activated oxygen molecules that can damage cells. Still others claim that capsaicin may prevent DNA damage and lung cancer due to cigarette smoke.

Over the years, the *Capsicum annum* or *Capsicum frutescens* herb has been used by alternative medicine practitioners as a remedy for a variety of conditions, such as upset stomach, menstrual cramps, headaches, shingles, diarrhea, loss of appetite, stomach ulcers, poor digestion, sore throat, itching, alcoholism, motion sickness, toothache, malaria, and yellow fever. Some practitioners also claim it can prevent colds, heart disease, and stroke; increase sexual potency; foster weight loss; and strengthen the heart.

What does it involve?

The capsaicin cream, ointment, gel, lotion, or stick is rubbed directly onto the skin over painful areas. Depending on the strength of the preparation, it may be recommended for use for as little as two days or as long as two months. It can be obtained with or without a prescription.

Capsicum is available in health food stores as a tonic, a capsule, or in tea. There are some recipes available over the Internet that advocate making a candy with cayenne pepper to relieve the pain of mouth sores caused by chemotherapy and radiation. Peppers are available fresh, canned, frozen, and dried in food stores.

What is the history behind it?

As far back as 5000 BC, people in South America ate meals prepared with hot peppers. Natives of Mexico and some Chinese (Hunan and Szechuan) are also known to have used hot peppers in many dishes and continue to do so. These cultures have also used hot peppers in herbal medicine to treat numerous conditions over the years.

While foods made with different kinds of peppers are popular in a variety of ethnic cuisines, it is only in recent years that interest in using capsaicin from hot peppers to manage pain and other symptoms or illnesses has grown. Medical researchers are now looking at the use of capsaicin as a possible cancer treatment.

What is the evidence?

Although there is little available research on the use of the whole *Capsicum* herb for people with cancer, capsaicin has been intensively researched for use on the skin. Extracted chemicals such as capsaicin are not the same as the whole plant, so study results of extracts are unlikely to be the same as studies using the whole plant.

A study in 1989 found topical capsaicin to have pain-relieving effects among 50 percent of a small group of women who had undergone mastectomy for breast cancer. A 1991 study concluded that capsaicin cream reduced the amount of pain caused by diabetic neuropathy (a nerve disorder). Nerve pain (also called neuropathic pain) is often experienced by patients after cancer surgery and may be felt as numbness, tingling, burning, shooting, or electric shock-like pain. In 1994, a review of previous research concluded that while topical capsaicin is not satisfactory as a therapy by itself, it may be used with other medicines to ease pain. A 2004 review of six clinical trials of patients with chronic long-term pain found that topical capsaicin was helpful to some. However, about a third of the patients using capsaicin had side effects that were not experienced by the placebo groups. Studies continue on new ways to use capsaicin for pain and itching.

A small 2006 study tested the effects on cholesterol of raw chili peppers. Out of twenty-seven test subjects, one group consumed raw chopped chilies every day for four weeks, and the other group consumed a bland diet. No differences in cholesterol were noted between the two groups.

In a pilot study conducted at the Yale University School of Medicine, oral capsaicin (mixed with taffy) reduced pain in eleven patients with mouth sores caused by chemotherapy or radiation therapy. For most of the patients, however, the pain relief was incomplete and did not last long. A later controlled study looked at larger doses of capsaicin for fifty patients with a condition called burning mouth syndrome. The researchers reported that some patients got relief from the mouth pain and burning, but more than 30 percent of patients taking capsaicin had fairly significant stomach pain. No patients in the placebo group had stomach complaints.

Studies have also been conducted to examine capsaicin's potential to relieve itching, reduce the size of nasal polyps, and protect against substances that cause cancer. However, researchers have found it difficult to conduct these studies because of the burning sensation caused by oral or topical use of capsaicin. The discomfort has caused some patients to stop using it. It also makes it difficult for researchers to conduct controlled studies of the drug, since the patient can often tell the active substance from the placebo.

Capsaicin has been shown to slow the growth of prostate cancer cells in laboratory studies and rodents. Researchers are looking into the use of capsaicin for prostate cancer in humans. Even though a treatment may look promising in animal and laboratory studies, further studies are required to find out whether the results apply to humans.

Available scientific research does not support claims for the effectiveness of capsicum or whole pepper supplements in preventing or curing cancer at this time. Claims that capsicum can help addiction, malaria, yellow fever, heart disease, stroke, weight loss, poor appetite, and sexual potency are not supported by available scientific evidence. The pepper extract capsaicin appears to have some value as a pain reliever, but its side effects limit its usefulness for some people.

Are there any possible problems or complications?

Cayenne and other peppers are considered safe to eat in moderate amounts for those who are not allergic to peppers. The FDA includes peppers on their "generally recognized as safe" list of food ingredients. However, capsicum supplements taken by mouth can cause stomach upset or diarrhea. Direct contact between peppers and the mouth or other mucous membranes can cause stinging, burning, or pain. Sweating, skin flushing, runny nose, and tears are also fairly common effects of taking capsicum supplements. Long-term use of supplements or chiles can cause stomach irritation.

Oleoresin of capsicum (OC), commonly called "pepper spray", is used in spray form as a way to incapacitate people in threatening situations. Usually the spray causes burning of the eyes, nose, mouth, and skin. Some people cough and have trouble breathing for a short time. Those with asthma or other breathing problems may have worse effects. Generally, pepper spray does not cause permanent damage, but there are exceptions, and deaths have been reported.

Some animal studies have shown that capsicum induced liver tumors and caused cancerous tumors (adenocarcinomas) of the intestine, although these effects have not been shown in humans.

Capsaicin in cream or other topical form often causes temporary stinging, burning, or itching when applied directly to the skin. In severe cases, blisters or rash may result. Capsaicin cream can increase the absorption of other substances through the skin, so other chemicals, lotions, and substances should be kept away from capsaicin-treated areas. Contact with eyes, mucous membranes, or broken skin should be avoided, as severe burning and irritation can occur. After applying the cream, wash hands thoroughly (unless applying to the hands). Some recommend using plastic gloves when applying the cream.

In addition, possible interactions between herbs and drugs or other herbs should be considered. Capsicum supplements may cause the body to absorb more theophylline (an asthma medicine) and acetaminophen (pain medicine). They can also interfere with or worsen side effects of certain blood pressure medicines and other drugs. Some combinations may be dangerous. Always tell your doctor and pharmacist about any herbs you are taking.

Those who are allergic to peppers should not take or use capsaicin or other pepper extracts. Children and women who are pregnant or breastfeeding should avoid taking this supplement internally. Relying on this type of treatment alone and avoiding or delaying conventional medical care for cancer may have serious health consequences.

This product is sold as a dietary supplement in the United States. Unlike companies that produce drugs (which must provide the FDA with results of detailed testing showing their product is safe and effective before the drug is approved for sale), the companies that make supplements do not have to show evidence of safety or health benefits to the FDA before selling their products. Supplement products without any reliable scientific evidence of health benefits may still be sold as long as the companies selling them do not claim the supplements can prevent, treat, or cure any specific disease. Some such products may not contain the amount of the herb or substance that is written on the label, and some may include other substances (contaminants). Though the FDA has written new rules to improve the quality of manufacturing processes for dietary supplements and the accurate listing of supplement ingredients, these rules do not take full effect until 2010. The new rules also do not address the safety of supplement ingredients or their effects on health when proper manufacturing techniques are used.

Most such supplements have not been tested to find out if they interact with medicines, foods, or other herbs and supplements. Even though some reports of interactions and harmful effects may be published, full studies of interactions and effects are not often available. Because of these limitations, any information on ill effects and interactions should be considered incomplete.

References

Ahuja KD, Ball MJ. Effects of daily ingestion of chilli on serum lipoprotein oxidation in adult men and women. *Br J Nutr.* 2006;96:239-242.

Berger A, Henderson M, Nadoolman W, Duffy V, Cooper D, Saberski L, Bartoshuk L. Oral capsaicin provides temporary relief for oral mucositis pain secondary to chemotherapy/radiation therapy. *J Pain Symptom Manage.* 1995;10:243-248.
Erratum in:
J Pain Symptom Manage. 1996;11:331.

Capsaicin. Memorial Sloan-Kettering Cancer Center Web site. http://www.mskcc.org/mskcc/html/69162.cfm. Accessed June 4, 2008.

Cayenne. Memorial Sloan-Kettering Cancer Center Web site. http://www.mskcc.org/mskcc/html/69167.cfm. Accessed June 4, 2008.

Commission on Life Sciences. *Carcinogens and Anticarcinogens in the Human Diet: A Comparison of Naturally Occurring and Synthetic Substances.* Washington, DC: National Academy Press; 1996:360.

Dini D, Bertelli G, Gozza A, Forno GG. Treatment of the post-mastectomy pain syndrome with topical capsaicin. *Pain.* 1993;54:223-226.

Ellison N, Loprinzi CL, Kugler J, Hatfield AK, Miser A, Sloan JA, Wender DB, Rowland KM, Molina R, Cascino TL, Vukov AM, Dhaliwal HS, Ghosh C. Phase III placebo-controlled trial of capsaicin cream in the management of surgical neuropathic pain in cancer patients. *J Clin Oncol.* 1997;15:2974-2980.

Fetrow CW, Avila JR. *Professional's Handbook of Complementary & Alternative Medicines.* Philadelphia, PA: Lippincott Williams & Wilkins; 2004.

Gagnier JJ, van Tulder MW, Berman B, Bombardier C. Herbal medicine for low back pain: a Cochrane review. *Spine.* 2007;32:82-92.

Gruenwald J. *PDR for Herbal Medicines.* 3rd ed. Montvale, NJ: Thomson PDR; 2004.

Johnson W Jr. Final report on the safety assessment of capsicum annuum extract, capsicum annuum fruit extract, capsicum annuum resin, capsicum annuum fruit powder, capsicum frutescens fruit, capsicum frutescens fruit extract, capsicum frutescens resin, and capsaicin. *Int J Toxicol.* 2007;26(suppl 1):3-106.

Mason L, Moore RA, Derry S, Edwards JE, McQuay HJ. Systematic review of topical capsaicin for the treatment of chronic pain. *BMJ.* 2004;328:991. Epub 2004 Mar 19.

Mori A, Lehmann S, O'Kelly J, Kumagai T, Desmond JC, Pervan M, McBride WH, Kizaki M, Koeffler HP. Capsaicin, a component of red peppers, inhibits the growth of androgen-independent, p53 mutant prostate cancer cells. *Cancer Res.* 2006;66:3222-3229.

Olajos EJ, Salem H. Riot control agents: pharmacology, toxicology, biochemistry and chemistry. *J Appl Toxicol.* 2001;21:355-391.

Petruzzi M, Lauritano D, De Benedittis M, Baldoni M, Serpico R. Systemic capsaicin for burning mouth syndrome: short-term results of a pilot study. *J Oral Pathol Med.* 2004;33:111-114.

Watson CP. Topical capsaicin as an adjuvant analgesic. *J Pain Symptom Manage.* 1994;9:425-433.

Watson CP, Evans RJ. The postmastectomy pain syndrome and topical capsaicin: a randomized trial. *Pain.* 1992;51:375-379.

CAT'S CLAW

Other common name(s): Una de Gato
Scientific/medical name(s): *Uncaria tomentosa*

Description

Cat's claw is a woody vine that winds its way up trees at high elevations in the Peruvian rain forests. The plant's name comes from the claw-like thorns that grow on the plant's stem, which can reach up to a hundred feet. The root, which can grow to the size of a watermelon, and the inside of the bark have traditionally been used in herbal remedies. Because of increased demand, the plant can now be harvested only above ground.

Overview

Cat's claw has been promoted as a remedy to boost the body's immune system, but available scientific evidence in humans does not support claims of immune-stimulating effects. Available scientific evidence also does not support cat's claw's effectiveness in preventing or treating cancer or any other disease. Cat's claw is associated with some serious side effects, although the extent of those effects is not known.

How is it promoted for use?

The most common claims for cat's claw are that it boosts the immune system and increases the body's ability to fight off infections, including yeasts, parasites, and herpes, as well as other viruses. The herb also is promoted as a remedy for arthritis, allergies, inflammatory bowel disorders, cancer, cardiovascular disease, diabetes, asthma, and menstrual disorders. South American folk medicine holds that cat's claw is a contraceptive, and some practitioners claim that it can significantly decrease AIDS-related symptoms.

What does it involve?

Cat's claw is taken by mouth and is available in capsules, tablets, tinctures, elixirs, and as a tea. Sometimes it can be found as a cream for application to the skin. Practitioner recommendations for how much to take vary widely. Some suggest a dose of 3,000 to 6,000 milligrams per day in pill form, or four strong cups of tea. Herbalists may prescribe up to 20 grams per day for seriously ill patients. Because herbs are not regulated in the United States, different brands of cat's claw may contain very different amounts of active ingredients.

What is the history behind it?

For centuries, South American native tribes have used cat's claw medicinally. Awareness of the herb grew in the United States and Europe during the 1970s, when an Austrian scientist, Klaus Kiplinger, traveled to the rain forests of Peru and learned about the plant from local priests. Kiplinger eventually received patents for isolating the active ingredients within the plant. Recently, cat's claw has become an extremely popular herbal supplement among consumers in the United States and Europe. Because demand for this herb has increased greatly in the past few years, the Peruvian government now forbids harvesting the roots of the plant. The same compounds are present in the bark as in the root, and so the plant is now harvested three feet above the ground. This preserves the plant so that it can be harvested again a few years later.

What is the evidence?

Rigorous scientific study of cat's claw in humans is not available. The reported positive effects of the herb are either anecdotal reports or the results of laboratory studies. In laboratory and animal studies, researchers have been able to identify certain substances in cat's claw that may lead to further discovery. Among these are chemicals called alkaloids. One Canadian laboratory study concluded that some of the alkaloids can stimulate the white blood cells of rats. Similar studies found that the alkaloids increase phagocytosis, the process in which white blood cells seek out and destroy invading germs. Also found in cat's claw were antioxidants—compounds that block the actions of free radicals, which can damage cells.

Certain alkaloids in cat's claw are thought to reduce inflammation, slow the heart rate, slow the growth of tumors, and possibly lower blood pressure. Human studies have not yet confirmed that cat's claw or its extracts have any of these effects. Peruvian researchers in the 1970s claimed that cat's claw was an effective treatment for children with leukemia, but available scientific evidence does not confirm those reports. Results of laboratory studies have been inconsistent. A 2006 study suggested this plant is not effective in killing leukemia cells and may actually help the leukemia cells to survive longer. A study published in 2007 suggested that chemicals from cat's claw might help kill cells from two forms of nervous-system cancer.

Available scientific evidence does not support claims that this herb can treat cancer or other diseases in people. Animal and laboratory studies may show promise, but further studies are necessary to find out whether the results apply to humans. Until clinical trials in humans are completed, the true value of cat's claw remains uncertain.

Are there any possible problems or complications?

More research is needed to be sure that cat's claw is safe. Thus far, animal studies suggest that it is unlikely to be very toxic to humans. Mild rash, lowered blood pressure, sleepiness, and diarrhea may be possible.

Herbalists warn that people who are taking blood pressure medicines, blood-thinning medications, hormones, or insulin should not take cat's claw. This herb may also have an effect on the way the body excretes drugs, so it is possible that it may raise the blood levels of certain sedatives and sleeping medicines. The potential interactions between herbs and other medications or herbs should be considered. Some combinations may be dangerous. Always tell your doctor and pharmacist about any herbs you are taking.

Other people who should not take cat's claw include those who have low blood pressure or an autoimmune disease (such as lupus or multiple sclerosis) or those who have had an organ or bone marrow transplant. Kidney failure has been reported in one person with lupus. Studies have also shown that cat's claw contains tannins, which, in large amounts may cause upset stomach or even kidney damage. Small children and women who are pregnant or breastfeeding should not use this herb. Relying on this type of treatment alone and avoiding or delaying conventional medical care for cancer may have serious health consequences.

This product is sold as a dietary supplement in the United States. Unlike companies that produce drugs (which must provide the FDA with results of detailed testing showing their product is safe and effective before the drug is approved for sale), the companies that make supplements do not have to show evidence of safety or health benefits to the FDA before selling their products. Supplement products without any reliable scientific evidence of health benefits may still be sold as long as the companies selling them do not claim the supplements can prevent, treat, or cure any specific disease. Some such products may not contain the amount of the herb or substance that is written on the label, and some may include other substances (contaminants). Though the FDA has written new rules to improve the quality of manufacturing processes for dietary supplements and the accurate listing of supplement ingredients, these rules do not take full effect until 2010. The new rules also do not address the safety of supplement ingredients or their effects on health when proper manufacturing techniques are used.

Most such supplements have not been tested to find out if they interact with medicines, foods, or other herbs and supplements. Even though some reports of interactions and harmful effects may be published, full studies of interactions and effects are not often available. Because of these limitations, any information on ill effects and interactions should be considered incomplete.

References

Cassileth B. *The Alternative Medicine Handbook: The Complete Reference Guide to Alternative and Complementary Therapies.* New York: W.W. Norton; 1998.

Cat's claw. Memorial Sloan-Kettering Cancer Center Web site. http://www.mskcc.org/mskcc/html/69166.cfm. Accessed June 4, 2008.

Garcia Prado E, Garcia Giminez MD, De la Puerta Vazquez R, Espartero Sanchez JL, Saenz Rodriguez MT. Antiproliferative effects of mitraphylline, a pentacyclic oxindole alkaloid of *Uncaria tomentosa* on human glioma and neuroblastoma cell lines. *Phytomedicine.* 2007;14:280-284.

Gruenwald J. *PDR for Herbal Medicines.* 3rd ed. Montvale, NJ: Thomson PDR; 2004.

Fetrow CW, Avila JR. *Professional's Handbook of Complementary & Alternative Medicines.* Philadelphia, PA: Lippincott Williams & Wilkins; 2004.

Herbal/plant therapies: cat's claw detailed scientific review. Complementary/Integrative Medicine Education Resources, The University of Texas M. D. Anderson Cancer Center Web site. http://www.mdanderson.org/departments/CIMER/display.cfm?id=A0AAF589-ECA2-11D4-810100508B603A14&method=displayFull. Accessed June 4, 2008.

Lemaire I, Assinewe V, Cano P, Awang DV, Arnason JT. Stimulation of interleukin-1 and -6 production in alveolar macrophages by the neotropical liana, *Uncaria tomentosa* (Uña de Gato). *J Ethnopharmacol.* 1999;64:109-115.

Moss R. *Herbs Against Cancer: History and Controversy.* New York: Equinox Press; 1998.

Riva L, Coradini D, Di Fronzo G, De Feo V, De Tommasi N, De Simmone F, Pizza C. The antiproliferative effects of Uncaria tomentosa extracts and fractions on the growth of breast cancer cell line. *Anticancer Res.* 2001;21:2457-2461.

Sandoval-Chacón M, Thompson JH, Zhang XJ, Liu X, Mannick EE, Sadowska-Krowicka H, Charbonnet RM, Clark DA, Miller MJ. Antiinflammatory actions of cat's claw: the role of NF-kappaB. *Aliment Pharmacol Ther.* 1998;12:1279-1289.

Spaulding-Albright N. A review of some herbal and related products commonly used in cancer patients. *J Am Diet Assoc.* 1997;97:S208-S215.

Styczynski J, Wysocki M. Alternative medicine remedies might stimulate viability of leukemic cells. *Pediatr Blood Cancer.* 2006;46:94-98.

Valerio LG Jr, Gonzales GF. Toxicological aspects of the South American herbs cat's claw (*Uncaria tomentosa*) and Maca (*Lepidium meyenii*): a critical synopsis. *Toxicol Rev.* 2005;24:11-35.

CELANDINE

Other common name(s): greater celandine, Ukrain, common celandine, tetterwort, celandine poppy

Scientific/medical name(s): *Chelidonium majus*

Description

The celandine plant, a member of the poppy family, grows in Europe and the temperate and subarctic regions of Asia. The roots, herb, and juice are used as remedies. Ukrain, promoted as a cancer drug, is a semisynthetic compound formed by chemically combining alkaloids from the celandine plant with thiophosphoric acid derivatives, including an older cancer treatment drug called thiotepa.

Overview

Available scientific evidence does not support claims that celandine is effective in treating cancer in humans. Small studies conducted mostly in eastern Europe found that Ukrain had some positive effects; however, substantial methodological limitations in these clinical trials limit the relevance of their results, which have not been rechecked to verify the treatment's safety and effectiveness. Celandine has been reported to cause hepatitis when used as an herbal preparation.

How is it promoted for use?

Celandine is promoted for use as a mild sedative, for the prevention of gallstones, and for the treatment of intestinal and digestive problems, liver disease, and eye irritation. Practitioners have used it on the skin to treat ringworm, warts, and corns. Supporters have also used celandine along with antiviral agents to treat herpes, human immunodeficiency virus, and the Epstein-Barr virus.

Proponents claim Ukrain, which contains celandine along with thiotepa (a chemotherapy drug) and other compounds, improves overall health for people who have many types of cancer including lung, colon, kidney, ovarian, breast, brain, pancreatic, and skin cancer. They further claim it helps people with cancer live longer by boosting the immune system and inhibiting tumor growth, without any major side effects. Ukrain supposedly causes cancer cells to die and leaves healthy cells undamaged. Proponents also claim that it protects cells from radiation damage, although strong scientific evidence supporting these claims is not available.

What does it involve?

Celandine is on the Commission E (Germany's regulatory agency for herbs) list of approved herbs for treatment of intestinal spasms. It can be bought in health food stores and over the Internet, and it is usually sold as a whole plant, although sellers sometimes offer just the top or the root. It is also available as an extract, tincture, or tea. The average dosage is 2 to 5 grams per day. It can be taken internally or used externally. A very dilute concentration is used in homeopathy, mainly as a liver remedy (see "Homeopathy," page 753).

Ukrain is administered through injection at doses ranging from 5 to 20 milligrams and can be given daily or up to every three days. Therapy can continue for ten to ninety days. Ukrain is available in Europe and Mexico, at some alternative therapy clinics in the United States, or through mail order.

What is the history behind it?

In folk medicine, celandine has long been believed to have disease-fighting effects. It was taken to reduce spasms and calm the patient, and it was thought to be helpful for asthma and gallbladder and liver disease. It was also used for treatment of polyps, lumps, cramps, gout, swelling, and many other conditions. It was especially popular in former Soviet states and as early as 1931 was claimed to be effective in treating some cases of cancer.

Ukrain, a chemical combination of compounds from the plant celandine and thiophosphoric acid, was first developed in 1978 by J. W. Nowicky, a native of the Ukraine and director of the Ukrain Anticancer Institute of Vienna, Austria. He first presented it at the 13th International Congress of Chemotherapy in Vienna in 1983. It is named after the country Ukraine.

What is the evidence?

Available scientific evidence does not support claims about the benefits of celandine. One compound extracted from celandine was recently tested in rats to find out whether it would help rheumatoid arthritis. While the study looked promising, more studies are needed to determine whether it will work in humans without producing serious side effects. It is important to note also that the whole herb would not be expected to produce the same effect as a purified extract.

There have been some case reports and small studies suggesting that treatment with Ukrain may decrease tumor size and improve overall health, including increasing appetite, reducing pain in joints, and reducing fever in people who have cancer. However, a 2005 review of all seven randomized controlled trials performed on Ukrain found they were generally weak studies. Methods and findings were not completely reported, and sample sizes were small. Response and survival rates in these studies were often higher than what is possible with the combination of chemotherapy drugs currently available in the United States. In addition, virtually all of the animal and human studies were published by researchers affiliated with the institution where Ukrain was developed. The size and methods of these studies are not considered by most cancer researchers to be sufficient for supporting the promoters' claims. Randomized clinical trials are needed to determine the safety and antitumor effects of Ukrain, if any, in humans.

Are there any possible problems or complications?

Researchers recently found that celandine may be responsible for many unexplained cases of hepatitis. The medical literature contains several reports of acute (sudden) hepatitis not caused by viruses, alcohol, or other drugs that improved after the herb was stopped. Celandine can cause rashes, itching, and serious allergic reactions in some people. The whole plant is reported as being at least mildly poisonous to humans, with the roots being the most toxic. The herb is reported to be poisonous to dogs and some farm animals. There are reports that Ukrain has produced pain, nausea, thirst, fever, and swelling or bleeding in the tumor area.

Women who are pregnant or breastfeeding should not use any form of this herb. Relying on this type of treatment alone and avoiding or delaying conventional medical care for cancer may have serious health consequences.

This product is sold as a dietary supplement in the United States. Unlike companies that produce drugs (which must provide the FDA with results of detailed testing showing their product is safe and effective before the drug is approved for sale), the companies that make supplements do not have to show evidence of safety or health benefits to the FDA before selling their products. Supplement products without any reliable scientific evidence of health benefits may still be sold as long as the companies selling them do not claim the supplements can prevent, treat, or cure any specific disease. Some such products may not contain the amount of the herb or substance that is written on the label, and some may include other substances (contaminants). Though the FDA has written new rules to improve the quality of manufacturing processes for dietary supplements and the accurate listing of supplement ingredients, these rules do not take full effect until 2010. The new rules also do not address the safety of supplement ingredients or their effects on health when proper manufacturing techniques are used.

Most such supplements have not been tested to find out if they interact with medicines, foods, or other herbs and supplements. Even though some reports of interactions and harmful effects may be published, full studies of interactions and effects are not often available. Because of these limitations, any information on ill effects and interactions should be considered incomplete.

References

Benninger J, Schneider HT, Schuppan D, Kirchner T, Hahn EG. Acute hepatitis induced by greater celandine (*Chelidonium majus*). *Gastroenterology.* 1999;117:1234-1237.

Blumenthal M, ed. *The Complete German Commission E Monographs: Therapeutic Guide to Herbal Medicines.* Austin, TX: American Botanical Council; 1998.

Boyko VN, Belski SN. The influence of the novel drug Ukrain on hemo- and immunopoiesis at the time of its maximum radioprotective effect. *Drugs Exp Clin Res.* 1998;24:335-337.

Boyko VN, Levshina YeV. A study of the influence of the novel drug Ukrain on in vivo effects of low-dose ionizing radiation. *Drugs Exp Clin Res.* 1998;24:339-341.

Chelidonium majus (celandine poppy). Provet Veterinary Web site. http://www.provet.co.uk. Accessed June 4, 2008.

Chelidonium majus – L. greater celandine. Plants for a Future Web site. http://www.pfaf.org/database/plants.php?Chelidonium+majus. Accessed June 4, 2008.

The effect of ukrain on cancer. Ukrin Web Site. http://www.ukrin.com. Accessed December 6, 2005. Content no longer available.

Ernst E, Schmidt K. Ukrain-a new cancer cure? A systematic review of randomised clinical trials. *BMC Cancer.* 2005;5:69.

Gruenwald J. *PDR for Herbal Medicines.* 3rd ed. Montvale, NJ: Thomson PDR; 2004.

Habermehl D, Kammerer B, Handrick R, Eldh T, Gruber C, Cordes N, Daniel PT, Plasswilm L, Bamberg M, Belka C, Jendrosserk V. Proapoptotic activity of Ukrain is based on *Chelidonium majus* L. alkaloids and mediated via a mitochondrial death pathway. *BMC Cancer.* 2006;6:14.

Lee YC, Kim SH, Roh SS, Choi HY, Seo YB. Suppressive effects of *Chelidonium majus* methanol extract in knee joint, regional lymph nodes, and spleen on collagen-induced arthritis in mice. *J Ethnopharmacol.* 2007;112:40-48. Epub 2007 Feb 2.

Stickel F, Pöschl G, Seitz HK, Waldherr R, Hahn EG, Schuppan D. Acute hepatitis induced by Greater Celandine (Chelidonium majus). *Scand J Gastroenterol.* 2003;38:565-568.

Uglianitsa KN, Nefyodov LI, Brzosko W. Evaluation of the efficacy of Ukrain in the treatment of breast cancer: clinical and laboratory studies. *Drugs Exp Clin Res.* 1998;24:231-239.

Ukrain. Memorial Sloan-Kettering Cancer Center Web site. http://www.mskcc.org/mskcc/html/69402.cfm. Accessed June 4, 2008.

CESIUM CHLORIDE

Other common name(s): high pH therapy
Scientific/medical name(s): CsCl

Description

Cesium chloride is the salt form of the element cesium. Cesium is a rare, naturally occurring element of alkali metal similar in chemical structure to lithium, sodium, and potassium. Radioactive cesium is used in some types of radiation therapy.

Overview

Radioactive cesium (cesium-137) is used in certain types of radiation therapy for cancer patients. However, available scientific evidence does not support claims that nonradioactive cesium chloride supplements have any effect on tumors. A few people have had life-threatening problems with heart rhythm, seizures, loss of consciousness, and electrolyte (blood chemistry) imbalances after taking cesium chloride.

How is it promoted for use?

Cesium can be absorbed by all cells, probably because of its similarity in chemical structure to potassium. Proponents claim the intracellular pH of tumor cells is usually very low, or acidic, compared with normal cells and that cesium chloride supplements raise the pH level of tumor cells to a normal level, which may slow the cancer's growth. Since proponents claim cesium chloride works by raising the pH of the tumor cells, its use in therapy has been called "high pH therapy."

What does it involve?

Cesium chloride supplements are available in pill form. Proponents suggest a dosage of 1 to 6 grams per day, sometimes dissolved in juice with other vitamins and minerals. Some practitioners give cesium chloride intravenously.

What is the history behind it?

Interest in cesium therapy began when scientists observed that certain regions of the world with low rates of certain types of cancer had a high concentration of alkali metals in the soil. As early as the 1920s, some researchers suggested cesium might be effective as an antitumor agent. However, further research starting in the 1930s suggested cesium had no effect on cancer cell growth. The use of cesium chloride for high pH therapy was first advanced in the 1980s.

What is the evidence?

Available scientific evidence does not support the claim that the intracellular pH of a cancer cell is any different than that of a normal cell or that malignant cells are more susceptible to toxic effects of high pH. Thus, the underlying principle behind high pH therapy remains unproven. Although it was observed that certain regions with low rates of cancer had a high concentration of alkali metals in the soil, it has never been shown that differences in other risk factors or protective factors were not involved, or that cesium provides any benefit in the prevention or treatment of cancer.

Studies conducted in several experimental tumor models in the 1980s found that the use of cesium or cesium chloride led to decreased tumor growth and fewer deaths in certain mice with cancerous tumors, such as those with sarcoma or breast cancer. In animal studies, chronic ingestion of cesium caused serious blood and neuromuscular side effects and even death. Animal and laboratory studies may show a substance has toxic effects, but further studies are necessary to determine whether the results apply to humans. More research is needed to determine the risks and safety of cesium. The benefit of cesium or cesium chloride for people with cancer, if any, is unknown.

Are there any possible problems or complications?

In a case report from 1984, one person described his own experiences after taking cesium chloride for thirty-six days. He took 3 grams of cesium chloride, dissolved in fluid, after his morning and evening meals, which consisted of an alternative dietary regimen (for example, restricted to wheat bran and certain grain products during the first three weeks of the study). He describes an "initial general feeling of well-being and heightened sense perception" [*Pharmacol Biochem Behav.* 1984; 21(suppl 1)] as well as nausea, diarrhea, and tingling in his lips, hands, and feet. However, a case report such as this is very different from a clinical trial involving many patients and is not helpful in deciding on a safe dose of cesium. Another person, who may be younger, older, smaller, or less healthy than this individual, may not do well with this dose.

In fact, several recent case reports have described serious side effects in people who have cancer and have taken similar doses of cesium chloride, including life-threatening problems with heart rhythm, seizures, loss of consciousness, and electrolyte imbalances. The acute and chronic toxicity of this substance is not fully known or understood. Consuming large amounts of cesium could result in nausea, diarrhea, disturbed heart rhythm, loss of consciousness, or even death. Based on results of animal studies, women who are pregnant or breastfeeding should avoid taking cesium chloride supplements. Relying on this type of treatment alone and avoiding or delaying conventional medical care for cancer may also have serious health consequences.

This product is sold as a dietary supplement in the United States. Unlike companies that produce drugs (which must provide the FDA with results of detailed testing showing their product is safe and effective before the drug is approved for sale), the companies that make supplements do not have to show evidence of safety or health benefits to the FDA before selling their products. Supplement products without any reliable scientific evidence of health benefits may still be sold as long as the companies selling them do not claim the supplements can prevent, treat, or cure any specific disease. Some such products may not contain the amount of the herb or substance that is written on the label, and some may include other substances (contaminants). Though the FDA has written new rules to improve the quality of manufacturing processes for dietary supplements and the accurate listing of supplement ingredients, these rules do not take full effect until 2010. The new rules also do not address the safety of supplement ingredients or their effects on health when proper manufacturing techniques are used.

Most such supplements have not been tested to find out if they interact with medicines, foods, or other herbs and supplements. Even though some reports of interactions and harmful effects may be published,

full studies of interactions and effects are not often available. Because of these limitations, any information on ill effects and interactions should be considered incomplete.

References

Cesium chloride. Memorial Sloan-Kettering Cancer Center Web site. http://www.mskcc.org/mskcc/html/69172.cfm. Accessed June 4, 2008.

Dalal AK, Harding JD, Verdino RJ. Acquired long QT syndrome and monomorphic ventricular tachycardia after alternative treatment with cesium chloride for brain cancer. *Mayo Clin Proc.* 2004:79(8);1065-1069.
Erratum in:
Mayo Clin Proc. 2004:79(9);1215

El-Domeiri AA, Messiha FS, Hsia WC. Effect of alkali metal salts on sarcoma I in A/J mice. *J Surg Oncol.* 1981;18:423-429.

Lyon AW, Mayhew WJ. Cesium toxicity: a case of self-treatment by alternate therapy gone awry. *Ther Drug Monit.* 2003;25:114-116.

Messiha FS. Developmental toxicity of cesium in the mouse. *Gen Pharmacol.* 1994;25:395-400.

Messiha FS, Stocco DM. Effect of cesium and potassium salts on survival of rats bearing Novikoff hepatoma. *Pharmacol Biochem Behav.* 1984;21 Suppl 1:31-34.

Neulieb R. Effect of oral intake of cesium chloride: a single case report. *Pharmacol Biochem Behav.* 1984;21(suppl 1):15-16.

Pinsky C, Bose R. Pharmacological and toxicological investigations of cesium. *Pharmacol Biochem Behav.* 1984;21 (suppl 1):17-23.

Pinter A, Doran P, Newman D. Cesium-induced torsades de pointes. *N Engl J Med.* 2002:346;383-384.

Samadani U, Marcotte P. Zero efficacy with cesium chloride self-treatment for brain cancer. *Mayo Clin Proc.* 2004;79:1588.

Sartori HE. Nutrients and cancer: an introduction to cesium therapy. *Pharmacol Biochem Behav.* 1984;21(suppl 1):7-10.

CHAMOMILE

Other common name(s): German chamomile, Hungarian chamomile
Scientific/medical name(s): *Matricaria chamomilla, Matricaria recutita, Chamomilla recutita*

Description

Chamomile is a daisy-like flower, a member of the family *Asteraceae* (previously called *Compositae*). The active compounds in German and Hungarian chamomile are extracted and used in herbal remedies. Other varieties of the plant, such as Roman or English Chamomile *(Chamaemelum nobile)*, which contain similar compounds, are not used as often for herbal remedies.

Overview

Chamomile has not been found to be useful in reducing the side effects of cancer treatment. Available scientific evidence does not support claims of chamomile's effectiveness for sedation, reducing inflammation, and treating intestinal cramps. These benefits have not been proven in human clinical trials, and the use of chamomile has resulted in many allergic reactions.

How is it promoted for use?

In traditional folk medicine, chamomile has been promoted as a treatment for a long list of ailments. Today, it is most commonly promoted as a sedative to induce sleep and to soothe gastrointestinal discomfort caused by spasms and inflammation. Some proponents also claim chamomile calms the mind, eases stress, reduces pain from swollen joints and rheumatoid arthritis, speeds the healing of wounds, and reduces skin inflammation caused by sunburn, rashes, eczema, and dermatitis. The herb is also promoted to treat menstrual disorders, migraine headaches, eye irritation, and hemorrhoids.

What does it involve?

Commission E (Germany's regulatory agency for herbs) has approved the use of German chamomile for gastrointestinal spasms and skin and mucous membrane inflammation. Proponents recommend steeping chamomile in hot water for five to ten minutes to make a tea, to be taken three or four times a day. It is also available in capsules and liquid extracts. For treatment of skin conditions, bandages containing chamomile are sometimes placed over wounds. Ointments and pastes of chamomile are also used for skin conditions. Less often, chamomile is taken as a capsule, tablet, or as a tincture, a solution of the chamomile components dissolved in alcohol.

What is the history behind it?

Chamomile has been used in herbal remedies for thousands of years. The Anglo-Saxons believed that it was one of nine sacred herbs given to humans by the god Woden. The herb has also earned a place of high regard in some systems of traditional medicine.

What is the evidence?

Research has failed to show the effectiveness of chamomile in managing the side effects of cancer treatment. In a randomized clinical trial, researchers concluded that chamomile did not decrease stomatitis (inflammation of the mouth) caused by the cancer drug 5-fluorouracil. Another randomized clinical trial found that radiation-induced skin reactions were not improved in areas treated with chamomile. Chamomile spray was no more effective than a placebo spray of salt solution in reducing sore throat after surgical anesthesia.

Animal studies have suggested that chamomile is effective in inducing sleep and reducing inflammation and intestinal cramps; however, these effects have not been clearly demonstrated in humans. In a small clinical study, chamomile extract was found to be effective in inducing deep sleep in ten of twelve people who were about to undergo cardiac catheterization. But according to Commission E, clinical evidence does not support the use of chamomile as a sedative.

Are there any possible problems or complications?

Some researchers report that allergic reactions to chamomile are relatively common and can result in symptoms such as abdominal cramps, itching, skin rashes, and even throat swelling that can cause serious problems with breathing. Using chamomile as an eyewash has resulted in red inflamed eyes and swollen eyelids in those who are sensitive to it. People who have severe allergies to echinacea (purple coneflower), chrysanthemums, asters, sunflowers, zinnias, dandelions, sagebrush, yarrow, tansy, ragweed, mugwort, or other members of the *Asteraceae* family should use chamomile with caution, if at all. People who are allergic to celery, feverfew, or birch pollen may have a higher risk for reacting to chamomile.

Chamomile may interact with blood-thinning medications such as warfarin (Coumadin). People taking these medications should consult their doctors before using chamomile. Women who are pregnant or breastfeeding should not use this herb. Relying on this type of treatment alone and avoiding or delaying conventional medical care for cancer may have serious health consequences.

This product is sold as a dietary supplement in the United States. Unlike companies that produce drugs (which must provide the FDA with results of detailed testing showing their product is safe and effective before the drug is approved for sale), the companies that make supplements do not have to show evidence of safety or health benefits to the FDA before selling their products. Supplement products without any reliable scientific evidence of health benefits may still be sold as long as the companies selling them do not claim the supplements can prevent, treat, or cure any specific disease. Some such products may not contain the amount of the herb or substance that is written on the label, and some may include other substances (contaminants). Though the FDA has written new rules to improve the quality of manufacturing processes for dietary supplements and the accurate listing of supplement ingredients, these rules do not take full effect until 2010. The new rules also do not address the safety of supplement ingredients or their effects on health when proper manufacturing techniques are used.

Most such supplements have not been tested to find out if they interact with medicines, foods, or other herbs and supplements. Even though some reports of interactions and harmful effects may be published, full studies of interactions and effects are not often available. Because of these limitations, any information on ill effects and interactions should be considered incomplete.

References

Blumenthal M, ed. *The Complete German Commission E Monographs: Therapeutic Guide to Herbal Medicines.* Austin, TX: American Botanical Council; 1998.

Chamomile (German). Memorial Sloan-Kettering Cancer Center Web site. http://www.mskcc.org/mskcc/html/69174.cfm. Accessed June 4, 2008.

Chamomile. New Zealand Dermatological Society Web site. http://dermnetnz.org/dermatitis/plants/chamomile.html. Accessed June 4, 2008.

Gruenwald J. *PDR for Herbal Medicines.* 3rd ed. Montvale, NJ: Thomson PDR; 2004.

Fidler P, Loprinzi CL, O'Fallon JR, Leitch M, Lee JK, Haynes DL, Novotny P, Clemens-Schutjer D, Bartel J, Michalak LC. Prospective evaluation of a chamomile mouthwash for prevention of 5-FU-induced oral mucositis. *Cancer.* 1996;77:522-525.

Jensen-Jarolim E, Reider N, Fritsch R, Breiteneder H. Fatal outcome of anaphylaxis to camomile-containing enema during labor: a case study. *J Allergy Clin Immunol.* 1998;102:1041-1042.

Kyokong O, Charuluxananan S, Muangmingsuk V, Rodanant O, Subornsug K, Punyasang W. Efficacy of chamomile-extract spray for prevention of post-operative sore throat. *J Med Assoc Thai.* 2002;85(suppl 1):S180-S185.

McKay DL, Blumberg JB. A review of the bioactivity and potential health benefits of chamomile tea (*Matricaria recutita* L.). *Phytother Res.* 2006;20:519-530.

Miller LG. Herbal medicinals: selected clinical considerations focusing on known or potential drug-herb interactions. *Arch Intern Med.* 1998;158:2200-2211.

Natural Standard. Herbal/plant therapies: chamomile (*Matricaria recutita, Chamaemelum nobile*) Complementary/Integrative Medicine Education Resources, The University of Texas M. D. Anderson Cancer Center Web site. http://www.mdanderson.org/departments/cimer/display.cfm?id=5E66445A-0ADF-4329-991BD62BFF53EAAF&method=displayFull. Accessed June 4, 2008.

O'Hara M, Kiefer D, Farrell K, Kemper K. A review of 12 commonly used medicinal herbs. *Arch Fam Med.* 1998;7:523-536.

Reider N, Sepp N, Fritsch P, Weinlich G, Jensen-Jarolim E. Anaphylaxis to chamomile: clinical features and allergen cross-reactivity. *Clin Exp Allergy.* 2000;30:1436–1443.

Rycroft RJ. Recurrent facial dermatitis from chamomile tea. *Contact Dermatitis.* 2004;48:229.

Subiza J, Subiza JL, Hinojosa M, Garcia R, Jerez M, Valdivieso R, Subiza E. Anaphylactic reaction after the ingestion of chamomile tea: a study of cross-reactivity with other composite pollens. *J Allergy Clin Immunol.* 1989;84:353-358.

CHAPARRAL

Other common name(s): greasewood, creosote bush
Scientific/medical name(s): *Larrea divericata coville, Larrea tridentata (DC) coville*

Description

Chaparral is an herb that comes from the leaves of the creosote bush, an evergreen desert shrub. The term "chaparral" refers to a group of plants dominated by evergreen shrubs that have small, stiff leaves and grow in dense clusters to heights of four to eight feet in the American West and Southwest.

Overview

Chaparral is considered a dangerous herb that can cause irreversible, life-threatening liver damage and kidney damage. The U.S. Food and Drug Administration (FDA) has cautioned against the internal use of chapparal. Research has not found it to be an effective treatment for cancer or any other disease. A study of nordihydroguaiaretic acid (NDGA), one of the chemicals in chaparral, concluded that it was not useful in treating people with cancer, although studies continue.

How is it promoted for use?

Proponents claim that chaparral can help relieve pain, reduce inflammation, aid congestion, increase urine elimination, and slow the aging process. It is also promoted as an anticancer agent and an antioxidant (a compound that blocks the action of free radicals, activated oxygen molecules that can damage cells). Some researchers think NDGA might make other anticancer drugs more effective, but this theory still needs to be tested through animal studies and clinical trials of people who have cancer.

What does it involve?

Chaparral is distributed in capsule or tablet form. Chaparral also can be made into a bitter and unpleasant-tasting tea or a tincture, a solution of chemicals from chaparral leaves dissolved in alcohol. Chaparral is also sometimes found with other herbs in a variety of teas.

What is the history behind it?

Native Americans used chaparral as an herbal remedy. They heated the leaves and applied them to the skin to treat wounds, bronchitis, coughs, skin disorders, venereal sores, warts, blemishes, and ringworm. Heated stems were inserted into tooth cavities to relieve pain, and the leaves and stems were boiled to make tea to relieve rheumatism and other conditions, including colds, bronchitis, digestive problems, and cancer.

According to anecdotal reports, chaparral tea was used widely in the United States from the late 1950s to the 1970s as an alternative anticancer agent. Experimental studies in the 1960s showed that chaparral could cause problems with kidney and liver function. The growth of interest in alternative medicine led to increased use of chaparral in the 1980s. By the early 1990s, there had been many reports of chaparral-linked illnesses, and the FDA issued a warning, resulting in the voluntary removal of many chaparral products from stores. Despite many concerns and warnings, chaparral has become more readily available again and is still advertised and sold on the Internet.

What is the evidence?

Available scientific evidence does not support the idea that chaparral can prevent or slow the growth of cancer in humans, nor does it support chaparral as effective in treating other medical conditions. Some preliminary laboratory studies have indicated that one of the chemicals in chaparral, NDGA, may possess anticancer properties. However, available scientific evidence has not confirmed these findings.

Studies of NDGA have had conflicting results. According to a 1990 government report, some researchers reported that NDGA inhibited cancer growth in animals. Others found that low levels of NDGA actually stimulated the growth of some types of tumor cells, although higher concentrations had the opposite effect. More recent cell culture studies using cancer cells grown in the laboratory suggest NDGA may make other anticancer drugs more effective, and researchers continue to look into the potential uses of purified NDGA. While these studies show some promise, further studies would be necessary to determine whether the results apply to humans.

In 1970, researchers from the University of Utah published results of a clinical study sponsored by the National Cancer Institute on chaparral tea and NDGA. People with advanced, incurable cancer drank chaparral tea or took doses of pure NDGA by mouth. Of the forty-five people who were evaluated, four experienced a decrease in the size of their tumors. The regression lasted between ten days and twenty months. However, tumors grew larger in others treated with chaparral. Overall, the authors concluded that chaparral tea was not an effective anticancer agent.

One case study reported that severe hepatitis developed in a sixty-year-old woman who had taken chaparral for ten months. She eventually required a liver transplant. In a later review of eighteen case reports of adverse reactions associated with taking chaparral, researchers concluded that the herb is linked with irreversible liver damage and liver failure.

Are there any possible problems or complications?

Although chaparral is still widely available, the FDA has recommended since 1968 that it not be taken internally. Chaparral is highly toxic and has been reported to cause severe and permanent liver disease that can be fatal. It has also been linked to kidney damage, including cysts in the kidney and kidney failure.

Chaparral may cause dangerous interactions with a number of other medicines and herbs. Blood-thinning medications (anticoagulants), nonsteroidal anti-inflammatory medicines (such as aspirin, ibuprofen, and naproxen), antidiabetic drugs, and certain antidepressants (MAO inhibitors) may cause problems while taking chaparral. Always tell your doctor and pharmacist about any herbs you are taking.

Other side effects of chaparral can include fatigue, stomach pain, diarrhea, weight loss, fever, itching, rash, and allergic reactions. This herb should be avoided, especially by women who are pregnant or breastfeeding. Relying on this type of treatment alone and avoiding or delaying conventional medical care for cancer may have serious health consequences.

This substance has not been thoroughly tested to find out how it interacts with medicines, foods, or dietary supplements. Even though some reports of interactions and harmful effects may be published, full studies of interactions and effects are not often available. Because of these limitations, any information on ill effects and interactions should be considered incomplete.

References

Chaparral (Larrea tridentata (DC) Coville, Larrea divaricata Cav) & Nordihydroguaiaretic acid (NDGA). Medline Plus Web site. http://www.nlm.nih.gov/medlineplus/druginfo/natural/patient-chaparral.html. Accessed April 12, 2007. Content no longer available.

Chaparral. Memorial Sloan-Kettering Cancer Center Web site. http://www.mskcc.org/mskcc/html/69175.cfm. Accessed June 4, 2008.

Ding XZ, Kuszynski CA, El-Metwally TH, Adrian TE. Lipoxygenase inhibition induced apoptosis, morphological changes, and carbonic anhydrase expression in human pancreatic cancer cells. *Biochem Biophys Res Commun.* 1999;266:392-399.

Fetrow CW, Avila JR. *Professional's Handbook of Complementary & Alternative Medicines.* Philadelphia, PA: Lippincott Williams & Wilkins; 2004.

Gordon DW, Rosenthal G, Hart J, Sirota R, Baker AL. Chaparral ingestion. The broadening spectrum of liver injury caused by herbal medications. *JAMA.* 1995;273:489-490.

Natural Standard. Herbal/plant therapies: chaparral (*Larrea tridentata* (DC) Coville, *Larrea divaricata* (Cav) & nordihydroguaiaretic acid (NDGA). Complementary/Integrative Medicine Education Resources, The University of Texas M. D. Anderson Cancer Center Web site. http://www.mdanderson.org/departments/cimer/display.cfm?id=5A5EF4F0-CF19-4FD1-9B40FD8546A616D9&method=displayFull. Accessed June 4, 2008.

Sheikh NM, Philen RM, Love LA. Chaparral-associated hepatotoxicity. *Arch Intern Med.* 1997;157:913-919.

Smart CR, Hogle HH, Vogel H, Broom AD, Bartholomew D. Clinical experience with nordihydroguaiaretic acid—"chaparrel tea" in the treatment of cancer. *Rocky Mt Med J.* 1970;67:39-43.

Soriano AF, Helfrich B, Chan DC, Heasley LE, Bunn PA Jr, Chou TC. Synergistic effects of new chemopreventive agents and conventional cytotoxic agents against human lung cancer cell lines. *Cancer Res.* 1999;59:6178-6184.

US Congress, Office of Technology Assessment. *Unconventional Cancer Treatments: OTA-H-405.* Washington, DC: US Government Printing Office; 1990.

CHINESE HERBAL MEDICINE

Other common name(s): traditional Chinese medicine, TCM, Chinese herbs, Oriental medicine

Scientific/medical name(s): none

Description

Chinese herbal medicine is a major aspect of traditional Chinese medicine, which focuses on restoring a balance of energy, body, and spirit to maintain health rather than treating a particular disease or medical condition. Herbs are used with the goal of restoring balance by nourishing the body.

Overview

Because of the large number of Chinese herbs used and the different uses recommended by practitioners, it is difficult to comment on Chinese herbal medicine as a whole. There may be some individual herbs or extracts that play a role in the prevention and treatment of cancer and other diseases when combined with conventional treatment. However, more research is needed to determine the effectiveness of these individual substances.

How is it promoted for use?

Chinese herbal medicine is not based on conventional Western concepts of medical diagnosis and treatment. It treats patients' main complaints or the patterns of their symptoms rather than the underlying causes. Practitioners attempt to prevent and treat imbalances, such as those caused by cancer and other diseases, with complex combinations of herbs, minerals, and plant extracts.

Chinese herbal medicine uses a variety of herbs in different combinations to restore balance to the body, such as astragalus, ginkgo, ginseng, green tea, and Siberian ginseng. Herbal preparations are said to prevent and treat hormone disturbances, infections, breathing disorders, and a vast number of other ailments and diseases. Some practitioners claim herbs have the power to prevent and treat a variety of types of cancer.

Most Chinese herbalists do not claim to cure cancer. They use herbal medicine with conventional treatments prescribed by oncologists, such as radiation therapy and chemotherapy. They claim that herbal remedies can help ease the side effects of conventional cancer therapies, control pain, improve quality of life, strengthen the immune system, and in some cases, stop tumor growth and spread.

One aspect of Chinese herbal medicine aims to restore or strengthen immunity and resistance to disease. Treatments undertaken with this goal are called Fu Zheng or Fu Zhen and are given as complementary therapy intended to reduce the side effects from conventional Western anticancer treatments.

What does it involve?

In China, more than thirty-two hundred herbs and three hundred mineral and animal extracts are used in more than four hundred different formulas. Herbal formulations may consist of four to twelve different ingredients, to be taken in the form of teas, powders, pills, tinctures, or syrups.

Chinese herbal remedies are usually made up of a number of herbs and mineral and animal extracts. Typically, one or two herbs are included that are said to have the greatest effect on the problem being treated. Other ingredients in the formula treat minor aspects of the problem, direct the formula to specific parts of the body, and help the other herbs work more efficiently.

With the increase in popularity of herbal medicine, many Chinese herbs are now sold individually and in formulas. In the United States, Chinese herbs and herbal formulas may be purchased in health food stores, some pharmacies, and from herbal medicine practitioners.

Before choosing a mixture of herbs for a patient, the traditional Chinese practitioner will typically ask about symptoms and examine the patient, often focusing on the skin, hair, tongue, eyes, pulse, and voice, in order to detect imbalances in the body.

What is the history behind it?

Native cultures all over the world have traditionally used herbs to maintain health and treat illnesses. Chinese herbal medicine developed as part of Chinese culture from tribal roots. By 200 BC, traditional Chinese medicine was firmly established, and by the first century AD, a listing of medicinal herbs and herbal formulations and their uses had been developed.

The classic Chinese book on medicinal herbs was written during the Ming Dynasty (1152-1578) by Li Shi-Zhen. It listed nearly two thousand herbs and extracts. By 1990, the latest edition of *The Pharmacopoeia of the People's Republic of China* listed more than five hundred single herbs or extracts and nearly three hundred complex formulations.

As Western conventional medicine spread to the East, some traditional Chinese medical practices began to be regarded as folklore. However, since 1949, the Chinese government has supported the use of both traditional and Western medicine. Chinese herbal medicine first came to widespread attention in the United States in the 1970s, when President Richard Nixon visited China. Today, at least thirty states license practitioners of Oriental medicine and more than twenty-five colleges of Oriental medicine exist in the United States.

What is the evidence?

Some herbs and herbal formulations have been evaluated in animal, laboratory, and human studies in both the East and the West with wide-ranging results. Research results vary widely depending on the specific herb, but several have shown activity against cancer cells in laboratory dishes and in some animals.

There is some evidence from randomized clinical trials that some Chinese herbs may contribute to longer survival rates, reduction of side effects, and lower risk for recurrence for some types of cancer, especially when combined with conventional treatment. Many of these studies, however, are published in Chinese, and some of them do not list the specific herbs that were tested. Some of these journal articles do not describe how the studies were conducted completely enough to determine whether they use methods comparable to those used in Western clinical research. However, there are some notable exceptions, such as PC-SPES, a mixture including several Chinese herbs that has been studied in considerable detail in U.S. clinical trials (see "PC-SPES," page 450). More controlled research is needed to determine the role of Chinese herbal medicine in cancer treatment and prevention.

Are there any possible problems or complications?

Because of the variety of herbs used in Chinese herbal medicine, there is a potential for negative interactions with prescribed drugs. Some herbal preparations contain other ingredients that are not always identified. The U.S. Food and Drug Administration (FDA) has issued a statement warning diabetics to avoid several specific brands of Chinese herbal products because they illegally contain the prescription diabetes drugs glyburide and phenformin. FDA warnings have been issued for PC-SPES, and production of that product was stopped because it contained the prescription drugs indomethaicin, diethylstilbestrol, and warfarin.

Similar concerns have been raised about Chinese herbal products for other diseases, which have been found to contain toxic contaminants and prescription drugs such as diazepam (Valium). Tests of Chinese herbal remedies by the California Department of Health found that nearly one third contained prescription drugs or were contaminated with toxic metals such as mercury, arsenic, and lead. Concerns about Chinese herbal products have been raised in other countries as well. The Japanese Ministry of Health, Labour, and Welfare reported that some Chinese herbal products contained contaminants that caused severe and sometimes fatal liver and thyroid problems.

Of the more than five thousand medicinal plant species in China, a small number are potentially toxic to the human body. Toxic herbs may mistakenly be harvested and shipped for herbal medicines and can cause harmful reactions in those who take the medicines. In addition, the herbal formulas used are often complex and difficult for manufacturers and practitioners to formulate correctly. For example, in the case of an herbal product intended to promote weight loss, manufacturers confused two Chinese herbs with similar names and mistakenly used the wrong one, which resulted in severe kidney damage that was fatal in some cases.

Any herb can cause allergic reactions in a few people. Those who are allergic to certain plants, including some plant-based foods, may be more likely to react to herbs.

Although the long history of traditional Chinese herbal medicine is sometimes interpreted as evidence of safety, it is important to note that many of these herbs are no longer produced and used as they were in the past. An herb may have been used safely under the supervision of a traditional practitioner. However, if the same herbs are used in higher doses or in doses of different concentrations, perhaps over a longer period and without medical guidance, the risks involved in taking those herbs change. In addition, toxic substances or prescription drugs can be introduced during the manufacturing process, either intentionally or inadvertently.

Practitioners of traditional Chinese medicine licensed by a state board can provide advice on the safest sources for herbs. Because some herbs used in traditional Chinese medicine may cause dangerous interactions with conventional medications, patients should talk with their doctors and pharmacists before using any of the herbs. Relying on this type of treatment alone and avoiding or delaying conventional medical care for cancer may have serious health consequences.

These substances may have not been thoroughly tested to find out how they interact with medicines, foods, or dietary supplements. Even though some reports of interactions and harmful effects may be published, full studies of interactions and effects are not often available. Because of these limitations, any information on ill effects and interactions should be considered incomplete.

References

Au AM, Ko R, Boo FO, Hsu R, Perez G, Yang Z. Screening methods for drugs and heavy metals in Chinese patent medicines. *Bull Environ Contam Toxicol.* 2000;65:112-119.

Boik J. *Cancer and Natural Medicine: A Textbook of Basic Science and Clinical Research.* Princeton, MN: Oregon Medical Press; 1995.

Cole MR, Fetrow CW. Adulteration of dietary supplements. *Am J Health-Syst Pharm.* 2003;60:1576-1580.

Ergil KV, Kramer EJ, Ng AT. Chinese herbal medicines. *West J Med.* 2002;176:275-279.

Ko RJ. Adulterants in Asian patent medicines. *N Engl J Med.* 1998;339:847.

Marcus DM, Grollman AP. Botanical medicines—the need for new regulations. *N Engl J Med.* 2002;347:2073-2076.

National Institutes of Health. *Alternative Medicine: Expanding Medical Horizons: A Report to the National Institutes of Health on Alternative Medical Systems and Practices in the United States.* Washington, DC: US Government Printing Office; 1994. NIH publication 94-066.

Traditional Chinese medicine. University of Maryland Medical Center Web site. http://www.umm.edu/altmed/articles/chinese-medicine-000363.htm. Updated December 1, 2002. Accessed June 4, 2008.

CHLORELLA

Other common name(s): sun chlorella, green algae
Scientific/medical name(s): *Chlorella pyrenoidosa, Chlorella vulgaris*

Description

Chlorella is a single-celled freshwater alga. These algae contain large amounts of chlorophyll, the chemical that gives plants their green color. Chlorophyll is an essential compound for photosynthesis, the process by which plants convert light into chemical energy. Chlorophyll is also available in green leafy vegetables.

Overview

Chlorella is widely used in Japan for a variety of health conditions; however, available scientific studies do not support its effectiveness for preventing or treating cancer or any other disease in humans.

How is it promoted for use?

Chlorella is promoted for a wide range of herbal remedies. Proponents claim it kills several types of cancer, fights bacterial and viral infections, enhances the immune system, increases the growth of beneficial germs in the digestive tract, lowers blood pressure and cholesterol levels, and promotes healing of intestinal ulcers, diverticulosis, and Crohn's disease. It is said to "cleanse" the blood, digestive system, and liver.

Supporters state that chlorella supplements increase the level of albumin in the body. Albumin is a protein normally present in the bloodstream, and promoters claim it is protective against diseases such as cancer, diabetes, arthritis, AIDS, pancreatitis, cirrhosis, hepatitis, anemia, and multiple sclerosis. Chlorella is said to prevent cancer through its ability to cleanse the body of toxins and heavy metals. Some Web sites describe it as the perfect food, saying that it regulates blood sugar, kills cancer cells, strengthens the immune system, and even "reverses the aging cycle." Available scientific evidence does not support these claims. Because of this lack of evidence, the U.S. Food and Drug Administration (FDA) has warned the proprietors of at least one Web site to stop making unproven statements about chlorella's benefits.

Chlorella contains vitamin C and carotenoids, both of which are antioxidants (see "Vitamin A and Beta Carotene," page 529, and "Vitamin C," page 538). Antioxidants are compounds that block the action of free radicals, activated oxygen molecules that can damage cells. Chlorella is also reported to contain high concentrations of B-complex vitamins (see "Vitamin B Complex," page 534).

What does it involve?

Chlorella is available as a tablet, liquid extract, and powder. Some herbalists recommend 2 to 3 grams per day, though higher doses may be suggested for "detoxification." A few people take up to 10 or 15 grams (2 to 3 teaspoons) per day. Although it may be taken on its own, many supporters suggest mixing the powdered form of chlorella into foods made with flour, such as bread or cookies.

What is the history behind it?

Chlorella was discovered in the late nineteenth century. Due to its high protein concentration and rapid growth rate, chlorella was investigated after World War II as a possible commercial food source. In the 1960s, some investigators claimed that the algae decreased the side effects of chemotherapy and slowed the growth of some cancer cells. Most of the research has been conducted in Japan, where chlorella is a top-selling dietary supplement.

What is the evidence?

Available scientific evidence does not support claims that chlorella is effective against cancer or other diseases in humans. Limited laboratory and animal research suggests that these algae may have some anticancer properties. Chlorella powder may inhibit the activity of some molecules involved in the growth of cancer cells.

One investigation concluded that a protein extract from one type of chlorella prevented the spread of cancer cells in mice. Another study in mice suggested that the extract reduced the side effects of chemotherapy treatment without affecting the potency of anticancer medications. A 2001 study from Brazil showed that an extract of chlorella prolonged the survival of mice that were injected with tumor cells. However, study results for extracted chemicals might not be consistent with studies using the whole plant. Further studies are needed to determine whether the results apply to humans.

In 2003, a supplement derived from chlorella was given to healthy adults to learn whether it boosted immune response to the flu shot. The study found there was no significant difference in antibodies between the group that received the chlorella supplements and the one that did not.

Are there any possible problems or complications?

Although chlorella appears to be safe in those who are not allergic, no research has been done in humans to learn whether it causes negative side effects or what can be expected from long-term use. If hives or a rash develops, stop taking chlorella and seek medical attention immediately. Relying on this type of treatment alone and avoiding or delaying conventional medical care for cancer may have serious health consequences.

This product is sold as a dietary supplement in the United States. Unlike companies that produce drugs (which must provide the FDA with results of detailed testing showing their product is safe and effective before the drug is approved for sale), the companies that make supplements do not have to show evidence of safety or health benefits to the FDA before selling their products. Supplement products without any reliable scientific evidence of health benefits may still be sold as long as the companies selling them do not claim the supplements can prevent, treat, or cure any specific disease. Some such products may not contain the amount of the herb or substance that is written on the label, and some may include other substances (contaminants). Though the FDA has written new rules to improve the quality of manufacturing processes for dietary supplements and the accurate listing of supplement ingredients, these rules do not take full effect until 2010. The new rules also do not address the safety of supplement ingredients or their effects on health when proper manufacturing techniques are used.

Most such supplements have not been tested to find out if they interact with medicines, foods, or other herbs and supplements. Even though some reports of interactions and harmful effects may be published, full studies of interactions and effects are not often available. Because of these limitations, any information on ill effects and interactions should be considered incomplete.

References

Barrett S. Mercola gets second warning letter. Consumer Health Digest #06-41. October 11, 2006. National Council Against Health Fraud Web site. http://www.ncahf.org/digest06/06-41.html. Accessed June 4, 2008.

Cheng FC, Lin A, Feng JJ, Mizoguchi T, Takekoshi H, Kubota H, Kato Y, Naoki Y. Effects of chlorella on activities of protein tyrosine phosphatases, matrix metalloproteinases, caspases, cytokine release, B and T cell proliferations, and phorbol ester receptor binding. *J Med Food.* 2004;7:146-152.

Halperin SA, Smith B, Nolan C, Shay J, Kralovec J. Safety and immunoenhancing effect of a *Chlorella*-derived dietary supplement in healthy adults undergoing influenza vaccination: randomized, double-blind, placebo-controlled trial. *CMAJ.* 2003;169:111-177.

Justo GZ, Silva MR, Queiroz ML. Effects of the green algae *Chlorella vulgaris* on the response of the host hematopoietic system to intraperitoneal ehrlich ascites tumor transplantation in mice. *Immunopharmacol Immunotoxicol.* 2001;23:119-132.

Konishi F, Mitsuyama M, Okuda M, Tanaka K, Hasegawa T, Nomoto K. Protective effect of an acidic glycoprotein obtained from culture of *Chlorella vulgaris* against myelosuppression by 5-fluorouracil. *Cancer Immunol Immunother.* 1996;42:268-274.

Tanaka K, Yamada A, Noda K, Hasegawa T, Okuda M, Shoyama Y, Nomoto K. A novel glycoprotein obtained from *Chlorella vulgaris* strain CK22 show antimetastatic immunopotentiation. *Cancer Immunol Immunother.* 1998;45:313-320.

CLOVES

Other common name(s): clove oil, oil of cloves (Eugenol)
Scientific/medical name(s): *Syzygium aromaticum, Caryophyllum aromaticum, Eugenia caryophyllata, Eugenia aromatica*

Description

The clove is an aromatic spice that grows as an evergreen tree in the tropical regions of Asia and South America. The oil extracted from the plant, leaves, flower buds, and fruit itself is used in herbal remedies and some dental practices.

Overview

Available scientific evidence does not support claims that cloves or clove oil is effective in treating or preventing cancer or any other disease. Some dentists and patients report that clove oil may relieve gum and tooth pain and may be useful as a topical antiseptic in mouthwash; however, there is limited scientific evidence for this claim.

How is it promoted for use?

Some proponents claim that cloves and clove oil, when taken internally, relieve nausea and vomiting, improve digestion, fight intestinal parasites, stimulate uterine contractions, ease arthritis inflammation, stop migraine headaches, and ease symptoms of colds and allergies. Practitioners of traditional Chinese medicine sometimes treat hiccups and impotence with cloves. Clove oil is also used in aromatherapy. Some practitioners claim that a mixture of cloves, black walnut hulls, and wormwood can cure cancer.

What does it involve?

Cloves are available in capsule or powder form or as a whole herb. Pure and diluted clove oil can also be purchased.

What is the history behind it?

Cloves and clove oil were reportedly used in Chinese medicine as early as 600 AD. Cloves have long been a part of various folk medicine traditions around the world. Clove oil has been used more recently by some dentists, who swab it inside patients' mouths to lessen the pain of anesthetic injections. People also applied it inside the mouth to help toothaches. Today, cloves are also used as an ingredient in baking and cooking and in perfumes, cigarettes, mouthwash, and toothpaste.

What is the evidence?

Clove oil has been approved for use in dentistry as a topical anesthetic by Commission E, Germany's regulatory agency for herbs. However, no well-controlled clinical studies have been done to evaluate the potential germ-killing and anticancer properties of cloves or clove oil in humans. A small controlled study published in 2006 compared clove gel with a numbing gel to lessen the pain of injections in the mouth. The researchers found that people who were given a placebo gel had more pain than those who received clove gel or numbing gel. The pain levels of those who received the numbing medicine and those who were given clove gel were about the same. Further studies are needed to be sure this is a reliable effect.

Two recent laboratory studies do suggest that clove and clove extracts may be antioxidants. Antioxidants are compounds that block the action of free radicals, activated oxygen molecules that can damage cells.

Very limited laboratory studies conducted in other countries suggest that clove oil may fight bacteria and prevent seizures. One recent study compared the oils from several herbs to find out how well they stopped the growth of certain germs. Clove oil was very effective at stopping the bacteria, yeasts, and molds that were tested. Along these lines, a Japanese study in mice suggested that a clove preparation taken by mouth might help reduce the severity of yeast infections in the mouth.

A 2006 study suggested that cloves contain chemicals that might reduce development of lung cancer in mice treated with cancer-causing chemicals. Another laboratory study suggested that compounds taken from cloves show promise as potential anticancer agents. However, study results of clove extracts will not necessarily be the same as studies using the raw plant. Likewise, while laboratory studies may show promise, further studies are needed to find out whether the results apply to humans.

Are there any possible problems or complications?

Cloves are generally considered safe, although a relatively small number of people may be allergic to eugenol, their main active ingredient. Severe reactions may occur in these people. Those known to be allergic to clove or balsam of Peru should avoid using cloves in any form, including inhaling the smoke from clove cigarettes.

Taking in large amounts of cloves or clove oil may cause nausea, vomiting, abdominal pain, diarrhea, burns in the mouth and throat, sore throat, seizures, difficulty breathing, rapid heartbeat, sleepiness, intestinal bleeding, and liver or kidney failure. More serious effects have been reported in young children, even with small doses. Clove supplements may cause bleeding in those taking medicine to stop blood clots (blood thinners). Use of clove supplements during pregnancy is not recommended.

Excessive application of undiluted clove oil on or near the teeth may cause irritation or damage to the gums or mouth and may damage the dental pulp, the soft core of the tooth, made up of living soft tissue and cells. It should be used for tooth and gum conditions only under the supervision of a dentist. Undiluted clove oil may cause skin irritation, rashes, or even burns.

Clove cigarettes, also known as kreteks, deliver more nicotine, carbon monoxide, and tar than regular cigarettes. In addition to having the same health risks as regular cigarettes, clove cigarettes may also increase the risk for suddenly developing life-threatening fluid build-up in the lungs, as well as serious pneumonia.

Relying on this type of treatment alone and avoiding or delaying conventional medical care for cancer may have serious health consequences.

This product is sold as a dietary supplement in the United States. Unlike companies that produce drugs (which must provide the FDA with results of detailed testing showing their product is safe and effective before the drug is approved for sale), the companies that make supplements do not have to show evidence of safety or health benefits to the FDA before selling their products. Supplement products without any reliable scientific evidence of health benefits may still be sold as long as the companies selling them do not claim the supplements can prevent, treat, or cure any specific disease. Some such products may not contain the amount of the herb or substance that is written on the label, and some

may include other substances (contaminants). Though the FDA has written new rules to improve the quality of manufacturing processes for dietary supplements and the accurate listing of supplement ingredients, these rules do not take full effect until 2010. The new rules also do not address the safety of supplement ingredients or their effects on health when proper manufacturing techniques are used.

Most such supplements have not been tested to find out if they interact with medicines, foods, or other herbs and supplements. Even though some reports of interactions and harmful effects may be published, full studies of interactions and effects are not often available. Because of these limitations, any information on ill effects and interactions should be considered incomplete.

References

Abdel-Wahhab MA, Aly SE. Antioxidant property of *Nigella sativa* (black cumin) and *Syzygium aromaticum* (clove) in rats during aflatoxicosis. *J Appl Toxicol.* 2005;25:218-223.

Alqareer A, Alyahya A, Andersson L. The effect of clove and benzocaine versus placebo as topical anesthetics. *J Dent.* 2006;34:747-750.

Banerjee S, Panda CK, Das S. Clove (*Syzygium aromaticum* L.), a potential chemopreventive agent for lung cancer. *Carcinogenesis.* 2006;27:1645-1654.

Clove (*Eugenia aromatica*) and clove oil (eugenol). Aetna InteliHealth Web site. http://www.intelihealth.com/IH/ihtIH?d=dmtContent&c=351409. Updated June 15, 2005. Accessed June 13, 2008.

Eugenol oil overdose. Medline Plus Web site. www.nlm.nih.gov/medlineplus/ency/article/002647.htm. Accessed June 4, 2008.

Fetrow CW, Avila JR. *Professional's Handbook of Complementary & Alternative Medicines.* Philadelphia, PA: Lippincott Williams & Wilkins; 2004.

Gruenwald J. *PDR for Herbal Medicines.* 3rd ed. Montvale, NJ: Thomson PDR; 2004.

Guidottii TL, Laing L, Prakash UB. Clove cigarettes. The basis for concern regarding health effects. *West J Med.* 1989;151:220-228.

Lee KG, Shibamoto T. Inhibition of malonaldehyde formation from blood plasma oxidation by aroma extracts and aroma components isolated from clove and eucalyptus. *Food Chem Toxicol.* 2001;39:1199-1204.

López P, Sánchez C, Batlle R, Nerín C. Solid- and vapor-phase antimicrobial activities of six essential oils: susceptibility of selected foodborne bacterial and fungal strains. *J Agric Food Chem.* 2005;53:6939-6946.

Pérez C, Anesini C. Antibacterial activity of alimentary plants against *Staphylococcus aureus* growth. *Am J Chin Med.* 1994;22:169-174.

Popular natural remedies, part XVII. Wright State University Pharmacy Web site. http://www.wright.edu/admin/fredwhite/pharmacy/popular_nremedies17.html. Accessed June 4, 2008.

Pourgholami MH, Kamalinejad M, Javadi M, Majzoob S, Sayyah M. Evaluation of the anticonvulsant activity of the essential oil of *Eugenia caryophyllata* in male mice. *J Ethnopharmacol.* 1999;64:167-171.

Taguchi Y, Ishibashi H, Takizawa T, Inoue S, Yamaguchi H, Abe S. Protection of oral or intestinal candidiasis in mice by oral or intragastric administration of herbal food, clove (*Syzygium aromaticum*) [Abstract]. *Nippon Ishinkin Gakkai Zasshi.* 2005;46:27-33.

Zheng GQ, Kenney PM, Lam LK. Sesquiterpenes from clove (*Eugenia caryophyllata*) as potential anticarcinogenic agents. *J Nat Prod.* 1992;55:999-1003.

COMFREY

Other common name(s): blackwort, bruisewort, common comfrey, knitbone, slippery root
Scientific/medical name(s): *Symphytum officinale*

Description

Comfrey is a fast-growing herb native to Europe and temperate parts of Asia. It now grows in North America as well. The roots and leaves are used in herbal remedies.

Overview

Although comfrey has been used in folk medicine for many years to help heal wounds, sprains, and fractures, there have been no studies in humans to prove that it is useful. Available scientific evidence does not support the idea that comfrey is effective in treating cancer. It is not considered safe for internal use due to toxic effects on the liver. There are several varieties of comfrey, some of which contain more toxic compounds than others.

How is it promoted for use?

Comfrey has been promoted mainly to speed the healing of wounds, sprains, bruises, and bone fractures and to reduce inflammation and swelling related to these injuries. Comfrey has also been used to treat a number of other ailments, including ulcers, gallstones, arthritis, diarrhea, colitis, cough, pleurisy, and pneumonia. A mouthwash made from comfrey is sometimes used for gum disease, hoarseness, and sore throat. Some proponents also claim comfrey has anticancer properties.

What does it involve?

Ointments, salves, and creams that contain comfrey are available for external use. Compresses and poultices are made from the crushed roots and leaves of comfrey or from liquid extracts pressed out of the plant. They are placed directly on bruises, wounds, or sprains, are covered with a dressing, and are replaced daily until healing occurs. For internal use, dried comfrey root or leaves are sometimes prepared as a tea.

In 2001, the U.S. Food and Drug Administration (FDA) asked manufacturers of dietary supplements to remove products containing comfrey from the market because of its potential to cause liver damage. However, whole leaves and roots and extracts of both are still available. Most comfrey capsules now contain whole-leaf comfrey. Comfrey can also be purchased to grow at home.

Comfrey has been approved by Commission E (Germany's regulatory agency for herbs) to be sold only in preparations that supply no more than 100 micrograms per day if applied to the skin and no more than 1 microgram of pyrrolizidine alkaloids (toxic compounds in comfrey) if taken by mouth. This is a tiny amount. For comparison, one baby aspirin has 80,000 micrograms (or 80 milligrams) of aspirin.

What is the history behind it?

It is reported that comfrey has been used since about 400 BC for wound healing, inflammation, gout, ulcers, gangrene, burns, sprains, and fractures. It also was eaten as a vegetable, much like spinach. In folk medicine, comfrey has been used to treat conditions such as arthritis, colitis, diarrhea, gallstones, and pleurisy. A few practitioners tried using comfrey to treat cancer in the twentieth century.

What is the evidence?

Available scientific evidence does not support claims that comfrey is useful in curing cancer or any other disease. A few recent studies that looked at European creams made from comfrey and comfrey extracts suggested they might be helpful in treating lower back pain, arthritis, and muscle aches when applied to the skin of the affected area. At least one study suggested that very high concentrations of the herb were more helpful than lower concentrations.

When taken internally, comfrey can cause severe liver damage. Several studies have shown that comfrey contains toxic compounds called pyrrolizidine alkaloids, or PAs, which can cause severe liver damage. Animal studies have also shown that exposure to these chemicals leads to the development of liver tumors.

Are there any possible problems or complications?

The internal use of comfrey is not considered safe. Experts strongly warn consumers not to eat or drink anything that contains comfrey. This herb should be avoided, especially by women who are pregnant or breastfeeding. The U.S. Pharmacopeia (the U.S. compendium of quality control tests and information on drugs) reports comfrey should not be used on broken skin because it may be absorbed into the body.

In July 2001, the FDA advised supplement manufacturers to remove products containing comfrey from the market and alert customers to stop using these products immediately because of the serious health hazards associated with pyrrolizidine alkaloids. The Federal Trade Commission has also taken action against unsafe products containing comfrey. Severe liver damage and even deaths have occurred with long-term use. Kidney damage is also possible.

Common comfrey can be easily mistaken for other plants in the same family, such as Russian comfrey or prickly comfrey, both of which contain even higher levels of the pyrrolizidine alkaloid toxin. Poisonings have also been reported when foxglove or other toxic plants have been mistaken for comfrey.

Allergic reactions to comfrey, while rare, are possible. Relying on this type of treatment alone and avoiding or delaying conventional medical care for cancer may have serious health consequences.

This substance has not been thoroughly tested to find out how it interacts with medicines, foods, or dietary supplements. Even though some reports of interactions and harmful effects may be published, full studies of interactions and effects are not often available. Because of these limitations, any information on ill effects and interactions should be considered incomplete.

References

Blumenthal M, ed. *The Complete German Commission E Monographs: Therapeutic Guide to Herbal Medicines.* Austin, TX: American Botanical Council; 1998.

FDA advises dietary supplement manufacturers to remove comfrey products from the market. July 6, 2001. Center for Food Safety and Applied Nutrition. US Food and Drug Administration Web site. http://www.cfsan.fda.gov/~dms/dspltr06.html. Accessed June 4, 2008.

Foodborne pathogenic microorganisms and natural toxins handbook: pyrrolizidine alkaloids. January 1992. Center for Food Safety and Applied Nutrition. US Food and Drug Administration Web site. http://www.cfsan.fda.gov/~mow/chap42.html. Accessed June 4, 2008.

Comfrey. British Columbia Cancer Agency Web site. http://www.bccancer.bc.ca/PPI/UnconventionalTherapies/Comfrey.htm. Updated February 2000. Accessed June 4, 2008.

Comfrey. Memorial Sloan-Kettering Cancer Center Web site. http://www.mskcc.org/mskcc/html/69190.cfm. Accessed June 4, 2008.

Comfrey. University of Maryland Medical Center Web site. http://www.umm.edu/altmed/ConsHerbs/Comfreych.html. Updated March 15, 2007. Accessed June 4, 2008.

D'Anchise R, Bulitta M, Giannetti B. Comfrey extract ointment in comparison to diclofenac gel in the treatment of acute unilateral ankle sprains (distortions). *Arzneimittel-Forschung.* 2007;57:712-716.

Grube B, Grünwald J, Krug L, Staiger C. Efficacy of a comfrey root (Symphyti offic. radix) extract ointment in the treatment of patients with painful osteoarthritis of the knee: results of a double-blind, randomised, bicenter, placebo-controlled trial. *Phytomedicine.* 2007;14:2-10.

Gruenwald J. *PDR for Herbal Medicines.* 3rd ed. Montvale, NJ: Thomson PDR; 2004.

Fetrow CW, Avila JR. *Professional's Handbook of Complementary & Alternative Medicines.* Philadelphia, PA: Lippincott Williams & Wilkins; 2004.

Kucera M, Barna M, Horàcek O, Kàlal J, Kucera A, Hladìkova M. Topical symphytum herb concentrate cream against myalgia: a randomized controlled double-blind clinical study. *Adv Ther.* 2005;22:681-692.

Ridker PM, McDermott WV. Comfrey herb tea and hepatic veno-occlusive disease. *Lancet.* 1989;1:657-658.

Teynor TM, Putnam DH, Doll JD, Kelling KA, Oelke EA, Undersander DJ, Oplinger ES. Comfrey. Alternative Field Crops Manual Web site. http://www.hort.purdue.edu/newcrop/afcm/comfrey.html. Updated November 17,1997. Accessed June 4, 2008.

COPPER

Other common name(s): none

Scientific/medical name(s): Cu, cupric oxide, copper sulfate, copper gluconate, copper picolinate, cupric acetate, alkaline copper carbonate

Description

Copper is a required nutrient. It is found naturally in foods such as seafood, liver, green vegetables, whole grains, wheat bran, lentils, and nuts. Copper helps regulate blood pressure and heart rate and is needed to absorb iron from the gut. It is used to make many important compounds in the body.

Overview

Some laboratory and animal studies have found that copper has antioxidant properties and may have some anticancer effects. Other studies have found that high copper levels in the blood were linked with cancer and other diseases. More extensive human studies are needed to determine what role copper may play in the prevention or treatment of cancer.

How is it promoted for use?

There are claims that copper aids in the healing process, helps to expel toxins from the body, and helps prevent heart problems. Copper is also used in some preparations of Iscador, a commercially prepared mistletoe extract sold as a complementary therapy in Europe for tumors of the liver, gallbladder, stomach, and kidneys.

There are also claims that copper actually promotes cancer growth. Proponents of this theory recommend a diet low in copper and the use of chelating agents that bind to copper and promote its elimination from the body (see "Chelation Therapy," page 717).

What does it involve?

Copper supplements are available in pill or capsule form. Copper is often added to vitamin supplements. However, most people are able to get enough copper in their bodies by eating balanced meals. Fruits and vegetables can provide up to 30 percent of a person's total copper intake. Some copper is also present in drinking water, and copper pipes can leach extra copper into the water they carry.

The Recommended Dietary Allowance (RDA) for copper is 0.9 milligrams per day for most adults, 1 milligram for pregnant women, and 1.3 milligrams for women who are breastfeeding. The RDA is enough to meet the needs of most people in these groups. Some people may not get enough copper from foods, especially if they take zinc supplements, which can partly block copper absorption. Large doses of vitamin C supplements can also block copper uptake. People who take zinc supplements or large doses of vitamin C may need to take extra copper to absorb enough. Those with malabsorption diseases or malnutrition may also need extra copper.

What is the history behind it?

While research into the antioxidant properties of copper is quite recent, healing properties have long been attributed to copper in folk medicine. Some people wear copper bracelets, for example, to help with arthritis. Today, many multivitamins and other herbal and mineral supplements include copper.

What is the evidence?

Copper is a trace mineral that is needed for many important body processes. Animal studies have shown that copper is useful in maintaining antioxidant defenses. Antioxidants block the actions of free radicals, activated oxygen molecules that can damage cells. While the role of copper in the cancer process is still unclear, copper complexes have been shown to have anticancer properties in laboratory studies.

Other laboratory and animal studies suggest that high copper levels may be linked to liver cancer and brain tumors. More recently, many studies have shown that patients' blood copper levels are higher with several types of cancer and other diseases. To add to the confusion, blood tests can show high copper levels even when there is little copper in the tissues. These high copper levels may be due to injury, disease, or inflammation.

Because copper is needed to form new blood vessels, and because cancer needs new blood vessels in order to grow, some researchers are interested in copper's possible impact on cancer. One group of researchers looked at whether a copper-lowering drug could help patients with advanced kidney cancer. Some patients' cancer stopped growing during the six-month treatment period. A few people had low white blood counts during treatment, requiring that treatment be stopped until they recovered. This was a small study, and further research is needed to find out whether copper can help more people with advanced cancer.

Another study noted high copper levels in the blood of people who died of heart disease. It is not known whether the laboratory tests accurately reflected copper levels in the body tissue or exactly what caused the high levels. In contrast, a recent study gave copper supplements to healthy women with no signs of copper deficiency. Their cholesterol and triglyceride levels improved, as did some other markers of heart disease risk. This small study did not look at actual heart disease, however. Further research is required to determine whether copper can affect heart disease risk.

Many people wear copper bracelets for their arthritis, and some people report improvements in their arthritis symptoms. However, available scientific evidence does not support claims that the bracelets are effective. A gel form of copper salicylate (an aspirin–copper compound) was found to be no more effective at relieving pain than sham gel, although the copper gel produced more rashes. Further research may help determine whether any form of copper might be helpful in arthritis treatment.

One laboratory study showed that the white blood cells of men who had been on a low-copper diet did not attack germs as effectively as they had when the same men were receiving enough copper. An older study in a group of children recovering from malnutrition showed that those who got copper supplements had significantly fewer lung infections than those who got sham supplements. While severe copper deficiency is known to result in poorer immune function, further studies are needed to find out what effect, if any, milder deficiency might have. These studies are hindered by the fact that copper levels in the blood do not always reflect nutritional status.

There is some evidence that trace metals, including copper, iron, and zinc, may have a role in forming the brain plaque associated with Alzheimer's disease. However, there is not enough evidence to define the role of copper in this process.

At this time, it is hard to say how each nutrient or nutrient combination affects a person's risk for cancer. On the other hand, large observational epidemiologic studies have shown that those whose diets are high in vegetables and low in animal fat, meat, and/or calories have lower risks for some of the most common types of cancer. Until more is known about this relationship, the American Cancer Society recommends eating a variety of healthful foods—with most of them coming from plant sources—rather than relying on supplements. Supplements may be helpful for some people, such as pregnant women, women of childbearing age, and people with restricted food intakes. If a supplement is taken, the best choice for most people is a balanced multivitamin/mineral supplement that contains no more than 100 percent of the "Daily Value" of most nutrients.

Are there any possible problems or complications?

Copper toxicity is rare, and copper supplements are considered safe when taken in recommended amounts. However, adults are advised not to take more than 10 milligrams per day because of increased risk for liver damage. The maximum recommended dosage is lower for children, depending on age. Copper overdose can cause serious problems such as liver damage, kidney failure, coma, and death. Early symptoms of overdose may include nausea, vomiting, diarrhea, abdominal pain, problems with coordination or movement, and sleepiness. There may also be behavioral problems, such as trouble concentrating or emotional disturbances.

People with Wilson's disease (a genetic disorder that allows copper to build up in the body) should not take copper supplements or multivitamins containing copper. Diabetics should also avoid these supplements because copper can affect blood sugar levels.

Problems may also happen when a person has too little copper. Copper is required for iron to be absorbed into the body and is necessary for babies to develop normally. Osteoporosis can develop in infants and adults with too little copper. In adults, low copper levels can result in anemia and low white blood cell counts. Low copper levels in adults have been reported to cause muscle spasms in the legs and trouble walking.

Copper can interfere with some medicines. Talk with your doctor or pharmacist about all medicines, herbs, and supplements you are taking. Relying on this type of treatment alone and avoiding or delaying conventional medical care for cancer may have serious health consequences.

This product is sold as a dietary supplement in the United States. Unlike companies that produce drugs (which must provide the FDA with results of detailed testing showing their product is safe and effective before the drug is approved for sale), the companies that make supplements do not have to show

evidence of safety or health benefits to the FDA before selling their products. Supplement products without any reliable scientific evidence of health benefits may still be sold as long as the companies selling them do not claim the supplements can prevent, treat, or cure any specific disease. Some such products may not contain the amount of the herb or substance that is written on the label, and some may include other substances (contaminants). Though the FDA has written new rules to improve the quality of manufacturing processes for dietary supplements and the accurate listing of supplement ingredients, these rules do not take full effect until 2010. The new rules also do not address the safety of supplement ingredients or their effects on health when proper manufacturing techniques are used.

Most such supplements have not been tested to find out if they interact with medicines, foods, or other herbs and supplements. Even though some reports of interactions and harmful effects may be published, full studies of interactions and effects are not often available. Because of these limitations, any information on ill effects and interactions should be considered incomplete.

References

Araya M, Olivares M, Pizarro F, Méndez MA, González M, Uauy R. Supplementing copper at the upper level of the adult dietary recommended intake induces detectable but transient changes in healthy adults. *J Nutr.* 2005;135:2367-2371.

Bügel S, Harper A, Rock E, O'Conner JM, Bonham MP, Strain JJ. Effect of copper supplementation on indices of copper status and certain CVD risk markers in young healthy women. *Br J Nutr.* 2005;94:231-236.

Cassileth B. *The Alternative Medicine Handbook: The Complete Reference Guide to Alternative and Complementary Therapies.* New York: W.W. Norton; 1998.

Castillo-Durán C, Fisberg M, Valenzuela A, Egaña JI, Uauy R. Controlled trial of copper supplementation during the recovery from marasmus. *Am J Clin Nutr.* 1983;37:898-903.

Copper. PDRhealth Web site. http://www.pdrhealth.com/drug_info/nmdrugprofiles/nutsupdrugs/cop_0083.shtml. Accessed June 4, 2008.

Davis CD, Feng Y. Dietary copper, manganese and iron affect the formation of aberrant crypts in colon of rats administered 3,2'-dimethyl-4-aminobiphenyl. *J Nutr.* 1999;129;1060-1067.

DiSilvestro RA, Sakamoto K, Milner JA. No effects of low copper intake on rat mammary tissue superoxide dismutase 1 activity and mammary chemical carcinogenesis. *Nutr Cancer.* 1998;31:218-220.

Eaton-Evans J, Mellwrath EM, Jackson WE, McCartney H, Strain JJ. Copper supplementation and the maintenance of bone mineral density in middle-aged women. *J Trace Elem Exp Med.* 1996;9:87-94.

Finefrock AE, Bush AI, Doraiswamy PM. Current status of metals as therapeutic targets in Alzheimer's disease. *J Am Geriatr Soc.* 2003;51:1143-1148.

Ford ES. Serum copper concentration and coronary heart disease among US adults. *Am J Epidemiol.* 2000;151:1182-1188.

Kelley DS, Daudu PA, Taylor PC, Mackey BE, Turnlund JR. Effects of low-copper diets on human immune response. *Am J Clin Nutr.* 1995;62:412-416.

Kumar N, Gross JB Jr, Ahlskog JE. Copper deficiency myelopathy produces a clinical picture like subacute combined degeneration. *Neurology.* 2004;63:33-39.

Higdon J. Copper. Linus Pauling Institute Micronutrient Information Center. Oregon State University Web site. http://lpi.oregonstate.edu/infocenter/minerals/copper/. Updated July 2007. Accessed June 4, 2008.

Mártin-Lagos F, Navarro-Alarcón M, Terrés-Martos C, López-G de la Serrana H, López-Martínez MC. Serum copper and zinc concentrations in serum from patients with cancer and cardiovascular disease. *Sci Total Environ.* 1997;204:27-35.

Milne DB, Nielsen FH. Effects of a diet low in copper on copper-status indicators in postmenopausal women. *Am J Clin Nutr.* 1996;63:358-364.

Percival SS. Copper and immunity. *Am J Clin Nutr.* 1998;67:1064S-1068S.

Redman BG, Esper P, Pan Q, Dunn RL, Hussain HK, Chenevert T, Brewer GJ, Merajver SD. Phase II trial of tetrathiomolybdate in patients with advanced kidney cancer. *Clin Cancer Res.* 2003;9:1666-1672.

Renault E, Deschatrette J. Alterations of rat hepatoma cell genomes induced by copper deficiency. *Nutr Cancer.* 1997;29:242-247.

Scheinberg IH, Sternlieb I. Wilson disease and idiopathic copper toxicosis. *Am J Clin Nutr.* 1996;63:842S-845S.

Shackel NA, Day RO, Kellett B, Brooks PM. Copper-salicylate gel for pain relief in osteoarthritis: a randomised controlled trial. *Med J Aust.* 1997;167:134-136.

Spencer JW, Jacobs JJ. *Complementary/Alternative Medicine: An Evidence-Based Approach.* St. Louis, MO: Mosby; 1999.

Strain JJ. Putative role of dietary trace elements in coronary heart disease and cancer. *Br J Biomed Sci.* 1994;51:241-251.

US Congress, Office of Technology Assessment. *Unconventional Cancer Treatments: OTA-H-405.* Washington, DC: US Government Printing Office; 1990.

Wu T, Sempos CT, Freudenheim JL, Muti P, Smit E. Serum iron, copper and zinc concentrations and risk of cancer mortality in US adults. *Ann Epidemiol.* 2004;14:195-201.

ECHINACEA

Other common name(s): purple coneflower, Kansas snakeroot, black sampson, sampson root

Scientific/medical name(s): *Echinacea purpurea, Echinacea angustifolia, Echinacea pallida*

Description

Echinacea is a wild herb that grows primarily in the Great Plains and eastern regions of North America. It is also cultivated in Europe. Three different species of the plant are used in herbal remedies—*Echinacea purpurea*, *Echinacea angustifolia*, and *Echinacea pallida*. *Echinacea purpurea* is the species most frequently used for research and treatment. Liquid extracts are made from the leaves and roots or from the whole plant.

Overview

Although echinacea has been widely promoted to help fight colds and flu, there is little scientific evidence that it is effective in preventing, shortening the duration, or relieving the symptoms of these infections. Available scientific evidence does not support claims that echinacea increases resistance to cancer or relieves the side effects of chemotherapy or radiation therapy. Long-term use of echinacea is linked with some side effects as well as potential interference with anesthesia and certain medicines.

How is it promoted for use?

Echinacea is promoted mainly as a treatment for colds, the flu, and other respiratory infections. In Germany, echinacea is a common over-the-counter medication, and more than three hundred echinacea products are reportedly sold. Commission E (Germany's regulatory agency for herbs) approved echinacea for treating respiratory infections, urinary tract infections, and poorly healing wounds.

Supporters claim echinacea boosts the body's immune system by stimulating the activity of immune system cells called macrophages, which attack and consume invading organisms, including cancer cells. Some claim that the herb stimulates the anticancer activity of natural killer cells (a type of white blood cell) and therefore could be used as a supplement to chemotherapy or radiation therapy.

What does it involve?

Echinacea is available in capsule and liquid form; however, there is controversy over its usefulness in liquid form. Although dosages may vary, most practitioners recommend 900 milligrams per day for no longer than eight weeks to boost the immune system. An injectable form is also available outside the United States.

What is the history behind it?

Echinacea has long been used in herbal remedies by Native Americans. In the nineteenth century, it became a commonly prescribed tonic and was billed as a natural remedy for infections and inflammation. The herb's use in the United States has surged along with interest in natural medicine. In the United States, products labeled as echinacea can be completely different chemical preparations, because of the variety of possible species and plant parts, various extraction methods, and the addition of other plant extracts.

What is the evidence?

Many practitioners and patients, particularly in Europe but also in the United States, are convinced that echinacea has the ability to enhance the immune system and fight off infections from colds and the flu. Although a few laboratory studies suggest that some chemicals found in echinacea might increase the activity of immune system cells, human studies have generally concluded that echinacea is not effective in preventing, shortening the duration of, or relieving the symptoms of these infections.

A few human studies suggested that there might be some benefit, but reviews of these studies have found that most tested too few patients or had flaws in the study design that limited the accuracy of their results. Several larger, more recent, and more rigorously conducted studies have found no benefit for children or adults.

In a recent study sponsored by the National Center for Complementary and Alternative Medicine, approximately four hundred volunteers were given a standard amount of cold virus. These volunteers were randomly assigned to receive one of three possible treatments: echinacea starting one week before infection, echinacea starting at the time of infection, or a placebo. The volunteers were isolated in hotel rooms to reduce other sources of infection. The researchers found that echinacea was not effective in preventing colds or reducing either their duration or the severity of symptoms reported by the volunteers. The researchers even measured the amount of nasal mucus in each volunteer, the number of immune system cells in their noses, and the levels of an immune system hormone in their noses. None of the measurements was influenced by echinacea.

A 2006 review of twenty-two studies concluded that echinacea does not appear to be effective in preventing colds. It also noted that some studies of *Echinacea purpurea* suggested it may have some value in treating colds if given shortly after symptoms develop, but the results were not fully consistent.

In terms of how people with cancer use echinacea, the consensus of available scientific evidence does not support claims that echinacea increases resistance to cancer or reduces the immune suppression resulting from chemotherapy.

Are there any possible problems or complications?

Although echinacea is relatively safe, some natural medicine practitioners caution that it may cause liver damage or suppress the immune system if used for more than eight weeks. They urge people taking medications known to cause liver toxicity, such as anabolic steroids, amiodarone (a drug for heart rhythm problems), and the chemotherapy drugs methotrexate and ketoconazole, to avoid echinacea use. Echinacea may also interact with other drugs. Some of these combinations may be dangerous. Always tell your doctor and pharmacist about any herbs or supplements you are taking.

Most practitioners recommend that people with autoimmune disorders such as multiple sclerosis or human immunodeficiency virus, people with leukemia, and women who are pregnant or breastfeeding not take echinacea. Careful observation of volunteers who have participated in clinical studies of echinacea have found that serious side effects are uncommon. The most frequent side effects are headache, dizziness, nausea, constipation, and abdominal pain. Rashes may occur, especially in children. Serious allergic reactions to echinacea have been reported rarely, including itching, trouble breathing, swelling of the face or throat, rash, and wheezing. They are more likely in people who have other allergies or asthma. Relying on this type of treatment alone and avoiding or delaying conventional medical care for cancer may have serious health consequences.

This product is sold as a dietary supplement in the United States. Unlike companies that produce drugs (which must provide the FDA with results of detailed testing showing their product is safe and effective before the drug is approved for sale), the companies that make supplements do not have to show evidence of safety or health benefits to the FDA before selling their products. Supplement products without any reliable scientific evidence of health benefits may still be sold as long as the companies selling them do not claim the supplements can prevent, treat, or cure any specific disease. Some such products may not contain the amount of the herb or substance that is written on the label, and some may include other substances (contaminants). Though the FDA has written new rules to improve the quality of manufacturing processes for dietary supplements and the accurate listing of supplement ingredients, these rules do not take full effect until 2010. The new rules also do not address the safety of supplement ingredients or their effects on health when proper manufacturing techniques are used.

Most such supplements have not been tested to find out if they interact with medicines, foods, or other herbs and supplements. Even though some reports of interactions and harmful effects may be published, full studies of interactions and effects are not often available. Because of these limitations, any information on ill effects and interactions should be considered incomplete.

References

Barrett BP, Brown RL, Locken K, Maberry R, Bobula JA, D'Alessio D. Treatment of the common cold with unrefined echinacea. A randomized, double-blind, placebo-controlled trial. *Ann Intern Med.* 2002;137:939-946.

Blumenthal M, ed. *The Complete German Commission E Monographs: Therapeutic Guide to Herbal Medicines.* Austin, TX: American Botanical Council; 1998.

Brinkeborn RM, Shah DV, Degenring FH. Echinaforce and other Echinacea fresh plant preparations in the treatment of the common cold. A randomized, placebo controlled, double-blind clinical trial. *Phytomedicine.* 1999;6:1-6.

Echinacea. Memorial Sloan-Kettering Cancer Center Web site. http://www.mskcc.org/mskcc/html/69209.cfm. Updated July 11, 2007. Accessed June 4, 2008.

Grimm W, Müller HH. A randomized controlled trial of the effect of fluid extract of *Echinacea purpurea* on the incidence and severity of colds and respiratory infections. *Am J Med.* 1999;106:138-143.

Kolata G. Study says echinacea has no effect on colds. *New York Times.* July 28, 2005.

Linde K, Barrett B, Wölkart K, Bauer R, Melchart D. Echinacea for preventing and treating the common cold. *Cochrane Database Syst Rev.* 2006;(1):CD000530.

Miller LG. Herbal medicinals: selected clinical considerations focusing on known or potential drug-herb interactions. *Arch Intern Med.* 1998;158:2200-2211.

Modarai M, Gertsch J, Suter A, Heinrich M, Kortenkamp A. Cytochrome P450 inhibitory action of Echinacea preparations differs widely and co-varies with alkylamide content. *J Pharm Pharmacol.* 2007;59:567-573.

Natural Standard. Herbal/plant therapies: Echinacea (*Echinacea angustifolia* DC, *Echinacea pallida, Echinacea purpurea*). Complementary/Integrative Medicine Education Resources, The University of Texas M. D. Anderson Cancer Center Web site. http://www.mdanderson.org/departments/cimer/display.cfm?id=3323E433-E473-4529-A34548F383CD19F5&method=displayFull. Accessed June 4, 2008.

O'Neil J, Hughes S, Lourie A, Zweifler J. Effects of echinacea on the frequency of upper respiratory tract symptoms: a randomized, double-blind, placebo-controlled trial. *Ann Allergy Asthma Immunol.* 2008;100:384-388.

Sampson W. Studying herbal remedies. *N Engl J Med.* 2005;353:337-339.

Taylor JA, Weber W, Standish L, Quinn H, Goesling J, McGann M, Calabrese C. Efficacy and safety of echinacea in treating upper respiratory tract infections in children: a randomized controlled trial. *JAMA.* 2003;290:2824-2830.

Turner RB, Bauer R, Woelkart K, Hulsey TC, Gangemi JD. An evaluation of *Echinacea angustifolia* in experimental rhinovirus infections. *N Engl J Med.* 2005;353:341-348.

ELEUTHERO

Other common name(s): Siberian ginseng, devil's shrub, devil's root, touch-me-not
Scientific/medical name(s): *Eleutherococcus senticosus, Acanthopanax senticosus*

Description

Eleuthero is a shrub that grows in Siberia, China, Korea, and Japan. The dried root and other underground parts of the plant are used in herbal remedies for a variety of conditions. It is a distant relative of true (*Panax*) ginseng (which includes Asian ginseng and American ginseng), but it does not belong to the *Panax* group of herbs. It was previously sold in the United States as "Siberian ginseng," but a 2002 U.S. law forbade the "ginseng" label. The name "eleuthero" is now more commonly used.

Overview

Some studies have suggested eleuthero may help boost energy or have other beneficial effects, but the research is far from conclusive, and more studies are needed. Available scientific evidence does not support eleuthero as an effective way to treat cancer or reduce the side effects of chemotherapy or radiation therapy.

How is it promoted for use?

Proponents of eleuthero claim that it boosts the immune system, increases energy and physical prowess, improves concentration and memory, and speeds recovery from illness. Some practitioners claim that the herb regulates blood pressure, reduces inflammation, has a restorative effect on many organs, and lowers blood sugar levels.

Some claim eleuthero can help with cancer-related fatigue. There are also claims that it helps chemotherapy drugs work better and that it reduces the toxic effects of chemotherapy and radiation therapy.

What does it involve?

Eleuthero is on the Commission E (Germany's regulatory agency for herbs) list of approved herbs, and the supplements are available as tablets and liquid extracts. The powdered or cut root can be brewed as a tea. An average dose is 2 to 3 grams per day. Typically, it is taken regularly for six to eight weeks, followed by a one- to two-week break before starting again.

What is the history behind it?

Eleuthero has been used in traditional Chinese medicine for thousands of years to treat rheumatism, weak liver and kidneys, and low energy levels and to prevent respiratory tract infections, including colds and the flu. Herbalists have long prescribed eleuthero for menopausal complaints, weakness in elderly people, physical and mental stress, trouble sleeping caused by anxiety, and even to treat cancer.

Eleuthero did not come into widespread use until the middle of the twentieth century, at a time when supplies of *Panax* ginseng were low. Russian and Chinese scientists found eleuthero seemed to have some of the same properties as *Panax* ginseng and could be grown faster. Athletes from the former Soviet Union used it because they believed it enhanced athletic performance during competitions. After the Chernobyl nuclear reactor disaster, Russian and Ukrainian citizens reportedly received the herb to counter the effects of radiation poisoning, though that benefit was not proven. It is still widely used in Russia and other Asian countries and has gained popularity in Western countries as well.

What is the evidence?

Eleuthero does not contain ginsenosides, the compounds found in Asian and American ginseng that are thought to be responsible for the plants' medicinal effects. Eleuthero contains other compounds, called eleutherosides, some of which may act like estrogen or other steroid hormones.

Research on the possible medicinal properties of eleuthero has been conducted mainly in Russia and other Asian countries. Few studies of eleuthero have been published in conventional peer-reviewed medical journals.

Some laboratory studies in cell cultures and animals have suggested that eleuthero may have immune-boosting properties. Whether these effects occur in people is unclear. The consensus of available scientific evidence does not show the herb is effective in treating cancer in humans or that it can reduce the side effects of chemotherapy.

One small study found that eleuthero was no better than a placebo in reducing chronic fatigue over the course of a few months, although there were indications it might be better among people whose fatigue was less severe. The study authors concluded that further research in this area may be warranted.

The evidence that eleuthero supplements enhance athletic ability is mixed. A recent review of eight clinical trials in humans found that while three studies suggested improved physical endurance, these studies had flaws in the way they were conducted. The five remaining studies, which were more scientifically sound, did not find a strong benefit.

Are there any possible problems or complications?

The health risks of eleuthero have not been firmly established, although major side effects from usual doses seem to be rare. Some cases of headache, diarrhea, nervousness, and trouble sleeping have been reported.

Eleuthero may raise blood pressure and increase heart rate, so people with high blood pressure or heart disease should talk with their doctors before taking it. It may also lower blood sugar levels, which may be important to people taking medicine for diabetes.

Eleuthero may alter the amount of time it takes for bleeding to stop. This could be an issue if it is taken before surgery or if a person is taking drugs that can affect blood clotting, such as aspirin or warfarin (Coumadin). Other interactions with drugs or other herbs may be possible. Tell your doctor and pharmacist about any herbs and supplements you are taking.

Eleuthero has not been well studied in women who are pregnant or breastfeeding. People with allergies to eleuthero or related plants should avoid this herb. Relying on this type of treatment alone and avoiding or delaying conventional medical care for cancer may have serious health consequences.

This product is sold as a dietary supplement in the United States. Unlike companies that produce drugs (which must provide the FDA with results of detailed testing showing their product is safe and effective before the drug is approved for sale), the companies that make supplements do not have to show evidence of safety or health benefits to the FDA before selling their products. Supplement products without any reliable scientific evidence of health benefits may still be sold as long as the companies selling them do not claim the supplements can prevent, treat, or cure any specific disease. Some such products may not contain the amount of the herb or substance that is written on the label, and some may include other substances (contaminants). Though the FDA has written new rules to improve the quality of manufacturing processes for dietary supplements and the accurate listing of supplement ingredients, these rules do not take full effect until 2010. The new rules also do not address the safety of supplement ingredients or their effects on health when proper manufacturing techniques are used.

Most such supplements have not been tested to find out if they interact with medicines, foods, or other herbs and supplements. Even though some reports of interactions and harmful effects may be published, full studies of interactions and effects are not often available. Because of these limitations, any information on ill effects and interactions should be considered incomplete.

References

Blumenthal M, ed. *The Complete German Commission E Monographs: Therapeutic Guide to Herbal Medicines.* Austin, TX: American Botanical Council; 1998.

Goulet ED, Dionne IJ. Assessment of the effects of eleutherococcus senticosus on endurance performance. *Int J Sport Nutr Exerc Metab.* 2005;15:75-83.

Gruenwald J. *PDR for Herbal Medicines.* 3rd ed. Montvale, NJ: Thomson PDR; 2004.

Hartz AJ, Bentler S, Noyes R, Hoehns J, Logemann C, Sinift S, Butani Y, Wang W, Brake K, Ernst M, Kautzman H. Randomized controlled trial of Siberian ginseng for chronic fatigue. *Psychol Med.* 2004;34:51-61.

Siberian ginseng. Memorial Sloan-Kettering Cancer Center Web site. http://www.mskcc.org/mskcc/html/69379.cfm. Updated July 17, 2007. Accessed June 6, 2008.

ENERCEL

Other common name(s): previously known as Hansi
Scientific/medical name(s): none

Description

Enercel is an herbal preparation consisting of very small dilutions from plants of the desert and rain forests, such as cactus *(Cacti grandiflora)*, aloe, arnica, lachesis, and licopodium, in a 2 percent to 8 percent alcohol base.

Overview

Available scientific evidence does not support claims that Enercel or Enercel Plus is effective in treating cancer or any other disease.

How is it promoted for use?

Proponents claim that Enercel enhances the immune system, prevents and stops the progression of some types of cancer, increases tolerance of side effects from chemotherapy and radiation therapy, and effectively treats chronic fatigue syndrome, AIDS, and asthma.

The proprietors of Enercel claim that the remedy works for asthma, stroke, Bell's palsy, and numerous other disorders. They claim that more than 150,000 people with cancer have reported positive responses with Enercel treatment. Currently, the company is licensed in El Salvador.

What does it involve?

Enercel is taken by mouth in drop form, by nasal mist, through a nebulizer, or by injection. The basic formula includes about ten components, the proportions of which are adjusted according to the condition being treated and whether the drug will be delivered orally or by injection. The U.S. Food and Drug Administration (FDA) has not approved Enercel injections.

What is the history behind it?

Hansi, the original formula, was claimed to have been developed by an Argentine biologist, Juan Jose Hirschmann, PhD, who introduced his formula in Buenos Aires in 1990.

What is the evidence?

Available scientific evidence does not support claims that Enercel or Enercel Plus is effective in treating cancer or any other disease. No studies testing this treatment could be found in the National Library of Medicine's PubMed database of medical journal articles. One Web site promoting Enercel-Hansi includes a page with the heading "Studies." Although the page includes experimental methods, results, and conclusions that are formatted to resemble a medical or scientific journal article, the authors provide no information regarding whether the manuscripts were ever published in any peer-reviewed journal. Because publication in such journals is considered standard practice among medical researchers, therapeutic claims that are promoted directly to the public and not subjected to the scrutiny of scientific experts cannot be considered reliable evidence.

Are there any possible problems or complications?

Not enough is known about Enercel to determine whether it is safe for humans. Relying on this type of treatment alone and avoiding or delaying conventional medical care may have serious health consequences.

This product is sold as a dietary supplement in the United States. Unlike companies that produce drugs (which must provide the FDA with results of detailed testing showing their product is safe and effective before the drug is approved for sale), the companies that make supplements do not have to show evidence of safety or health benefits to the FDA before selling their products. Supplement products without any reliable scientific evidence of health benefits may still be sold as long as the companies selling them do not claim the supplements can prevent, treat, or cure any specific disease. Some such products may not contain the amount of the herb or substance that is written on the label, and some may include other substances (contaminants). Though the FDA has written new rules to improve the quality of manufacturing processes for dietary supplements and the accurate listing of supplement ingredients, these rules do not take full effect until 2010. The new rules also do not address the safety of supplement ingredients or their effects on health when proper manufacturing techniques are used.

Most such supplements have not been tested to find out if they interact with medicines, foods, or other herbs and supplements. Even though some reports of interactions and harmful effects may be published, full studies of interactions and effects are not often available. Because of these limitations, any information on ill effects and interactions should be considered incomplete.

References

Enercel. Enercel Web site. http://www.enercel.com/layout.htm. Accessed April 17, 2007. Site discontinued.

Enercel. Enercel Web site. http://www.enercel.org. Accessed June 20, 2008.

Enercel. Manufacturer's product information. Enercel Web site. http://www.enercel.com. Accessed December 21, 2005. Site discontinued.

Studies. Hansi-Enercel Web site. http://www.prescriptionhelp.ws/page4.html. Accessed June 20, 2008.

ESSIAC TEA

Other common name(s): Essiac, Flor Essence, Tea of Life, Herbal Essence, Vitalitea
Scientific/medical name(s): none

Description

Essiac is a mixture of herbs that are combined to make a tea. The original formula included burdock root *(Arctium lappa L.)*, slippery elm inner bark *(Ulmus fulva Michx.)*, sheep sorrel *(Rumex acetosella L.)*, and Indian rhubarb root *(Rheum palmatum L.)*. Watercress *(Nasturtium officinale R.Br.)*, blessed thistle *(Cnicus benedictus L.)*, red clover *(Trifolium pratense L.)*, and kelp *(Laminaria digitata [Hudson] Lamx.)* were added to later recipes for a product sold as Flor Essence.

Overview

There have been no published clinical trials in conventional medical journals showing the effectiveness of Essiac in the treatment of cancer. Some of the specific herbs contained in the mixture have shown some anticancer effects in laboratory experiments. However, most laboratory studies of Essiac have found no effectiveness against cancer cells, and one reported that it increases growth of breast cancer cells. Available scientific evidence does not support its use for the treatment of cancer in humans.

How is it promoted for use?

Promoters claim Essiac strengthens the immune system, improves well-being, relieves pain, increases appetite, reduces tumor size, and extends survival. Some also claim that it cleanses the blood, promotes cell repair, restores energy levels, and detoxifies the body. The herbs contained in Essiac are claimed to relieve inflammation, lubricate bones and joints, stimulate the stomach, and eliminate excess mucus in organs, tissues, lymph glands, and nerve channels.

It was originally claimed Essiac worked by changing tumors into normal tissue. Proponents claimed a tumor would become larger and harder after a few doses of Essiac, then would soften, shrink, and be discharged by the body.

Essiac and Flor Essence are also promoted to treat AIDS and a variety of digestive system problems.

What does it involve?

Essiac is available in dry and liquid formulas, and methods of preparation and dosage vary by manufacturer. Some recommend spring or nonfluoridated water, and most require refrigeration after brewing. A typical dose is 1 ounce taken one to three times per day. Practitioners advise that Essiac tea should be taken on an empty stomach, two hours before or after meals, for a period of at least one to two years. The manufacturer of Flor Essence recommends 1 to 12 ounces of tea daily.

Essiac and Flor Essence are available through mail-order outlets and can also be purchased in the United States in health food stores as a dietary supplement and as a health tonic in Canada.

What is the history behind it?

In 1922, a public health nurse named Rene Caisse from Ontario, Canada learned about Essiac from a patient. The patient claimed to have recovered from breast cancer by taking an Indian herbal tea developed by an Ojibwa medicine man. She obtained the recipe and reportedly treated her aunt's stomach cancer with the tea. In 1924, Caisse opened a clinic and began to offer cancer patients the herbal mixture, which she named Essiac (her last name spelled backward). She treated thousands of patients using her secret formula as a tea and as an injection. Canadian medical authorities investigated the clinic in 1938 and concluded that there was little evidence for the effectiveness of Essiac. Caisse gave her four-herb formula to a manufacturer in Toronto in 1977, one year before her death, with the intent of having it tested and sold for a reasonable cost.

Memorial Sloan-Kettering Cancer Center conducted animal testing of Essiac in 1959 and the mid-1970s, but no antitumor effects were verified. In 1983, Canadian federal health officials requested that Essiac be tested by the U.S. National Cancer Institute (NCI), which found no evidence of anticancer activity in animal studies. Canadian health officials reviewed eighty-six case studies and concluded that there was no evidence that Essiac slowed the progression of cancer. They noted that there were few serious side effects, however, and that people may have benefited psychologically from the treatment.

What is the evidence?

Although there have been many testimonials, there have been no clinical trials testing the effectiveness of Essiac or Flor Essence. Reviews of medical records of people who have been treated with Essiac do not support claims that this product helps people with cancer live longer or that it relieves their symptoms.

Animal studies conducted at Memorial Sloan-Kettering Cancer Center and the NCI from the 1950s through the 1980s concluded that Essiac was not effective. The majority of subsequent studies have confirmed these findings. A recent laboratory study found that Essiac and Flor Essence actually increased growth of breast cancer cells. Flor Essence has not been tested as a cancer treatment in humans.

Some components of Essiac and Flor Essence have been tested individually in laboratory and animal studies. Some of these studies identified substances with antitumor or anti-inflammatory properties. However, these results cannot be interpreted as evidence of effectiveness in humans. To the contrary, the available scientific information indicates that these products are not helpful.

Are there any possible problems or complications?

Serious side effects are uncommon. Essiac may cause headache, nausea, diarrhea or constipation, vomiting, low blood sugar, liver damage, and kidney damage. Rarely, serious allergic reactions have been reported.

In addition, the potential interactions between Essiac and other drugs and herbs should be considered. Some of these combinations may be dangerous. Always tell your doctor and pharmacist about any herbs you are taking. Relying on this type of treatment alone and avoiding or delaying conventional medical care for cancer may have serious health consequences.

This product is sold as a dietary supplement in the United States. Unlike companies that produce drugs (which must provide the FDA with results of detailed testing showing their product is safe and effective before the drug is approved for sale), the companies that make supplements do not have to show evidence of safety or health benefits to the FDA before selling their products. Supplement products without any reliable scientific evidence of health benefits may still be sold as long as the companies selling them do not claim the supplements can prevent, treat, or cure any specific disease. Some such products may not contain the amount of the herb or substance that is written on the label, and some may include other substances (contaminants). Though the FDA has written new rules to improve the quality of manufacturing processes for dietary supplements and the accurate listing of supplement ingredients, these rules do not take full effect until 2010. The new rules also do not address the safety of supplement ingredients or their effects on health when proper manufacturing techniques are used.

Most such supplements have not been tested to find out if they interact with medicines, foods, or other herbs and supplements. Even though some reports of interactions and harmful effects may be published, full studies of interactions and effects are not often available. Because of these limitations, any information on ill effects and interactions should be considered incomplete.

References

Eberding A, Madera C, Xie S, Wood CA, Brown PN, Guns ES. Evaluation of the antiproliferative effects of Essiac on in vitro and in vivo models of prostate cancer compared to paclitaxel. *Nutr Cancer.* 2007;58:188-196.

Essiac. Memorial Sloan-Kettering Cancer Center Web site. http://www.mskcc.org/mskcc/html/69215.cfm. Accessed June 4, 2008.

Essiac/Flor-Essence (PDQ®). National Cancer Institute Web site. http://www.cancer.gov/cancertopics/pdq/cam/essiac/healthprofessional/allpages. Accessed June 4, 2008.

Herbal/plant therapies: Essiac detailed scientific review. Complementary/Integrative Medicine Education Resources, The University of Texas M. D. Anderson Cancer Center Web site. http://www.mdanderson.org/departments/CIMER/display.cfm?id=03F2CD11-EE0F-11D4-810200508B603A14&method=displayFull. Accessed June 4, 2008.

Kulp KS, Montgomery JL, Nelson DO, Cutter B, Latham ER, Shattuck DL, Klotz DM, Bennett LM. Essiac and Flor-Essence herbal tonics stimulate the in vitro growth of human breast cancer cells. *Breast Cancer Res Treat.* 2006;98:249-259. Epub 2006 Mar 16.

Seely D, Kennedy DA, Myers SP, Cheras PA, Lin D, Li R, Cattley T, Brent PA, Mills E, Leonard BJ. In vitro analysis of the herbal compound Essiac. *Anticancer Res.* 2007;27:3875-3882.

Zick SM, Sen A, Feng Y, Green J, Olatunde S, Boon H. Trial of Essiac to ascertain its effect in women with breast cancer (TEA-BC). *J Altern Complement Med.* 2006;12:971-980.

EVENING PRIMROSE

Other common name(s): Evening Primrose Oil
Scientific/medical name(s): *Oenothera biennis*

Description

Evening primrose is a flowering plant originally native to North America that now grows throughout much of Europe and parts of Asia. It blooms every other year, and its large, fragrant yellow flowers open at dusk and remain open through the night. In Germany, the plant is called "night candle" for this reason. The oil extracted from the ripe seeds and the fresh plant are used in herbal remedies.

Overview

Available scientific evidence does not support evening primrose oil as an effective treatment for preventing or treating cancer. Some studies suggest it may help with certain types of skin rashes, such as eczema and atopic dermatitis, although further research is needed to confirm this. Whereas the essential fatty acids found in evening primrose play a role in health and disease, larger clinical studies are needed to find out whether they are useful in treating cancer or other conditions.

How is it promoted for use?

Evening primrose is promoted as an herbal remedy for a very broad range of conditions, including dermatitis, premenstrual syndrome, menopausal symptoms, eczema, inflammation, hyperactivity in children, high cholesterol, asthmatic cough, upset stomach, psoriasis, rheumatoid arthritis, and diabetic nerve damage. Some proponents also believe the plant has anticancer properties. Some claims of evening primrose's health benefits are based on the fact that the oil extracted from the seeds and plant contains gamma-linolenic acid (GLA), an essential omega-6 fatty acid. GLA is thought to play a key role in many biological processes. Omega-6 fatty acids are different from omega-3 fatty acids (see "Gamma-Linolenic Acid," page 744, and "Omega-3 Fatty Acids," page 659).

What does it involve?

The oil can be purchased in capsules, gelcaps, and a less commonly available liquid form, and the powdered plant can be purchased and made into a tea. Daily doses of evening primrose oil have ranged from two to sixteen capsules of 500 milligrams in clinical trials, although in one study up to thirty-six capsules per day were used.

What is the history behind it?

In folk medicine, evening primrose has been used to treat asthma, gastrointestinal disorders, whooping cough, and symptoms associated with premenstrual syndrome. The scientific name of the plant, *Oenothera biennis*, comes from the two Greek words, *oinos* ("wine") and *thera* ("hunt"), because eating the roots was once believed to increase a person's appetite for wine. Folklore also says that evening primrose counters the effects of drinking too much wine. Use of evening primrose as an herbal remedy is relatively recent. Scientific research regarding its healing properties began in the 1980s.

What is the evidence?

Available scientific evidence does not support claims that evening primrose oil has any effect on cancer. Most research has been conducted in laboratory settings or involved small numbers of patients. One laboratory study concluded that evening primrose oil might help slow the growth of breast cancer cells. Other laboratory studies have found that evening primrose oil slowed the growth of skin cancer cells, and a diet enriched with evening primrose oil was thought to enhance the body's ability to fight tumors. However, further studies are needed to learn whether the results apply to humans.

Research into the use of evening primrose oil for other conditions has been mixed. Some research evidence suggests that it may help symptoms of rheumatoid arthritis over the long term, although more information is needed. Studies that tested evening primrose oil taken by mouth for the skin conditions atopic dermatitis and eczema showed conflicting results. Results of studies of evening primrose oil for treating premenstrual syndrome, menopause symptoms, breast pain, and psoriasis have been either mixed or not favorable. Most research has been conducted in laboratory settings or involved small numbers of patients. In late 2002, the United Kingdom withdrew the prescription forms of fatty acid that were made from evening primrose because of lack of evidence of its effectiveness. A recent review concluded that evening primrose is not effective as a treatment for menopausal symptoms. Large-scale clinical trials involving humans are needed to find out the value of evening primrose in treating any illness.

Are there any possible problems or complications?

No major health hazards have been identified with taking evening primrose. Headaches, bloating, and indigestion are reported as possible side effects. One article reported that the fatty acid in primrose oil (GLA) might lower seizure thresholds, so it should not be used in people who have seizures. It may also increase the seizure risk in those who are taking medicines for schizophrenia.

There are also reports that GLA may slow the blood's ability to clot. Evening primrose oil can cause problems if taken with herbs or medicines that slow blood clotting (such as blood-thinning medications like warfarin). In addition, the potential interactions between oil of evening primrose and other drugs and herbs should be considered. Some of these combinations may be dangerous. Always tell your doctor and pharmacist about any herbs you are taking. Women who are pregnant or breastfeeding should not use this herb. Relying on this type of treatment alone and avoiding or delaying conventional medical care for cancer may have serious health consequences.

This product is sold as a dietary supplement in the United States. Unlike companies that produce drugs (which must provide the FDA with results of detailed testing showing their product is safe and effective before the drug is approved for sale), the companies that make supplements do not have to show

evidence of safety or health benefits to the FDA before selling their products. Supplement products without any reliable scientific evidence of health benefits may still be sold as long as the companies selling them do not claim the supplements can prevent, treat, or cure any specific disease. Some such products may not contain the amount of the herb or substance that is written on the label, and some may include other substances (contaminants). Though the FDA has written new rules to improve the quality of manufacturing processes for dietary supplements and the accurate listing of supplement ingredients, these rules do not take full effect until 2010. The new rules also do not address the safety of supplement ingredients or their effects on health when proper manufacturing techniques are used.

Most such supplements have not been tested to find out if they interact with medicines, foods, or other herbs and supplements. Even though some reports of interactions and harmful effects may be published, full studies of interactions and effects are not often available. Because of these limitations, any information on ill effects and interactions should be considered incomplete.

References

Belch JJ, Ansell D, Madhok R, O'Dowd A, Sturrock RD. Effects of altering dietary essential fatty acids on requirements for non-steroidal anti-inflammatory drugs in patients with rheumatoid arthritis: a double blind placebo controlled study. *Ann Rheum Dis.* 1988;47:96-104.

Bown D. *Encyclopedia of Herbs & Their Uses.* New York: DK Publishing Inc; 1995.

Cheema D, Coomarasamy A, El-Toukhy T. Non-hormonal therapy of post-menopausal vasomotor symptoms: a structured evidence-based review. *Arch Gynecol Obstet.* 2007;276:463-469.

Epogam and Efamast (gamolenic acid) withdrawal of marketing authorisations. CMO's Update: a communication to all doctors from the Chief Medical Officer. 2002;34:2. Department of Health Web site. http://www.dh.gov.uk/en/Publicationsandstatistics/Lettersandcirculars/CMOupdate/DH_4003840.

Evening primrose. Drug Digest Web site. http://www.drugdigest.org/DD/DVH/HerbsWho/ 0,3923, 4010|Evening%20Primrose,00.html. Accessed June 4, 2008.

Evening primrose oil. Memorial Sloan-Kettering Cancer Center Web site. http://www.mskcc.org/mskcc/html/69216.cfm. Accessed June 4, 2008.

Fetrow CW, Avila JR. *Professional's Handbook of Complementary & Alternative Medicines.* Philadelphia, PA: Lippincott Williams & Wilkins; 2004.

Goyal A, Mansel RE; Efamast Study Group. A randomized multicenter study of gamolenic acid (Efamast) with and without antioxidant vitamins and minerals in the management of mastalgia. *Breast J.* 2005;11:41-47.

Gruenwald J. *PDR for Herbal Medicines.* 3rd ed. Montvale, NJ: Thomson PDR; 2004.

Kleijnen J. Evening primrose oil. *BMJ.* 1994;309:824-825.

Miller LG. Herbal medicinals: selected clinical considerations focusing on known or potential drug-herb interactions. *Arch Intern Med.* 1998;158:2200-2211.

Muñoz SE, Lopez CB, Valentich MA, Eynard AR. Differential modulation by dietary n-6 or n-9 unsaturated fatty acids on the development of two murine mammary gland tumors having different metastatic capabilities. *Cancer Lett.* 1998;126:149-155.

Muñoz SE, Piegari M, Guzmán CA, Eynard AR. Differential effects of dietary *Oenothera, Zizyphus mistol,* and corn oils, and essential fatty acid deficiency on the progression of a murine mammary gland adenocarcinoma. *Nutrition.* 1999;15:208-212.

FLAXSEED

Other common name(s): flaxseed oil, linseed, lint bells, linum
Scientific/medical name(s): *Linum usitatissimum*

Description

Flax is an annual plant cultivated for its fiber, which is used in making linen. Flaxseed and its oil are used in herbal remedies.

Overview

Flaxseed and its oil have been promoted since the 1950s as dietary nutrients with anticancer properties. Most of the evidence of flaxseed's ability to prevent the growth or spread of cancer has come from a few studies in animals. Only recently has there been some clinical evidence suggesting that flaxseed supplements, along with a diet low in fat, may be useful in men with early-stage prostate cancer. Controlled clinical studies are needed to determine its usefulness in preventing or treating cancer in humans.

How is it promoted for use?

Herbalists promote the use of flaxseed for constipation, abdominal problems, breathing problems, sore throat, eczema, menstrual problems, and arthritis. The oil extracted from flaxseeds is said to lower cholesterol levels, boost the immune system, and prevent cancer. Flaxseed oil is high in alpha-linolenic acid, an omega-3 fatty acid that is thought to have beneficial effects against cancer when consumed.

Recently, attention has also focused on the flaxseed itself, which is a rich source of lignans, compounds that can act as antiestrogens or as weak estrogens. It is thought that lignans may play a role in preventing estrogen-dependent cancers, such as some types of breast cancer. Lignans may also function as antioxidants and, through mechanisms that are not yet fully understood, may slow cell growth. When flaxseeds are consumed, the lignans are activated by bacteria in the intestine.

What does it involve?

Flaxseed is available in flour, meal, and seed form. It may be found in some multigrain breads, cereals, breakfast bars, and muffins. The toasted seeds are sometimes mixed into bread dough or sprinkled over salads, yogurt, or cereal. Flaxseed meal can be used in the same way. Flaxseed oil is available in many health food stores in liquid form and is sometimes mixed into cottage cheese or other foods. The oil is also available in softgel capsules.

What is the history behind it?

Flaxseed was cultivated by the Babylonians in 3000 BC. A German biochemist, Johanna Budwig, first brought attention to flaxseed oil as a treatment in the 1950s through a diet she devised for cancer patients. The diet was a strict regimen that avoided sugar, animal fats, salad oil, meats, butter, and margarine. The patients were given flaxseed oil, mixed with cottage cheese and milk, and meals high in fruits, vegetables, and fiber. She claimed that within three months, some patients on this diet had smaller tumors, some had no tumors left, and all felt better.

What is the evidence?

Most of the evidence for the anticancer effects of flaxseed and flaxseed oil comes from research using laboratory animals or cells grown in laboratory dishes. In one cell culture study, flaxseed lignans reduced stickiness and movement of breast cancer cells, both properties related to the cancer's ability to spread or metastasize. Researchers have also found that a diet supplemented with flaxseed may reduce the formation, growth, or spread of prostate cancer, breast cancer, and melanoma in mice. Flaxseed reduced formation of precancerous colon polyps in one study of rats, but in another study had no effect on the formation of intestinal cancer in mice. In a 2007 report, flaxseed reduced growth of breast cancer cells in mice and enhanced the effectiveness of tamoxifen, a conventional drug for hormonal therapy.

There have been some small studies of the effects of flaxseed in humans. A small study of fifteen men found that a low-fat diet supplemented with flaxseed lowered their blood prostate-specific antigen (PSA) levels and slowed the growth of benign prostate cells, suggesting that it might be useful in reducing risk for prostate cancer. Another study of twenty-five men with prostate cancer found that a low-fat diet along with ground flaxseed reduced serum testosterone, slowed the growth rate of cancer cells, and increased the death rate of cancer cells.

More research in humans is needed to determine the usefulness of flaxseed in cancer treatment and prevention. While animal and laboratory studies show promise, further studies are needed to determine whether the results apply to humans.

Are there any possible problems or complications?

The immature pods of flaxseed are poisonous and should never be used. Flaxseeds and flaxseed oil can spoil if they are not kept refrigerated. They should be protected from light, heat, air, and moisture.

Some possible side effects include diarrhea, gas, and nausea. Flaxseed oil should not be used with other laxatives or stool softeners. People who have inflammatory bowel disease or narrowing of the intestine, esophagus, or stomach should avoid flaxseed. Flaxseed is also not recommended by some doctors for people with diabetes.

Some medicines and supplements may not be absorbed properly if they are taken at the same time as flaxseed. For this reason, some doctors recommend taking medications one or two hours before or after taking flaxseed.

Flaxseed may also interfere with x-rays taken after a barium enema, and some doctors recommend avoiding taking flaxseed before undergoing this test. In addition, the potential interactions between flaxseed and other drugs and herbs should be considered. Some of these combinations may be dangerous. Always tell your doctor and pharmacist about any herbs you are taking.

A few severe allergic reactions to flaxseed have been reported. Those allergic to other plants may be more likely to be allergic to flax. Relying on this type of treatment alone and avoiding or delaying conventional medical care for cancer may have serious health consequences.

This product is sold as a dietary supplement in the United States. Unlike companies that produce drugs (which must provide the FDA with results of detailed testing showing their product is safe and effective before the drug is approved for sale), the companies that make supplements do not have to show evidence of safety or health benefits to the FDA before selling their products. Supplement products without any reliable scientific evidence of health benefits may still be sold as long as the companies selling them do not claim the supplements can prevent, treat, or cure any specific disease. Some such products may not contain the amount of the herb or substance that is written on the label, and some may include other substances (contaminants). Though the FDA has written new rules to improve the quality of manufacturing processes for dietary supplements and the accurate listing of supplement ingredients, these rules do not take full effect until 2010. The new rules also do not address the safety of supplement ingredients or their effects on health when proper manufacturing techniques are used.

Most such supplements have not been tested to find out if they interact with medicines, foods, or other herbs and supplements. Even though some reports of interactions and harmful effects may be published,

full studies of interactions and effects are not often available. Because of these limitations, any information on ill effects and interactions should be considered incomplete.

References

Basch E, Bent S, Collins J, Dacey C, Hammerness P, Harrison M, Smith M, Szapary P, Ulbricht C, Vora M, Weissner W; Natural Standard Resource Collaboration. Flax and flaxseed oil (Linum usitatissimum): a review by the Natural Standard Research Collaboration. *J Soc Integr Oncol.* 2007;5:92-105.

Bergman Jungeström M, Thompson LU, Dabrosin C. Flaxseed and its lignans inhibit estradiol-induced growth, angiogenesis, and secretion of vascular endothelial growth factor in human breast cancer xenografts in vivo. *Clin Cancer Res.* 2007;13:1061-1067.

Chen J, Hui E, Ip T, Thompson LU. Dietary flaxseed enhances the inhibitory effect of tamoxifen on the growth of estrogen-dependent human breast cancer (MCF-7) in nude mice. *Clin Cancer Res.* 2004;10:7703-7711.

Chen J, Power KA, Mann J, Cheng A, Thompson LU. Flaxseed alone or in combination with tamoxifen inhibits MCF-7 breast tumor growth in ovariectomized athymic mice with high circulating levels of estrogen. *Exp Biol Med.* 2007;232:1071-1080.

Chen J, Stavro PM, Thompson LU. Dietary flaxseed inhibits human breast cancer growth and metastasis and downregulates expression of insulin-like growth factor and epidermal growth factor receptor. *Nutr Cancer.* 2002;43:187-192.

Chen J, Wang L, Thompson LU. Flaxseed and its components reduce metastasis after surgical excision of solid human breast tumor in nude mice. *Cancer Lett.* 2006;234:168-175.

Demark-Wahnefried W, Price DT, Polascik TJ, Robertson CN, Anderson EE, Paulson DF, Walther PJ, Gannon M, Vollmer RT. Pilot study of dietary fat restriction and flaxseed supplementation in men with prostate cancer before surgery: exploring the effects on hormonal levels, prostate-specific antigen, and histopathologic features. *Urology.* 2001;58:47-52.

Demark-Wahnefried W, Robertson CN, Walther PJ, Polascik TJ, Paulson DF, Vollmer RT. Pilot study to explore effects of low-fat, flaxseed-supplemented diet on proliferation of benign prostatic epithelium and prostate-specific antigen. *Urology.* 2004;63:900-904.

Flaxseed. Memorial Sloan-Kettering Cancer Center Web site. http://www.mskcc.org/mskcc/html/69220.cfm. Accessed June 4, 2008.

Haggans CJ, Hutchins AM, Olson BA, Thomas W, Martini MC, Slavin JL. Effect of flaxseed consumption on urinary estrogen metabolites in postmenopausal women. *Nutr Cancer.* 1999;33:188-195.

Lin X, Gingrich JR, Bao W, Li J, Haroon ZA, Demark-Wahnefried W. Effect of flaxseed supplementation on prostatic carcinoma in transgenic mice. *Urology.* 2002;60:919-924.

Natural Standard. Herbal/plant therapies: flaxseed and flaxseed oil (*Linum usitatissimum*). Complementary/Integrative Medicine Education Resources, The University of Texas M. D. Anderson Cancer Center Web site. http://www.mdanderson.org/departments/cimer/display.cfm?id=0D86E843-44DF-4766-9D743BA1FE8B9877&method=displayFull. Accessed June 4, 2008.

Yan L, Yee JA, Li D, McGuire MH, Thompson LU. Dietary flaxseed supplementation and experimental metastasis of melanoma cells in mice. *Cancer Lett.* 1998;124:181-186.

FLOWER REMEDIES

Other common name(s): Bach remedies, Bach flower remedies
Scientific/medical name(s): none

Description

Flower remedies are prepared by picking certain plants or flowers in full bloom and leaving them in water for two to four hours in the sun. Alternately, the plants may be picked and boiled for half an hour. The liquid is then preserved with brandy and further diluted so that very small amounts of the original plant solution remain in the final formula. Thirty-eight different flowers are used to make the original thirty-nine remedies.

Overview

Available scientific evidence does not support claims that flower remedies are effective in treating cancer or any other disease. Many people report that flower remedies are helpful for stabilizing emotions. However, available scientific studies have shown no health benefits when compared with placebo treatments.

How is it promoted for use?

Proponents claim that flower remedies ease stress and reduce negative emotions, which in turn stimulates the body's healing processes to help fight illness. Proponents believe that physical illness is caused by underlying emotional problems or disorders. They do not claim that flower remedies cure diseases, only that they help the body's natural defenses so that the body can heal itself. Supporters suggest that flower remedies can help improve sleep, reduce stress, calm fears, ease childbirth, reduce anxiety, and lessen skeletal and muscular pain.

There are seven categories of emotional problems that supporters believe can be affected by flower remedies. These include fear, uncertainty, general disinterest, loneliness, oversensitivity to influences and ideas, despondency or despair, and overconcern for the welfare of others. Flower remedies are said to be safe for everyone, even family pets.

What does it involve?

Usually, two to four drops of flower essence preparation are placed directly under the tongue several times a day. A few drops can also be put into a glass of water or juice and sipped three to four times a day. Very small or even undetectable amounts of the flower extract remain in the final remedy formula. The patient or practitioner chooses the flower essences based on the patient's emotional condition.

The original thirty-nine remedies consisted of thirty-eight individual flower essences and a solution called "rescue remedy," which is a combination of five flower essences. Rescue remedy can be used to deal with emotional trauma or emergency situations. This remedy comes in a spray bottle so it can be sprayed into the mouth and in a cream that can be used on the wrists, neck, or ankles.

What is the history behind it?

In the 1930s, an English homeopathic physician named Edward Bach developed the theory that the successful treatment of negative emotions would heal illness. His ideas in this area were shared by others who believed in the connection between mind and body and that emotional health influenced physical health. Bach believed flowers were one key to strengthening the mind-body link and that flower essences could soothe emotions.

Since Bach's time, more flowers have been added to the original thirty-eight, reportedly following the same general principles he outlined.

What is the evidence?

Despite numerous personal reports claiming flower remedies improve health, available scientific evidence does not support claims that the treatment results in any measurable positive results beyond that of placebo treatment. Some specific studies have tested for the effect of flower remedies on attention deficit disorder and anxiety. A 2005 study in Israel tested the remedies to see whether they helped attention deficit disorder in children. It found that there was no difference between the effects of the remedies compared with placebo. In Germany, a group of researchers compared the flower remedies to a placebo to see whether the remedies helped test anxiety. While there was no difference between the placebo and flower essence groups, both groups reported a significant decrease in test anxiety. It appears that both the sham treatment and the flower essences produced a placebo effect.

Are there any possible problems or complications?

There are no known harmful effects reported with the ingestion of flower remedies. People taking medications such as metronidazole (Flagyl) or disulfiram (Antabuse) may have nausea and vomiting if they use a brandy- or alcohol-based form of the remedies. Those who wish to avoid alcohol entirely should not use flower remedies. Allergies to the plants might produce reactions if enough of the flower extract is present in the remedy, although no reports of this have been found in the medical literature to date. Relying on this type of treatment alone and avoiding or delaying conventional medical care for cancer may have serious health consequences.

This product is sold as a dietary supplement in the United States. Unlike companies that produce drugs (which must provide the FDA with results of detailed testing showing their product is safe and effective before the drug is approved for sale), the companies that make supplements do not have to show evidence of safety or health benefits to the FDA before selling their products. Supplement products without any reliable scientific evidence of health benefits may still be sold as long as the companies selling them do not claim the supplements can prevent, treat, or cure any specific disease. Some such products may not contain the amount of the herb or substance that is written on the label, and some may include other substances (contaminants). Though the FDA has written new rules to improve the quality of manufacturing processes for dietary supplements and the accurate listing of supplement ingredients, these rules do not take full effect until 2010. The new rules also do not address the safety of supplement ingredients or their effects on health when proper manufacturing techniques are used.

Most such supplements have not been tested to find out if they interact with medicines, foods, or other herbs and supplements. Even though some reports of interactions and harmful effects may be published, full studies of interactions and effects are not often available. Because of these limitations, any information on ill effects and interactions should be considered incomplete.

References

Bach flower remedies. Aetna InteliHealth Web site. http://www.intelihealth.com/IH/ihtIH?d=dmtContent&c=358740. Accessed June 4, 2008.

Barrett S. Questionable "self-help" products. Quackwatch Web site. http://www.quackwatch.org/01QuackeryRelatedTopics/mentprod.html. Updated August 18, 2004. Accessed June 4, 2008.

Ernst E. "Flower remedies": a systematic review of the clinical evidence. *Wien Klin Wochenschr.* 2002;114:963-966.

Kaptchuk TJ. The placebo effect in alternative medicine: can the performance of a healing ritual have clinical significance? *Ann Intern Med.* 2002;136:817-825.

Pintov S, Hochman M, Livne A, Heyman E, Lahat E. Bach flower remedies used for attention deficit hyperactivity disorder in children—a prospective double blind controlled study. *Eur J Paediatr Neurol.* 2005;9:395-398. Epub 2005 Oct 27.

Walach H, Rilling C, Engelke U. Efficacy of Bach-flower remedies in test anxiety: a double-blind, placebo-controlled, randomized trial with partial crossover. *J Anxiety Disord.* 2001;15:359-366.

FOLIC ACID

Other common name(s): folate, folacin, vitamin B9
Scientific/medical name(s): pteroylglutamic acid

Description

Folic acid, or folate, is a B vitamin found in many vegetables, beans, fruits, and whole grains and in fortified breakfast cereals. It helps the body build and maintain DNA and is important in helping the body make new cells, especially red blood cells.

Overview

Low levels of folic acid in the blood have been linked with higher rates of colorectal cancer and some other types of cancer, as well as with certain birth defects. It is not clear whether consuming high amounts of folic acid—from the diet or through supplements—can lower cancer risk in average people or how much folic acid might be needed to be helpful. These issues are being studied. High doses of folic acid can interfere with the effectiveness of some chemotherapy drugs, such as methotrexate.

How is it promoted for use?

Folic acid, or folate, is a B vitamin. It is promoted mainly as part of a healthy diet to reduce the risk for neural tube birth defects such as spina bifida and anencephaly, some types of cancer, and heart disease. It has also been studied for use in Alzheimer's disease and chronic fatigue syndrome. While evidence of its ability to reduce neural tube defects in infants when taken by the mother before and during pregnancy is fairly strong, its effects against other conditions are still under study.

What does it involve?

The terms "folate" and "folic acid" are often used interchangeably, although they are slightly different. Folate is a naturally occurring vitamin found in dark leafy green vegetables, citrus fruits, liver, and in smaller amounts in many other foods (broccoli, beans, peas, eggs, etc.). Folic acid is a manmade form of this vitamin and is actually easier for the body to absorb and use. Folic acid is found in fortified grain-based cereals and breads, and supplements are available in tablet and powder form in drug stores and health food stores. Most multivitamins contain folic acid.

In the United States, the current Dietary Reference Intake (DRI) of folic acid is 400 micrograms per day for adolescents and adults, 500 micrograms per day for women who are breastfeeding, and 600 micrograms per day for pregnant women.

What is the history behind it?

Folic acid was first identified in the 1930s as a substance that helped prevent anemia (low red blood cell levels) during pregnancy. It is named after the Latin word for leaf (*folium*), because it was first isolated from spinach and other green leafy vegetables.

The first studies that looked at the connection between folic acid and cancer took place in the 1960s and 1970s. After noting that cells from the cervix in folate-deficient women looked similar to cervix cells showing early signs of cancer, researchers began to suspect a link between the two. By the 1990s, observational studies found that certain types of cancer, such as cervical and colorectal cancer, were more likely to develop in people with lower blood levels of folic acid.

The importance of folic acid in preventing neural tube birth defects led the U.S. Food and Drug Administration (FDA) to require that grain-based foods, cereals, and dietary supplements be enriched with folate starting in 1998. Neural tube defects are a type of birth defect in which the brain, spinal cord, or their protective coverings do not fully develop. These defects occur early in fetal development. Spina bifida is one of the more common types of neural tube defects.

What is the evidence?

How folic acid might affect cancer risk is not exactly clear. Cells need folic acid to make and repair DNA when they divide to create new cells, and it may be involved in how cells turn certain genes on and off. Scientists believe low levels of folic acid can lead to changes in the chemicals that affect DNA, which may alter how well cells can repair themselves or divide without making mistakes. These changes might in turn lead to cancer.

Some observational epidemiologic studies have found a link between lower intake of folic acid and higher risk for certain types of cancer. But these studies were done at different times and looked at different populations around the world, which can make it difficult to compare findings and draw conclusions. The United States has enriched grain products with folate since 1998. Therefore, it is likely that far fewer Americans are now folic acid–deficient than was the case in the past (or is the case now in other countries). Therefore, it is difficult to know how the results from previous studies might apply to people today, as the current baseline folic acid levels here are likely higher.

Several observational epidemiologic studies have found that folic acid may be linked to a lower risk for colon cancer. A large study that tracked nurses in the United States from 1980 to 1994 reported that the women with a high intake of folic acid were much less likely to get colon cancer than those with a lower intake. An even larger study involving both men and women found a weaker link overall but noted that folic acid was more likely to be helpful in those who had two or more alcoholic drinks a day.

Studies of folic acid and breast cancer have had mixed results. The large study of nurses mentioned above found that folic acid intake did not affect breast cancer risk overall, but women who had one or more alcoholic drinks a day and took in enough folic acid had lower breast cancer risk than those who did not. A 2003 study of more than sixty-six thousand older women showed that women who drank more alcohol were more likely to have breast cancer. In this study, however, the drinkers with higher folic acid intakes did not have less breast cancer.

Some observational epidemiologic studies have found folic acid is linked to lower rates of ovarian cancer in women who have at least one drink a day, but research in this area is not conclusive. Some research has also suggested that folic acid may be linked to lower risk for cancers of the pancreas, esophagus, and stomach. Further research is needed to clarify these findings.

Whether folic acid works against cancer may also depend on when it is taken. Some researchers think that folic acid may not be helpful, and could even be harmful, in people who already have cancer or precancerous conditions. For example, two randomized, controlled trials found that folic acid supplements had no effect on existing precancerous conditions of the cervix.

Overall, the evidence that folic acid can help prevent cancer is promising but not conclusive. Further research involving randomized, controlled clinical trials is needed to determine what effect folic acid may have on the development of cancer.

At this time, it is hard to say how each nutrient or nutrient combination affects a person's risk for cancer. On the other hand, studies of large groups of people have shown that those whose diets are high in vegetables and low in animal fat, meat, and/or calories have lower risks for some of the most common types of cancer. Until more is known about this relationship, the American Cancer Society recommends eating a variety of healthful foods—with most of them coming from plant sources—rather than relying on supplements. Supplements may be helpful for some people, such as pregnant women, women of childbearing age, and people with restricted food intakes. If a supplement is taken, the best choice for most people is a balanced multivitamin/mineral supplement that contains no more than 100 percent of the "Daily Value" of most nutrients.

Are there any possible problems or complications?

Folic acid is considered a safe and necessary dietary nutrient. Because it is a water-soluble vitamin, most excess folic acid is excreted in the urine. However, if taken in extremely large doses, it may cause symptoms such as upset stomach or trouble sleeping. Folic acid can also mask symptoms of vitamin B12 deficiency by correcting the anemia caused by low vitamin B12 levels. However, vitamin B12 deficiency can cause nervous system damage, which folic acid cannot correct. In fact, high doses of folic acid can worsen the nervous system damage, and continued B12 deficiency can allow the damage to become permanent. High doses of folic acid may also interfere with the effectiveness of the chemotherapy drug methotrexate and similar drugs. Always tell your doctor and pharmacist about any supplements and herbs you are taking. Relying on the use of supplements alone and avoiding or delaying conventional medical care for cancer may have serious health consequences.

This product is sold as a dietary supplement in the United States. Unlike companies that produce drugs (which must provide the FDA with results of detailed testing showing their product is safe and effective before the drug is approved for sale), the companies that make supplements do not have to show evidence of safety or health benefits to the FDA before selling their products. Supplement products without any reliable scientific evidence of health benefits may still be sold as long as the companies selling them do not claim the supplements can prevent, treat, or cure any specific disease. Some such products may not contain the amount of the herb or substance that is written on the label, and some may include other substances (contaminants). Though the FDA has written new rules to improve the quality of manufacturing processes for dietary supplements and the accurate listing of supplement ingredients, these rules do not take full effect until 2010. The new rules also do not address the safety of supplement ingredients or their effects on health when proper manufacturing techniques are used.

Most such supplements have not been tested to find out if they interact with medicines, foods, or other herbs and supplements. Even though some reports of interactions and harmful effects may be published, full studies of interactions and effects are not often available. Because of these limitations, any information on ill effects and interactions should be considered incomplete.

References

Dietary supplement fact sheet: folate. Office of Dietary Supplements Web site. http://ods.od.nih.gov/factsheets/folate.asp#h8. Acccssed June 4, 2008.

Feigelson HS, Jonas CR, Robertson AS, McCullough ML, Thun MJ, Calle EE. Alcohol, folate, methionine, and risk of incident breast cancer in the American Cancer Society Cancer Prevention Study II Nutrition Cohort. *Cancer Epidemiol Biomarkers Prev.* 2003;12:161-164.

Folic acid—easy to read. The National Women's Health Information Center Web site. http://www.womenshealth.gov/faq/Easyread/folic-etr.htm. Accessed June 20, 2008.

Folic acid. PDRhealth Web site. http://www.pdrhealth.com/drug_info/nmdrugprofiles/nutsupdrugs/fol_0110.shtml. Accessed June 4, 2008.

Giovannucci E, Stampfer MJ, Colditz GA, Hunter DJ, Fuchs C, Rosner BA, Speizer FE, Willett WC. Multivitamin use, folate, and colon cancer in women in the Nurses' Health Study. *Ann Intern Med.* 1998;129:517-524.

Jacobs EJ, Connell CJ, Patel AV, Chao A, Rodriguez C, Seymour J, McCullough ML, Calle EE, Thun MJ. Multivitamin use and colon cancer mortality in the Cancer Prevention Study II cohort (United States). *Cancer Causes Control.* 2001;12:927-934.

Kushi LH, Byers T, Doyle C, Bandera EV, McCullough M, McTiernan A, Gansler T, Andrews KS, Thun MJ; American Cancer Society 2006 Nutrition and Physical Activity Guidelines Advisory Committee. American Cancer Society guidelines on nutrition and physical activity for cancer prevention: reducing the risk of cancer with healthy food choices and physical activity. *CA Cancer J Clin.* 2006;56:254-281.

Larsson SC, Giovannucci E, Wolk A. Dietary folate intake and incidence of ovarian cancer: the Swedish Mammography Cohort. *J Natl Cancer Inst.* 2004;96:396-402.

Mason JB, Levesque T. Folate: effects on carcinogenesis and the potential for cancer chemoprevention. *Oncology (Williston Park).* 1996;10:1727-1744.

MRC Vitamin Study Research Group. Prevention of neural tube defects: results of the Medical Research Council Vitamin Study. *Lancet.* 1991;338:131-137.

Zhang S, Hunter DJ, Hankinson SE, Giovannucci EL, Rosner BA, Colditz GA, Speizer FE, Willett WC. A prospective study of folate intake and the risk of breast cancer. *JAMA.* 1999;281:1632-1637.

GERMANIUM

Other common name(s): germanium sesquioxide, germanium 132, organic germanium, vitamin O; other forms of organic and inorganic germanium

Scientific/medical name(s): bis-carboxyethyl germanium sesquioxide, Ge-132

Description

Germanium is a mineral. Small amounts of organic germanium are found in some plant-based foods. Inorganic germanium is mined and widely used as a semiconductor in the electronics industry. Both organic and inorganic germanium have been sold as dietary supplements, though the organic forms are more commonly used today. Ge-132 is a synthetic form of organic germanium.

Overview

Available scientific evidence does not support claims that germanium supplements are effective in preventing or treating cancer in humans, and there are numerous reports showing that they may be harmful. A study conducted by the U.S. Food and Drug Administration (FDA) reported that supplements containing germanium present a potential hazard to humans. As a result, the FDA has banned its import as a food supplement. However, the amount of germanium naturally found in foods does not appear to be toxic.

How is it promoted for use?

Proponents claim germanium can be used to treat leukemia and cancers of the lung, bladder, larynx, breast, and uterus. They also claim it can help neurosis, asthma, diabetes, hypertension, cardiac insufficiency, Parkinson's disease, neuralgia, chronic fatigue, hepatitis, and cirrhosis of the liver. Supporters say germanium stimulates the body's production of interferon, a naturally occurring anticancer agent, and helps the immune system by boosting the activity of natural killer cells, a type of white blood cell that attacks invading germs.

What does it involve?

Germanium supplements are available in powdered form and in capsules ranging from 35 to 500 milligrams. There is no standardized dose. These supplements are available in health food stores and over the Internet.

What is the history behind it?

The late Dr. Kazuhiko Asai of Japan began investigating the biological properties of germanium after reading reports from Russia that said the mineral had tremendous therapeutic value. In 1969, Dr. Asai founded the Asai Germanium Research Institute. He reported that he had developed a way to produce germanium that was chemically identical to the germanium extracted from plants. Dr. Asai also found that germanium was present in many common herbal remedies, including ginseng, garlic, comfrey, and aloe.

Dr. Otto Warburg, a Nobel Prize winning biochemist, stated that germanium helped to increase the delivery of oxygen to cells. He believed that boosting the oxygen supply to healthy cells slowed the growth of tumors.

What is the evidence?

Available scientific evidence does not support claims that germanium supplements promote health or increase the body's production of interferon. It also does not support the claim that germanium is an essential nutrient in animals or humans.

A study conducted by the FDA found at least thirty-one cases of kidney failure linked to germanium products. Nine deaths have also been reported. Most of these effects were from inorganic forms of germanium, but the FDA has also found severe kidney damage in people taking organic germanium.

Because of the way it is processed, organic germanium is easily contaminated with inorganic germanium, which appears to be more toxic than the organic form. It is uncertain whether the kidney damage and other toxic effects reported in people who took organic germanium were actually caused by the supplement's contamination with inorganic germanium. Because of this problem with purity, products containing germanium of any sort can pose a hazard to humans.

In the early 1980s, small studies were done using germanium on people with various types of cancer. In the first study, even those who received the lowest doses had toxic effects, and none of the patients got better. Later, a group of twenty-five patients were given spirogermanium (a form of organic germanium) three times a week for two weeks. Most patients got worse, and toxic side effects were common. Because of these results—many toxic effects and little effect on the cancer—studies on spirogermanium were stopped.

Are there any possible problems or complications?

Germanium supplements may pose a danger for humans. Scientists warn that inorganic germanium may cause permanent kidney failure, and even supplements labeled as organic may be contaminated with inorganic germanium. At least nine deaths have been reported. While organic germanium appears to have less toxicity than inorganic germanium, it has caused kidney damage and liver changes. Other reported effects include anemia, poor appetite, weight loss, nausea, vomiting, tiredness, muscle weakness, skin rashes, and numbness in the hands and feet due to nerve damage. The toxic effects build up over time and get worse the longer this mineral is taken.

Germanium may interfere with certain other medicines and may make seizures worse. Drugs that can cause kidney problems may be more likely to cause harm if taken with germanium. Very little testing during pregnancy has been reported, but at least one form of germanium caused ill effects on fetuses in animal tests. Women who are pregnant or breastfeeding should not take germanium. Germanium is not recommended for anyone because of its potential for serious health hazards. Relying on this type of treatment alone and avoiding or delaying conventional medical care for cancer may have serious health consequences.

This product is sold as a dietary supplement in the United States. Unlike companies that produce drugs (which must provide the FDA with results of detailed testing showing their product is safe and effective before the drug is approved for sale), the companies that make supplements do not have to show evidence of safety or health benefits to the FDA before selling their products. Supplement products without any reliable scientific evidence of health benefits may still be sold as long as the companies selling them do not claim the supplements can prevent, treat, or cure any specific disease. Some such products may not contain the amount of the herb or substance that is written on the label, and some may include other substances (contaminants). Though the FDA has written new rules to improve the quality of manufacturing processes for dietary supplements and the accurate listing of supplement ingredients, these rules do not take full effect until 2010. The new rules also do not address the safety of supplement ingredients or their effects on health when proper manufacturing techniques are used.

Most such supplements have not been tested to find out if they interact with medicines, foods, or other herbs and supplements. Even though some reports of interactions and harmful effects may be published, full studies of interactions and effects are not often available. Because of these limitations, any information on ill effects and interactions should be considered incomplete.

References

Expert Group on Vitamins and Minerals 2003. Risk assessment: germanium. Food Standards Agency Web site. http://www.food.gov.uk/multimedia/pdfs/evm_germanium.pdf. Accessed June 4, 2008.

Gerber GB, Leonard A. Mutagenicity, carcinogenicity and teratogenicity of germanium compounds. *Mutat Res.* 1997;387:141-146.

Germanium. Memorial Sloan-Kettering Cancer Center Web site. http://www.mskcc.org/mskcc/html/69232.cfm. Accessed June 4, 2008.

Germanium. National Products Association Web site. http://www.naturalproductsassoc.org/site/PageServer?pagename=rr_bg_germanium. Accessed June 4, 2008.

Germanium. PDRhealth Web site. http://www.pdrhealth.com/drug_info/nmdrugprofiles/nutsupdrugs/ger_0119.shtml. Accessed June 4, 2008.

Memorandum in response to new dietary ingredient notification, November 13, 2002. US Food and Drug Administration Web site. http://www.fda.gov/ohrms/DOCKETS/dockets/95s0316/95s-0316-rpt0155-01-vol113.pdf. Accessed June 4, 2008.

Tao SH, Bolger PM. Hazard assessment of germanium supplements. *Regul Toxicol Pharmacol.* 1997;25:211-219.

GINGER

Other common name(s): ginger root
Scientific/medical name(s): *Zingiber officinale*

Description

Ginger is a plant native to Southeast Asia that is also grown in the United States, China, India, and various tropical regions. The root is usually the part of the plant used in herbal remedies.

Overview

Ginger has a long history as an herbal remedy for upset stomach, motion sickness, and loss of appetite, as well as being used as a pungent spice for cooking. Some controlled studies in humans show ginger reduces nausea and vomiting from some causes. Most clinical studies of ginger have tested the use of this herb for nausea associated with pregnancy or following surgery. Very little is known about its effectiveness in relieving nausea and vomiting from chemotherapy.

There are a number of conventional medicines for nausea and vomiting associated with chemotherapy. Available scientific evidence does not support claims that ginger can add to the effectiveness of these medicines. However, some people with cancer find that the taste or aroma of beverages and foods containing ginger helps soothe their nausea.

Ginger may interfere with blood clotting and should be used by cancer patients only after talking about it with their doctors. This concern applies mostly to people whose clotting function is already weakened by their cancer or its treatment or to people having surgery.

How is it promoted for use?

Ginger has been used to control or prevent nausea, vomiting, and motion sickness; as an anti-inflammatory (a drug that reduces pain and swelling); a cold remedy; an aid to digestion; a remedy for intestinal gas; and to help relieve nausea in cancer patients who are having chemotherapy. Some proponents have also claimed ginger is able to keep tumors from developing, even though available scientific evidence does not support this claim.

What does it involve?

Ginger has been approved by Commission E (Germany's regulatory agency for herbs) for indigestion and the prevention of motion sickness. Ginger is available as a dried or fresh root, as a tea, in powder form, as a liquid extract, as a tincture, in tablets, in capsules, and in candied form. Many parents give their children ginger ale to settle an upset stomach, but the soft drink often does not contain much ginger, and some ales have artificial flavoring in them instead of ginger.

Fresh or dried ginger root is used in cooking and in preparing herbal remedies. A broad range of daily doses of ginger is reported, from 250 milligrams to 1 gram. For the treatment of nausea, the usual dose is 250 milligrams to 1 gram of powdered ginger taken with a liquid several times per day.

What is the history behind it?

The root of the ginger plant has been used in cooking and as an herbal remedy since ancient times. The ancient Greeks ate ginger wrapped in bread to prevent nausea from a huge feast. For many centuries, Chinese sailors have taken ginger to avoid sea sickness. A proverb from ancient India maintains that everything good can be found in ginger. Its traditional role in herbal medicine has been as a remedy for nausea, motion sickness, heartburn, vomiting, stomach cramps, and loss of appetite.

What is the evidence?

According to some, but not all, controlled studies in humans, ginger reduces nausea. Most studies also show that ginger reduces motion sickness and severe vomiting in early pregnancy. Although some clinicians warn that using ginger during pregnancy or breastfeeding in amounts beyond that eaten in foods might cause harmful effects, there is no objective evidence of harm to the mother, fetus, or infant.

Studies of ginger's ability to reduce nausea and vomiting associated with surgery have had mixed results. At least three studies found ginger had no effect on nausea and vomiting after surgery, while other studies have found a significant decrease in nausea and vomiting when ginger was given before the operation. These inconsistencies may be due to the difficulty in measuring symptoms of nausea.

The chemotherapy drug cisplatin can cause nausea, vomiting, and delayed emptying of the stomach. Indian researchers found that extracts from ginger helped to speed up stomach emptying in dogs and rats that were given cisplatin chemotherapy. However, extracted chemicals or substances are different from the raw plant. Thus, study results of extracts will not necessarily have the same result as studies using the raw plant. In a clinical trial of patients receiving cisplatin, addition of ginger to standard drugs for nausea did not reduce this symptom.

While ginger may be effective in treating nausea and vomiting associated with some cancer treatments, it may also interfere with blood clotting. This side effect could be life threatening to some patients receiving chemotherapy.

Recent preliminary results in animals show some effect in slowing or preventing tumor growth. While these results are not well understood, they warrant further investigation. However, it is too early in the research process to say whether ginger will have the same effect in humans.

Are there any possible problems or complications?

People who have cancer should talk to their doctor before taking ginger, because it has the potential to interfere with blood clotting and prolong bleeding time. There is some disagreement in published studies about the likelihood of this side effect. The risk for serious bleeding may be higher if the person is taking blood-thinning medications such as warfarin (Coumadin) or a medicine that can lower his or her level of platelets (blood cells that help the blood to clot) or interfere with platelet function. In rare cases, some people have experienced an allergic reaction to ginger. Ginger has also been reported to cause occasional rashes, heartburn, and mild stomach upset. Relying on this type of treatment alone and avoiding or delaying conventional medical care for cancer may have serious health consequences.

This product is sold as a dietary supplement in the United States. Unlike companies that produce drugs (which must provide the FDA with results of detailed testing showing their product is safe and effective before the drug is approved for sale), the companies that make supplements do not have to show evidence of safety or health benefits to the FDA before selling their products. Supplement products without any reliable scientific evidence of health benefits may still be sold as long as the companies selling them do not claim the supplements can prevent, treat, or cure any specific disease. Some such products may not contain the amount of the herb or substance that is written on the label, and some may include other substances (contaminants). Though the FDA has written new rules to improve the quality of manufacturing processes for dietary supplements and the accurate listing of supplement ingredients, these rules do not take full effect until 2010. The new rules also do not address the safety of supplement ingredients or their effects on health when proper manufacturing techniques are used.

Most such supplements have not been tested to find out if they interact with medicines, foods, or other herbs and supplements. Even though some reports of interactions and harmful effects may be published, full studies of interactions and effects are not often available. Because of these limitations, any information on ill effects and interactions should be considered incomplete.

References

Blumenthal M, ed. *The Complete German Commission E Monographs: Therapeutic Guide to Herbal Medicines.* Austin, TX: American Botanical Council; 1998.

Borrelli F, Capasso R, Aviello G, Pittler MH, Izzo AA. Effectiveness and safety of ginger in the treatment of pregnancy-induced nausea and vomiting. *Obstet Gynecol.* 2005;105:849-856.

Ginger. Memorial Sloan-Kettering Cancer Center Web site. http://www.mskcc.org/mskcc/html/69234.cfm. Accessed June 4, 2008.

Gruenwald J. *PDR for Herbal Medicines.* 3rd ed. Montvale, NJ: Thomson PDR; 2004.

Janssen PL, Meyboom S, van Staveren WA, de Vegt F, Katan MB. Consumption of ginger (Zingiber officinale roscoe) does not affect ex vivo platelet thromboxane production in humans. *Eur J Clin Nutr.* 1996;50:772-774.

Lumb AB. Effect of dried ginger on human platelet function. *Thromb Haemost.* 1994;71:110-111.

Manusirivithaya S, Sripramote M, Tangjitgamol S, Sheanakul C, Leelahakorn S, Thavaramara T, Tangcharoenpanich K. Antiemetic effect of ginger in gynecologic oncology patients receiving cisplatin. *Int J Gynecol Cancer.* 2004;14:1063-1069.

Miller LG. Herbal medicinals: selected clinical considerations focusing on known or potential drug-herb interactions. *Arch Intern Med.* 1998;158:2200-2211.

Natural Standard. Herbal/plant therapies: ginger (*Zingiber officinale* Roscoe). Complementary/Integrative Medicine Education Resources, The University of Texas M. D. Anderson Cancer Center Web site. http://www.

mdanderson.org/departments/cimer/display.cfm?id=82CB5C51-25BC-4E47-B40D13CCB176AE64&method=displayFull. Accessed June 4, 2008.

O'Hara MA, Kiefer D, Farrell K, Kemper K. A review of 12 commonly used medicinal herbs. *Arch Fam Med.* 1998;7:523-536.

Shalansky S, Lynd L, Richardson K, Ingaszewski A, Kerr C. Risk of warfarin-related bleeding events and supratherapeutic international normalized ratios associated with complementary and alternative medicine: a longitudinal analysis. *Pharmacotherapy.* 2007;27:1237-1247.

Sharma SS, Gupta YK. Reversal of cisplatin-induced delay in gastric emptying in rats by ginger (*Zingiber officinale*). *J Ethnopharmacol.* 1998;62:49-55.

Smith C, Crowther C, Willson K, Hotham N, McMillian V. A randomized controlled trial of ginger to treat nausea and vomiting in pregnancy. *Obstet Gynecol.* 2004;103:639-645.

Tavlan A, Tuncer S, Erol A, Reisli R, Aysolmaz G, Otelcioglu S. Prevention of postoperative nausea and vomiting after thyroidectomy: combined antiemetic treatment with dexamethasone and ginger versus dexamethasone alone. *Clinical Drug Investig.* 2006;26:209-214.

GINKGO

Other common name(s): ginkgo biloba, maidenhair tree, EGb 761
Scientific/medical name(s): *Ginkgo biloba*

Description

Ginkgo is an extract of leaves from the ginkgo tree, one of the world's oldest surviving species of tree, which comes from China, Japan, and Korea. Ginkgo is used as a dietary supplement in the United States for a variety of conditions.

Overview

Ginkgo has shown some benefit in the treatment of mild to moderate dementia. Other studies have shown that it can help improve blood circulation and flow to the brain. Few side effects have been reported, but it has the potential to interfere with blood clotting, anesthesia, and some medications. Available scientific evidence does not support claims that it is effective in preventing or treating cancer in humans.

How is it promoted for use?

Ginkgo is promoted as an aid to memory and concentration. It is believed to stimulate blood circulation and the flow of oxygen to the brain. Widely used in Europe, the extract has also become popular in the United States. Claims include improved memory and vision in the elderly and a slowing of the progression of Alzheimer's disease and dementia.

Ginkgo is sometimes promoted for tinnitus (ringing in the ears), sudden deafness, dizziness, altitude sickness, and intermittent claudication (cramp-like pain in the lower legs caused by poor circulation). In addition, ginkgo has been used as a treatment for a blood vessel disorder known as Raynaud's disease, in which the toes or fingers turn cool and pale when exposed to cold because of insufficient blood supply. European and Asian doctors have also used ginkgo in stroke patients to attempt to limit tissue damage to the brain.

Although ginkgo is not usually promoted as a cancer treatment, herbalists note that it contains some substances that may prove to have activity against cancer, including flavonoids, which are thought to be anti-inflammatory, and proanthocyanidins, which are antioxidants. It also contains a compound called ginkgolide B, which may counteract a body chemical called platelet-activating factor (PAF) that is thought to promote tumor growth.

What does it involve?

Ginkgo leaf extract is on the Commission E (Germany's regulatory agency for herbs) list of approved herbs and can be taken by mouth in pill or liquid form. The average dose of ginkgo extract is 120 to 240 milligrams per day, usually divided into two to three doses. Proponents usually do not recommend the crude, dried leaf preparations because they claim this preparation does not contain enough of the active ingredients.

What is the history behind it?

Chinese herbalists have used the fruit of the ginkgo tree for about four thousand years as a remedy for asthma, coughs, and allergic reactions. Cooked ginkgo seeds are also sometimes eaten after the pulp has been removed from the outside. In the past few decades, an extract of ginkgo leaves has been used in Western medicine, first in Europe and more recently in the United States, because it is supposed to help memory, brain function, and blood circulation.

What is the evidence?

The possible effects of ginkgo leaf extract in preventing or treating cancer have not been well studied. Some small studies done in Asia have suggested that ginkgo extract may affect cancer cells in culture dishes and laboratory animals, but no studies have been done to show it can prevent or treat cancer in humans. A few small studies have looked at adding ginkgo to other treatments in cancer patients, but the results have not been conclusive. More research is needed in this area.

Ginkgo leaf extract appears to improve blood flow to the brain. Some, but not all, studies have found positive results from ginkgo extract on memory. Most randomized, controlled studies have found that ginkgo extract can improve cognitive and social function in patients with mild to moderate dementia resulting from Alzheimer's disease or problems with blood circulation in the brain. Results of its effects on memory and concentration in people without dementia have been mixed.

Some studies have found ginkgo leaf extract may have modest benefits in patients with claudication or sudden hearing loss. A 2004 review of studies concluded that there was not enough evidence to support claims that ginkgo can help tinnitus.

Are there any possible problems or complications?

Ginkgo leaf extract is generally considered safe. Some possible side effects include headache, mild stomach upset, and diarrhea. Because of its potential to block platelet-activating factor, ginkgo is not recommended for people using aspirin, other nonsteroidal anti-inflammatory drugs (such as ibuprofen), or blood-thinning medications such as warfarin (Coumadin). Doctors often advise stopping the use of ginkgo extract several days before surgery. People with seizure disorders should not use ginkgo because it may reduce the effects of seizure medication. Potential interactions between ginkgo and other drugs and herbs should be considered. Some combinations may be dangerous. Always tell your doctor and pharmacist about any herbs you are taking.

Allergic reactions to gingko have been reported, including severe skin reactions with blistering. People who react to poison ivy, mango, cashews, and sumac may be more likely to react to ginkgo.

Uncooked ginkgo fruit or seed can cause more serious problems, including vomiting, seizures, and loss of consciousness. The seed contains a toxin that is reportedly inactivated by cooking. Poisoning from eating the seeds has been reported in adults and children, sometimes resulting in death. The uncooked fruit and seed are also more likely to cause allergic rashes and intestinal irritation than the leaf extract.

This herb has not been studied in women who are pregnant or breastfeeding. Relying on this type of treatment alone and avoiding or delaying conventional medical care for cancer may have serious health consequences.

This product is sold as a dietary supplement in the United States. Unlike companies that produce drugs (which must provide the FDA with results of detailed testing showing their product is safe and effective before the drug is approved for sale), the companies that make supplements do not have to show evidence of safety or health benefits to the FDA before selling their products. Supplement products

without any reliable scientific evidence of health benefits may still be sold as long as the companies selling them do not claim the supplements can prevent, treat, or cure any specific disease. Some such products may not contain the amount of the herb or substance that is written on the label, and some may include other substances (contaminants). Though the FDA has written new rules to improve the quality of manufacturing processes for dietary supplements and the accurate listing of supplement ingredients, these rules do not take full effect until 2010. The new rules also do not address the safety of supplement ingredients or their effects on health when proper manufacturing techniques are used.

Most such supplements have not been tested to find out if they interact with medicines, foods, or other herbs and supplements. Even though some reports of interactions and harmful effects may be published, full studies of interactions and effects are not often available. Because of these limitations, any information on ill effects and interactions should be considered incomplete.

References

Birks J, Grimley EV, Van Dongen M. Ginkgo biloba for cognitive impairment and dementia. *Cochrane Database Syst Rev.* 2002;(4):CD003120.

Blumenthal M, ed. *The Complete German Commission E Monographs: Therapeutic Guide to Herbal Medicines.* Austin, TX: American Botanical Council; 1998.

Ginkgo. Memorial Sloan-Kettering Cancer Center Web site. http://www.mskcc.org/mskcc/html/69235.cfm. Updated February 29, 2008. Accessed June 4, 2008.

Ginkgo. National Center for Complementary and Alternative Medicine Web site. http://nccam.nih.gov/health/ginkgo/. Updated May 27, 2008. Accessed January 6, 2009.

Gruenwald J. *PDR for Herbal Medicines.* 3rd ed. Montvale, NJ: Thomson PDR; 2004.

Hasegawa S, Oda Y, Ichiyama T, Hori Y, Furukawa S. Ginkgo nut intoxication in a 2-year-old male. *Pediatr Neurol.* 2006;35:275-276.

Hilton M, Stuart E. Ginkgo biloba for tinnitus. *Cochrane Database Syst Rev.* 2004;(2):CD003852.

Le Bars PL, Katz MM, Berman N, Itil TM, Freedman AM, Schatzberg AF. A placebo-controlled, double-blind, randomized trial of an extract of Ginkgo biloba for dementia. North American (EGb) Study Group. *JAMA.* 1997;278:1327-1332.

Miwa H, Iijima M, Tanaka S, Mizuno Y. Generalized convulsions after consuming a large amount of gingko nuts. *Epilepsia.* 2001;42:280-281.

Natural Standard. Herbal/plant therapies: ginkgo (*Ginkgo biloba* L.). Complementary/Integrative Medicine Education Resources, The University of Texas M. D. Anderson Cancer Center Web site. http://www.mdanderson.org/departments/cimer/display.cfm?id=6bf16f2a-7c12-4546-8b39271278bdf215&method=displayfull. Accessed June 4, 2008.

Sierpina VS, Wollschlaeger B, Blumenthal M. Ginkgo biloba. *Am Fam Physician.* 2003;68:923-926.

Suzuki R, Kohno H, Sugie S, Sasaki K, Yoshimura T, Wada K, Tanaka T. Preventive effects of extract of leaves of ginkgo (Ginkgo biloba) and its component bilobalide on azoxymethane-induced colonic aberrant crypt foci in rats. *Cancer Lett.* 2004;210:159-169.

Ye B, Aponte M, Dai Y, Li L, Ho MC, Vitonis A, Edwards D, Huang TN, Cramer DW. *Ginkgo biloba* and ovarian cancer prevention: epidemiological and biological evidence. *Cancer Lett.* 2007;251:43-52. Epub 2006 Dec 27.

Zeng X, Liu M, Yang Y, Li Y, Asplund K. Ginkgo biloba for acute ischaemic stroke. *Cochrane Database Syst Rev.* 2005;(4):CD003691.

GINSENG

Other common name(s): Panax ginseng, Asian ginseng, Oriental ginseng, Chinese ginseng, Japanese ginseng, Korean ginseng, American ginseng, man root

Scientific/medical name(s): *Panax ginseng* C. A. Meyer, *Panax quinquefolius*

Description

Asian ginseng (*Panax ginseng*) is a perennial plant grown in China, Korea, Japan, and Russia. American ginseng (*Panax quinquefolius*), a plant with similar properties, is grown mainly in the United States. The dried roots of the plants are used in some traditional medicines to treat a variety of conditions, including cancer. The ginseng plants of the *Panax* group discussed here should not be confused with Siberian ginseng (eleuthero), which has different properties (see page 337).

Overview

Available scientific evidence does not support claims that ginseng is effective in preventing or treating cancer in humans. Studies done in the laboratory suggest some substances in ginseng may have anticancer properties, and some observational epidemiologic studies in Asia link it to lower cancer risk. Clinical trials are still needed to determine whether it is effective in people. Ginseng should be used cautiously, as it can cause undesirable side effects in high doses and may even be dangerous when taken with certain medicines or if the patient is undergoing surgery.

How is it promoted for use?

Ginseng is an ancient herb that is claimed to help the body prevent and fight diseases, including cancer. Promoters claim ginseng enhances athletic performance and provides energy to people who are stressed or fatigued. It is sometimes used during recovery from illness. There are also claims ginseng relieves depression and anxiety, protects the heart, strengthens digestive functions, prevents hardening of the arteries, stabilizes blood pressure and insulin levels, helps with erectile dysfunction, and even delays the effects of aging.

What does it involve?

Ginseng is available as a powder, capsule, or tea or is sometimes sold already mixed with foods. There is no standard dosage; however, Commission E (Germany's regulatory agency for herbs) suggests taking 1 to 2 grams per day of ginseng root for up to three months.

There is some variation in quality and strength among ginseng products. Since it is expensive, some packagers may dilute it or substitute less expensive ingredients to make it affordable to the consumer. Some ginseng products from areas of the world such as Siberia, Alaska, and Brazil are mislabeled. True ginseng has the word *Panax* as part of its Latin, or scientific, name. A 1978 study of fifty-four ginseng products found that one quarter of them contained no ginseng at all, although the content of products may be more reliable today.

What is the history behind it?

The Chinese have been using ginseng for thousands of years as an herbal remedy. Early Chinese books listing curative foods claimed ginseng could enlighten the mind and increase wisdom. The Chinese also used ginseng to treat ailments of the digestive and respiratory systems, nervous disorders, and diabetes; to keep the elderly warm in winter; and to increase energy and improve memory. The life-prolonging effects of ginseng were first described during China's Liang Dynasty (220–589 AD).

North American ginseng was discovered growing in the mountains of Quebec by a Jesuit priest in the early 1700s. It was soon exported to China, where its medicinal value was appreciated. Other variations of ginseng are grown in Korea and Japan. Ginseng was not used in Western medicine until the 1950s, when scientists in the Soviet Union began studying its health benefits and concluded that it was an "adaptogen"—that is, something that helps the body adapt to outside stresses and ward off disease. The Vietcong used it extensively to treat gunshot wounds during the Vietnam War.

In 1978, Taik-Koo Yun, MD, from the Korea Cancer Center Hospital in Seoul, began to conduct observational epidemiologic studies to investigate whether ginseng had anticancer properties. He has published articles arguing that ginseng can prevent most cancers, but he is not certain how this occurs. He has encouraged more worldwide study of this herb.

What is the evidence?

Ginseng has been known for three thousand years, but despite a good deal of research, scientists still are not certain whether the herb can help prevent or treat cancer. Most studies of ginseng have been done in China and Korea, and only recently has it received more research attention in Western countries.

The medicinal effects of ginseng are thought to be due to a group of about two dozen substances in the root called ginsenosides, which resemble steroid hormones. In laboratory research using cell cultures and animals, some ginsenosides have been shown to boost the immune system or slow the growth of cancer cells. Some may also have anti-inflammatory and antioxidant effects. Whether these properties will translate into anticancer activity in humans is still not clear, as few human studies have been done.

Several case-control studies done in Korea have found that people who took ginseng extract seemed to have a lower risk for cancer overall. One recent Chinese study suggested that women with breast cancer who used ginseng before their diagnosis survived longer than those who did not. The same study found that the women who used ginseng during treatment reported better quality of life than those who did not. These studies were not the most scientifically convincing, however, and the authors point out that further research is needed to determine the true benefit of ginseng both in cancer prevention and for people who have cancer. Researchers are looking at ginseng's potential to improve the effectiveness of other cancer treatments, such as chemotherapy, and are studying its effects on cancer-related fatigue.

The benefits of ginseng for other medical conditions have not been shown conclusively, although research is ongoing. Many studies of this herb have suffered from design problems, and results have been contradictory. Some scientists have found that it raises blood pressure while others have reported that it lowers blood pressure. In some studies, ginsenosides seem to act as stimulants, but in others they seem to work as sedatives. The only conclusions that can be reached with any certainty at this time are that ginseng is a complex herb and that its medicinal effects are not clearly defined.

A systematic review of randomized clinical trials evaluated the evidence of ginseng root extract's effectiveness. Based on data from sixteen studies, the researchers concluded that ginseng root extract had not been shown to have a significant effect on physical performance, diabetes, herpes infections, psychomotor performance, cognitive function, or the immune system. More research into its medicinal properties is needed.

Are there any possible problems or complications?

Ginseng is generally considered safe, although there are some possible side effects, especially at higher doses. Side effects may include increased heart rate, nausea, headaches, trouble sleeping, and restlessness. Possible effects in women may include swollen breasts and vaginal bleeding. Ginseng may lower blood sugar levels, a side effect that could be of particular importance to people taking medicine for diabetes.

Because ginseng may have steroid hormone-like effects, some doctors caution against its use in women who have had breast or endometrial cancer. Not enough study has been done to show whether ginseng is safe for women who are pregnant or breastfeeding. Women who fall into these groups should speak with their doctors before taking ginseng.

Ginseng can have an effect on how long it takes for bleeding to stop. This side effect could be an issue if ginseng is taken before surgery or if the patient is taking drugs that affect blood clotting, such as aspirin or warfarin (Coumadin).

Ginseng may cause headaches and tremors, and it can cause manic episodes if used with antidepressants known as MAOIs, such as phenelzine (Nardil). Relying on this type of treatment alone and avoiding or delaying conventional medical care for cancer may have serious health consequences.

This product is sold as a dietary supplement in the United States. Unlike companies that produce drugs (which must provide the FDA with results of detailed testing showing their product is safe and effective before the drug is approved for sale), the companies that make supplements do not have to show evidence of safety or health benefits to the FDA before selling their products. Supplement products without any reliable scientific evidence of health benefits may still be sold as long as the companies selling them do not claim the supplements can prevent, treat, or cure any specific disease. Some such products may not contain the amount of the herb or substance that is written on the label, and some may include other substances (contaminants). Though the FDA has written new rules to improve the quality of manufacturing processes for dietary supplements and the accurate listing of supplement ingredients, these rules do not take full effect until 2010. The new rules also do not address the safety of supplement ingredients or their effects on health when proper manufacturing techniques are used.

Most such supplements have not been tested to find out if they interact with medicines, foods, or other herbs and supplements. Even though some reports of interactions and harmful effects may be published, full studies of interactions and effects are not often available. Because of these limitations, any information on ill effects and interactions should be considered incomplete.

References

Blumenthal M, ed. *The Complete German Commission E Monographs: Therapeutic Guide to Herbal Medicines.* Austin, TX: American Botanical Council; 1998.

Cui Y, Shu XO, Gao YT, Cai H, Tao MH, Zheng W. Association of ginseng use with survival and quality of life among breast cancer patients. *Am J Epidemiol.* 2006;163:645-653. Epub 2006 Feb 16.

Ginseng (American). Memorial Sloan-Kettering Cancer Center Web site. http://www.mskcc.org/mskcc/html/69236.cfm. Updated September 26, 2007. Accessed June 5, 2008.

Ginseng (Asian). Memorial Sloan-Kettering Cancer Center Web site. http://www.mskcc.org/mskcc/html/69237.cfm. Updated September 17, 2007. Accessed June 5, 2008.

Gruenwald J. *PDR for Herbal Medicines.* 3rd ed. Montvale, NJ: Thomson PDR; 2004.

Natural Standard. Herbal/plant therapies: ginseng (American ginseng, Asian ginseng, Chinese ginseng, Korean red ginseng, *Panax ginseng*: Panax spp. including *P. ginseng* C.C. Meyer and *P. quinquefolius* L., excluding *Eleutherococcus senticosus*). Complementary/Integrative Medicine Education Resources, The University of Texas M. D. Anderson Cancer Center Web site. http://www.mdanderson.org/departments/cimer/display.cfm?id=DB3FF279-E763-49C4-9A0F41944C3503AF&method=displayFull. Accessed June 5, 2008.

O'Hara M, Kiefer D, Farrell K, Kemper K. A review of 12 commonly used medicinal herbs. *Arch Fam Med.* 1998;7:523-536.

Spaulding-Albright N. A review of some herbal and related products commonly used in cancer patients. *J Am Diet Assoc.* 1997;97:S208-S215.

Vogler BK, Pittler MH, Ernst E. The efficacy of ginseng. A systematic review of randomized clinical trials. *Eur J Clin Pharmacol.* 1999;55:567-575.

Yun TK, Choi SY, Yun HY. Epidemiological study on cancer prevention by ginseng: are all kinds of cancers preventable by ginseng? *J Korean Med Sci.* 2001;16(suppl):S19-S27.

GLYCONUTRIENTS

Other common name(s): glyconutritionals, Ambrotose, Glycentials, and others
Scientific/medical name(s): mannose, galactose, fucose, xylose, glucose, sialic acid, N-acetylglucosamine, N-acetylgalactosamine

Description

Glyconutrients refers to a group of eight sugars, or monosaccharides, that are used by cells in the body to make two important types of molecules: glycoproteins (proteins with sugar molecules attached) and glycolipids (lipids with sugar molecules attached). These molecules are important in the communication that occurs between cells. In recent years, various combinations of these sugars have been sold as dietary supplements with a supposed wide range of health benefits.

Overview

Glyconutrients can all be made by the human body. Available scientific evidence does not support claims that people are deficient in these sugars or that dietary supplements containing them can prevent, treat, or cure cancer or any other disease.

How is it promoted for use?

Glyconutrients are often promoted as being "essential sugars," in much the same terms as the essential amino acids—in other words, as sugars that the body cannot do without. Proponents of supplements containing glyconutrients claim that people are often deficient in these sugars. While it is true that these sugars are needed for signaling between cells, they do not have to be ingested in supplement form. The human body can make them from nutrients normally found in food.

Promoters claim that glyconutrient supplements have a wide range of helpful effects, including improving memory and sleep, lessening anxiety and depression, and lowering blood pressure and cholesterol levels. They are also claimed to help retain muscle mass, reduce body fat, aid in wound healing, and reduce symptoms from autoimmune disorders such as allergies and arthritis. Perhaps the biggest claim for these products is that they help boost the immune system, which in turn is supposed to help the body defend against a range of diseases, including cancer.

What does it involve?

The sugars sold as glyconutrients are found in many plant sources, but mixtures of glyconutrients are more commonly sold as dietary supplements in capsule or powder form. Each brand may have different ingredients, so there is no standard dosage.

What is the history behind it?

Researchers began studying glycoproteins and glycolipids in the middle of the twentieth century and, over time, have learned the structure and functions of many of these molecules. Their importance in signaling between cells has become clear in the last few decades, although many of the details of their actions remain to be worked out. Although proponents of glyconutrient supplements claim that people are deficient in some of the sugars used to make glycoproteins, researchers have found that the human body can make these substances on its own. Glyconutrients as dietary supplements have only become popular in the last decade or so, in large part because of aggressive promotion by marketing companies.

What is the evidence?

There is a wealth of laboratory evidence that glycoproteins are important in communication between cells and that this in turn may affect body systems such as the immune system. However, other than the rare exception of people with certain inherited genetic diseases, available scientific evidence does not suggest that people are deficient in the sugars considered "glyconutrients." Available evidence does not support claims that such deficiencies lead to disease. There are no reliable, controlled studies in the medical literature that show that taking glyconutrient supplements has any effect on cancer or other disorders. The few individual case reports mentioned by promoters of glyconutrient supplements have appeared mainly in obscure medical journals or cannot be found in published medical literature. More rigorous scientific studies are needed to clarify any possible benefit from taking such supplements.

Are there any possible problems or complications?

It is unclear whether rigorous safety testing has been done on dietary supplements containing glyconutrients. The ingredients come mainly from plant sources, and there appear to be few side effects other than possible allergic reactions to the plants used in the supplements. Relying on this type of treatment alone and avoiding or delaying conventional medical care for cancer may have serious health consequences.

This product is sold as a dietary supplement in the United States. Unlike companies that produce drugs (which must provide the FDA with results of detailed testing showing their product is safe and effective before the drug is approved for sale), the companies that make supplements do not have to show evidence of safety or health benefits to the FDA before selling their products. Supplement products without any reliable scientific evidence of health benefits may still be sold as long as the companies selling them do not claim the supplements can prevent, treat, or cure any specific disease. Some such products may not contain the amount of the herb or substance that is written on the label, and some may include other substances (contaminants). Though the FDA has written new rules to improve the quality of manufacturing processes for dietary supplements and the accurate listing of supplement ingredients, these rules do not take full effect until 2010. The new rules also do not address the safety of supplement ingredients or their effects on health when proper manufacturing techniques are used.

Most such supplements have not been tested to find out if they interact with medicines, foods, or other herbs and supplements. Even though some reports of interactions and harmful effects may be published, full studies of interactions and effects are not often available. Because of these limitations, any information on ill effects and interactions should be considered incomplete.

References

Barrett S. Mannatech claims criticized. Consumer Health Digest #06-44. October 31, 2006. National Council Against Health Fraud Web site. http://www.ncahf.org/digest06/06-44.html. Accessed June 5, 2008.

Glyconutrients. Memorial Sloan-Kettering Cancer Center Web site. http://www.mskcc.org/mskcc/html/70468.cfm. Updated December 18, 2007. Accessed June 5, 2008.

Greenberg H. Texas Attorney General probing Mannatech. Commentary: focus on health claims for nutritional supplements. October 26, 2006. Marketwatch Web site. http://www.marketwatch.com/news/story/story.aspx?siteid=mktw&guid=%7B50E126AD-F88B-4070-BA5E-635DDD72B298%7D. Accessed June 5, 2008.

GOLDENSEAL

Other common name(s): eye balm, eye root, goldsiegel, ground raspberry, Indian dye, Indian paint, jaundice root, yellow paint, yellow puccoon, yellow root

Scientific/medical name(s): *Hydrastis canadensis*

Description

Goldenseal is a bitter herb related to the buttercup. It is native to the eastern United States, although it can be grown elsewhere. Goldenseal takes its name from the golden-yellow scars that appear at the top of the root when the stem is broken off, which resemble an old-fashioned wax letter seal. The roots and rootstock, or rhizomes, of the plant are used in herbal remedies.

Overview

Available scientific evidence does not support claims that goldenseal is effective in treating cancer or other diseases. Goldenseal can have toxic side effects, and high doses can cause death. Some supplements sold as goldenseal contain other herbs and compounds that can make their effects unpredictable. Two chemicals in the herb (berberine and hydrastine) have been studied for use as medical treatments.

How is it promoted for use?

Practitioners promote the use of goldenseal for a wide variety of conditions, including digestive problems such as peptic ulcers and colitis, urinary tract irritation, constipation, poor appetite, bleeding after childbirth, painful menstruation, eczema, itching, ringing in the ears, tuberculosis, cancer, and other ailments. Some claim goldenseal stimulates the immune system, and some recommend it for colds. Goldenseal has been used on the skin to treat wounds, herpes sores, and other skin conditions. It is sometimes made into a tea and used as a mouthwash or as a douche.

Berberine, a chemical contained in goldenseal, is said to fight off infection caused by some bacteria, fungi, and yeast and can act as a mild sedative. Some claim that berberine is more effective than aspirin for reducing fevers. Another chemical in goldenseal, hydrastine, is said to reduce blood pressure. Some people believe that goldenseal helps mask drugs in the urine so they cannot be detected on drug screening tests.

What does it involve?

Goldenseal can be taken internally as a capsule, extract, tincture, or tea. Suppliers also grind the root and sell the powder, which can be prepared in different ways. The amount of goldenseal recommended depends on how it is prepared (for example, tincture versus dried root).

Proponents use tooth powder and mouthwash made from goldenseal to treat tooth and gum infections. They also apply the powder to cold sores and skin wounds. Some use a goldenseal solution in ear drops, douches, and eye drops for conjunctivitis (inflammation of the eye). Salves made from goldenseal are used for eczema and psoriasis.

What is the history behind it?

For centuries some Native American tribes have used goldenseal for medicinal purposes. It was taken as a stimulant and used for stomach ulcers. Mouth sores and irritated eyes were washed with goldenseal solutions. It was also used as a face paint and as a dye for clothing. The herb later became an important ingredient in American folk medicine. It was made into an eyewash and into a tea to treat sores in the mouth and throat.

By 1900, it had been harvested nearly to extinction and is still considered an endangered species. It is currently grown in the United States in limited quantities. Possibly because of the small supply, some sellers substitute or mix goldenseal with other herbs that also contain berberine.

There can be wide variation among products sold as goldenseal. A study published in 2003 looked for the main goldenseal compounds in twenty different goldenseal products from different marketers. Hydrastine content ranged from none (0 percent) to 3 percent, and berberine ranged from less than 1 percent to nearly 6 percent in product samples. Another study published in 2003 tested goldenseal powder obtained from three different suppliers. It found that the samples contained varying amounts of the goldenseal compounds. One of the samples contained compounds that are not found in goldenseal.

What is the evidence?

Available scientific evidence does not support the use of goldenseal for cancer or any other medical condition in humans. There has been limited testing of goldenseal for other conditions. In one animal study, goldenseal appeared to stimulate the immune system.

The National Center for Complementary and Alternative Medicine, part of the National Institutes of Health, recommended that the National Toxicology Program (NTP) test goldenseal for its potential to cause developmental problems and/or cancer of the reproductive system. To date, no findings on reproductive effects have been published by the NTP. However, a group of researchers in Australia studied the effect of goldenseal on the outcomes of rat pregnancies. No ill effects were found, although the researchers caution that false results could have happened because of goldenseal's poor absorption when the herb is taken by mouth. In other words, it is possible that the rats did not actually absorb enough of the herb for it to have an effect.

Two of the chemicals in goldenseal—berberine and hydrastine—have been studied for some time. Laboratory research seemed to show that berberine stopped some cancer cells from reproducing, but this effect did not carry over when it was tested in animals. Later laboratory tests showed promise with one type of brain cancer, but animal studies have not been completed. Studies in the laboratory have shown that direct contact with berberine helps stop bacteria and some types of fungus from growing. Animal studies suggest that it may also reduce certain types of diarrhea. In addition, berberine has been studied for its blood-thinning and heart stimulant properties in animals.

Hydrastine, another component of goldenseal, may raise blood pressure. Animal studies have suggested it may help with stabilizing diabetes. Further studies are needed to determine whether the results apply to humans. In addition, it is important to remember that herb extracts would not be expected to have the same effect as the whole herb.

Are there any possible problems or complications?

Goldenseal may produce toxic effects, including digestive complaints, nervousness, depression, constipation, rapid heartbeat, diarrhea, stomach cramps and pain, mouth ulcers, nausea, seizures, vomiting, and central nervous system depression. High doses may cause breathing problems, paralysis, and even death. Long-term use may lead to vitamin B deficiency, hallucinations, and delirium.

Berberine, one of the active compounds in goldenseal, can disrupt heart rhythm. This compound can also cause jaundice in newborns, a condition marked by yellowed skin and eyes that is sometimes linked to deafness or brain damage. Goldenseal may have an unpredictable effect on blood pressure, since different compounds in it have opposite effects on blood pressure. People with high blood pressure or heart disease may be more likely to be harmed by goldenseal than people without these conditions.

If hives, a rash, or shortness of breath develops, stop taking goldenseal and seek medical attention immediately. Potential interactions between goldenseal and other drugs and herbs should also be considered. Always tell your doctor and pharmacist about any herbs and supplements you are taking.

Berberine is known to reduce sperm motility in bulls, but it is unknown whether it affects fertility in humans. Men who are trying to have children may wish to avoid goldenseal until human studies are done. There are also concerns that high doses of goldenseal might tighten the womb in pregnant women and cause miscarriage or early labor. Women who are pregnant or breastfeeding should not use goldenseal unless further studies show it to be safe.

Goldenseal applied to the skin may make it more sensitive to the sun, so avoid sunlight and artificial sunlight while using it. If sunlight is unavoidable, cover up or use sunscreen.

Relying on this type of treatment alone and avoiding or delaying conventional medical care for cancer may have serious health consequences.

This product is sold as a dietary supplement in the United States. Unlike companies that produce drugs (which must provide the FDA with results of detailed testing showing their product is safe and effective before the drug is approved for sale), the companies that make supplements do not have to show evidence of safety or health benefits to the FDA before selling their products. Supplement products without any reliable scientific evidence of health benefits may still be sold as long as the companies selling them do not claim the supplements can prevent, treat, or cure any specific disease. Some such products may not contain the amount of the herb or substance that is written on the label, and some may include other substances (contaminants). Though the FDA has written new rules to improve the quality of manufacturing processes for dietary supplements and the accurate listing of supplement ingredients, these rules do not take full effect until 2010. The new rules also do not address the safety of supplement ingredients or their effects on health when proper manufacturing techniques are used.

Most such supplements have not been tested to find out if they interact with medicines, foods, or other herbs and supplements. Even though some reports of interactions and harmful effects may be published, full studies of interactions and effects are not often available. Because of these limitations, any information on ill effects and interactions should be considered incomplete.

References

Davis JM, McCoy JA. Commercial goldenseal cultivation. Department of Horticultural Science, College of Agriculture & Life Sciences. North Carolina State University Web site. http://www.ces.ncsu.edu/depts/hort/hil/hil-131.html. Updated July 2000. Accessed June 5, 2008.

Edwards DJ, Draper EJ. Variations in alkaloid content of herbal products containing goldenseal. *J Am Pharm Assoc.* 2003;43:419-423.

Fetrow CW, Avila JR. *Professional's Handbook of Complementary & Alternative Medicines.* Philadelphia, PA: Lippincott Williams & Wilkins; 2004.

Goldenseal. Memorial Sloan-Kettering Cancer Center Web site. http://www.mskcc.org/mskcc/html/69241.cfm. Updated December 19, 2007. Accessed June 5, 2008.

Goldenseal. National Center for Complementary and Alternative Medicine Web site. http://nccam.nih.gov/health/goldenseal/. Updated May 27, 2008. Accessed June 5, 2008.

Gruenwald J. *PDR for Herbal Medicines.* 3rd ed. Montvale, NJ: Thomson PDR; 2004.

Gurley BJ, Gardner SF, Hubbard MA, Williams DK, Gentry WB, Khan IA, Shah A. In vivo effects of goldenseal, kava kava, black cohosh, and valerian on human cytochrome P450 1A2, 2D6, 2E1, and 3A4/5 phenotypes. *Clin Pharmacol Ther.* 2005;77:415-426.

Gurley BJ, Swain A, Hubbard MA, Hartsfield F, Thaden J, Williams DK, Gentry WB, Tong Y. Supplementation with goldenseal (*Hydrastis canadensis*), but not kava kava (*Piper methysticum*), inhibits human CYP3A activity in vivo. *Clin Pharmacol Ther.* 2008:83:61-69.

Inbaraj JJ, Kukielczak BM, Bilski P, Sandvik SL, Chignell CF. Photochemistry and photocytotoxicity of alkaloids from Goldenseal (*Hydrastis canadensis* L.) 1. Berberine. *Chem Res Toxicol.* 2001;14:1529-1534.

Rehman J, Dillow JM, Carter SM, Chou J, Le B, Maisel AS. Increased production of antigen-specific immunoglobulins G and M following in vivo treatment with the medicinal plants Echinacea angustifolia and Hydrastis canadensis. *Immunol Lett.* 1999;68:391-395.

Tice R. Goldenseal (*Hydrastis canadensis* L.) and two of its constituent alkaloids berberine [2086-83-1] and hydrastine [118-08-1] review of toxicological literature. November 1997. National Toxicology Program Web site. http://ntp.niehs.nih.gov/ntp/htdocs/Chem_Background/ExSumPdf/Goldenseal.pdf. Accessed June 5, 2008.

Weber HA, Zart MK, Hodges AE, Molloy HM, O'Brien BM, Moody LA, Clark AP, Harris RK, Overstreet JD, Smith CS. Chemical comparison of goldenseal (*Hydrastis canadensis* L.) root powder from three commercial suppliers. *J Agric Food Chem.* 2003;51:7352-7358.

Yao M, Ritchie HE, Brown-Woodman PD. A reproductive screening test of goldenseal. *Birth Defects Res B Dev Reprod Toxicol.* 2005;74:399-404.

GOTU KOLA

Other common name(s): centella, pennywort, Madekassol
Scientific/medical name(s): *Centella asiatica, Hydrocotyle asiatica*

Description

Gotu kola is a swamp plant that grows naturally in Madagascar, India, Sri Lanka, Indonesia, and many parts of South Africa. Its dried leaves and stems are used in herbal remedies. The active compounds in gotu kola are called saponins, or triterpenoids. Gotu kola is also used in Ayurvedic and Chinese medicine to treat skin wounds. Gotu kola is not related to the kola (cola) nut and contains no caffeine or stimulants.

Overview

Some clinical trials have looked at the use of gotu kola and its compounds in people with poor blood flow, usually in the legs. These limited studies suggest that gotu kola may help reduce swelling in the legs and feet, although more scientific studies are needed. Other research that has looked at gotu kola in humans has been limited by small numbers of patients and problems in study methods. Although at least one laboratory study of tumor cells showed reduced cell growth with gotu kola, available scientific evidence does not support claims of its effectiveness for treating cancer or any other disease in humans.

How is it promoted for use?

Proponents claim that gotu kola possesses numerous curative qualities. Some practitioners maintain that gotu kola reduces fever and relieves congestion caused by colds and upper respiratory infections. Some women use gotu kola for birth control, and some herbalists claim that gotu kola is an antidote for poisonous mushrooms and arsenic poisoning. Some believe that it can be applied externally to treat snakebites, herpes, fractures, and sprains.

In some folk medicine traditions, gotu kola is used to treat syphilis, rheumatism, leprosy, mental illness, and epilepsy. It is also used to stimulate urination and to relieve physical and mental exhaustion, diarrhea, eye diseases, inflammation, asthma, high blood pressure, liver disease, dysentery, urinary tract infections, eczema, and psoriasis. Some manufacturers of the herbal supplement claim gotu kola can be used to treat cancer as well.

What does it involve?

Gotu kola is available as a capsule, eye drop, extract, powder, and ointment and can be purchased from health food stores and over the Internet. Dried gotu kola can be made into a tea. Recommended dosage depends on the condition being treated.

What is the history behind it?

Gotu kola has a long history in the folk medicines of India, Indonesia, Sri Lanka, and Madagascar and is still widely used in these countries today. It has been used for generations in India to promote relaxation, improve memory, and aid meditation. In traditional Chinese medicine, the herb is believed to promote longevity. The Chinese name for gotu kola translates to "fountain of youth." A Sri Lankan legend says that elephants have long lives because they eat gotu kola.

What is the evidence?

Animal and laboratory studies of gotu kola have shown promising results for some uses, but further research is needed to determine its benefits for humans. One group of gotu kola compounds that has been extracted and tested in clinical trials is called total triterpenic fraction of *Centella asiatica* (TTFCA). A few clinical trials in humans have suggested that extracts of gotu kola and TTFCA, when taken by mouth, were more helpful than a placebo at reducing swelling of the legs and feet due to varicose veins and poor circulation, a condition called chronic venous insufficiency. It seemed to reduce the "leakage" of blood vessels that seems to contribute to swelling. Further research is needed to determine whether these results will hold true. It is also important to remember that extracted chemicals such as TTFCA are not the same as the herb itself. Studies of extracts may not show the same results as studies using the raw plant.

One study in India reported that gotu kola extract slowed the development of tumors in mice and increased their life span. Other studies with rats showed that gotu kola extract had calming effects and prevented ulcers. Animal studies have shown that gotu kola, when applied to the skin or taken by mouth, seems to promote collagen production in wounds, which contributes to healing.

Laboratory studies showed that fresh gotu kola juice slowed the growth of tumor cells, but not as much as more purified extracts from the plant. Laboratory studies have also suggested that extracts of gotu kola could be useful in the treatment of scleroderma and for the prevention and treatment of Alzheimer's disease. A small number of laboratory studies conducted in India and Europe suggest that an ointment or gel made from gotu kola may speed wound healing. None of these studies have been done on humans, although some of the wound-healing studies also looked promising in rodent tests.

Although animal and laboratory studies look promising for some of these uses, further studies are necessary to determine whether the results hold true for humans. More well-controlled research is needed to understand whether gotu kola will play any role in cancer treatment.

Are there any possible problems or complications?

Gotu kola is generally considered safe; however there are no large clinical studies in humans to fully document side effects. When used on the skin, possible side effects include a burning sensation, itching, or allergic rash. Stomach irritation and nausea have been observed when the herb is taken by mouth. Drowsiness has been reported, especially when the herb is taken in larger doses. High doses of gotu kola have been reported to increase blood sugar and raise cholesterol levels. A few cases of hepatitis (liver inflammation) have been reported in people taking gotu kola. It may increase sensitivity to the sun, so avoid sunlight or use sunscreen while taking it. This herb can cause allergic reactions in some people. Gotu kola impairs fertility in mice, but human effects are less well known.

In addition, the potential interactions between gotu kola and other drugs and herbs should be considered. Some of these combinations may be dangerous. Always tell your doctor and pharmacist about any herbs you are taking.

Women who are pregnant or breastfeeding should not use this herb. Relying on this type of treatment alone and avoiding or delaying conventional medical care for cancer may have serious health consequences.

This product is sold as a dietary supplement in the United States. Unlike companies that produce drugs (which must provide the FDA with results of detailed testing showing their product is safe and effective before the drug is approved for sale), the companies that make supplements do not have to show evidence of safety or health benefits to the FDA before selling their products. Supplement products without any reliable scientific evidence of health benefits may still be sold as long as the companies selling them do not claim the supplements can prevent, treat, or cure any specific disease. Some such products may not contain the amount of the herb or substance that is written on the label, and some may include other substances (contaminants). Though the FDA has written new rules to improve the quality of manufacturing processes for dietary supplements and the accurate listing of supplement ingredients, these rules do not take full effect until 2010. The new rules also do not address the safety of supplement ingredients or their effects on health when proper manufacturing techniques are used.

Most such supplements have not been tested to find out if they interact with medicines, foods, or other herbs and supplements. Even though some reports of interactions and harmful effects may be published, full studies of interactions and effects are not often available. Because of these limitations, any information on ill effects and interactions should be considered incomplete.

References

Awang DV. Gotu kola. *Can Pharm J.* 1998;131:42-46.

Babu TD, Kuttan G, Padikkala J. Cytotoxic and anti-tumour properties of certain taxa of Umbelliferae with special reference to *Centella asiatica* (L.) Urban. *J Ethnopharmacol.* 1995;48:53-57.

Fetrow CW, Avila JR. *Professional's Handbook of Complementary & Alternative Medicines.* Philadelphia, PA: Lippincott Williams & Wilkins; 2004.

Gnanapragasam A, Ebenezar KK, Sathish V, Govindaraju P, Devaki T. Protective effect of *Centella asiatica* on antioxidant tissue defense system against adriamycin induced cardiomyopathy in rats. *Life Sci.* 2004;76:585-597.

Gotu kola. Memorial Sloan-Kettering Cancer Center Web site. http://www.mskcc.org/mskcc/html/69242.cfm. Updated December 18, 2007. Accessed June 5, 2008.

Gruenwald J. *PDR for Herbal Medicines.* 3rd ed. Montvale, NJ: Thomson PDR; 2004.

Jorge OA, Jorge AD. Hepatotoxicity associated with the ingestion of *Centella asiatica. Rev Esp Enferm Dig.* 2005;97:115-124.

Pointel JP, Boccalon H, Cloarec M, Ledevehat C, Joubert M. Titrated extract of Centella asiatica (TECA) in the treatment of venous insufficiency of the lower limbs. *Angiology.* 1987;38:46-50.

Sunilkumar, Parameshwaraiah S, Shivakumar HG. Evaluation of topical formulations of aqueous extract of Centella asiatica on open wounds in rats. *Indian J Exp Biol.* 1998;36:569-572.

Veerendra Kumar MH, Gupta YK. Effect of *Centella asiatica* on cognition and oxidative stress in an intracerebroventricular streptozotocin model of Alzheimer's disease in rats. *Clin Exp Pharmacol Physiol.* 2003;30:336-342.

GREEN TEA

Other common name(s): green tea extract, Chinese tea
Scientific/medical name(s): *Camellia sinensis*

Description

Green tea is a drink made from the steamed and dried leaves of the *Camellia sinesis* plant, a shrub native to Asia. Black tea is also made from this plant, but unlike green tea, black tea is made from leaves that have been fermented. Fermentation may reduce the levels of some compounds, such as antioxidants, in the tea.

Overview

Some researchers believe green tea may protect against certain types of cancer because it contains antioxidants. However, results from human studies have been mixed. More research is needed to determine the role of green tea in cancer prevention.

How is it promoted for use?

Green tea is widely consumed in Japan, China, and other Asian nations and is becoming more popular in Western nations. Some reports indicate green tea may have the ability to help prevent cancers of the skin, esophagus, stomach, colon, pancreas, lung, bladder, prostate, and breast.

Green tea contains chemicals known as polyphenols, which have antioxidant properties. The major group of polyphenols in green tea are called catechins, and the most important catechin seems to be epigallocatechin-3-gallate (EGCG). EGCG may cause cancer cells to die in much the same way that normal cells do. This effect is important because cancer cells are different from normal cells in that they do not die when they should—they continue to grow and spread.

Herbalists use green tea and extracts of its leaves for stomach problems, vomiting, and diarrhea and to reduce tooth decay, blood pressure, cholesterol levels, and blockages of the blood vessels in the heart that can lead to heart attacks. Green tea is also promoted as preventing certain bacterial infections. In recent years, some researchers have suggested that black tea may also be effective in cancer prevention. These claims are currently being studied.

What does it involve?

The typical amount of green tea consumed varies widely, and it is not clear how much might be needed for beneficial effects. Three cups a day or more is the amount typically taken in Asian countries. Green tea is usually brewed using one to two teaspoons of the dried tea in a cup of boiling water or is steeped for three to fifteen minutes. Bottles and cans of prepared green tea are sold under a variety of brand names, often with additional ingredients.

Green tea extract is also available in capsule form. Three capsules of green tea extract a day is a common recommended dosage, but this dosage and its effects remain uncertain. There is wide variation in the contents of these extracts.

What is the history behind it?

The Chinese have been drinking green tea for at least three thousand years, and this beverage has been popular in some other Asian countries for at least a thousand years. In recent years, scientists have begun to study its health effects more closely in laboratory and animal studies and in observational human studies.

What is the evidence?

Many laboratory studies in cell cultures and animals have shown green tea acts against cancer cells. Test tube studies have suggested that compounds in the tea may help stop new blood vessels from forming, thereby cutting off the supply of blood to cancer cells. It is tempting to assume that it may therefore help prevent some cancers, but studies in humans have been mixed. Most human studies have been epidemiologic studies in East Asia, in which researchers compared tea drinkers with non-tea drinkers while trying to account for other lifestyle differences. These types of studies are complex, and it is often hard to draw firm conclusions from them.

Large observational epidemiologic studies in East Asia generally have not found that green tea drinkers have a lower risk for breast, stomach, or colon cancer than non-tea drinkers. One study found that Asian-American women who drink green tea regularly have a lower risk for breast cancer than those who do not. A Chinese study found that green tea drinking was linked to fewer cancers of the esophagus for people who did not smoke. On the other hand, a 2006

Japanese study showed that those with cancer of the esophagus were more likely to be green tea drinkers than those who did not have the cancer. Other studies of green tea's ability to prevent or treat lung, prostate, bladder, or other types of cancer have yielded similarly mixed results.

While the results of laboratory studies have been promising, at this time the available scientific evidence does not support claims that green tea can help prevent or treat any specific type of cancer in humans. Controlled, randomized clinical trials are needed to determine its effectiveness. Several studies are currently under way.

Are there any possible problems or complications?

Moderate intake of green tea is generally considered safe. Asians have consumed this tea for thousands of years with few dangerous side effects. However, some people may have allergic reactions and should stop drinking it if reactions occur. Drinking large amounts of tea may cause nutritional and other problems because of the caffeine content and the strong binding activities of the polyphenols, which can make it harder for the body to absorb certain medicines and iron supplements. Always tell your doctor and pharmacist about any herbs and supplements you are taking.

Possible effects from too much caffeine are the major concern with green tea. Too much caffeine can lead to nausea, trouble sleeping, and frequent urination. Because caffeine acts as a stimulant, people with irregular heartbeats or who have anxiety attacks should be cautious in its use.

Women who are pregnant or breastfeeding should not drink green tea in large amounts. Caffeine can cross the placenta and affect the fetus and can also be passed along in breast milk. Relying on this type of treatment alone and avoiding or delaying conventional medical care for cancer may have serious health consequences.

This product is sold as a dietary supplement in the United States. Unlike companies that produce drugs (which must provide the FDA with results of detailed testing showing their product is safe and effective before the drug is approved for sale), the companies that make supplements do not have to show evidence of safety or health benefits to the FDA before selling their products. Supplement products without any reliable scientific evidence of health benefits may still be sold as long as the companies selling them do not claim the supplements can prevent, treat, or cure any specific disease. Some such products may not contain the amount of the herb or substance that is written on the label, and some may include other substances (contaminants). Though the FDA has written new rules to improve the quality of manufacturing processes for dietary supplements and the accurate listing of supplement ingredients, these rules do not take full effect until 2010. The new rules also do not address the safety of supplement ingredients or their effects on health when proper manufacturing techniques are used.

Most such supplements have not been tested to find out if they interact with medicines, foods, or other herbs and supplements. Even though some reports of interactions and harmful effects may be published, full studies of interactions and effects are not often available. Because of these limitations, any information on ill effects and interactions should be considered incomplete.

References

Baliga MS, Meleth S, Katiyar SK. Growth inhibitory and antimetastatic effect of green tea polyphenols on metastasis-specific mouse mammary carcinoma 4T1 cells in vitro and in vivo systems. *Clin Cancer Res.* 2005;11:1918-1927.

Gao YT, McLaughlin JK, Blot WJ, Ji BT, Dai Q, Fraumeni JF Jr. Reduced risk of esophageal cancer associated with green tea consumption. *J Natl Cancer Inst.* 1994;86:855-858.

Green tea. Memorial Sloan-Kettering Cancer Center Web site. http://www.mskcc.org/mskcc/html/69247.cfm. Updated August 14, 2007. Accessed June 5, 2008.

Gruenwald J. *PDR for Herbal Medicines.* 3rd ed. Montvale, NJ: Thomson PDR; 2004.

Ishikawa A, Kuriyama S, Tsubono Y, Fukao A, Takahashi H, Tachiya H, Tsuji I. Smoking, alcohol drinking, green tea consumption and the risk of esophageal cancer in Japanese men. *J Epidemiol.* 2006;16:185-192.

Jatoi A, Ellison N, Burch PA, Sloan JA, Dakhil SR, Novotny P, Tan W, Fitch TR, Rowland KM, Young CY, Flynn PJ. A phase II trial of green tea in the treatment of patients with androgen independent metastatic prostate carcinoma. *Cancer.* 2003;97:1442-1446.

Ji BT, Chow WH, Hsing AW, McLaughlin JK, Dai Q, Goa YT, Fraumeni JF Jr. Green tea consumption and the risk of pancreatic and colorectal cancers. *Int J Cancer.* 1997;70:255-258.

Jian L, Xie LP, Lee AH, Binns CW. Protective effect of green tea against prostate cancer: a case-control study in southeast China. *Int J Cancer.* 2004;108:130-135.

Kurahashi N, Sasazuki S, Iwasaki M, Inoue M, Tsugane S; JPHC Study Group. Green tea consumption and prostate cancer risk in Japanese men: a prospective study. *Am J Epidemiol.* 2008;167:71-77.

Kuriyama S, Shimazu T, Ohmori K, Kikuchi N, Nakaya N, NishinoY, Tsubono Y, Tsuji I. Green tea consumption and mortality due to cardiovascular disease, cancer, and all causes in Japan: the Ohsaki study. *JAMA.* 2006;296:1255-1265.

Nagano J, Kono S, Preston DL, Mabuchi K. A prospective study of green tea consumption and cancer incidence, Hiroshima and Nagasaki (Japan). *Cancer Causes Control.* 2001;12:501-508.

Natural Standard. Herbal/plant therapies: green tea (*Camellia sinensis*). Complementary/Integrative Medicine Education Resources, The University of Texas M. D. Anderson Cancer Center Web site. http://www.mdanderson.org/departments/cimer/display.cfm?id=41513F0E-8ECA-46B8-BA633C9453373584&method=displayFull. Accessed June 5, 2008.

Nihal M, Ahmad N, Mukhtar H, Wood GS. Anti-proliferative and proapoptotic effects of (-)-epigallocatechin-3-gallate on human melanoma: possible implications for the chemoprevention of melanoma. *Int J Cancer.* 2005;114:513-521.

Pisters KM, Newman RA, Coldman B, Shin DM, Khuri FR, Hong WK, Glisson BS, Lee JS. Phase I trial of oral green tea extract in adult patients with solid tumors. *J Clin Oncol.* 2001;19:1830-1838.

Steele VE, Kelloff GJ, Balentine D, Boone CW, Mehta R, Bagheri D, Sigman CC, Zhu S, Sharma S. Comparative chemopreventive mechanisms of green tea, black tea and selected polyphenol extracts measured by in vitro bioassays. *Carcinogenesis.* 2000;21:63-67.

Sun CL, Yuan JM, Koh WP, Yu MC. Green tea, black tea and breast cancer risk: a meta-analysis of epidemiological studies. *Carcinogenesis.* 2006;27:1310-1315. Epub 2005 Nov 25.

Suzuki Y, Tsubono Y, Nakaya N, Koizumi Y, Suzuki Y, Shibuya D, Tsuji I. Green tea and the risk of colorectal cancer: pooled analysis of two prospective studies in Japan. *J Epidemiol.* 2005;15:118-124.

Suzuki Y, Tsubono Y, Nakaya N, Suzuki Y, Koizumi Y, Tsuji I. Green tea and the risk of breast cancer: pooled analysis of two prospective studies in Japan. *Br J Cancer.* 2004;90:1361-1363.

Tsubono Y, Nishino Y, Komatsu S, Hsieh CC, Kanemura S, Tsuji I, Nakatsuka H, Fukao A, Satoh H, Hisamichi S. Green tea and the risk of gastric cancer in Japan. *N Engl J Med.* 2001;344:632-636.

Wu AH, Yu MC, Tseng CC, Hankin J, Pike MC. Green tea and risk of breast cancer in Asian Americans. *Int J Cancer.* 2003;106:574-579.

HOXSEY HERBAL TREATMENT

Other common name(s): Hoxsey method, Hoxsey treatment, Hoxsey herbs, Hoxsey herbal therapy, Hoxsey formula

Scientific/medical name(s): none

Description

The Hoxsey herbal treatment is a regimen that includes the use of two types of herbal mixtures: a "brown tonic" to be taken by mouth and a paste, salve, or yellow powder for external use. Both the paste and the powder are caustic, meaning they can burn the skin (see "Cancer Salves," page 171).

Overview

Available scientific evidence does not support claims that the Hoxsey herbal treatment is effective in treating cancer, and there have been no clinical trials of the treatment published in conventional medical journals. In some animal studies, a few of the herbs contained in the Hoxsey formula were studied separately and showed some anticancer activity. It is not known whether the combination of herbs taken by mouth has harmful effects. The paste made for external application can severely burn, scar, and disfigure the skin.

How is it promoted for use?

The Hoxsey herbal treatment is specifically promoted to treat people with cancer. People who use the tonic claim that it removes toxins from the body, strengthens the immune system, and enhances the body's ability to absorb and excrete, or get rid of, tumors. The external treatment is used to treat skin cancer. It is supposed to keep cancer from spreading and help destroy cancer cells. Those who use the Hoxsey treatment say that it restores the body's chemistry to a normal state.

What does it involve?

The herbal tonic for internal use contains a combination of supplements and herbs that may include pokeweed, burdock root, licorice, barberry, buckthorn bark, stillingia root, red clover, prickly ash bark, potassium iodide, and cascara. The components depend on when it was made, for whom, and the clinic in which it was made. The pastes or salves for external use may contain antimony trisulfide, zinc chloride, and blood root, and the powder consists of arsenic sulfide, sulfur, and talc. The external preparation is rubbed directly onto tumors. Internal and external dosages vary depending on the patient and whether the tumor is inside the body or on the skin. The Hoxsey herbal treatment is no longer legal in the United States, although it can be obtained through clinics in Mexico. Adapted versions of the formula are being used by some naturopathic practitioners in the United States.

In addition to the herbs and other ingredients described above, the Hoxsey treatment now also includes antiseptic douches and washes, laxative tablets, and nutritional supplements. Food restrictions are now part of the treatment as well, and patients undergoing this treatment may not be allowed pork, vinegar, tomatoes, pickles, carbonated drinks, alcohol, bleached flour, sugar, and most salt.

What is the history behind it?

The Hoxsey herbal treatment is one of the oldest alternative cancer treatments in the United States. Its controversial history dates back to the 1920s, when Harry Hoxsey, who had no medical training, began marketing a mixture of herbs that he believed would treat cancer. Hoxsey claimed that his great grandfather, John Hoxsey, developed the first version of the herbal formula in 1840 when he noticed a tumor that had developed on one of his horse's legs. The animal began eating some of the wild plants growing in the meadow, and within a short time the tumor disappeared. John Hoxsey gathered the herbs and mixed them with old home remedies used for cancer.

Harry's father, a veterinarian, was the first to use the herbal formula to treat people with cancer. Harry, however, was the one who attracted fame and fortune through self-promotion, publicity, and sensational claims. He even conducted public healing sessions using his herbal concoction. Hoxsey opened his first clinic in Taylorville, Illinois, in the 1920s, and at one point operated clinics in seventeen states. He claimed that at their peak his clinics treated tens of thousands of cancer patients every year. Hoxsey was convicted and fined numerous times for practicing medicine without a license and moved his clinics from state to state to avoid legal problems.

In 1936, Hoxsey opened a clinic in Dallas, Texas, that became one of the largest privately owned cancer centers in the world. In 1949, Hoxsey sued the editor of the prestigious *Journal of the American Medical Association* for libel and slander after the journal called him a fraud. Hoxsey won the case, but the judge awarded him only $1.

By 1960, after battling Hoxsey for a decade, the U.S. Food and Drug Administration (FDA) finally banned the sale of the Hoxsey herbal treatment in the United States and forced Hoxsey to close all clinics in the United States. In 1963, one of Hoxsey's nurses set up a clinic in Tijuana, Mexico. Just before her death in 1999, the clinic was taken over by her sister and still operates today. Hoxsey himself was found to have prostate cancer in 1967. When he did not respond to his own treatment, Hoxsey underwent conventional surgery. He died seven years later.

What is the evidence?

Available scientific evidence does not support claims that the Hoxsey herbal treatment has any value in the treatment of cancer in humans. In 1946, the National Cancer Institute reviewed seventy-seven case reports of Hoxsey's patients and concluded that none of them met the criteria for scientific evaluation.

Experts from The University of Texas M. D. Anderson Cancer Center have reviewed all four published human studies of the Hoxsey herbal treatment. One study was published in a pamphlet provided by the Tijuana clinic and simply contains a description of nine patients who received the treatment. It concluded that the treatment is effective, even though most of the Hoxsey-treated patients received standard cancer treatment in addition to the Hoxsey treatment. Seven additional cases were reviewed in a book, which concludes that patients "got well when they weren't supposed to" (Ausubel, 2000); that is, they had a dismal prognosis but were cured by the Hoxsey treatment. The cases described in the book, however, include some in which the cancer was not confirmed by biopsy and several in which patients also received conventional treatment. A study published in the *Journal of Naturopathic Medicine* involved thirty-nine people with various types of cancer who took the Hoxsey herbal treatment. Ten patients died after an average of fifteen months, and twenty-three never completed the study. Six patients claimed to be disease-free after four years. A study reporting outcomes of 149 patients registering at the Hoxsey clinic during the first three months of 1992 was published in 2001 in the *Journal of Alternative and Complementary Medicine*. Seventeen patients were still alive, sixty-eight had died, and information regarding the remaining sixty-four was not available. The researchers concluded that the value of the treatment could not be evaluated because follow-up for so many patients was incomplete. None of these four studies contains convincing evidence of effectiveness.

According to a 1990 report from the U.S. Congressional Office of Technology Assessment, the National Advisory Cancer Council studied many of Hoxsey's patient records and learned that biopsies were not performed on most of the patients, so there was no confirmation that they actually had cancer. In a separate review, the National Cancer Institute investigated four hundred patients who were reported as cured by Hoxsey. Patients or their families were interviewed, and all records were carefully reviewed. These patients fell into three groups: those who had been treated but were not confirmed to have had cancer, those who had received successful conventional cancer treatment before seeing Hoxsey, and those who had cancer and had died of it or were still alive with evidence of cancer. Out of the four hundred cases, not one case of a Hoxsey cure could be documented.

To collect some reliable information, a carefully controlled study of the Hoxsey tonic was performed on mice with tumors. There was no difference in tumor size and growth between the treated and untreated mice. The main ingredient in the tonic, potassium iodide, had been tested already and found to be useless in cancer treatment.

In some animal studies, a few of the individual herbs contained in the Hoxsey treatment showed some anticancer activity. Further studies are needed to determine whether the results apply to humans.

Are there any possible problems or complications?

Some of the ingredients in the internal formula, such as buckthorn, can cause nausea, vomiting, diarrhea, anxiety, and trembling. Cascara can also cause diarrhea. Pokeweed is a poisonous plant that can cause side effects such as nausea, vomiting, diarrhea, abdominal cramps, and heart block (a blockage of the electrical impulses that stimulate the heart to contract), and has caused deaths in children. Red clover may increase the risk for bleeding for people who take blood-thinning medications such as warfarin (Coumadin). It also has estrogen-like activity, which means it should be avoided by women with estrogen receptor–positive breast tumors. Taking iodine in large amounts over a long period of time can cause inflamed salivary glands, skin outbreaks, and impotence. The paste made for external use can severely burn, scar, and disfigure the skin.

Interactions with other drugs may occur. For example, potassium iodide can cause problems in those taking lithium or blood-thinning medications. Potential interactions between the Hoxsey herbs and other drugs and herbs should be considered. Some of these combinations may be dangerous. Always tell your doctor and pharmacist about any herbs you are taking.

People with allergies to any of the ingredients may experience severe reactions to the internal or external formulas. If hives, rashes, or shortness of breath develop, stop taking the herbs and seek medical attention immediately.

Women who are pregnant or breastfeeding should not use this treatment in any form. Relying on this type of treatment alone and avoiding or delaying conventional medical care for cancer may have serious health consequences.

These substances may have not been thoroughly tested to find out how they interact with medicines, foods, or dietary supplements. Even though some reports of interactions and harmful effects may be published, full studies of interactions and effects are not often available. Because of these limitations, any information on ill effects and interactions should be considered incomplete.

References

American Cancer Society. Questionable methods of cancer management: 'nutritional' therapies. *CA Cancer J Clin.* 1993;43:309-319.

American Cancer Society. Unproven methods of cancer management: Hoxsey Method/Bio-Medical Center. *CA Cancer J Clin.* 1990;40:51-55.

Austin S, Baumgartner E, DeKadt S. Long-term follow-up of cancer patients using Contreras, Hoxsey and Gerson therapies. *J Naturopathic Med.* 1994;5:74-76.

Ausubel K. *When Healing Becomes a Crime.* Rochester, VT: Healing Arts Press; 2000. Quoted by: Hoxsey herbal therapy. The University of Texas M. D. Anderson Cancer Center Web site.

Herbal/plant therapies: Hoxsey. Complementary/Integrative Medicine Education Resources, The University of Texas M. D. Anderson Cancer Center Web site. http://www.mdanderson.org/departments/CIMER/display.cfm?id=A0AAFDBB-ECA2-11D4-810100508B603A14&method=displayFull. Accessed June 5, 2008.

Hoxsey herbal therapy. Memorial Sloan-Kettering Cancer Center Web site. http://www.mskcc.org/mskcc/html/69258.cfm. Updated August 31, 2007. Accessed June 5, 2008.

National Institutes of Health. *Alternative Medicine: Expanding Medical Horizons: A Report to the National Institutes of Health on Alternative Medical Systems and Practices in the United States.* Washington, DC: US Government Printing Office; 1994. NIH publication 94-066.

Spaulding-Albright N. A review of some herbal and related products commonly used in cancer patients. *J Am Diet Assoc.* 1997;97:S208-S215.

US Congress, Office of Technology Assessment. *Unconventional Cancer Treatments: OTA-H-405.* Washington, DC: US Government Printing Office; 1990.

INDIAN SNAKEROOT

Other common name(s): snakeroot, rauwolfia, rauvolfia, serpentwood, reserpine
Scientific/medical name(s): *Rauwolfia serpentina*

Description

Indian snakeroot is a plant that grows in India, Thailand, and other parts of Asia, South America, and Africa. There are more than one hundred species of Indian snakeroot. *Rauwolfia serpentina* is the most commonly used species in herbal remedies. Reserpine, a chemical found in the roots, is responsible for most of the plant's effects on the body.

Overview

Available scientific evidence does not support claims that Indian snakeroot is effective in treating cancer, liver disease, or mental illness. It also has many dangerous side effects and is likely to increase the risk for cancer. The drug reserpine, which is extracted from snakeroot, is used in conventional medicine to treat high blood pressure and agitation.

How is it promoted for use?

According to its proponents, Indian snakeroot lowers high blood pressure (hypertension), eases anxiety and tension, reduces fever, stops diarrhea and dysentery, and can be used to treat some psychiatric illnesses. Some believe that Indian snakeroot stops or interferes with the growth of cancer cells. A few herbalists recommend that it not be used at all because of its hazardous effects.

What does it involve?

Indian snakeroot is on the Commission E (Germany's regulatory agency for herbs) list of approved herbs for treating mild hypertension. In the United Kingdom, it is available by prescription only. In the United States, Indian snakeroot supplements are available as tablets, as powder, or in liquid form. Ground or powdered Indian snakeroot can also be brewed as a tea.

Rauwolfia is also offered as a homeopathic remedy (see "Homeopathy," page 753), using extremely diluted solutions of the herb. Little or no actual snakeroot is ingested when the homeopathic remedy is used.

Reserpine, which is extracted from the rauwolfia root, is a prescription drug approved by the U.S. Food and Drug Administration (FDA). It may be given as a pill or injection. For the prescription medicine reserpine, the daily adult dose is less than 1 milligram per day.

What is the history behind it?

References to Indian snakeroot were found in Hindu texts dating back to 600 BC. A tea made from the plant has been used for centuries in India for treating insanity, hysteria, and restlessness. Mahatma Gandhi reportedly drank Indian snakeroot tea regularly.

In Western medicine, reserpine was commonly prescribed by physicians for many years to treat high blood pressure and to calm agitated people. However, other equally effective drugs with fewer side effects have since taken its place.

In India, pastes made from the plant are applied as antidotes to bites from venomous reptiles such as snakes. Extracts are sometimes taken as a remedy for constipation, liver diseases, and rheumatism. African serpentwood (*Rauwolfia vomitoria*), a plant from the same family as Indian snakeroot, has long been used in traditional African medicine to calm mentally disturbed patients.

What is the evidence?

The drug reserpine, which is extracted from Indian snakeroot, is widely known to be an effective tranquilizer and treatment for high blood pressure. Recent studies suggest that Indian snakeroot contains some substances that can reduce the growth of cancer cells in laboratory dishes and in mice, but no human studies have been reported. The consensus of available scientific evidence does not support claims that traditional preparations of Indian snakeroot can treat liver disease or cancer.

Are there any possible problems or complications?

Indian snakeroot is linked with many side effects, including decreased heart rate, low blood pressure, decreased sex drive and performance, increased appetite, weight gain, swelling, stomach complaints, diarrhea, stuffy nose, nightmares, hallucinations, stomach or intestinal ulcers, poor coordination, dizziness, and dry mouth. Indian snakeroot can also impair physical abilities and occasionally cause depression severe enough that the person loses touch with reality.

People who have had depression, asthma, heart problems, peptic ulcers or ulcerative colitis, and women who have had breast cancer should not take Indian snakeroot. Indian snakeroot should also be avoided by people taking sleeping pills, appetite suppressants, heart medicines, and antipsychotic drugs because of the chance of increased blood pressure, increased heart rate, or uncontrollable muscle movements. When taken with alcohol, it increases impairment and sleepiness. In addition, other potential interactions between Indian snakeroot and other drugs and herbs should be considered. Some of these combinations may be dangerous. Always tell your doctor and pharmacist about any herbs you are taking.

Rauwolfia may affect the fetus in unknown ways. It is known to pass into breast milk. Women who are pregnant or breastfeeding should not use this herb.

The prescription drug reserpine can interact with other medicines, such as cold remedies, heart medicines, sedatives, and mental health drugs called MAO inhibitors. Talk with your doctor or pharmacist about all medicines and supplements you are taking. Reserpine is also known to cause cancer in mice, and at least one observational study showed that people who had been treated with it had slightly higher cancer rates. Because of this, it is listed as a probable cancer-causing substance by the National Toxicology Program. Since reserpine is a component of snakeroot, it is expected that snakeroot may have some similar effects if enough of it is taken.

Some people can become allergic to rauwolfia. Relying on this type of treatment alone and avoiding or delaying conventional medical care for cancer may have serious health consequences.

This product is sold as a dietary supplement in the United States. Unlike companies that produce drugs (which must provide the FDA with results of detailed testing showing their product is safe and effective before the drug is approved for sale), the companies that make supplements do not have to show evidence of safety or health benefits to the FDA before selling their products. Supplement products without any reliable scientific evidence of health benefits may still be sold as long as the companies selling them do not claim the supplements can prevent, treat, or cure any specific disease. Some such products may not contain the amount of the herb or substance that is written on the label, and some may include other substances (contaminants). Though the FDA has written new rules to improve the quality of manufacturing processes for dietary supplements and the accurate listing of supplement ingredients, these rules do not take full effect until 2010. The new rules also do not address the safety of supplement ingredients or their effects on health when proper manufacturing techniques are used.

Most such supplements have not been tested to find out if they interact with medicines, foods, or other herbs and supplements. Even though some reports of interactions and harmful effects may be published, full studies of interactions and effects are not often available. Because of these limitations, any information on ill effects and interactions should be considered incomplete.

References

Bemis DL, Capodice JL, Gorroochurn P, Katz AE, Buttyan R. Anti-prostate cancer activity of a beta-carboline alkaloid enriched extract from *Rauwolfia vomitoria. Int J Oncol.* 2006;29:1065-1073.

Blumenthal M, ed. *The Complete German Commission E Monographs: Therapeutic Guide to Herbal Medicines.* Austin, TX: American Botanical Council; 1998.

Bown D. *New Encyclopedia of Herbs & Their Uses.* New York: DK Publishing Inc; 2001.

Fetrow CW, Avila JR. *Professional's Handbook of Complementary & Alternative Medicines.* Springhouse, PA: Springhouse Corp; 1999.

Gruenwald J. *PDR for Herbal Medicines.* 3rd ed. Montvale, NJ: Thomson PDR; 2004.

Grossman E, Messerli FH, Goldbourt U. Carcinogenicity of antihypertensive therapy. *Curr Hypertens Rep.* 2002;4:195-201.

Indian Snakeroot. PDRhealth Web site. http://www.pdrhealth.com/drugs/altmed/altmed-mono.aspx?contentFileName=ame0238.xml&contentName=Indian+Snakeroot. Accessed June 5, 2008.

Reserpine. Drugs Web site. http://www.drugs.com/pro/reserpine.html. Updated May 2006. Accessed June 6, 2008.

Reserpine: CAS RN 50-55-5. Hazardous Substances Data Bank Web site. http://toxnet.nlm.nih.gov/cgi-bin/sis/search/f?./temp/~gIIMg3:1. Accessed June 18, 2008.

KAMPO

Other common name(s): Japanese herbal therapy
Scientific/medical name(s): none

Description

Kampo is the name for a traditional Japanese herbal medicine system that involves the use of more than 210 different herbal preparations in fixed combinations. Kampo is a Japanese name for Chinese herbal medicine, although the Japanese form is now quite different from its Chinese origins. Kampo herbal mixtures made in Japan are standardized to ensure quality and consistency.

Overview

Despite the popularity of kampo among Japanese physicians and patients, available scientific evidence does not support claims that Japanese herbal preparations are effective in preventing or treating cancer in humans. At least one kampo compound shows promise against pancreatic cancer in an animal study, but human testing is needed. There is some evidence that certain kampo compounds might be helpful for other diseases, and a small study suggested that a kampo extract called TJ14 might help reduce diarrhea from irinotecan chemotherapy.

How is it promoted for use?

Proponents claim that the kampo preparations Juzen-taiho-to and Hochu-ekki-to boost the anticancer activities of a type of white blood cell called a natural killer cell. The remedy Sho-saiko is claimed to enhance the function of macrophages, a type of white blood cell that attacks cancer cells. Proponents also say that some kampo remedies are more effective than conventional methods for treating chronic prostatitis (inflammation of the prostate gland). Practitioners of kampo claim that these herbal formulas can be used to treat many other conditions such as constipation, gastritis, irritable bowel syndrome, allergies, arthritis, and hypertension.

What does it involve?

Kampo practitioners may prescribe one or more herbal mixtures. The formula selected depends on the patient's particular complaint and condition. Unlike Western medicine, kampo does not give names to diseases but describes the patient as deviating in some way from a healthy balance. A patient's illness is diagnosed based on a concept called "sho," which involves the practitioner visually observing the patient, listening to the sounds made by his or her body, smelling and touching the patient, and questioning the patient. Signs and symptoms are then interpreted according to the ancient theories of the eight disease states (two of which are yin and yo, called yin and yang in Chinese medicine) and three substances (such as qi, the life energy of the unified body and spirit). The interpretation of the patient's symptoms depends a great deal on the intuition, experience, and observation skills of the practitioner. The kampo preparation is chosen based on the diagnosis, and it is intended to help the patient return to a balanced state. The patient may have to take part in several sessions or visits with the practitioner, in which changes may be made in the herb prescriptions as the patient's symptoms change. Western diagnoses such as lung cancer or high blood pressure are not considered as part of this process.

What is the history behind it?

Kampo evolved from traditional Chinese herbal medicine and dates back more than fifteen hundred years. Kampo changed in different ways from Chinese herbal medicine over the years, however, becoming simpler and more practical than its Chinese counterpart.

When Western medicine was introduced in Japan between 1868 and 1912, the popularity of kampo declined. By 1883, Japanese law had decreed that no kampo physicians could be officially licensed as medical doctors. Interest in kampo began to be revived in 1928 and was further bolstered when people saw harmful side effects of Western drugs such as thalidomide, which caused severe birth defects. By 1976, the Japanese government had approved 147 types of kampo herbal extracts to be covered by national health insurance. In 1988, the Japanese herbal medicine industry began to regulate the production of kampo preparations to ensure quality and consistency. In 1993, the Ministry of Education in Japan approved the establishment of the

Department of Japanese Oriental (Kampo) Medicine at Toyama Medical and Pharmaceutical University, which grants university degrees in kampo.

Today about three-fourths of physicians in Japan prescribe kampo medications, and kampo is practiced alongside Western medicine. There are more than 210 prescription and over-the-counter kampo drugs officially approved by the Japanese government, some of which are covered by Japanese health insurance.

What is the evidence?

Very little scientific research has been done on kampo as a cancer therapy, and available evidence does not support claims that Japanese herbal preparations cure cancer or slow its growth in humans. In one animal study conducted in Japan, researchers concluded that the kampo preparations Juzen-taiho-to and Shimotsu-to significantly reduced the spread of colon cancer cells to the liver and of melanoma cells to the lungs. A 2006 laboratory study tested about five hundred compounds used in kampo to determine what effect they might have on cancer cells in a test tube. The cancer cells were kept in a nutrient solution to mimic the conditions in which they are able to grow in the body. The researchers identified a chemical called arctigenin in the kampo herb *Arctium lappa* that slowed the growth of pancreatic tumor cells. They also tested it in mice and found that it slowed cancer growth there as well. Other researchers have found additional substances in kampo herbs that show promise based on studies of cancer cells in laboratory dishes or animals. However, no studies have convincingly shown that kampo remedies stop or slow the spread of cancer in humans.

One small study from 2003 looked at the effect of kampo on diarrhea resulting from a type of chemotherapy called irinotecan. Patients taking a kampo medicine called TJ14 had less severe diarrhea than the control group.

Most studies of kampo have been done in Japan, with mixed results. Because many of these studies did not always use rigorous scientific methods, the results must be considered preliminary. One 2005 study compared hormone replacement therapy with gui-zhi-fu-ling-wan, a kampo medicine, to determine whether it helped hot flashes in women after menopause. Blood flow measurements under the jaw found that both treatments significantly reduced blood flow to the face. Another study by the same researchers suggested that another kampo remedy, xiong-gui-taio-xue-yin, helped reduce symptoms of depression and nervousness in women after childbirth. Because this study did not use a placebo, the effect of expectation, sometimes called the placebo effect, may have played a role in the results.

Another Japanese study tested a remedy called toki-shakuyaku-san against iron supplements for women with mild to moderate anemia. While both groups reported improved symptoms, only the women who received iron had improved blood counts.

Most of the studies looking at kampo are preliminary and have not used strict scientific methods. Carefully controlled randomized clinical trials are needed to test claims that kampo is effective against cancer and other disease or that it improves general health and well-being. The compounds that have shown promise in laboratory and animal studies need further study to determine whether they work for humans and whether they can be used without too many ill effects.

Are there any possible problems or complications?

Little is known about kampo's safety, since no controlled research has been done to learn about possible side effects. Allergic reactions to the herbs used in kampo have been reported. Some kampo products contain ephedrine, which has been banned in the United States because of its ability to cause heart attacks, strokes, and sudden death. Women who are pregnant or breastfeeding should not use kampo.

Kampo preparations produced outside Japan may differ from the Japanese products in content and preparation. The effectiveness of some herbs used in kampo can be affected by grapefruit and grapefruit juice. In addition, the potential interactions between kampo herbs and other drugs and herbs should be considered. Some of these combinations may be dangerous. Always tell your doctor and pharmacist about any herbs or supplements you are taking. Relying on this type of treatment alone and avoiding or delaying conventional medical care for cancer may have serious health consequences.

These substances may have not been thoroughly tested to find out how they interact with medicines, foods, or dietary supplements. Even though some reports of interactions and harmful effects may be published, full studies of interactions and effects are not often available. Because of these limitations, any information on ill effects and interactions should be considered incomplete.

References

Akase T, Akase T, Onodera S, Jobo T, Matsushita R, Kaneko M, Tashiro S. A comparative study of the usefulness of toki-shakuyaku-san and an oral iron preparation in the treatment of hypochromic anemia in cases of uterine myoma [Abstract]. *Yakugaku Zasshi.* 2003;123:817-824.

Awale S, Lu J, Kalauni SK, Kurashima Y, Tezuka Y, Kadota S, Esumi H. Identification of arctigenin as an antitumor agent having the ability to eliminate the tolerance of cancer cells to nutrient starvation. *Cancer Res.* 2006;66:1751-1757.

Efferth T, Miyachi H, Bartsch H. Pharmacogenomics of a traditional Japanese herbal medicine (Kampo) for cancer therapy. *Cancer Genomics Proteomics.* 2007;4:81-91.

Ikegami F, Fujii Y, Satoh T. Toxicological considerations of Kampo medicines in clinical use. *Toxicology.* 2004;198:221-228.

Mori K, Kondo T, Kamiyama Y, Kano Y, Tominaga K. Preventive effect of Kampo medicine (Hangeshashin-to) against irinotecan-induced diarrhea in advanced non-small-cell lung cancer. *Cancer Chemother Pharmacol.* 2006;51:403-406. Epub 2003 Apr 9.

Onishi Y, Yamaura T, Tauchi K, Sakamoto T, Tsukada K, Nunome S, Komatsu Y, Saiki I. Expression of the anti-metastatic effect induced by Juzen-taiho-to is based on the content of Shimotsu-to constituents. *Biol Pharm Bull.* 1998;21:761-765.

Ross C. New life for old medicine. *Lancet.* 1993;342(8869):485-486.
Erratum in:
Lancet. 1993;342(8873):752.

Terasawa K. Evidence-based reconstruction of kampo medicine: part I—is kampo CAM? *Evid Based Complement Alternat Med.* 2004;1:11-16. http://ecam.oxfordjournals.org/cgi/content/full/1/1/11. Accessed August 14, 2008.

Terasawa K. Evidence-based reconstruction of kampo medicine: part II—the concept of sho. *Evid Based Complement Alternat Med.* 2004;1:119-123. http://ecam.oxfordjournals.org/cgi/content/full/1/2/119. Accessed August 14, 2008.

Terasawa K. Evidence-based reconstruction of kampo medicine: part III—how should kampo be evaluated? *Evid Based Complement Alternat Med.* 2004;1:219-222. http://ecam.oxfordjournals.org/cgi/content/full/1/3/219. Accessed August 14, 2008.

Ushiroyama T, Ikeda A, Sakuma K, Ueki M. Comparing the effects of estrogen and an herbal medicine on peripheral blood flow in post-menopausal women with hot flashes: hormone replacement therapy and gui-zhi-fu-ling-wan, a Kampo medicine [Abstract]. *Am J Chin Med.* 2005;33:259-267.

Yafune A, Cyong JC. Population pharmacokinetic analysis of ephedrine in Kampo prescriptions: a study in healthy volunteers and clinical use of the pharmacokinetic results [Abstract]. *Int J Clin Pharmacol Res.* 2001;21:95-102.

KAVA

Other common name(s): kava-kava, kavalactones
Scientific/medical name(s): *Piper methysticum*

Description

Kava is a large shrub with broad, heart-shaped leaves, a member of the same family as black pepper (the *Piperaceae* family). It is native to many Pacific islands, including New Guinea, Fiji, Tahiti, Samoa, Tonga, and Hawaii. The roots of the plant are used in herbal remedies and for ceremonies or rituals.

Overview

Some studies support the use of kava for reducing anxiety, and it is widely used to help with sleep. It may have several effects on the brain, some of which are similar to prescription tranquilizers. The safe dosage of kava needed to reduce anxiety is uncertain. Reports of more than fifty cases of severe liver impairment in people taking kava supplements have led several countries to ban or restrict sales of kava. Some of the patients had liver transplants and some died. Side effects appear to increase with larger doses taken over longer periods of time. Kava appears to increase the effects of some medicines and can interfere with anesthesia as well.

How is it promoted for use?

Kava supplements are promoted mainly for anxiety, nervous tension, stress, restlessness, and, at higher doses, sleeplessness. Many users say the herb improves mood and brings on a sense of well-being, relaxation, and even euphoria.

In South Pacific folk medicine, a drink made from the kava root has been used to treat uterine inflammation, headaches, colds, rheumatism, and menopausal symptoms. In these traditional settings, the kava root is chewed, ground, or beaten, then soaked in cold water or coconut milk. Users drink the liquid to relieve headaches, restore vigor, promote urination, soothe upset stomachs, ease symptoms of asthma and tuberculosis, and cure fungal infections. Some users believe that kava inhibits the growth of the gonorrhea bacteria. The leaves and branches of the kava plant are sometimes applied to the skin. Kava creams are used to soothe stings and inflamed skin.

Kava is not promoted as an anticancer treatment. While its reputation for easing mild anxiety may be of interest to people with cancer, there are many effective prescription medicines and many nonmedical treatments (including complementary mind–body methods) for anxiety that patients can discuss with their doctors.

What does it involve?

Kava is available as a tablet, capsule, cream, and as a powder, which can be made into tea or mixed with other drinks. Daily doses range from 50 to 240 milligrams of kavalactones (the active ingredient in kava). For anxiety, it may be taken several times a day. For sleep, it is taken about an hour before bedtime.

Kava dietary supplements are made by using solvents to extract kavalactones from kava roots. There are reports that some manufacturers have also used the peelings from kava stems, which contain a possible toxin. Differences in quality and type of ingredients and methods of extraction mean that the kava used as a dietary supplement is not the same as the kava used in the traditional Fijian, Samoan, and Tongan cultures. There is some question about whether the differences between the plant as used traditionally and kava dietary supplements may account for the rare but extreme cases of toxicity that have been linked to supplements.

Because of reports of liver failure caused by kava supplements, Germany, France, the United Kingdom, the Netherlands, Canada, and Switzerland have all banned or restricted kava. The U.S. Food and Drug Administration (FDA) and the Centers for Disease Control and Prevention have issued warnings about liver failure to U.S. consumers.

What is the history behind it?

The people of the South Pacific have used kava socially, ceremonially, and medicinally for thousands of years. A beverage prepared from the kava root is traditionally offered to visiting royalty and dignitaries and served at meetings of village elders. The drink is also often shared at social gatherings.

Accounts of kava first came to the West from the English naval officer Captain James Cook, who encountered the plant during a trip to Polynesia in the 1770s. Interest in kava spread quickly. Kava first underwent medical investigation in the 1860s and by the end of the nineteenth century, kava preparations were available in German pharmacies.

What is the evidence?

Kava has been the focus of dozens of medical studies, some of which support claims made about the herb's usefulness for mild anxiety. Kava appears to ease symptoms of tension, nervousness, and stress. In recent studies, patients with varying levels of anxiety took kava extract, and many reported relief within days or weeks. It does not appear to be very effective in those with moderate to severe anxiety.

Some researchers have found that kava compares well to prescription anti-anxiety medicines. In clinical studies, it caused few side effects and did not appear to be addictive. One study showed that kava did not impair reaction time and even improved concentration. In comparison, common prescription drugs for anxiety slow reaction time. In other recent clinical trials, however, kava was no more effective than placebo in treating anxiety or insomnia.

Exactly how kava works is still uncertain. Some scientists think that kava works in the brain in a similar way to the group of prescription tranquilizers called benzodiazepines. In addition, it appears to block dopamine, which may explain how it can produce a sensation of pleasure. It may also act in other parts of the brain and other organs.

More research is needed on long-term use and safe dosing. Studies are also needed to find out whether the cases of liver failure were caused by the way the kava was processed or by the kava root itself, and whether the problem can be addressed so that these serious effects can be avoided in the future.

Are there any possible problems or complications?

In rare cases, kava can lead to liver failure and other life-threatening problems. Even moderate use can lead to abnormal organ function, including increased levels of liver enzymes. According to the FDA, people who have had liver problems and those taking medications that may affect the liver, such as cholesterol-lowering drugs, should check with their doctors before taking kava. The FDA further recommends that kava be stopped if symptoms of liver disease, such as jaundice (marked by brown urine and yellowing of the eyes or skin) occur. Other symptoms of liver disease include nausea, vomiting, light-colored stools, unusual tiredness, weakness, stomach pain, and loss of appetite. People who drink alcohol regularly have a higher risk for liver damage.

Kava may affect reflexes and judgment, so it should not be used by people driving or operating heavy machinery. Other side effects of kava include severe involuntary movements, headache, upset stomach, drowsiness, trouble breathing, poor appetite, weight loss, scaly skin, red eyes, abnormal blood cells, blood in the urine, poor coordination, and muscle weakness. Kava may worsen symptoms in people who have Parkinson's disease, seizures, depression, or bipolar disorder. Studies have not been done on children or women who are pregnant or breastfeeding, and no safety data is available. Although rare, some allergic reactions to kava have been reported.

Kava should not be taken with drugs that cause drowsiness, such as anti-anxiety medicines, muscle relaxants, sedatives, pain relievers, or alcohol, because of the risk for extreme drowsiness or even unconsciousness. People taking antidepressants or drugs that affect dopamine (such as haloperidol, risperidone, metoclopramide, or l-dopa) should not use kava. Those taking blood-thinning medications may have increased risk for bleeding. Because of its potential to interact with anesthetics, people who are planning to have surgery should stop taking it for two to three weeks before surgery. In addition, other potential interactions between kava and other drugs and herbs should be considered. Always tell your doctor and pharmacist about any herbs you are taking.

A safe dosage of kava has not been determined. Kava should not be taken for more than four weeks unless recommended by a doctor. Relying on this type of treatment alone and avoiding or delaying conventional medical care for cancer may have serious health consequences.

This product is sold as a dietary supplement in the United States. Unlike companies that produce drugs (which must provide the FDA with results of detailed testing showing their product is safe and effective before the drug is approved for sale), the companies that make supplements do not have to show evidence of safety or health benefits to the FDA before selling their products. Supplement products without any reliable scientific evidence of health benefits may still be sold as long as the companies

selling them do not claim the supplements can prevent, treat, or cure any specific disease. Some such products may not contain the amount of the herb or substance that is written on the label, and some may include other substances (contaminants). Though the FDA has written new rules to improve the quality of manufacturing processes for dietary supplements and the accurate listing of supplement ingredients, these rules do not take full effect until 2010. The new rules also do not address the safety of supplement ingredients or their effects on health when proper manufacturing techniques are used.

Most such supplements have not been tested to find out if they interact with medicines, foods, or other herbs and supplements. Even though some reports of interactions and harmful effects may be published, full studies of interactions and effects are not often available. Because of these limitations, any information on ill effects and interactions should be considered incomplete.

References

Blumenthal M, ed. *The Complete German Commission E Monographs: Therapeutic Guide to Herbal Medicines.* Austin, TX: American Botanical Council; 1998.

Bressler R. Interactions between kava and prescription medications. *Geriatrics.* 2005;60;24-25.

Cerrato PL. Natural tranquilizers? *RN.* 1998;61:61-62.

Connor KM, Payne V, Davidson JR. Kava in generalized anxiety disorder: three placebo-controlled trials. *Int Clin Psychopharmacol.* 2006;21:249-253.

Cupp MJ. Herbal remedies: adverse effects and drug interactions. *Am Fam Physician.* 1999;59:1239-1245.

Ernst E. Herbal remedies for anxiety - a systematic review of controlled clinical trials. *Phytomedicine.* 2006;13:205-208. Epub 2005 Aug 15.

Gruenwald J. *PDR for Herbal Medicines.* 3rd ed. Montvale, NJ: Thomson PDR; 2004.

Jacobs BP, Bent S, Tice JA, Blackwell T, Cummings SR. An internet-based randomized, placebo-controlled trial of kava and valerian for anxiety and insomnia. *Medicine (Baltimore).* 2005;84:197-207.

Kava: a human health risk assessment. Technical report series no. 30, June 2004. Food Standards Australia New Zealand Web site. http://www.foodstandards.gov.au/_srcfiles/30_Kava.pdf. Accessed June 6, 2008.

Kava. Memorial Sloan-Kettering Cancer Center Web site. http://www.mskcc.org/mskcc/html/69272.cfm. Updated September 17, 2007. Accessed June 6, 2008.

Kava. University of Washington Department of Family Medicine Web site. http://www.fammed.washington.edu/predoctoral/CAM/images/kava.pdf. Accessed June 5, 2008.

Overton A. Kava: Case. Utox Update. Utah Poison Control Center. 2001;3:1-2.

Pittler MH, Ernst E. Kava extract for treating anxiety. *Cochrane Database Syst Rev.* 2003;(1):CD003383.

Wong AH, Smith M, Boon HS. Herbal remedies in psychiatric practice. *Arch Gen Psychiatry.* 1998;55:1033-1044.

LARCH

Other common name(s): larch arabinogalactan, American larch, Eastern larch, European larch, common larch, tamarack

Scientific/medical name(s): *Larix occidentalis, Larix laricina, Larix decidua, Larix europaea*

Description

A member of the pine family, the larch tree has the unusual quality of losing its needles each fall. Several types of larch tree grow in central Europe, North America, northern Russia, and Siberia. The bark and its resin are used in herbal remedies. An extract of larch called arabinogalactan is sold as an herbal remedy and fiber supplement.

Overview

Larch arabinogalactan is approved by the U.S. Food and Drug Administration (FDA) as a food additive and fiber supplement. However, available scientific evidence does not support claims that larch bark is effective in treating cancer or any other disease in humans. Early laboratory evidence suggested that larch arabinogalactan may stimulate the immune system. However, a more recent study in mice contradicts this finding. Further studies are needed to identify other uses for larch in humans.

How is it promoted for use?

Proponents believe that larch can be used to treat bronchitis, colds, and other respiratory conditions. Arabinogalactan is promoted to stimulate the immune system and increase the effectiveness of some drugs, including chemotherapy medications. Some claim that the compound also inhibits the spread of cancer to the liver. Larch resin is recommended to be applied to the skin for wounds and scrapes.

What does it involve?

The extract arabinogalactan is a type of complex sugar, called a polysaccharide or glycan, that the body cannot digest. Arabinogalactans are also found in some common foods such as tomatoes, wheat, carrots, certain mushrooms, and other plants. The food additive gum arabic is a type of arabinogalactan.

Larch arabinogalactan is available as a fiber supplement in powder form. It can be mixed with water or juice or sprinkled on food. It can also be bought in capsule and tablet form. Larch resin is available in ointments, lotions, and oils, often in blends with other herbs and oils, for application to the skin.

What is the history behind it?

The bark of the larch tree has been used in various folk medicine traditions to treat rheumatism, jaundice, skin problems, and as a poultice for wounds, swelling, and burns. Native Americans used the needles and inner bark to make a tea to treat coughs and constipation. Resin from the bark was used by Native Americans as a chewing gum and to relieve indigestion. The resin was also used to treat kidney and lung disorders and as a dressing for burns and sores.

Larch arabinogalactan was first isolated from the bark of the larch tree in 1992, although this substance is also available from other plant sources. The FDA has approved arabinogalactan from both the Eastern and the Western larch as a food additive, so that it can be used in foods as an emulsifier, stabilizer, thickener, moisture retainer, binder, and for other purposes. It is also approved as a fiber supplement.

What is the evidence?

In one laboratory study, researchers at the University of Minnesota concluded that larch arabinogalactan is a safe source of dietary fiber and may be effective in boosting the immune system. The research was sponsored, however, by the company that owns the patent to the extract. Another laboratory study done in Germany found that arabinogalactan from the Western larch stimulated the action of a type of white blood cell called natural killer cells.

More recently, a brief animal study looked at white blood cells that serve important immune functions. The researchers found that arabinogalactan actually seemed to suppress production of some of these white blood cells, seeming to contradict the results of the earlier study. With daily injections of arabinogalactan, the mice had fewer white blood cells in the bone marrow after a week. Levels of natural killer cells went back to normal after two weeks of injections. Immune cells in the spleen were mostly present in normal numbers, although the levels of some types of immune cells were lower in the spleen even when they were normal in the bone marrow. Further studies are necessary to determine whether arabinogalactan helps human immune function.

A 2004 human study compared larch arabinogalactan with rice starch to determine whether it improved cholesterol, triglycerides, and sugar levels. At the end of six months, there were no differences between the group that received rice starch and the group that received arabinogalactan.

Little scientific information is available on the effects of larch resin mixtures on human skin. It may have antiseptic, or germ-killing, properties.

Are there any possible problems or complications?

Larch has been approved by Germany's Commission E for external use, and is recommended for colds, coughs, and bronchitis. The *Larix* genus is listed in the FDA's Poisonous Plant Database, although reports of toxic effects were not found in the medical literature. Kidney damage might occur if the bark is ingested or if the oils are spread over a large area of the body and absorbed through the skin.

Larch allergies have not been reported; however, rashes, hives, and contact dermatitis have occurred in people working with some species of larch. It is possible that many of these reactions are due to contact with lichens that grow on the bark of the larch rather than the larch itself.

The larch extract arabinogalactan is generally recognized as safe and is approved by the FDA as a food additive and fiber supplement. However, it contains galactose, a type of sugar, and people who require a low-galactose diet should avoid arabinogalactan. Those with lactose intolerance should use the supplement with caution. Relying on this type of treatment alone and avoiding or delaying conventional medical care for cancer may have serious health consequences.

This product is sold as a dietary supplement in the United States. Unlike companies that produce drugs (which must provide the FDA with results of detailed testing showing their product is safe and effective before the drug is approved for sale), the companies that make supplements do not have to show evidence of safety or health benefits to the FDA before selling their products. Supplement products without any reliable scientific evidence of health benefits may still be sold as long as the companies selling them do not claim the supplements can prevent, treat, or cure any specific disease. Some such products may not contain the amount of the herb or substance that is written on the label, and some may include other substances (contaminants). Though the FDA has written new rules to improve the quality of manufacturing processes for dietary supplements and the accurate listing of supplement ingredients, these rules do not take full effect until 2010. The new rules also do not address the safety of supplement ingredients or their effects on health when proper manufacturing techniques are used.

Most such supplements have not been tested to find out if they interact with medicines, foods, or other herbs and supplements. Even though some reports of interactions and harmful effects may be published, full studies of interactions and effects are not often available. Because of these limitations, any information on ill effects and interactions should be considered incomplete.

References

Adams J. University of Minnesota researchers uncover immune-boosting fiber. *Minnesota Daily.* January 7,1999.

Blumenthal M, ed. *The Complete German Commission E Monographs: Therapeutic Guide to Herbal Medicines.* Austin, TX: American Botanical Council; 1998.

Bown D. *New Encyclopedia of Herbs & Their Uses.* New York: DK Publishing Inc; 2001.

Center for Food Safety and Applied Nutrition. Agency response letter: GRAS notice no. GRN 000084. February 19, 2002. US Food and Drug Administration Web site. http://www.cfsan.fda.gov/~rdb/opa-g084.html. Accessed June 6, 2008.

Currier NL, Lejtenyi D, Miller SC. Effect over time of in-vivo administration of the polysaccharide arabinogalactan on immune and hemopoietic cell lineages in murine spleen and bone marrow. *Phytomedicine.* 2003;10:145-153.

Gruenwald J. *PDR for Herbal Medicines.* 3rd ed. Montvale, NJ: Thomson PDR; 2004.

Hauer J, Anderer FA. Mechanism of stimulation of human natural killer cytotoxicity by arabinogalactan from Larix occidentalis. *Cancer Immunol Immunother.* 1993;36:237-244.

Larch arabinogalactan. PDRhealth Web site. http://www.pdrhealth.com/drug_info/nmdrugprofiles/nutsupdrugs/lar_0320.shtml. Accessed April 23, 2007. Content no longer available.

Larch. PDRhealth Web site. http://www.pdrhealth.com/drugs/altmed/altmed-mono.aspx?contentFileName=ame0368.xml&contentName=Larch. Accessed June 6, 2008.

Larix laricina. US Department of Agriculture Forest Service Web site. http://www2.fpl.fs.fed.us/TechSheets/SoftwoodNA/pdf_files/larixlariceng.pdf. Accessed June 6, 2008.

Lichens. DermNet NZ Web site. http://www.dermnetnz.org/dermatitis/plants/lichen.html. Updated March 18, 2008. Accessed June 6, 2008.

Marett R, Slavin JL. No long-term benefits of supplementation with arabinogalactan on serum lipids and glucose. *J Am Diet Assoc.* 2004;104:636-639.

Robinson RR, Feirtag J, Slavin JL. Effects of dietary arabinogalactan on gastrointestinal and blood parameters in healthy human subjects. *J Am Coll Nutr.* 2001;20:279-285.

LICORICE

Other common name(s): sweet root, licorice root
Scientific/medical name(s): gan cao, *Glycyrrhiza glabra, Glycyrrhiza uralensis*

Description

Licorice is a perennial plant that grows in southern Europe, Asia, and the Mediterranean. The dried roots and underground stems of the plant are used in herbal remedies.

Overview

Licorice root is an ingredient in many traditional Chinese herbal remedies. It also has been used in other countries to treat a wide variety of health problems. However, it is linked to some fairly serious side effects. Whole-herb licorice can cause an imbalance of fluid and the mineral potassium in the body, which can lead to heart rhythm problems, high blood pressure, muscle weakness, and even paralysis. While recent laboratory research has identified some components that might be useful in cancer prevention or treatment, there is almost no information available about their effectiveness in humans. More research is needed to find out whether licorice extract has any role in cancer prevention or treatment.

How is it promoted for use?

Licorice is promoted to treat peptic ulcers, eczema, skin infections, cold sores, menopausal symptoms, liver disease, respiratory ailments, inflammatory problems, chronic fatigue syndrome, AIDS, and even cancer. It has also been promoted to relieve symptoms of Addison's disease, lower cholesterol and triglyceride levels, strengthen the immune system, and treat hepatitis.

Many food products are widely available that contain traces of licorice. Some licorice candy sold in the United States is actually flavored with anise and does not contain licorice. Glycyrrhizin (an active ingredient from the plant) is used as a flavoring in candy, gum, cookies, beverages, and cough syrup. Licorice is also used as a flavoring for tobacco products.

What does it involve?

Licorice is packaged as capsules, as tablets, and as a liquid extract. It can be purchased at grocery stores, health food stores, or pharmacies. According to Commission E (Germany's regulatory agency for herbs), the recommended dosage ranges from 200 to 600 milligrams for no more than four weeks for peptic ulcers. Licorice is also an ingredient in many traditional Chinese herbal formulations. The best known of these are herbal products for prostate cancer treatment such as PC-HOPE and PC-CARE (see page 448). Because of its side effects, glycyrrhizin is removed from many licorice formulas. This is called deglycyrrhizinated licorice (DGL).

What is the history behind it?

Licorice extract has been used in traditional Chinese medicine for centuries. The Chinese used it as a mild laxative and to help regulate the heartbeat in those with heart problems. Traditional Chinese herbalists often prescribe licorice with the intent of helping other herbs to work better together and promoting absorption of herbs. It was also used for medicinal purposes in ancient Egypt, Greece, and Rome.

What is the evidence?

Some research suggests that licorice can promote healing of peptic ulcers. However, most of the evidence is from older studies, smaller case series, and laboratory studies. Licorice is less effective than conventional prescription and over-the-counter medications for ulcers.

Laboratory studies have identified several substances in licorice that may help prevent DNA mutations, inhibit tumor formation, or even kill cancer cells. For example, licochalcone-A, glabridin, and licocoumarone have been tested using cancer cells growing in laboratory dishes, and preliminary studies indicate that these chemicals can stop the growth of or even kill breast cancer, prostate cancer, and leukemia cells. In studies with mice, glycyrrhizin and glycyrrhizic acid reduced formation of skin, colon, liver, uterine, and breast cancers.

Although results of animal studies suggest some chemicals from licorice might be useful in preventing or treating some forms of cancer, no human clinical trials of licorice supplements or substances from licorice have been reported. Licorice is an ingredient in PC-SPES, an herbal product for prostate cancer treatment, and although there have been several clinical trials of PC-SPES, they do not address whether licorice contributed to its benefits.

Glycyrrhizin may be useful as a treatment for chronic hepatitis, and a Japanese study found that patients with chronic hepatitis C who took this supplement had lower risk for liver cancer. However, this study asked patients to remember and report whether they had used the supplement in the past. This kind of study is considered less reliable than a clinical trial that randomly assigns patients to various treatments and follows the patients over time.

Are there any possible problems or complications?

Regular consumption of licorice has been shown to cause headaches, lethargy, water retention, high blood pressure, and muscle weakness. In extremely large amounts, it can cause paralysis and heart failure. People with high blood pressure, irregular heartbeat, or cardiovascular, kidney, or liver diseases should avoid licorice unless given under a doctor's supervision. Use of DGL, or deglycyrrhizinated licorice, helps to avoid the risk for more serious side effects.

Studies in laboratory animals have suggested that licorice may cause birth defects. Women who are pregnant should not use licorice. Most herbalists also recommend that women who are breastfeeding avoid this supplement.

In addition, the potential interactions between licorice and other drugs and herbs should be considered. For example, licorice can cause problems for patients taking heart medicines, steroids, diuretics, or insulin. Blood-thinning medications and hormone therapy can interact with licorice and even DGL. Some of these combinations may be dangerous. Always tell your doctor and pharmacist about any herbs you are taking. Relying on this type of treatment alone and avoiding or delaying conventional medical care for cancer may have serious health consequences.

This product is sold as a dietary supplement in the United States. Unlike companies that produce drugs (which must provide the FDA with results of detailed testing showing their product is safe and effective before the drug is approved for sale), the companies that make supplements do not have to show evidence of safety or health benefits to the FDA before selling their products. Supplement products without any reliable scientific evidence of health benefits may still be sold as long as the companies selling them do not claim the supplements can prevent, treat, or cure any specific disease. Some such products may not contain the amount of the herb or substance that is written on the label, and some may include other substances (contaminants). Though the FDA has written new rules to improve the quality of manufacturing processes for dietary supplements and the accurate listing of supplement ingredients, these rules do not take full effect until 2010. The new rules also do not address the safety of supplement ingredients or their effects on health when proper manufacturing techniques are used.

Most such supplements have not been tested to find out if they interact with medicines, foods, or other herbs and supplements. Even though some reports of interactions and harmful effects may be published, full studies of interactions and effects are not often available. Because of these limitations, any information on ill effects and interactions should be considered incomplete.

References

Arase Y, Ikeda K, Murashima N, Chayama K, Tsubota A, Koida I, Suzuki Y, Saitoh S, Kobayashi M, Kumada H. The long term efficacy of glycyrrhizin in chronic hepatitis C patients. *Cancer.* 1997;79:1494-1500.

Blumenthal M, ed. *The Complete German Commission E Monographs: Therapeutic Guide to Herbal Medicines.* Austin, TX: American Botanical Council; 1998.

Davis EA, Morris DJ. Medicinal uses of licorice through the millennia: good and plenty of it. *Mol Cell Endocrinol.* 1991;78:1-6.

Edwards CR. Lessons from licorice. *N Engl J Med.* 1991;325:1242-1243.

Fu Y, Hsieh TC, Guo J, Kunicki J, Lee MY. Darzynkiewicz Z, Wu JM. Licochalcone-A, a novel flavonoid isolated from licorice root (*Glycyrrhiza glabra*), causes G2 and late-G1 arrests in androgen-independent PC-3 prostate cancer cells. *Biochem Biophys Res Commun.* 2004;322:263-270.

Izzo AA, Di Carlo G, Borrelli F, Ernst E. Cardiovascular pharmacotherapy and herbal medicines: the risk of drug interaction. *Int J Cardiol.* 2005;98:1-14.

Licorice. Guide to medicinal and aromatic plants. Purdue University Web site. http://www.hort.purdue.edu/newcrop/med-aro/factsheets/LICORICE.html. Updated December 6, 1997. Accessed June 6, 2008.

Licorice. Memorial Sloan-Kettering Cancer Center Web site. http://www.mskcc.org/mskcc/html/69281.cfm. Updated August 14, 2007. Accessed June 6, 2008.

Miyake K, Tango T, Ota Y, Mitamura K, Yoshiba M, Kako M, Hayashi S, Ikeda Y, Hayashida N, Iwabuchi S, Sato Y, Tomi T, Funaki N, Hashimoto N, Umeda T, Miyazaki J, Tanaka K, Endo Y, Suzuki H. Efficacy of Stronger Neo-Minophagen C compared between two doses administered three times a week on patients with chronic viral hepatitis. *J Gastroenterol Hepatol.* 2002;17:1198-1204.

Niwa K, Lian Z, Onogi K, Yun W, Tang L, Mori H, Tamaya T. Preventive effects of glycyrrhizin on estrogen-related endometrial carcinogenesis in mice. *Oncol Rep.* 2007;17:617-622

Sigurjonsdottir HA, Manhem K, Axelson M, Wallerstedt S. Subjects with essential hypertension are more sensitive to the inhibition of 11 beta-HSD by liquorice. *J Hum Hypertens.* 2003;17:125-131.

Suzuki F, Schmitt DA, Utsunomiya T, Pollard RB. Stimulation of host resistance against tumors by glycyrrhizin, an active component of licorice roots. *In Vivo.* 1992;6:589-596.

Tamir S, Eizenberg M, Somjen D, Stern N, Shelach R, Kaye A, Vaya J. Estrogenic and antiproliferative properties of glabridin from licorice in human breast cancer cells. *Cancer Res.* 2000;60:5704-5709.

Wang ZY, Nixon DW. Licorice and cancer. *Nutr Cancer.* 2001;39:1-11.

MARIJUANA

Other common name(s): pot, grass, cannabis, weed, hemp
Scientific/medical name(s): *Cannabis sativa*, delta-9-tetrahydrocannabinol (THC)

Description

Cannabis sativa is an annual plant that grows wild in warm and tropical climates throughout the world and is cultivated commercially. The leaves and buds of the plant have been used in herbal remedies for centuries. Scientists have identified sixty-six biologically active ingredients, called cannabinoids, in marijuana. The most potent of these is thought to be the chemical delta-9-tetrahydrocannabinol, or THC, although other active substances are being tested.

Overview

The cannabinoid drug THC has been approved by the U.S. Food and Drug Administration (FDA) for use in relieving nausea and vomiting and increasing appetite in people with cancer and AIDS. Testing of other marijuana extracts is still in the early stages. Results are mixed in studies of marijuana use for muscle tremors and spasticity in people with multiple sclerosis or Parkinson's disease.

How is it promoted for use?

THC is promoted to relieve pain, control nausea and vomiting, and stimulate appetite in people with cancer and AIDS. Researchers also report that THC decreases pressure within the eyes, thereby reducing the severity of glaucoma.

Some supporters claim that marijuana has antibacterial properties, inhibits tumor growth, and enlarges the airways, which may ease the severity of asthma attacks. Others claim that marijuana can be used to control seizures and muscle spasms in people who have epilepsy and spinal cord injuries.

What does it involve?

THC has been available by prescription (as dronabinol) in pill or suppository form since 1985. Several pharmaceutical companies are also developing a form of THC that would be delivered through an inhaler. Some research studies use a liquid cannabis-based extract that is sprayed in the mouth to deliver marijuana compounds.

In raw form, marijuana is most commonly smoked in pipes or homemade cigarettes. It is also eaten directly or mixed with foods. Raw marijuana is illegal in the United States and is not approved by the FDA for medical uses.

What is the history behind it?

Marijuana has been described in Indian and Chinese medical texts for more than three thousand years. It was used to treat conditions such as beriberi, constipation, gout, malaria, rheumatism, and absent-mindedness, as well as depression, insomnia, vomiting, tetanus, and coughs. In the Middle Ages, herbalists used it externally to relieve muscle and joint pain. In the mid-1800s, the plant was mentioned as a treatment for gonorrhea and angina (chest pains related to heart disease). It was also used to treat intestinal pain, cholera, epilepsy, strychnine poisoning, bronchitis, whooping cough, and asthma. Marijuana is legal in many parts of Asia and the Middle East but illegal in most Western countries.

In the last few years, marijuana has been the subject of extensive medical research. However, political and legal controversies surrounding its status as an illegal substance, as well as concerns about potentially harmful side effects, have hampered the process of scientific inquiry in many countries, including the United States. Despite this, researchers continue to study marijuana's potential medical applications.

The prescription drug dronabinol is made from an active ingredient of marijuana. It is available for patients with chemotherapy-related nausea and vomiting that does not respond to usual treatments. It is also used for people with AIDS and patients experiencing severe weight loss, sometimes called wasting.

What is the evidence?

Much of the research on marijuana has been centered on cannabinoids, the best known active ingredients in marijuana, and THC, the cannabinoid thought to be the most potent. Marijuana and its extracts have been studied for their effects on nausea and vomiting related to chemotherapy, appetite, glaucoma, neuropathic pain, and spasticity in patients with multiple sclerosis. Research findings have been mixed.

One review of studies published between 1975 and 1996 concluded that oral THC is as effective or more effective than commonly used prescription drugs for reducing nausea associated with chemotherapy. The reviewers also concluded that cannabinoids may be useful at low doses to improve appetite in patients with AIDS. They found that THC reduces eye pressure in people who have glaucoma. None of the studies, however, showed that THC or other ingredients in marijuana addressed the underlying causes of glaucoma. They reported that marijuana may cause toxic side effects, and the benefits of THC must be carefully weighed against its potential risks. They concluded that the evidence did not support smoking marijuana as a medication and that additional research was needed.

Further research into marijuana's benefit for nausea and vomiting has had conflicting results. A review suggested that cannabinoids did not work better than standard treatment when used with chemotherapy known to produce severe vomiting.

Another comprehensive review of marijuana studies found there was not enough persuasive evidence to recommend marijuana as a treatment for nausea. However, a more recent study concluded that specific chemicals in marijuana, or synthetic copies of those chemicals, may prove helpful to some patients with certain illnesses or symptoms, including nausea.

A 2006 study of people with advanced cancer and weight loss found that neither cannabis extract nor low doses of THC improved appetite significantly better than placebo. Over the six-week period, all three groups reported improved appetite. However, doses used in this study were low and were not increased over time as is usually done with THC. A 2005 study in New York compared dronabinol and marijuana in people with human immunodeficiency virus who had smoked marijuana previously. The researchers noted that both improved food intake in people who had severe weight loss due to their illness.

A 2004 study looked at people with multiple sclerosis (MS) using cannabis-based liquid extract. This liquid extract contained both THC and cannabidiol, which has different activity from THC. The patients receiving the extract reported less spasticity than those on placebo. In contrast, a small study that looked at arm tremors in people with MS compared the liquid marijuana extract with placebo. It found no measurable difference in tremor between people getting the extract and those on placebo.

A small early study of CT-3, a substance related to delta-9-THC, looked at people with neuropathic pain (pain related to the nerves of the body). It tested CT-3 against a placebo and found that patients reported lower pain levels three hours after receiving the CT-3 compared with placebo.

The most in-depth investigation into the medical use of marijuana was authorized by the U.S. Government in 1997. The Office of National Drug Control Policy commissioned the Institute of Medicine (IOM) to assess the potential health benefits and risks of marijuana. The IOM is an independent research body affiliated with the National Academy of Sciences. The IOM issued its final report in 1999 and offered several conclusions regarding marijuana's usefulness.

First, it found that scientific data indicated that cannabinoids, particularly THC, have some potential to relieve pain, control nausea and vomiting, and stimulate appetite. Cannabinoids probably affect control of movement and memory, but their effects on the immune system are unclear. It found that some of the effects of cannabinoids, such as reduced anxiety, sedation, and euphoria, may be helpful for certain patients and situations and undesirable for others. Based on the many studies reviewed, researchers also found that smoking marijuana delivers harmful substances and may be an important risk factor in the development of lung diseases and certain types of cancer. The IOM stated that because marijuana contains a number of active compounds, it cannot be expected to provide precise effects unless the individual components are isolated.

More recently, scientists reported that cannabidiol, one of the chemicals found in marijuana, slows growth of breast cancer cells growing in laboratory dishes. However, this substance has not yet been tested in humans or even in animals that have cancer. Cannabidiol levels in marijuana are low, so any benefit from this compound would require use of a purified and concentrated form.

Are there any possible problems or complications?

Smoking or eating raw marijuana can cause a number of effects, including feelings of euphoria, short-term memory loss, difficulty in completing complex tasks, changes in the perception of time and space, sleepiness, anxiety, confusion, and inability to concentrate. In studies, cannabinoids have been linked with dizziness, depression, paranoia, and hallucinations. Other side effects include low blood pressure, rapid heartbeat, and heart palpitations. Instances of death are rare. A review of studies looked at cannabinoid use in chemotherapy patients and found that one in eleven would stop using it because of side effects.

Many researchers agree that marijuana contains known carcinogens, or chemicals that can cause cancer. Results of epidemiologic studies of marijuana and cancer risk have been inconsistent, and most recent epidemiologic studies have not found a substantial effect on cancer risk. However, some researchers caution that these studies are difficult to conduct, as some people may not be truthful about illegal habits such as smoking marijuana, and that negative results should not be interpreted as convincing evidence of safety. They caution that smoking marijuana may decrease reproductive function, cause lung disease, and increase the risk for cancer of the lungs, mouth, and tongue. It may also suppress the body's immune system and increase the risk for leukemia in children whose mothers smoke marijuana during pregnancy. Women who are pregnant or breastfeeding should not use marijuana.

The symptoms of a marijuana overdose include nausea, vomiting, hacking cough, disturbances to heart rhythms, and numbness in the limbs. Chronic use can also lead to laryngitis, bronchitis, and general apathy. With chronic use, the ability to learn and remember new information may become impaired.

Although it is rare, severe shutdown of blood circulation to the arms or legs has been reported in young people who smoked marijuana. In some cases, it was so severe that amputation was required. Marijuana may also serve as a trigger for heart attack on rare occasions, usually within an hour of smoking. Allergic reactions, some severe, have been reported.

Dronabinol, the prescription drug form of THC, also can cause complications. People with heart problems may have trouble with increased heart rate, decreased blood pressure, and fainting. Dronabinol can cause mood changes or a feeling of being "high" that is uncomfortable for some people. It can also worsen depression, mania, or other mental illness, and it may increase some effects of sedatives, sleeping pills, or alcohol, such as sleepiness and poor coordination.

Driving, operating machinery, or engaging in hazardous activities that require clear thinking and good coordination are not recommended until dronabinol's effects are known. People taking dronabinol should be under the supervision of a responsible adult at all times when they start taking the medication and after any dose adjustments.

Like marijuana, dronabinol should not be used during breastfeeding because the drug is concentrated in breast milk and is passed to the baby. It is not recommended during pregnancy. People who have had emotional illnesses, paranoia, or hallucinations may become worse when taking dronabinol or marijuana. Older patients may have more problems with side effects and are usually started on lower doses. Relying on this type of treatment alone and avoiding or delaying conventional medical care for cancer may have serious health consequences.

This substance has not been thoroughly tested to find out how it interacts with medicines, foods, or dietary supplements. Even though some reports of interactions and harmful effects may be published, full studies of interactions and effects are not often available. Because of these limitations, any information on ill effects and interactions should be considered incomplete.

References

Barsky SH, Roth MD, Kleerup EC, Simmons M, Tashkin DP. Histopathologic and molecular alterations in bronchial epithelium in habitual smokers of marijuana, cocaine, and/or tobacco. *J Natl Cancer Inst.* 1998;90:1198-1205.

Bolla KI, Eldreth DA, Matochik JA, Cadet JL. Neural substrates of faulty decision-making in abstinent marijuana users. *Neuroimage.* 2005;26:480-492. Epub 2005 Mar 23.

Cannabis-In-Cachexia-Study-Group, Strasser F, Luftner D, Possinger K, Ernest G, Ruhstaller T, Meissner W, Ko YD, Schnelle M, Reif M, Cerny T. Comparison of orally administered cannabis extract and delta-9-tetrahydrocannabinol in treating patients with cancer-related anorexia-cachexia syndrome: a multicenter, phase III, randomized, double-blind, placebo-controlled clinical trial from the Cannabis-In-Cachexia-Study-Group. *J Clin Oncol.* 2006;24:3394-3400.

Disdier P, Granel B, Serratrice J, Constans J, Michon-Pasturel U, Hachulla E, Conri C, Devulder B, Swiader L, Piquet P, Branchereau A, Jouglard J, Moulin G, Weiller PJ. Cannabis arteritis revisited—ten new case reports. *Angiology.* 2001;52:1-5.

DuPont RL. Examining the debate on the use of medical marijuana. *Proc Assoc Am Physicians.* 1999;111:166-172.

Fox P, Bain PG, Glickman S, Carroll C, Zajicek J. The effect of cannabis on tremor in patients with multiple sclerosis. *Neurology.* 2004;62:1105-1109.

Gruenwald J. *PDR for Herbal Medicines.* 3rd ed. Montvale, NJ: Thomson PDR; 2004.

Haney M, Rabkin J, Gunderson E, Foltin RW. Dronabinol and marijuana in HIV(+) marijuana smokers: acute effects on caloric intake and mood. *Psychopharmacology (Berl).* 2005;181:170-178. Epub 2005 Oct 15.

Hashibe M, Morgenstern H, Cui Y, Tashkin DP, Zhang ZF, Cozen W, Mack TM, Greenland S. Marijuana use and the risk of lung and upper aerodigestive tract cancers: results of a population-based case-control study. *Cancer Epidemiol Biomarkers Prev.* 2006;15:1829-1834

Joy JE, Watson SJ Jr, Benson JA Jr., eds. *Marijuana and Medicine: Assessing the Science Base.* Washington, DC: National Academy Press; 1999.

Kalb C. No green light yet: a long-awaited report supports medical marijuana. So now what? *Newsweek.* 1999;133:35.

Karst M, Salim K, Burstein S, Conrad I, Hoy L, Schneider U. Analgesic effect of the synthetic cannabinoid CT-3 on chronic neuropathic pain: a randomized controlled trial. *JAMA.* 2003;290:1757-1762.

Marijuana use in supportive care for cancer patients. National Cancer Institute Web site. http://www.cancer.gov/cancertopics/factsheet/Support/marijuana. Updated December 12, 2000. Accessed June 6, 2008.

McAllister SD, Christian RT, Horowitz MP, Garcia A, Desprez PY. Cannabidiol as a novel inhibitor of Id-1 gene expression in aggressive breast cancer cells. *Mol Cancer Ther.* 2007;6:2921-2927.

Mehra R, Moore BA, Crothers K, Tetrault J, Fiellin DA. The association between marijuana smoking and lung cancer: a systematic review. *Arch Intern Med.* 2006;166:1359-1367.

Mittleman MA, Lewis RA, Maclure M, Sherwood JB, Muller JE. Triggering myocardial infarction by marijuana. *Circulation.* 2001;103:2805-2809.

Nahas G, Latour C. The human toxicity of marijuana. *Med J Aust.* 1992;156:495-497.

Schwartz RH, Voth EA, Sheridan MJ. Marijuana to prevent nausea and vomiting in cancer patients: a survey of clinical oncologists. *South Med J.* 1997;90:167-172.

Smigel K. Cancer problems lead list for potential marijuana research studies. *J Natl Cancer Inst.* 1997;89:1255.

Tramér MR, Carroll D, Campbell FA, Reynolds DJ, Moore RA, McQuay HJ. Cannabinoids for control of chemotherapy induced nausea and vomiting: quantitative systematic review. *BMJ.* 2001;323:16-21.

Voth EA, Schwartz RH. Medicinal applications of delta-9-tetrahydrocannabinol and marijuana. *Ann Intern Med.* 1997;126:791-798.

Wade DT, Makela P, Robson P, House H, Bateman C. Do cannabis-based medicinal extracts have general or specific effects on symptoms in multiple sclerosis? A double-blind, randomized, placebo-controlled study on 160 patients. *Mult Scler.* 2004;10:434-441.

Woolridge E, Barton S, Samuel J, Osorio J, Dougherty A, Holdcroft A. Cannabis use in HIV for pain and other medical symptoms. *J Pain Symptom Manage.* 2005;29:358-367.

MILK THISTLE

Other common name(s): Mary thistle, Marian thistle, holy thistle, lady thistle, silymarin
Scientific/medical name(s): *Silybum marianum*

Description

Milk thistle, a plant belonging to the same family as daisies, is native to the Mediterranean regions and grows in Europe, North America, South America, and Australia. The ripe seeds are used to make herbal remedies. They contain the antioxidant silymarin, which is thought to be responsible for milk thistle's helpful effects. Silymarin is a combination of three different compounds: silybinin (also called silybin or silibinin), silidyanin (also spelled silidianin), and silychristin (also spelled silichristin).

Overview

A few studies have suggested that silymarin, an antioxidant, may be useful for treating certain types of liver diseases in humans such as cirrhosis or chronic hepatitis. Most of the studies did not show improved survival, although laboratory tests showed an improvement in liver function in some. Larger randomized clinical trials are needed to determine whether these effects are reliable. Early studies in test tubes and laboratory animals have suggested that silymarin may help with cancer prevention and treatment. Human studies are needed to find out what role silymarin may play in preventing or treating cancer in people.

How is it promoted for use?

Proponents claim that milk thistle detoxifies and protects the liver and is an effective treatment for hepatitis C, jaundice, and cirrhosis. They also claim it strengthens the spleen and gallbladder, benefits people with diabetes, and slows the growth of certain types of cancer, including skin cancer, breast cancer, and prostate cancer. Some believe that milk thistle is an antidote for certain varieties of poisonous mushrooms.

Proponents also state that silymarin is a potent antioxidant. Antioxidants are compounds that block the action of activated oxygen molecules called free radicals, which can damage cells.

What does it involve?

Milk thistle supplements are made from the ripe seed, which is actually the fruit of the plant. The supplement is available as a capsule, tablet, powder, and liquid extract. Powdered milk thistle can be made into a tea. A typical daily dose ranges from 140 to 400 milligrams of silymarin, usually divided into two or three doses. The leaves, flower, roots, and stalk of the milk thistle plant contain very little silymarin and are usually not used in supplements.

What is the history behind it?

Milk thistle has been used for thousands of years in Europe as a liver restorative. It was recommended to treat malaria, melancholy, plague, and many other illnesses. It was also thought to reduce the effects of toxins such as poisonous mushrooms and alcohol on the liver. All parts of the milk thistle plant have been eaten as food in European countries, and its seeds have been made into a drink similar to coffee. Only recently have scientists begun to test its effectiveness in treating illness.

What is the evidence?

Silymarin has been studied extensively in the laboratory for the treatment of short-term and chronic liver diseases, and to a lesser extent for some types of cancer. Some research indicates that silymarin may be useful for treating certain liver diseases, particularly those caused by exposure to toxins. Commission E (Germany's regulatory agency for herbs) approved the use of milk thistle fruit (the part of the plant that contains silymarin) as a treatment for toxic liver disease and as supportive treatment for chronic inflammatory liver disease and cirrhosis of the liver.

One review of both clinical and laboratory research found that silymarin may be effective for patients with hepatitis, alcoholic liver disease, and cirrhosis. However, the researchers noted that all of the clinical trials were conducted outside of the United States, were difficult to interpret, involved small numbers of patients, and were not consistent in following scientific methods.

More recently, a group reviewed studies of the use of milk thistle for alcoholic or viral hepatitis and observed problems with study methods in most of them. For example, fewer than half of the studies were properly double-blinded, meaning participants or researchers might have been aware of which substance was being tested. In the clinical trials that were properly conducted, milk thistle did not show any effect.

Studies in laboratory mice have concluded that silymarin provided some protection against skin cancer caused by chemical carcinogens or ultraviolet radiation, possibly because of its antioxidant properties. Studies using cancer cells grown in a laboratory and animal studies found that silymarin reduced growth of breast, prostate, and cervical cancer cells. These test-tube studies also suggested that silymarin may be able to enhance the effectiveness of some chemotherapy drugs. Further studies are required to find out whether the results apply to humans. Preliminary clinical studies in cancer patients indicate that silymarin does not cause serious side effects. However, studies of anticancer activity in human patients have not been published as of 2008.

A study of rats given a type of chemotherapy that often harms the kidneys showed less kidney damage in rats that were also given silymarin. Again, human studies are needed to learn whether this effect might also happen in people.

Are there any possible problems or complications?

Silymarin is generally considered safe. A few people have reported stomach upset such as nausea, abdominal pain, diarrhea, and vomiting, although this is thought to have been due to contamination of the supplement with outside substances, not the silymarin itself. Large doses of silymarin may have a laxative effect. Allergic reactions are rare but may be more common among people who are allergic to plants in the same family, such as ragweed, chrysanthemums, marigolds, and daisies. Anyone who has hives, shortness of breath, dizziness, or swelling in the mouth or throat after taking silymarin should call emergency services right away. Studies have not been done to test silymarin's safety in children or in pregnant or breastfeeding women.

In general, antioxidant supplements are not recommended during chemotherapy or radiation therapy for cancer, since they may block some of the cancer-killing effects of these treatments.

In addition, the potential interactions between silymarin and other drugs and herbs should be considered. Some of these combinations may be dangerous. Always tell your doctor and pharmacist about any herbs you are taking. Relying on this type of treatment alone and avoiding or delaying conventional medical care for cancer may have serious health consequences.

This product is sold as a dietary supplement in the United States. Unlike companies that produce drugs (which must provide the FDA with results of detailed testing showing their product is safe and effective before the drug is approved for sale), the companies that make supplements do not have to show evidence of safety or health benefits to the FDA before selling their products. Supplement products without any reliable scientific evidence of health benefits may still be sold as long as the companies selling them do not claim the supplements can prevent, treat, or cure any specific disease. Some such products may not contain the amount of the herb or substance that is written on the label, and some may include other substances (contaminants). Though the FDA has written new rules to improve the quality of manufacturing processes for dietary supplements and the accurate listing of supplement ingredients, these rules do not take full effect until 2010. The new rules also do not address the safety of supplement ingredients or their effects on health when proper manufacturing techniques are used.

Most such supplements have not been tested to find out if they interact with medicines, foods, or other herbs and supplements. Even though some reports of interactions and harmful effects may be published, full studies of interactions and effects are not often available. Because of these limitations, any information on ill effects and interactions should be considered incomplete.

References

Agency for Healthcare Research and Quality. *Milk Thistle: Effects on Liver Disease and Cirrhosis and Clinical Adverse Effects.* Rockville, MD: Agency for Healthcare Research and Quality; 2000. AHRQ Publication No. 01-E024.

National Center for Biotechnology Information Web site. http://www.ncbi.nlm.nih.gov/books/bv.fcgi?rid=hstat1.section.29172. Accessed June 6, 2008.

Blumenthal M, ed. *The Complete German Commission E Monographs: Therapeutic Guide to Herbal Medicines.* Austin, TX: American Botanical Council; 1998.

Crops: milk thistle. Manitoba Agriculture, Food and Rural Initiatives Web site. http://www.gov.mb.ca/agriculture/crops/medicinal/bkq00s15.html. Updated March 2006. Accessed June 6, 2008.

Fetrow CW, Avila JR. *Professional's Handbook of Complementary & Alternative Medicines.* Springhouse, PA: Springhouse Corp; 1999.

Flora K, Hahn M, Rosen H, Benner K. Milk thistle (Silybum marianum) for the therapy of liver disease. *Am J Gastroenterol.* 1998;93:139-143.

Gruenwald J. *PDR for Herbal Medicines.* 3rd ed. Montvale, NJ: Thomson PDR; 2004.

Langenfeld J. Milk thistle. Creighton University School of Medicine Complementary and Alternative Medicine Web site. http://altmed.creighton.edu/MilkThistle/. Accessed June 6, 2008.

Lawenda BD, Kelly KM, Ladas EJ, Sagar SM, Vickers A, Blumberg JB. Should supplemental antioxidant administration be avoided during chemotherapy and radiation therapy? *J Natl Cancer Inst.* 2008;100:773-783.

Milk thistle. Memorial Sloan-Kettering Cancer Center Web site. http://www.mskcc.org/mskcc/html/69303.cfm. Updated August 7, 2007. Accessed June 6, 2008.

Milk thistle. National Cancer Institute Web site. http://www.cancer.gov/cancertopics/pdq/cam/milkthistle/HealthProfessional/page1. Updated March 20, 2008. Accessed July 31, 2008.

Milk thistle. National Center for Complementary and Alternative Medicine Web site. http://nccam.nih.gov/health/milkthistle/milkthistle.pdf. Created September 2005. Accessed June 6, 2008.

Rambaldi A, Jacobs BP, Iaquinto G, Gluud C. Milk thistle for alcoholic and/or hepatitis B or C virus liver diseases. *Cochrane Database Syst Rev.* 2005;(2):CD003620.

Singh RP, Agarwal R. Mechanisms and preclinical efficacy of silibinin in preventing skin cancer. *Eur J Cancer.* 2005;41:1969-1979.

Singh RP, Deep G, Chittezhath M, Kaur M, Dwyer-Nield LD, Malkinson AM, Agarwal R. Effect of silibinin on the growth and progression of primary lung tumors in mice. *J Natl Cancer Inst.* 2006;98:846-855.

Singh RP, Mallikarjuna GU, Sharma G, Dhanalakshmi S, Tyagi AK, Chan DC, Agarwal C, Agarwal R. Oral silibinin inhibits lung tumor growth in athymic nude mice and forms a novel chemocombination with doxorubicin targeting nuclear factor kappaB-mediated inducible chemoresistance. *Clin Cancer Res.* 2004;10:8641-8647.

Tyagi AK, Agarwal C, Chan DC, Agarwal R. Synergistic anti-cancer effects of silibinin with conventional cytotoxic agents doxorubicin, cisplatin and carboplatin against human breast carcinoma MCF-7 and MDA-MB468 cells. *Oncol Rep.* 2004;11:493-499.

van Erp NP, Baker SD, Zhao M, Rudek MA, Guchelaar HJ, Nortier JW, Sparreboom A, Gelderblom H. Effect of milk thistle (*Silybum marianum*) on the pharmacokinetics of irinotecan. *Clin Cancer Res.* 2005;11:7800-7806.

Zi X, Grasso AW, Kung HJ, Agarwal R. A flavonoid antioxidant, silymarin, inhibits activation of erbB1 signaling and induces cyclin-dependent kinase inhibitors, G1 arrest, and anticarciniogenic effects in human prostate carcinoma DU145 cells. *Cancer Res.* 1999;59:622-632.

MISTLETOE

Other common name(s): all heal, bird lime, devil's fuge, golden bough, Iscador, Eurixor, Helixor, Isorel, Iscucin, Plenosol, ABNOBAviscum

Scientific/medical name(s): *Viscum album, Viscum coloratum*

Description

Mistletoe is a semiparasitic plant that grows on several species of trees native to Great Britain, Europe, and western Asia. It differs from the mistletoe found in the United States. The plant's leaves and twigs are used in herbal remedies; the berries are not used.

Overview

A number of laboratory experiments suggest mistletoe may have the potential to treat cancer, but these results have not yet been reflected in clinical trials. Available evidence from well-designed clinical trials does not support claims that mistletoe can improve length or quality of life.

How is it promoted for use?

Proponents claim that mistletoe stimulates the immune system, helping the body fight more efficiently against cancer and other diseases. Mistletoe extracts are promoted as a remedy for a many types of cancer, including cancer of the cervix, ovary, breast, stomach, colon, and lung and as a treatment for leukemia, sarcoma, and lymphoma. Supporters claim mistletoe extract injected directly into or near a tumor can slow and possibly reverse the growth of cancer cells, even in advanced cases of cancer.

Promoters also claim mistletoe can lower blood pressure, decrease heart rate, relax spasms, and relieve symptoms of arthritis and rheumatism. It is further claimed to have sedative effects and is promoted to relieve the side effects of chemotherapy and radiation therapy.

What does it involve?

Commission E (Germany's regulatory agency for herbs) has approved mistletoe as palliative therapy—therapy intended to treat symptoms, not cure disease—for malignant tumors. The herb is prepared as a whole plant extract to be injected and is not used orally. The plant itself is poisonous and is not safe to eat. Mistletoe extracts are injected under the skin near the tumor. Daily injections are often given before and after surgery, chemotherapy, or radiation therapy and may continue for ten to fourteen days. Mistletoe injections promoted to prevent cancer may involve three to seven injections a week over several months to several years.

What is the history behind it?

Mistletoe is surrounded by fascinating myths and legends dating back many centuries. More than two thousand years ago, the Druids (members of the educated class among the ancient Celts in Europe) used mistletoe in many religious rituals. Their name for mistletoe meant "all healer," because they believed it had magical powers. Today, its name in Brittany, Wales, Scotland, and Ireland (*an t'uil*) still translates the same. The tradition of kissing under mistletoe dates back to a Scandinavian myth in which the plant becomes a symbol of love.

The liquid extract of the mistletoe plant has been used as an alternative method to treat cancer for more than seventy-five years. Modern research on mistletoe began in 1916 with Rudolph Steiner, PhD. Steiner combined spiritual and scientific approaches to medicine and to the treatment of cancer in particular. He believed that cancer formed when regulation of the body's physical or spiritual defenses faltered, and that mistletoe could reestablish that regulatory balance and fight back the tumor. Later researchers carried Steiner's beliefs further, contending that some of the chemicals in mistletoe could stop cancer growth and even kill cancer cells directly while enhancing the body's immune system.

Mistletoe injections are currently among the most widely used unconventional cancer treatments in Europe. Physicians in Switzerland, the Netherlands, and Great Britain commonly prescribe the treatment. In Europe, the most common commercial preparations are sold under the trade names Iscador and Helixor. Only the European species of the mistletoe plant is used for cancer treatment. Mistletoe injections are not available in the United States, except in clinical trials, because the drug is not approved for sale by the U.S. Food and Drug Administration (FDA).

What is the evidence?

Researchers have completed numerous studies of mistletoe and its effects on cancer. Carefully controlled human clinical studies have indicated that mistletoe does not have any significant effect on survival of people with cancer. A 2008 review of available clinical evidence concluded that the studies that reported improved survival had flaws in their design and could not be considered scientifically dependable. Two scientifically sound clinical trials of mistletoe suggested that mistletoe may improve quality of life among people with cancer, although positive conclusions were reported from many other studies believed to be flawed.

Mistletoe preparations vary widely depending on how they are made (for instance, whether they are extracted with water or alcohol solutions or fermented or nonfermented), the particular species from which they are obtained, and the season in which the plant was harvested. Researchers are working to identify the most important components in mistletoe, though they are thought currently to be the lectins, or proteins. A number of laboratory experiments suggest that mistletoe extracts may have some potential to combat and kill cancer cells, but these results have yet to be reflected in human trials. Laboratory experiments also hint that mistletoe increases the activity of lymphocytes, which are cells that attack invading organisms.

Are there any possible problems or complications?

In recommended doses, purified mistletoe extract is generally considered safe. Possible side effects include temporary redness at the injection site, headaches, fever, and chills. Rarely, in people allergic to mistletoe, a severe and potentially life-threatening condition called anaphylactic shock can develop.

Potentially dangerous interactions with conventional medicines are possible, particularly with some medications that are used for high blood pressure, irregular heart rhythm, and heart failure. Always tell your doctor and pharmacist about any herbs you are taking.

The mistletoe plant should not be eaten because all parts of it are poisonous. Consuming mistletoe has been known to cause seizures, coma, and death. Other symptoms of mistletoe toxicity include blurred vision, nausea and vomiting, stomach pain, diarrhea, slow or irregular heartbeat, low blood pressure, confusion, and drowsiness.

Women who are pregnant or breastfeeding should not use this herb. Relying on this type of treatment alone and avoiding or delaying conventional medical care for cancer may have serious health consequences.

This substance has not been thoroughly tested to find out how it interacts with medicines, foods, or dietary supplements. Even though some reports of interactions and harmful effects may be published, full studies of interactions and effects are not often available. Because of these limitations, any information on ill effects and interactions should be considered incomplete.

References

Blumenthal M, ed. *The Complete German Commission E Monographs: Therapeutic Guide to Herbal Medicines.* Austin, TX: American Botanical Council; 1998.

Dold U, Edler L, Mäurer HCh, et al, eds. *Adjuvant Cancer Therapy in Advanced Non-Small Cell Bronchial Cancer: Multicentric Controlled Studies To Test the Efficacy of Iscador and Polyerga* [in German]. Stuttgart, Germany: Georg Thieme Verlag; 1991.

Ernst E. Mistletoe as a treatment for cancer. *BMJ.* 2006;333:1282-1283.

Ernst E, Schmidt K, Steuer-Vogt MK. Mistletoe for cancer? A systematic review of randomised clinical trials. *Int J Cancer.* 2003;107:262-267.

Horneber MA, Bueschel G, Huber R, Linde K, Rostock M. Mistletoe therapy in oncology. *Cochrane Database Syst Rev.* 2008;(2):CD003297.

Kleeberg UR, Suciu S, Bröcker EB, Ruiter DJ, Chartier C, Liénard D, Marsden J, Schadendorf D, Eggermont AM; EORTC Melanoma Group in cooperation with the German Cancer Society (DKG). Final results of the EORTC 18871/DKG 80-1 randomised phase III trial. rIFN-alpha2b versus rIFN-gamma versus ISCADOR M versus observation after surgery in melanoma patients with either high-risk primary (thickness >3 mm) or regional lymph node metastasis. *Eur J Cancer.* 2004;40:390-402.

Mistletoe (European). Memorial Sloan-Kettering Cancer Center Web site. http://www.mskcc.org/mskcc/html/69305.cfm. Updated December 11, 2007. Accessed June 6, 2008.

Mistletoe extracts (PDQ®). National Cancer Institute Web site. http://www.nci.nih.gov/cancertopics/pdq/cam/mistletoe/HealthProfessional. Updated April 28, 2008. Accessed June 6, 2008.

Steuer-Vogt MK, Bonkowsky V, Ambrosch P, Scholz M, Neiss A, Strutz J, Hennig M, Lenarz T, Arnold W. The effect of an adjuvant mistletoe treatment programme in resected head and neck cancer patients: a randomized controlled clinical trial. *Eur J Cancer.* 2001;37:23-31.

US Congress, Office of Technology Assessment. *Unconventional Cancer Treatments: OTA-H-405*. Washington, DC: US Government Printing Office; 1990.

MOLYBDENUM

Other common name(s): none
Scientific/medical name(s): Mo, sodium molybdate, ammonium molybdate

Description

Molybdenum is a mineral that is present in very small quantities in the body. It is involved in many important biological processes, possibly including development of the nervous system, waste processing in the kidneys, and energy production in cells.

Overview

Molybdenum is an essential element in human nutrition, but its precise function and interactions with other chemicals are not well understood. Some evidence suggests that too little molybdenum in the diet may be responsible for some health problems. Molybdenum is used as a treatment in the rare cases of inherited metabolic diseases (such as Wilson's disease) in which the body cannot process copper. More research is needed to learn whether it may have a role in preventing cancer and other diseases. It has shown promise in animal studies in reducing the harmful effects of certain cancer drugs on the heart and lungs.

How is it promoted for use?

Proponents claim molybdenum is an antioxidant that prevents cancer by protecting cells from free radicals, destructive molecules that may damage cells. Some supporters also claim that molybdenum prevents anemia, gout, dental cavities, and sexual impotence.

What does it involve?

Food is the major source of molybdenum for most people. Common sources of molybdenum include legumes, such as beans, peas, and lentils; grains; leafy vegetables; liver; and nuts. However, the amount of molybdenum in plants varies according to the amount in the soil.

Humans require very small amounts of molybdenum, and deficiency appears to happen only under the most unusual circumstances. For example, molybdenum deficiency may appear in a person fed entirely through the veins for a very long time, or in a person with a genetic problem in which the body cannot use the molybdenum that is eaten in foods.

Molybdenum is sold as a supplement in some health food stores and over the Internet. It is sold as sodium molybdate or ammonium molybdate in capsule form, usually in combination with other nutrients. A typical dosage is 75 micrograms daily.

What is the history behind it?

Knowledge of molybdenum dates back to the Middle Ages. Pure molybdenum was first produced in 1893. Serious research into molybdenum's importance in the human body began only within the past couple of decades. In 2001, the U.S. Food and Nutrition Board established the Recommended Dietary Allowance (RDA) of molybdenum for most adults at 45 micrograms, with an RDA of 50 micrograms for women who are pregnant or breastfeeding.

What is the evidence?

A large, randomized study was conducted in Linxian, an area of north central China whose residents have very high rates of esophageal and stomach cancers. Researchers gave more than thirty thousand people one of several combinations of essential minerals and nutrients. One group received vitamin C and molybdenum. The scientists did not find any reductions in cancer mortality rates among those who received molybdenum. Some evidence suggested that the soil in Linxian, which contained low levels of molybdenum, may have led to the formation of chemicals in plants that increase the risk for cancers of the esophagus. More data are needed to find out whether there is a connection.

Tetrathiomolybdate (a form of molybdenum that is different from the forms used in dietary supplements) is being tested as a cancer treatment. It is known that molybdenum depletes copper in the body, and copper is required for new blood vessels to be formed. Some studies in mice show that tetrathiomolybdate might improve the response to breast cancer drugs, but human studies are required to find out whether this is true. Animal studies also suggest that tetrathiomolybdate might be helpful in reducing the heart and lung damage caused by some chemotherapy drugs. This possibility has not yet been studied in human clinical trials. In 2003, researchers did a small study on people with advanced kidney cancer. Researchers gave tetrathiomolybdate (a form of molybdenum) to fifteen patients to reduce the copper levels in their bodies. Even though no one had a remission of their cancer, four people's tumors stopped growing for six months. Some patients, however, had anemia (low red blood cell counts) or low white blood cell counts due to the lack of copper and had to have their molybdenum doses reduced. The researchers noted that this approach might be useful in combination with other cancer treatments and recommended large, well-controlled studies to better evaluate tetrathiomolybdate. However, a small 2006 study did not show a reduction in growth of advanced prostate cancer.

Studies in mice show that molybdenum might improve the response to breast cancer treatment drugs, but human studies are required to find out whether this is true. Animal studies also suggest that molybdenum might be helpful in reducing the heart and lung damage caused by some chemotherapy drugs. This possibility has not yet been studied in human clinical trials.

Are there any possible problems or complications?

In animals, molybdenum deficiency does not occur naturally and must be produced by a carefully controlled diet. Overdoses are extremely rare. Large amounts of molybdenum produce symptoms of copper deficiency in cattle, and taking too much supplemental molybdenum could produce the same symptoms in humans. Symptoms of too much molybdenum include tiredness, dizziness, rashes, low white blood cell counts, and anemia. High molybdenum levels are also linked to gout.

In workplaces where the mineral is processed, molybdenum dust can irritate the nose and throat and may cause coughing and wheezing. In workplace settings, prolonged exposure to high molybdenum levels has been linked to weakness, fatigue, headache, poor appetite, and muscle and joint pain.

Molybdenum deficiencies are very rare among humans; therefore most practitioners do not recommend supplements. Relying on this type of treatment alone and avoiding or delaying conventional medical care for cancer may have serious health consequences.

This product is sold as a dietary supplement in the United States. Unlike companies that produce drugs (which must provide the FDA with results of detailed testing showing their product is safe and effective before the drug is approved for sale), the companies that make supplements do not have to show evidence of safety or health benefits to the FDA before selling their products. Supplement products without any reliable scientific evidence of health benefits may still be sold as long as the companies selling them do not claim the supplements can prevent, treat, or cure any specific disease. Some such products may not contain the amount of the herb or substance that is written on the label, and some may include other substances (contaminants). Though the FDA has written new rules to improve the quality of manufacturing processes for dietary supplements and the accurate listing of supplement ingredients, these rules do not take full effect until 2010. The new rules also do not address the safety of supplement ingredients or their effects on health when proper manufacturing techniques are used.

Most such supplements have not been tested to find out if they interact with medicines, foods, or other herbs and supplements. Even though some reports of interactions and harmful effects may be published, full studies of interactions and effects are not often available. Because of these limitations, any information on ill effects and interactions should be considered incomplete.

References

Barceloux DG. Molybdenum. *J Toxicol.* 1999;37:231-237.
Erratum in:
J Toxicol. 2000;38:813.

Blot WJ, Li JY, Taylor PR, Guo W, Dawsey SM, Li B. The Linxian trials: mortality rates by vitamin-mineral intervention group. *Am J Clin Nutr.* 1995;62:1424S-1426S.

Brewer GJ, Ullenbruch MR, Dick R, Olivarez L, Phan SH. Tetrathiomolybdate therapy protects against bleomycin-induced pulmonary fibrosis in mice. *J Lab Clin Med.* 2003;141:210-216.

Cassileth B. *The Alternative Medicine Handbook: The Complete Reference Guide to Alternative and Complementary Therapies.* New York: W.W. Norton; 1998.

Food and Nutrition Board. Dietary reference intakes: elements. Institute of Medicine Web site. http://www.iom.edu/Object.File/Master/7/294/0.pdf. Accessed June 6, 2008.

Hassouneh B, Islam M, Nagel T, Pan Q, Merajver SD, Teknos TN. Tetrathiomolybdate promotes tumor necrosis and prevents distant metastases by suppressing angiogenesis in head and neck cancer. *Mol Cancer Ther.* 2007;6:1039-1045.

Henry NL, Dunn R, Merjaver S, Pan Q, Pienta KJ, Brewer G, Smith DC. Phase II trial of copper depletion with tetrathiomolybdate as an antiangiogenesis strategy in patients with hormone-refractory prostate cancer. *Oncology.* 2006;71:168-175.

Hou G, Dick R, Abrams GD, Brewer GJ. Tetrathiomolybdate protects against cardiac damage by doxorubicin in mice. *J Lab Clin Med.* 2005;146:299-303.

Kamangar F, Qiao YL, Yu B, Sun XD, Abnet CC, Fan JH, Mark SD, Zhao P, Dawsey SM, Taylor PR. Lung cancer chemoprevention: a randomized, double-blind trial in Linxian, China. *Cancer Epidemiol Biomarkers Prev.* 2006;15:1562-1564.

Molybdenum. Linus Pauling Institute Web site. http://lpi.oregonstate.edu/infocenter/minerals/molybdenum/. Updated April, 2007. Accessed August 6, 2008.

Molybdenum. PDRhealth Web site. http://www.pdrhealth.com/drug_info/nmdrugprofiles/nutsupdrugs/mol_0332.shtml. Accessed June 6, 2008.

Nakadaira H, Endoh K, Yamamoto M, Katoh K. Distribution of selenium and molybdenum and cancer mortality in Niigata, Japan. *Arch Environ Health.* 1995;50:374-380.

National Institute of Occupational Safety and Health. Molybdenum (soluble compounds, as MO). Centers for Disease Control and Prevention Web site. http://www.cdc.gov/niosh/idlh/moly-mo.html. Updated August 16, 1996. Accessed June 6, 2008.

Pan Q, Bao LW, Kleer CG, Brewer GJ, Merajver SD. Antiangiogenic tetrathiomolybdate enhances the efficacy of doxorubicin against breast carcinoma. *Mol Cancer Ther.* 2003;2:617-622.

Qu CX, Kamangar F, Fan JH, Yu B, Sun XD, Taylor PR, Chen BE, Abnet CC, Qiao YL, Mark SD, Dawsey SM. Chemoprevention of primary liver cancer: a randomized, double-blind trial in Linxian, China. *J Natl Cancer Inst.* 2007;99:1240-1247.

Rajagopalan KV. Molybdenum: an essential trace element in human nutrition. *Annu Rev Nutr.* 1988;8:401-427.

Redman BG, Esper P, Pan Q, Dunn RL, Hussain HK, Chenevert T, Brewer GJ, Merajver SD. Phase II trial of tetrathiomolybdate in patients with advanced kidney cancer. *Clin Cancer Res.* 2003;9:1666-1672.

MUGWORT

Other common name(s): ai ye, St. John's plant, common wormwood, wild wormwood

Scientific/medical name(s): *Artemisia vulgaris*

Description

Mugwort is a perennial plant that is a member of the daisy family and a relative of ragweed. It is native to Asia and Europe and now grows as a weed in North America. It can grow to six feet tall, with stalks of small reddish-brown or yellow flowers in summer. The dried leaves and roots of the plant are used in herbal remedies. Mugwort should not be confused with St. John's wort *(Hypericum perforatum)* or wormwood *(Artemisia absinthium)*, despite their similar names.

Overview

Available scientific evidence does not support claims that mugwort is effective in treating gastrointestinal problems or any other medical condition, including cancer.

How is it promoted for use?

Mugwort is promoted to treat stomach and intestinal disorders such as colic, persistent vomiting, diarrhea, constipation, flatulence, and cramps. The herb has also been promoted as a treatment for a wide range of other conditions, including headaches, nose bleeds, muscle spasms, epilepsy, circulatory problems, menopausal and menstrual complaints, chills, fever, rheumatism, asthma, dermatitis, dysentery, gout, and infertility. Proponents also claim mugwort oil has antibacterial and antifungal properties and can be used to treat worm infestations and snakebites.

Some proponents claim mugwort is a sedative and use it to treat neuroses, hysteria, general irritability, restlessness, insomnia, anxiety, mild depression, anorexia, and opium addiction.

Dried mugwort, or moxa, is used in moxibustion treatments to treat cancer (see "Moxibustion," page 223).

What does it involve?

Mugwort is available as a mixture of dried leaves and roots, an extract, tincture, tea, and in pill form. Mugwort can also be used as a poultice. It is also used in North American flower remedies and made into homeopathic preparations (see "Homeopathy," page 753). It is on the Commission E (Germany's regulatory agency for herbs) list of unapproved herbs. This means that it is not recommended for use because it has not been proven safe and effective.

What is the history behind it?

Herbalists have prescribed mugwort to treat many different conditions over the years. The Chinese have also used dried mugwort leaves (and sometimes leaves of other *Artemisia* species), or moxa, in moxibustion for centuries. In the Middle Ages in England, mugwort was sometimes worn on St. John's Eve and was thought to protect the wearer from evil possession. Young women were told to sew mugwort into a small piece of cloth and place it under their pillows to induce vivid dreams. In the 1830s, Portuguese sailors introduced mugwort to France, where it became popular as a treatment for blindness and other illnesses. Mugwort has also been used as a tea, a beer flavoring, and occasionally as a spice for meats.

What is the evidence?

Research on mugwort has focused on its properties related to allergic sensitivities, which are similar to those of the American ragweed. Little research has been done on the use of mugwort as a medical treatment, although an extract (artemisinin) from another member of the *Artemisia* family (*Artemisia annua*) is used in conventional medicine as a treatment for malaria. There have been only a few preliminary laboratory studies and case reports of the potential of *Artemisia* species in treating cancer, but most of these studies involve other *Artemisia* species (*Artemisia annua*, *Artemisia asiatica*, and *Artemisia princeps*) rather than mugwort. There is no convincing clinical evidence available to support any of the claims made for mugwort as a treatment for people with cancer, including claims about the anticancer effectiveness of moxibustion.

Are there any possible problems or complications?

Mugwort is generally considered safe. Mugwort pollen is known to cause hay fever. On rare occasions, it can cause reactions ranging from rashes to severe, life-threatening symptoms. Mugwort allergy also appears to be related to several food allergies. Women who are pregnant or breastfeeding should not use this herb. In addition, the potential interactions between mugwort and other drugs and herbs should be considered. Always tell your doctor and pharmacist about any herbs you are taking. Relying on this type of treatment alone and avoiding or delaying conventional medical care for cancer may have serious health consequences.

This product is sold as a dietary supplement in the United States. Unlike companies that produce drugs (which must provide the FDA with results of detailed testing showing their product is safe and effective before the drug is approved for sale), the companies that make supplements do not have to show evidence of safety or health benefits to the FDA before selling their products. Supplement products without any reliable scientific evidence of health benefits may still be sold as long as the companies selling them do not claim the supplements can prevent, treat, or cure any specific disease. Some such products may not contain the amount of the herb or substance that is written on the label, and some may include other substances (contaminants). Though the FDA has written new rules to improve the quality of manufacturing processes for dietary supplements and the accurate listing of supplement ingredients, these rules do not take full effect until 2010. The new rules also do not address the safety of supplement ingredients or their effects on health when proper manufacturing techniques are used.

Most such supplements have not been tested to find out if they interact with medicines, foods, or other herbs and supplements. Even though some reports of interactions and harmful effects may be published, full studies of interactions and effects are not often available. Because of these limitations, any information on ill effects and interactions should be considered incomplete.

References

Anliker MD, Borelli S, Wüthrich B. Occupational protein contact dermatitis from spices in a butcher: a new presentation of the mugwort-spice syndrome. *Contact Dermatitis.* 2002;46:72-74.

Berger TG, Dieckmann D, Efferth T, Schultz ES, Funk JO, Baur A, Schuler G. Artesunate in the treatment of metastatic uveal melanoma—first experiences. *Oncol Rep.* 2005;14:1599-1603.

Blumenthal M, ed. *The Complete German Commission E Monographs: Therapeutic Guide to Herbal Medicines.* Austin, TX: American Botanical Council; 1998.

Fetrow CW, Avila JR. *Professional's Handbook of Complementary & Alternative Medicines.* Philadelphia, PA: Lippincott Williams & Wilkins; 2004.

Gruenwald J. *PDR for Herbal Medicines.* 3rd ed. Montvale, NJ: Thomson PDR; 2004.

Hsu E. Reflections on the 'discovery' of the antimalarial qinghao. *British J Clin Pharmacol.* 2006;61:666-670.

Kim MJ, Kim DH, Na HK, Oh TY, Shin CY, Surh Ph D Professor YJ. Eupatilin, a pharmacologically active flavone derived from *Artemisia* plants, induces apoptosis in human gastric cancer (AGS) cells. *J Environ Pathol Toxicol Oncol.* 2005;24:261-269.

Kurzen M, Bayerl C, Goerdt S. Occupational allergy to mugwort [in German] [Abstract]. *J Dtsch Dermatol Ges.* 2003;1:285-290.

Lee HG, Yu KA, Oh WK, Baeg TW, Oh HC, Ahn JS, Jang WC, Kim JW, Lim JS, Choe YK, Yoon DY. Inhibitory effect of jaceosidin isolated from *Artemisia argyi* on the function of E6 and E7 oncoproteins of HPV 16. *J Ethnopharmacol.* 2005;98:339-343.

Mueller MS, Runyambo N, Wagner I, Borrmann S, Dietz K, Heide L. Randomized controlled trial of a traditional preparation of Artemisia annua L. (Annual Wormwood) in the treatment of malaria. *Trans R Soc Trop Med Hyg.* 2004;98:318-321.

Mugwort. PDRhealth Web site. http://www.pdrhealth.com/drug_info/nmdrugprofiles/herbaldrugs/101960.shtml. Accessed April 25, 2007. Content no longer available.

Sarath VJ, So CS, Won YD, Gollapudi S. Artemisia princeps var orientalis induces apoptosis in human breast cancer MCF-7 cells. *Anticancer Res.* 2007;27:3891-3898.

Wopfner N, Gadermaier G, Egger M, Asero R, Ebner C, Jahn-Schmid B, Ferreira F. The spectrum of allergens in ragweed and mugwort pollen. *Int Arch Allergy Immunol.* 2005;138:337-346. Epub 2005 Oct 24.

OLEANDER LEAF

Other common name(s): oleander, dogbane, laurier rose, rosebay, Anvirzel, Xenavex, SAOB-0401

Scientific/medical name(s): *Nerium oleander, Thevetia peruviana*

Description

Oleander is a poisonous evergreen shrub or small tree identified by its fragrant white, red, pink, or purple flowers and long slender, leathery leaves, which grow in pairs opposite each other or in whorls of three. It grows in mild climates or as an indoor plant. The active ingredients are extracted from the leaves, but all parts of the plant are poisonous.

Overview

Oleander extracts—in carefully controlled doses—are in the early phases of testing to find out whether they are effective in treating cancer. There have been numerous reports of poisoning and death from ingestion of oleander, oleander leaf tea, and its extracts. It has killed adults, children, pets, and livestock. Even a small amount of oleander can cause death due to its effects on the heart. Inhaling the smoke from burning oleander or eating honey made from its nectar can produce poisonous effects. Since such tiny amounts can cause death, oleander supplements and extracts from any part of the oleander plant should not be used except under the careful observation and controlled conditions of a clinical trial.

How is it promoted for use?

Even though oleander is poisonous, heavily diluted oleander preparations have been promoted to treat a variety of conditions including muscle cramps, asthma, corns, menstrual pain, epilepsy, paralysis, skin diseases, heart problems, and cancer. It has also been used in folk remedies as an insecticide and to kill rats.

What does it involve?

There is no established therapeutic dose of oleander extract. The oleander leaf is on the Commission E (Germany's regulatory agency for herbs) list of unapproved herbs. This means that it is not recommended for use because it has not been proven to be safe or effective. The plant parts are toxic, whether cooked, raw, or made into tea.

An injectable oleander extract with the brand name of Anvirzel was available at one time, but it has not been approved for marketing by the U.S. Food and Drug Administration (FDA). In March 2000, the FDA warned Anvirzel's manufacturers to stop promoting the product as safe and effective after it found misleading information on their Web site. The FDA noted that claims were being made based on preliminary and inconclusive data. A company cannot make such claims unless a drug has been fully tested and shown to be safe and effective.

What is the history behind it?

Although this plant is poisonous, products made from oleander have been used for centuries as herbal medicine. Historical records show that the Mesopotamians in the fifteenth century BC believed in the healing properties of oleander. The Babylonians used a mixture of oleander and licorice to treat hangovers. Pliny the Elder of ancient Greece wrote about the appearance and properties of oleander. Arab physicians first used oleander as a cancer treatment in the eighth century AD.

During the 1960s, Huseyin Z. Ozel, MD, a Turkish physician, began his studies of oleander as an anticancer treatment. He developed an oleander extract that he patented and trademarked in the United States and Europe as Anvirzel. He began his study because of folk traditions that suggested that an extract of oleander was effective against leukemia.

What is the evidence?

The effectiveness of oleander has not been proven. In test tube studies, oleandrin, one of the substances found in oleander extracts, caused apoptosis (a specific type of cell death) of prostate cancer cells. In other test tube studies, Anvirzel appeared to slow the growth of human bladder cancer cells, but human studies are needed to determine whether it will work in people. Very early studies of carefully dosed Anvirzel in people with cancer have not yet shown that it helps. Side effects included nausea and vomiting, aches, and redness at the injection site, but the drug did not appear to affect the cancer in these patients. One very early study of eighteen patients with advanced cancer was done primarily to determine the best dose of the drug. No measurable responses were noted in patients' cancer during this small study. Although there are claims that Anvirzel improves quality of life, reduces pain, increases energy, and causes cancer regression and remission, available scientific evidence does not support these claims.

Another company had planned to offer an oleander extract that could be placed under the tongue, which they named Xenavex. Phase I and Phase II clinical trials on Xenavex were announced in 2005 on people with non–small cell lung cancer. However, the clinical trials were not done, and the announcements were later removed from the federal clinical trials Web site. The company did not return calls or e-mails about the product.

Before any form of oleander can be recommended for human use, it must be thoroughly tested in people using the carefully controlled dosing and observation procedures used in clinical trials.

Are there any possible problems or complications?

The oleander plant is poisonous, and many people have died of heart failure or respiratory paralysis after eating parts of the plant or drinking tea made from it. Some of the symptoms and signs of oleander toxicity are nausea, vomiting, colic, appetite loss, dizziness, drowsiness, high potassium levels, dilated pupils, bloody diarrhea, seizures, loss of consciousness, slow or irregular pulse, and heart block—a blockage of the electrical impulses that stimulate the heart to contract. There have been reports of death occurring after oral and/or rectal administration of the extract from the plant. The FDA has received reports of at least two deaths linked to Anvirzel.

Skin irritation from contact with oleander has occurred and allergies are possible. One report observed that when oleander was taken by a pregnant woman twelve hours before delivery, her baby was affected with seizures and a slowed heart rate. No other cause for the seizures and low heart rate was found. This herb should be avoided, especially by children and women who are pregnant or breastfeeding. Relying on this type of treatment alone and avoiding or delaying conventional medical care for cancer may have serious health consequences.

This substance has not been thoroughly tested to find out how it interacts with medicines, foods, or dietary supplements. Even though some reports of interactions and harmful effects may be published, full studies of interactions and effects are not often available. Because of these limitations, any information on ill effects and interactions should be considered incomplete.

References

Blumenthal M, ed. *The Complete German Commission E Monographs: Therapeutic Guide to Herbal Medicines.* Austin, TX: American Botanical Council; 1998.

Clark RF, Selden BS, Curry SC. Digoxin-specific Fab fragments in the treatment of oleander toxicity in a canine model. *Ann Emerg Med.* 1991;20:1073-1077.

Davies MK, Mayne AJ. Oleander poisoning. *Arch Dis Child.* 2001;84:9.

Fetrow CW, Avila JR. *Professional's Handbook of Complementary & Alternative Medicines.* Philadelphia, PA: Lippincott Williams & Wilkins; 2004.

Gruenwald J. *PDR for Herbal Medicines.* 3rd ed. Montvale, NJ: Thomson PDR; 2004.

Lamm D, Ashish K, DeHaven J. Cytotoxic effect of Nerium oleander extract (Anvirzel) on bladder cancer cells. In: Program and abstracts of the American Society of Clinical Oncology (ASCO) annual meeting; May 15-19, 1999; Atlanta, Georgia. Abstract 1328.

Langford SD, Boor PJ. Oleander toxicity: examination of human and animal toxic exposures. *Toxicology.* 1996;109:1-13.

McConkey DJ, Lin Y, Nutt LK, Ozel HZ, Newman RA. Cardiac glycosides stimulate Ca2+ increases and apoptosis in androgen-independent, metastatic human prostate adenocarcinoma cells. *Cancer Res.* 2000;60:3807-3812.

Mekhail T, Kaur H, Ganapathi R, Budd GT, Elson P, Bukowski RM. Phase 1 trial of Anvirzel in patients with refractory solid tumors. *Invest New Drugs.* 2006;24:423-427.

Oleander (*Nerium oleander, Thevetia peruviana*). Aetna InteliHealth Web site. http://www.intelihealth.com/IH/ihtIH/WSIHW000/8513/31402/351437.html. Updated June 20, 2005. Accessed June 6, 2008.

Thilagar S, Thirumalaikolundusubramanian P, Gopalakrishnan S, Lakshmikandan R, Ayyappan A, Subramanian R. Possible yellow oleander toxicity in a neonate. *Indian Pediatr.* 1986;23:393.

Turan N, Akgün-Dar K, Kuruca SE, Kiliçaslan-Ayna T, Seyhan VG, Atasever B, Meriçli F, Carin M. Cytotoxic effects of leaf, stem and root extracts of Nerium oleander on leukemia cell lines and role of the p-glycoprotein in this effect. *J Exp Ther Oncol.* 2006;6:31-38.

US National Institutes of Health. Clinical trial announcement: a phase I/II multicenter, off-label, dose escalation study of Xenavex in patients with advanced (stage IIIB or IV) non-small cell lung cancer; for whom previous therapy has failed. ClinicalTrials.gov Web site. http://www.clinicaltrials.gov. Accessed October 18, 2005. Content no longer available.

ORTHOMOLECULAR MEDICINE

Other common name(s): megavitamin/megamineral therapy, nutritional medicine
Scientific/medical name(s): none

Description

Orthomolecular medicine is the use of high doses of vitamins, minerals, or hormones to prevent and treat a wide variety of conditions. The doses are well above the Recommended Dietary Allowance (RDA) and may be used along with special diets and conventional treatment.

Overview

Available scientific evidence does not support the use of orthomolecular therapy for most of the conditions for which it is promoted. However, vitamins, minerals, and other supplements have been and continue to be studied to determine whether they can help or prevent many types of illness. While some supplements have been shown to help certain conditions, a few have unexpectedly proven to be harmful. At this time, eating nutritious foods is the best proven strategy to get the vitamins, minerals, and nutrients that are needed for good health.

How is it promoted for use?

Orthomolecular medicine is promoted to help people with depression, schizophrenia, and other psychiatric illnesses; Parkinson's disease; shingles; irritable bowel syndrome; alcoholism; colds; heart disease; hay fever; pneumonia; bruises; acne; eczema; bug bites; cold sores; chronic fatigue syndrome; and many other health problems. Supporters believe poor nutrition and refined foods are at the root of many of these illnesses. Proponents of this therapy believe that conventional medicine is foreign to the body and potentially harmful. They prefer vitamins, minerals, enzymes, and other substances they consider to be "natural."

What does it involve?

Depending on the diagnosis, high doses of vitamin C, niacin, or other vitamins and minerals may be recommended. These are usually taken by mouth. The patient may be put on a diet free of refined sugar and white flour. The diet may follow other specific guidelines. In some cases, the practitioner may perform hair analysis, blood tests, or urine tests to learn the levels of certain minerals or vitamins in the person's body.

What is the history behind it?

The concept of orthomolecular medicine dates back to the early 1950s. Nobel Prize winner Linus Pauling, PhD, coined the term in 1968. Proponents believe that taking large doses of vitamins or nutrients could correct "biochemical abnormalities" and thereby reverse a wide variety of conditions such as alcoholism, allergies, arthritis, asthma, cancer, depression, epilepsy, heart disease, high blood pressure, hyperactivity, migraine headaches, mental retardation, and schizophrenia.

What is the evidence?

So far, most studies have shown that taking supplements is not as effective in cancer prevention as eating the foods that contain the vitamins or minerals. This may be because foods have helpful nutrients other than those being studied, because nutrients have different effects when combined than when consumed individually, or because of other factors.

In some cases, supplements are effective in correcting deficiencies. It has long been known, for instance, that iron supplements can help iron-deficiency anemia and that vitamin C supplements can correct scurvy. Both are examples of diseases caused by a deficiency of a vitamin or mineral. A few vitamins and minerals have been shown to have physical effects beyond correcting deficiencies. For example, supplements of nicotinic acid (a form of niacin, or vitamin B3) have been shown to help lower cholesterol levels in some people and have become part of standard medical treatment.

Research is still under way to learn more about the use of supplements to treat or prevent specific health conditions, including cancer.

Some studies have looked at the role of several antioxidants, alone or in combination, in the prevention and treatment of cancer and other diseases. Antioxidants are compounds that block the action of activated oxygen molecules called free radicals, which can damage cells. They are thought to reduce the risk for some types of cancer. Examples of antioxidants are vitamin C, vitamin E, and beta carotene (a precursor of vitamin A). Certain trace minerals such as selenium, copper, and zinc also act as antioxidants. Other studies have looked at minerals in the body such as potassium, magnesium, and calcium.

The antioxidants vitamin E, vitamin C, beta carotene, selenium, and zinc were given to French men and women over a seven-year period. Others were given a placebo over that same time period. The men who took the supplement combination seemed to have slightly lower cancer risk than those who took the placebo. However, the men began the study with lower levels of antioxidants in their bodies, especially levels of beta carotene and vitamins C and E. This may partly explain why they benefited more. The women who took the supplement had the same cancer risk as those who took the placebo.

A large clinical trial looked at whether beta carotene and retinol (a form of vitamin A) could help reduce cancer and deaths in people who were at high risk for lung cancer because of smoking or asbestos exposure. In 1996, the researchers found that the group receiving the vitamins had a higher risk for lung cancer, heart disease, and death. The study was stopped right away. Researchers continued to follow the groups to determine whether these effects continued beyond the study. The risk for heart disease dropped back to a normal level very quickly, but cancer risk stayed higher for several years.

One 2005 study looked at whether supplements might help prevent side effects of cancer treatment. Canadian researchers gave "natural" vitamin E and beta carotene to people undergoing radiation therapy for head and neck cancers. The researchers found that those who received the vitamins had fewer side effects from treatment. However, later on, those individuals had more recurrences of their cancer. This finding supports older information suggesting that antioxidant supplements taken during cancer treatment may decrease the treatment's effectiveness.

The HOPE TOO study followed up on patients with diabetes or vascular disease who had been studied in the 1990s. It found that there was no difference in cancer or blood vessel disease in the heart between those who received vitamin E and those who took placebo. Unexpectedly, those who received vitamin E had increased rates of heart failure compared with those who received the placebo.

Clinical trials using high doses of vitamins have been done for people with mental illnesses. Schizophrenic patients treated with vitamin C or vitamin B6 showed no improvement over those receiving a placebo. Children with attention deficit disorder who received high doses of vitamins C, B3, B5, and B6 proved no different from those receiving a placebo.

A 2007 review of sixty-eight studies of vitamin supplements concluded that people taking vitamin A and vitamin E supplements had shorter life expectancy than those who did not take these supplements. Vitamin C had no effect on longevity.

As studies continue, researchers are learning from these surprising findings. For example, researchers have found that supplement recommendations cannot be made based solely on observational studies. Nearly all of the large observational epidemiologic studies showed strong links between low intake of beta carotene in foods and higher rates of cancer. However, a subsequent clinical trial found that giving beta carotene supplements turned out to raise cancer risk—the opposite of what was expected. Also, researchers noted that the effects of some supplements take years to show up and that some effects take years to wear off after the supplements are stopped.

More nutrients are still being studied in controlled clinical trials, such as a study in which trace minerals are given to seriously ill patients to see whether survival is improved. One preliminary study suggests that the antioxidant lutein may help those with macular degeneration, a loss of vision in older people caused by poor circulation to the retina. More research is needed to find out whether this result will hold true in larger studies.

It is well known that nutrition is important to overall health. Poor nutrition may contribute to illness; for example, obesity is linked to diabetes and heart disease and raises the risk for some types of cancer. Healthy nutrition may contribute to good outcomes from illness. In one study, for example, women who ate low-fat diets after treatment for estrogen receptor–negative breast cancer were less likely to have recurrence of their cancer. However, vitamin or mineral supplements have not been proven to cure any type of cancer. Available scientific studies have not shown that orthomolecular medicine can help most of the conditions for which it is recommended.

At this time, it is hard to say how each nutrient or nutrient combination affects a person's risk for cancer. Studies of large groups of people have shown that those whose diets are high in vegetables and low in animal fat, meat, and/or calories have lower risks for some of the most common types of cancer. However, until more is known about this relationship, the American Cancer Society recommends eating a variety of healthful foods—with most of them coming from plant sources—rather than relying on supplements.

While it is best to get vitamins and minerals from foods, supplements may be helpful for some people, such as pregnant women, women of childbearing age, and people with restricted food intakes. If a supplement is taken, the best choice for most people is a balanced multivitamin/mineral supplement that contains no more than 100 percent of the "Daily Value" of most nutrients.

Are there any possible problems or complications?

Vitamin A, vitamin D, selenium, iron, magnesium, zinc, and other supplements can cause complications if too much is taken. Occasional deaths have been reported from iron or magnesium overdoses, mostly in children. Overdoses of minerals may also cause vomiting, diarrhea, hair loss, rashes, and diseases of the nails. Zinc and molybdenum can cause the body's copper levels to drop, which may cause anemia and low white blood cell counts. High doses of pyridoxine (vitamin B6) have been linked with reports of pain, numbness in the hands and legs, and trouble walking. Vitamin A overdoses can cause headache, drowsiness, irritability, vomiting, loss of hair and eyebrows, and peeling of the skin. Too much vitamin D can cause poor appetite, nausea, vomiting, weakness, itching, and permanent kidney damage.

Some supplements can raise the risk for cancer or heart disease. In addition, the potential interactions between supplements and drugs and herbs should be considered. Some of these combinations may be dangerous. Always tell your doctor and pharmacist about any supplements and herbs you are taking.

Antioxidant supplements can interfere with chemotherapy or radiation therapy. Patients who are in cancer treatment should consult with a knowledgeable physician before taking vitamins, minerals, or other supplements. Relying on this type of treatment alone and avoiding or delaying conventional medical care for cancer may have serious health consequences.

These substances may have not been thoroughly tested to find out how they interact with medicines, foods, or dietary supplements. Even though some reports of interactions and harmful effects may be published, full studies of interactions and effects are not often available. Because of these limitations, any information on ill effects and interactions should be considered incomplete.

References

Bairati I, Meyer F, Gélinas M, Fortin A, Nabid A, Brochet F, Mercier JP, Têtu B, Harel F, Abdous B, Vigneault E, Vass S, Del Vecchio P, Roy J. Randomized trial of antioxidant vitamins to prevent acute adverse effects of radiation therapy in head and neck cancer patients. *J Clin Oncol.* 2005;23:5805-5813. Epub 2005 Jul 18.

Bjelakovic G, Nikolova D, Gluud LL, Simonetti RG, Gluud C. Mortality in randomized trials of antioxidant supplements for primary and secondary prevention: systematic review and meta-analysis. *JAMA.* 2007;297:842-857.

Forman JP, Rimm EB, Stampfer MJ, Curhan GC. Folate intake and the risk of incident hypertension among US women. *JAMA.* 2005;293:320-329.

Galan P, Briançon S, Favier A, Bertrais S, Preziosi P, Faurer H, Arnaud J, Arnault N, Czernichow S, Mennen L, Hercberg S. Antioxidant status and risk of cancer in the SU.VI.MAX study: is the effect of supplementation dependent on baseline levels? *Br J Nutr.* 2005;94:125-132.

Haslam RH, Dalby JT, Rademaker AW. Effects of megavitamin therapy on children with attention deficit disorders. *Pediatrics.* 1984;74:103-111.

Hercberg S, Galan P, Preziosi P, Bertrais S, Mennen L, Malvy D, Roussel AM, Favier A, Briançon S. The SU.VI.MAX study: a randomized, placebo-controlled trial of the health effects of antioxidant vitamins and minerals. *Arch Intern Med.* 2004;164:2335-2342.

Goodman GE, Thornquist MD, Balmes J, Cullen MR, Meyskens FL, Omenn GS, Valanis B, Williams JH Jr. The Beta-Carotene and Retinol Efficacy Trial: incidence of lung cancer and cardiovascular disease mortality during 6-year follow-up after stopping beta-carotene and retinol supplements. *J Natl Cancer Inst.* 2004;96:1743-1750.

Kushi LH, Byers T, Doyle C, Bandera EV, McCullough M, McTiernan A, Gansler T, Andrews KS, Thun MJ; American Cancer Society 2006 Nutrition and Physical Activity Guidelines Advisory Committee. American Cancer Society guidelines on nutrition and physical activity for cancer prevention: reducing the risk of cancer with healthy food choices and physical activity. *CA Cancer J Clin.* 2006;56:254-281.

Lawenda BD, Kelly KM, Ladas EJ, Sagar SM, Vickers A, Blumberg JB. Should supplemental antioxidant administration be avoided during chemotherapy and radiation therapy? *J Natl Cancer Inst.* 2008;100:773-783.

Lerner V, Miodownik C, Kaptsan A, Cohen H, Loewenthal U, Kotler M. Vitamin B6 as add-on treatment in chronic schizophrenic and schizoaffective patients: a double-blind, placebo-controlled study. *J Clin Psychiatry.* 2002;63:54-58.

Lonn E, Bosch J, Yusuf S, Sheridan P, Pogue J, Arnold JM, Ross C, Arnold A, Sleight P, Probstfield J, Dagenais GR; HOPE and HOPE-TOO Trial Investigators. Effects of long-term vitamin E supplementation on cardiovascular events and cancer: a randomized controlled trial. *JAMA.* 2005;293:1338-1347.

McGuire JK, Kulkarni MS, Baden HP. Fatal hypermagnesemia in a child treated with megavitamin/megamineral therapy. *Pediatrics.* 2000;105:E18.

Merck manual. Merck Web site. http://www.merck.com/mmpe/index.html. Accessed June 23, 2008.

Morris CC. Pediatric iron poisonings in the United States. *South Med J.* 2000;93:352-358.

Richer S, Stiles W, Statkute L, Pulido J, Frankowski J, Rudy D, Pei K, Tsipursky M, Nyland J. Double-masked, placebo-controlled, randomized trial of lutein and antioxidant supplementation in the intervention of atrophic age-related macular degeneration: the Veterans LAST study (Lutein Antioxidant Supplementation Trial). *Optometry.* 2004;75:216-230.

Taylor PR, Greenwald P. Nutritional interventions and cancer prevention. *J Clin Oncol.* 2005;23:333-345.

PAU D'ARCO

Other common name(s): lapachol, lapacho, lapacho morado, lapacho Colorado, ipe roxo, ipes, taheebo, tahuari, trumpet bush, trumpet tree

Scientific/medical name(s): *Tabebuia impetiginosa, Tabebuia avellanedae, Tabebuia heptaphylla, Tabebuia ipê*

Description

Pau d'arco is a large tree that grows naturally in the rain forests of Central and South America. It may be cultivated in southern Florida. There are about one hundred species of the tree, which produces large flowers and can grow to 150 feet tall and six feet in diameter. *Tebebuia impetiginosa* produces purple or pink flowers, while other varieties produce yellow or white flowers. The inner bark of the tree is used in herbal remedies.

Overview

Laboratory and animal studies suggest that lapachol and other compounds extracted from or made from pau d'arco may have some effects against certain illnesses. However, available evidence from well-designed, controlled studies does not support this substance as an effective treatment for cancer in humans. Pau d'arco also has potentially dangerous side effects.

How is it promoted for use?

Pau d'arco is promoted as a cure for dozens of illnesses and medical conditions, including arthritis, ulcers, diabetes, and cancer. Proponents also claim that, when taken internally, pau d'arco relieves infections, reduces inflammation, promotes digestion, strengthens the immune system, flushes toxins from the body, and protects against cardiovascular disease and high blood pressure. Proponents also use it to treat lupus, osteomyelitis, Parkinson's disease, and psoriasis and to relieve pain. Some use the boiled bark externally as a poultice or use the strained liquid as a wash to treat skin inflammations, fungal infections, hemorrhoids, eczema, and wounds.

What does it involve?

Pau d'arco is available as a capsule, tablet, salve, liquid extract, powder, and tea from health food stores and over the Internet. Recommended dosage varies by manufacturer. When making tea, practitioners say the bark must be boiled or simmered for at least eight minutes to release the active ingredients, which do not dissolve easily in water.

What is the history behind it?

Tea made from pau d'arco is thought to have been popular among the ancient Incas and natives of the South American rain forests, who used it to cure disease and as a tonic to strengthen the body and improve overall health. Caribbean folk healers reportedly use the leaf and the bark to treat backaches, toothaches, and sexually transmitted diseases. The native tribes of Brazil used the tree to make bows for hunting. When the Portuguese colonized Brazil, they named the tree pau d'arco, which means "bow stick." The herb remains a popular Brazilian folk remedy.

New interest in pau d'arco arose in the mid-1960s, when a Brazilian physician claimed that the substance could relieve pain, increase the number of red blood cells, and cure numerous illnesses, including cancer. Since the early 1980s, the herb has been sold in health food stores in the United States, where it is promoted as a treatment for virtually every kind of medical complaint.

What is the evidence?

One of the active ingredients in pau d'arco that has been studied is called lapachol. In laboratory animals, lapachol was found to be effective against malaria and certain kinds of animal tumor cells, such as sarcoma, but it did not have an effect on other kinds of cancer, including leukemia and adenocarcinoma. Further studies are required to determine whether these results apply to humans.

There have been only a few studies on lapachol in humans. An uncontrolled study sponsored by the National Cancer Institute in the early 1970s found no toxic effects on liver or kidney tissue. However, lapachol did prevent blood from clotting, and doses thought to be high enough to affect tumors posed a serious risk for bleeding. Clotting function returned to normal when the drug was stopped. Based on these results, approval for lapachol as a new anticancer drug was not sought. Research in the area was discontinued. Canada subsequently banned the substance in 1985.

Pau d'arco contains at least twenty active compounds, including naphthaquinones (of which lapachol is one), anthraquinones, alkaloids, quercetin, and other flavonoids whose effects are not fully known. Unconfirmed tests showed that crude extracts of the tree bark stimulated the activity of immune system cells called macrophages. The substance also killed lung cancer cells and liver cancer cells grown in test tubes and reduced the rate of lung cancer spread in mice after surgery to remove the initial tumor. The bark extract also may kill bacteria or fungi. In a 2004 study, two compounds made from naphthaquinones showed promise in animal studies for malaria treatment. It is important to note, however, that studies of extracted compounds would not be expected to yield the same results as studies of the raw bark.

Are there any possible problems or complications?

Pau d'arco has some potentially serious side effects. Some of the chemicals in pau d'arco, such as hydroquinone, are known to be toxic. High doses taken internally may cause liver and kidney damage. In animal studies, birth defects and deaths occurred among rats whose mothers were given lapachol during pregnancy. Pau d'arco should be avoided, especially by women who are pregnant or breastfeeding.

Even low doses of pau d'arco can cause dizziness, nausea, vomiting, and diarrhea and can interfere with blood clotting. The resulting bleeding can cause anemia. In addition, pau d'arco, when taken by mouth, can interact with aspirin and blood-thinning medications, further increasing the risk for bleeding. It may also increase the risk for bleeding in people with hemophilia or other clotting disorders.

The bark of the tree can sensitize skin and has caused asthma in work settings where people are exposed to the wood dust. Allergic reactions are possible.

Twelve commercial pau d'arco products that were tested in Canada showed that only one contained lapachol, which normally makes up about 7 percent of pau d'arco, suggesting the products likely contained other substances.

The potential interactions between pau d'arco and other drugs and herbs should be considered. Some of these combinations may be dangerous. Always tell your doctor and pharmacist about any herbs you are taking. Relying on this type of treatment alone and avoiding or delaying conventional medical care for cancer may have serious health consequences.

This product is sold as a dietary supplement in the United States. Unlike companies that produce drugs (which must provide the FDA with results of detailed testing showing their product is safe and effective before the drug is approved for sale), the companies that make supplements do not have to show evidence of safety or health benefits to the FDA before selling their products. Supplement products without any reliable scientific evidence of health benefits may still be sold as long as the companies selling them do not claim the supplements can prevent, treat, or cure any specific disease. Some such products may not contain the amount of the herb or substance that is written on the label, and some may include other substances (contaminants). Though the FDA has written new rules to improve the quality of manufacturing processes for dietary supplements and the accurate listing of supplement ingredients, these rules do not take full effect until 2010. The new rules also do not address the safety of supplement ingredients or their effects on health when proper manufacturing techniques are used.

Most such supplements have not been tested to find out if they interact with medicines, foods, or other herbs and supplements. Even though some reports of interactions and harmful effects may be published, full studies of interactions and effects are not often available. Because of these limitations, any information on ill effects and interactions should be considered incomplete.

References

Algranti E, Mendonca EM, Ali SA, Kokron CM, Raile V. Occupational asthma caused by Ipe (Tabebuia spp) dust. *J Investig Allergol Clin Immunol.* 2005;15:81-83.

American Cancer Society. Questionable methods of cancer management: 'nutritional' therapies. *CA Cancer J Clin.* 1993;43:309-319.

Cassileth BR. Evaluating complementary and alternative therapies for cancer patients. *CA Cancer J Clin.* 1999;49:362-375.

de Andrade-Neto VF, Goulart MO, da Silva Filho JF, da Silva MJ, Pinto Mdo C, Pinto AV, Zalis MG, Carvalho LH, Krettli AU. Antimalarial activity of phenazines from lapachol, beta-lapachone and its derivatives against *Plasmodium falciparum* in vitro and *Plasmodium berghei* in vivo. *Bioorg Med Chem Lett.* 2004;14:1145-1149.

Dinnen RD, Ebisuzaki K. The search for novel anticancer agents: a differentiation-based assay and analysis of a folklore product. *Anticancer Res.* 1997;17:1027-1033.

Felício AC, Chang CV, Brandão MA, Peters VM, Guerra Mde O. Fetal growth in rats treated with lapachol. *Contraception.* 2002;66:289-293.

Fetrow CW, Avila JR. *Professional's Handbook of Complementary & Alternative Medicines.* Philadelphia, PA: Lippincott Williams & Wilkins; 2004.

Montbriand MJ. Past and present herbs used to treat cancer: medicine, magic, or poison? *Oncol Nurs Forum.* 1999;26:49-60; quiz 61-62.

Pau darco. Drug Digest Web site. http://www.drugdigest.org/DD/DVH/HerbsWho/0,3923,552793|Pau+D%27arco,00.html. Accessed June 6, 2008.

Pau d'arco. Memorial Sloan-Kettering Cancer Center Web site. http://www.mskcc.org/mskcc/html/69325.cfm. Updated January 8, 2008. Accessed June 6, 2008.

Pau d'arco/taheebo tea/lapacho/lapacho morado/ipe roxo/ipe/trumpet bush. BC Cancer Agency Web site. http://www.bccancer.bc.ca/HPI/UnconventionalTherapies/PauDArco.htm. Updated February 2000. Accessed June 6, 2008.

US Congress, Office of Technology Assessment. *Unconventional Cancer Treatments: OTA-H-405*. Washington, DC: US Government Printing Office; 1990.

Woo HJ, Choi YH. Growth inhibition of A549 human lung carcinoma cells by beta-lapachone through induction of apoptosis and inhibition of telomerase activity. *Int J Oncol.* 2005;26:1017-1023.

Woo HJ, Park KY, Rhu CH, Choi BT, Kim GY, Park YM, Choi YH. Beta-lapachone, a quinone isolated from Tabebuia avellanedae, induces apoptosis in HepG2 hepatoma cell line through induction of Bax and activation of caspase. *J Med Food.* 2006;9:161-168.

PC-SPES, PC-HOPE, AND PC-CARE

Other common name(s): PC-PLUS, Prostasol
Scientific/medical name(s): none

Description

PC-SPES was a formula consisting of eight herbs that contained a range of plant chemicals including flavonoids, alkanoids, polysaccharides, amino acids, and trace minerals such as selenium, calcium, magnesium, zinc, and copper. The eight herbs used were chrysanthemum, isatis, licorice, *Ganoderma lucidum*, *Panax pseudoginseng*, *Rabdosia rubescens*, saw palmetto, and skullcap (see "Licorice," page 410, and "Saw Palmetto," page 484), although other compounds were found in the formula.

"PC" stands for prostate cancer, and "SPES" is the Latin word for hope. PC-SPES was removed from the U.S. market in February 2002. The U.S. Food and Drug Administration (FDA) issued a warning for people to stop using the product because PC-SPES capsules were found to contain prescription drugs that could cause serious health problems.

Since then, several new herbal products for prostate cancer have been developed. The two most popular of these are PC-HOPE and PC-CARE. A similar product is Prostasol, previously sold as PC-PLUS. PC-HOPE includes the following ingredients: magnesium, sterolins, quercetin, "proprietary blend," Reishi (as *Ganoderma lucidum*), Baikal skullcap (as *Scutellaria baicalensis*), Rabdosia (as *Rabdosia rubescens Hara*), Dyer's woad (as *Isatis indigotica Fortune*), mum (as *Dendranthema morifolium Tzelev*), saw palmetto (as *Serenoa repens*), San-Qi ginseng (as *Panax notoginseng*), and licorice (as *Glycyrrhiza glabra*). The company that produces this product recommends starting with 2 to 6 tablets daily and gradually reducing the dose over a period of months.

The ingredients of PC-CARE are listed as "Proprietary Blend," Reishi, Baikal skullcap, *Rabdosia rubescens, Isatis indigotica*, chrysanthemum, saw palmetto, rye, and licorice. The company producing this product recommends 3 tablets daily.

Overview

Several carefully designed clinical trials found that PC-SPES was an effective treatment for patients with prostate cancer, including some whose cancer did not respond to conventional hormone therapy. Common side effects included breast enlargement and tenderness, hot flashes, and decreased libido. Blood clots were a less common but more serious side effect. However, because the production process for PC-SPES did not offer adequate protection against contamination, this product is no longer available.

Newer products, such as PC-HOPE and PC-CARE, contain many of the same ingredients as PC-SPES. However, because of limitations in the way herbal products are regulated in the United States, patients and clinicians cannot make any assumptions regarding the purity, safety, or effectiveness of these new products. More research is needed to evaluate them.

How is it promoted for use?

PC-SPES was promoted as a treatment for prostate cancer. Proponents claimed that the herbal preparation could prevent or delay the recurrence of prostate cancer, inhibit the growth of prostate tumors, lengthen the survival time of prostate cancer patients, improve the effectiveness of conventional treatments, and delay the need for treatment with chemotherapy. PC-HOPE, PC-CARE, and Prostasol (previously known as PC-PLUS) are promoted in similar ways.

What does it involve?

These herbal formulations for prostate cancer treatment come in capsules and are taken daily, in varying dosages. PC-SPES is no longer produced. PC-HOPE and PC-CARE are available in health food stores, from some nutritionists, and directly from manufacturers.

What is the history behind it?

PC-SPES was developed in the early 1990s by a chemist named Sophie Chen, PhD, who claimed to have developed the formula by integrating modern science and ancient Chinese herbal wisdom.

By the mid 1990s, the formula was widely promoted in the United States and was named PC-SPES. Production of PC-SPES was stopped in 2002 when it was found to be contaminated with varying amounts of three prescription drugs: warfarin (an anticoagulant), diethylstilbestrol (DES, an estrogen-like hormone), and indomethacin (an anti-inflammatory drug). PC-HOPE, PC-CARE, and Prostasol became popular after production of PC-SPES was halted.

What is the evidence?

PC-SPES has been carefully evaluated in several clinical trials. In virtually all of these studies, PC-SPES was found to be effective in reducing blood levels of prostate-specific antigen (PSA), a protein secreted by cancerous prostate cells that is widely used by doctors as a measure of whether prostate cancer is responding to treatment or continuing to grow and spread. Several studies also observed shrinking in tumors following treatment.

A randomized clinical trial comparing PC-SPES and DES was started before PC-SPES's problems with contamination were known, and results were published in 2004. DES is sometimes used as a hormonal treatment for prostate cancer that is no longer responding to treatments that block production or activity of male hormones. Although some of the PC-SPES tablets used in the study were later found to be contaminated with DES or other estrogenic prescription drugs, the herbal product was actually more effective than DES pills in lowering blood PSA levels and in delaying growth of the cancer. The men receiving PC-SPES were at lower risk for blood clots than those taking DES.

Prior to its removal from the market, laboratory studies of PC-SPES looked at how its ingredients blocked the growth of prostate cancer cells. Substances from some of the ingredients acted as phytoestrogens (estrogen-like substances found in plants) and blocked the growth of prostate cancer cells. Prostate cancer cells are fueled by androgens (male hormones) and slowed by estrogens (female hormones). Some ingredients may have helped to activate the immune system. Still others acted in ways not yet completely understood, but which appeared to involve mechanisms other than acting as estrogens.

A few laboratory studies of PC-HOPE and PC-CARE have been published, and these studies suggest they are active against prostate cancer cells. Two European clinical studies of PC-HOPE suggest it may improve patients' quality of life and lower their PSA levels. These two studies are summarized in press releases on the Internet, but as of mid-2008 the detailed results had not yet been published in medical journals.

Before PC-SPES was removed from the market, many prostate specialists considered it a reasonable option for treating men whose prostate cancers were androgen-independent, meaning they were no longer responding to treatments that block production or activity of male hormones. PC-SPES was not recommended for cancers that were still responding to conventional hormonal treatments or for men with localized prostate cancer that could be treated with surgery or radiation therapy.

The role of newer herbal formulations remains uncertain, because U.S. laws permit companies to sell these products without providing detailed information on safety and effectiveness (as would be required for new drugs). It will probably take a few years for prostate cancer researchers to complete clinical studies of PC-HOPE and PC-CARE similar to those they had done on PC-SPES.

Are there any possible problems or complications?

Side effects associated with the use of PC-SPES included increased breast size, nipple tenderness or pain, and reduced sex drive. There was also an increased risk for blood clots, which are potentially fatal. Since PC-HOPE, Prostasol, and PC-CARE are reported to be quite similar to PC-SPES, side effects may also be similar.

As with all herbs, allergic reactions are possible. In addition, the potential interactions between herbs and other drugs and herbs should be considered. Some of these combinations may be dangerous. Always tell your doctor and pharmacist about any herbs you are taking. Relying on this type of treatment alone and avoiding or delaying conventional medical care for cancer may have serious health consequences.

This product is sold as a dietary supplement in the United States. Unlike companies that produce drugs (which must provide the FDA with results of detailed testing showing their product is safe and effective before the drug is approved for sale), the companies that make supplements do not have to show evidence of safety or health benefits to the FDA before selling their products. Supplement products without any reliable scientific evidence of health benefits may still be sold as long as the companies selling them do not claim the supplements can prevent, treat, or cure any specific disease. Some such products may not contain the amount of the herb or substance that is written on the label, and some may include other substances (contaminants). Though the FDA has written new rules to improve the quality of manufacturing processes for dietary supplements and the accurate listing of supplement ingredients, these rules do not take full effect until 2010. The new rules also do not address the safety of supplement ingredients or their effects on health when proper manufacturing techniques are used.

Most such supplements have not been tested to find out if they interact with medicines, foods, or other herbs and supplements. Even though some reports of interactions and harmful effects may be published, full studies of interactions and effects are not often available. Because of these limitations, any information on ill effects and interactions should be considered incomplete.

References

Bigler D, Gulding KM, Dann R, Sheabar FZ, Conaway MR, Theodorescu D. Gene profiling and promoter reporter assays: novel tools for comparing the biological effects of botanical extracts on human prostate cancer cells and understanding their mechanisms of action. *Oncogene.* 2003;22:1261-1272.

de la Taille A, Buttyan R, Hayek O, Bagiella E, Shabsigh A, Burchardt M, Burchardt T, Chopin DK, Katz AE. Herbal therapy PC-SPES: in vitro effects and evaluation of its efficacy in 69 patients with prostate cancer. *J Urol.* 2000;164:1229-1234.

DiPaola RS, Zhang H, Lambert GH, Meeker R, Licitra E, Rafi MM, Zhu BT, Spaulding H, Goodin S, Toledano MB, Hait WN, Gallo MA. Clinical and biologic activity of an estrogenic herbal combination (PC-SPES) in prostate cancer. *N Engl J Med.* 1998;339:785-791.

Guns ES, Goldenberg SL, Brown PN. Mass spectral analysis of PC-SPES confirms the presence of diethylstilbestrol. *Can J Urol.* 2002;9:1684-1688; discussion 1689.

Ikezoe T, Chen S, Saito T, Asou H, Kyo T, Tanosaki S, Heber D, Taguchi H, Koeffler HP. PC-SPES decreases proliferation and induces differentiation and apoptosis of human acute myeloid leukemia cells. *Int J Oncol.* 2003;23:1203-1211.

Natural Standard. Herbal/plant therapies: PC-SPES. Complementary/Integrative Medicine Education Resources, The University of Texas M. D. Anderson Cancer Center Web site. http://www.mdanderson.org/departments/cimer/display.cfm?id=66d17404-09ad-443e-b865bcfc6b635507&method=displayfull. Accessed June 6, 2008.

Nelson PS, Montgomery B. Unconventional therapy for prostate cancer: good, bad or questionable? *Nat Rev Cancer.* 2003;3:845-858.

Oh WK, George DJ, Hackmann K, Manola J, Kantoff PW. Activity of the herbal combination, PC-SPES, in the treatment of patients with androgen-independent prostate cancer. *Urology.* 2001;57:122-126.

Oh WK, Kantoff PW, Weinberg V, Jones G, Rini BI, Derynck MK, Bok R, Smith MR, Bubley GJ, Rosen RT, DiPaola RS, Small EJ. Prospective, multicenter, randomized phase II trial of the herbal supplement, PC-SPES, and diethylstilbestrol in patients with androgen-independent prostate cancer. *J Clin Oncol.* 2004;22:3705-3712.

PC-SPES. Memorial Sloan-Kettering Cancer Center Web site. http://www.mskcc.org/mskcc/html/69326.cfm. Updated August 7, 2007. Accessed June 6, 2008.

PC-SPES (PDQ). National Cancer Institute Web site. http://www.nci.nih.gov/cancertopics/pdq/cam/pc-spes/HealthProfessional/page1. Updated April 23, 2008. Accessed June 6, 2008.

Pfeifer BL, Pirani JF, Hamann SR, Klippel KF. PC-SPES, a dietary supplement for the treatment of hormone-refractory prostate cancer. *BJU Int.* 2000;85:481-485.

Small EJ, Frohlich MW, Bok R, Shinohara K, Grossfeld G, Rozenblat Z, Kelly WK, Corry M, Reese DM. Prospective trial of the herbal supplement PC-SPES in patients with progressive prostate cancer. *J Clin Oncol.* 2000;18:3595-3603.

Sovak M, Seligson AL, Konas M, Hajduch M, Dolezal M, Machala M, Nagourney R. Herbal composition PC-SPES for management of prostate cancer: identification of active principles. *J Natl Cancer Inst.* 2002;94:1275-1281.

PEPPERMINT

Other common name(s): peppermint oil, mint, balm mint, brandy mint, green mint
Scientific/medical name(s): *Mentha piperita*

Description

Peppermint is a plant native to Europe and is now cultivated widely in the United States and Canada. The oil from the leaves and flowering tops of the plant is used in herbal remedies. Its main active ingredients are menthol and menthone.

Overview

Available scientific evidence does not support claims that peppermint oil is effective in treating side effects related to chemotherapy and radiation. However, there is some evidence that it may be effective in controlling nausea after surgery. Preliminary studies suggest that direct contact with peppermint oil may be helpful in reducing spasms in the esophagus and intestines during endoscopies and other procedures. There is mixed evidence that enteric-coated peppermint oil (supplements that are coated so that they are not absorbed by the body until they reach the small intestine) might be helpful in treating symptoms of irritable bowel syndrome such as cramps. It is known to worsen acid reflux in some people. Strong vapors of menthol or peppermint can cause breathing problems for some people, especially infants.

How is it promoted for use?

Proponents claim peppermint oil improves digestion and relieves intestinal ailments such as gas, indigestion, cramps, diarrhea, and symptoms of irritable bowel syndrome and food poisoning. Some say it has a soothing effect and reduces anxiety.

Sprays and inhalants containing peppermint oil are promoted to relieve sore throats, toothaches, colds, coughs, laryngitis, bronchitis, nasal congestion, and inflammation of the mouth and throat. Another reported use of peppermint oil is to apply it to the forehead and temples to relieve tension headaches. Some claim that salves made from menthol (one of the major active ingredients in peppermint) ease muscle pain and soreness associated with injuries, arthritis, rheumatism, and neuralgia. Menthol vapors are also believed to relieve respiratory and sinus congestion.

Aromatherapists claim the scent of peppermint improves concentration, stimulates the mind and body, decreases inflammation, improves digestion, and relieves stomach pain (see "Aromatherapy," page 57).

What does it involve?

Peppermint oil is the most frequently used form of the peppermint plant. The pure oil or a liquid extract containing the oil can be taken directly or swallowed in capsules. It is also made in enteric-coated capsules, which are designed to melt after they pass through the stomach. Peppermint is also available as a spray and inhalant for treating ailments of the throat, mouth, nose, sinuses, and lungs. The leaves are sometimes brewed as a tea.

Peppermint oil is on the Commission E (Germany's regulatory agency for herbs) list of approved herbs. Common dosages are 1 to 2 capsules three times a day for irritable bowel syndrome; 1 tablespoon of leaves in a cup of boiling water for tea, two or three times a day; 3 to 4 drops in hot water for inhalation; 1 percent to 5 percent essential oil for nasal ointments; and 5 percent to 20 percent essential oil for other ointments applied to the skin.

Many well-known commercial products also contain menthol in salve form, which is rubbed directly on the skin or has its vapors inhaled. Peppermint is often used to flavor toothpaste, mouthwash, cosmetics, chewing gum, candy, and pharmaceuticals.

What is the history behind it?

Peppermint may have been used as a digestive aid thousands of years ago in ancient Egypt. More recently, peppermint has been used as a folk remedy for vomiting, morning sickness, respiratory infections, and menstrual problems. Preparations containing menthol have a long history as a treatment for muscle soreness and pain, itching, and sunburn and to clear nasal congestion.

What is the evidence?

There are many anecdotal reports supporting the use of peppermint as a treatment for various digestive and breathing complaints. However, there is not enough scientific evidence available to conclude that peppermint lives up to all the claims made by proponents, especially its use as a treatment for stomach cancer or any other type of cancer.

Although available scientific evidence does not support claims that peppermint oil is effective in treating side effects related to chemotherapy and radiation therapy, it was found to be useful in controlling nausea after surgery. A randomized clinical trial in the United Kingdom found that patients who received peppermint oil before surgery had less nausea after surgery than those who did not.

In 2002, researchers discovered a nerve ending that responded to cold and to menthol. This may explain the cooling sensation from menthol, as well as its common use as an inhalant to reduce congestion in the nose. However, available studies do not yet show whether it actually "opens" the nose or improves breathing when a person has a cold.

There is debate about whether peppermint oil is effective in treating irritable bowel syndrome. Several randomized controlled trials suggest that enteric-coated peppermint may be helpful, but the studies have been small and have not followed the patients for very long. Well-designed larger studies are needed to determine whether this possibility holds true.

Some early evidence suggests that instilling peppermint oil into the colon during a barium enema (an x-ray test of the bowel) may reduce intestinal spasms and decrease the need for intravenous antispasm medications. A recent study suggests that taking peppermint oil by mouth can reduce intestinal spasms during barium enema examination. A Japanese study looked at introducing peppermint oil directly into the esophagus to reduce spasms in the muscle ring above the stomach during endoscopy. The researchers reported it worked more quickly than an injection of a standard antispasmodic medicine. However, additional well-controlled studies are needed to make definite conclusions. These results need to be checked in larger clinical trials before being routinely recommended.

Studies that looked at applying peppermint oil to the forehead and temples to help tension headaches suggested it might be useful in some people, but further studies are needed to determine whether this is truly helpful for tension headaches.

Aromatherapy using peppermint oil for nausea after surgery showed it to be no more effective than isopropyl alcohol or a salt water placebo. A gauze pad containing the liquid was placed under the patient's nose, and the patient was asked to breathe deeply through the nose and exhale through the mouth. Nausea scores were the same across the groups, and only 52 percent of patients required conventional medicines to control their nausea. Four out of five patients were satisfied with how their nausea was managed. In this case, the change in patients' breathing may have helped more than the aroma being tested.

Are there any possible problems or complications?

Peppermint is considered safe when taken by nonallergic people in normal doses. It can cause irritation when applied to the skin. Because peppermint may increase symptoms of acid reflux disease and hiatal hernia, people with these conditions are advised to avoid the herb. People with gallstones or liver damage should also use caution when using peppermint. Peppermint oil and menthol products should not be applied to the nose or face of an infant or small child since they could cause breathing problems. Rare cases of allergic rashes, hives, asthma, and other reactions have been reported in people who are sensitive to peppermint or its components.

Acid-reducing medicines may allow enteric-coated peppermint to be released before it leaves the stomach, which may reduce its effect on an irritable bowel. Peppermint oil may interact with other medicines as well, so it is helpful to talk with your doctor or pharmacist about all medicines and supplements that you are taking.

Menthone (which makes up around 20 percent of peppermint oil) was given to rats for four weeks by mouth. It affected kidney and liver function, and very high doses caused cyst-like spaces in the brainstem. In other animal studies, large does have caused weakness, seizures, and brain damage. Menthol is considered to be the most toxic component of peppermint oil. As little as two grams are thought to be fatal in some, although people have survived higher doses. In work settings, those who handle menthol are cautioned that it can cause irritation of the eyes. Eyes should be thoroughly flushed if contact occurs. For skin contact, wash with soap and water. Stomach upset with pain, vomiting, vertigo, drowsiness, and coma may result from ingestion, and death may occur because of lung failure.

Peppermint oil should not be taken by injection; a recent report describes the case of a young woman who had serious lung damage after intravenous injection of peppermint oil. She survived but required intensive care and the support of a breathing machine for thirteen days. Taking any type of oil by injection can cause serious effects, including death.

Peppermint oils, when taken by mouth, can affect the way that other drugs are absorbed by the body and may interfere with antacids, medications for high blood pressure, and others. Mint salves and creams can cause the ingredients in other creams and ointments to be absorbed more quickly. Other potential interactions between peppermint and other drugs and herbs should be considered. Some of these combinations may be dangerous. Always tell your doctor and pharmacist about any herbs you are taking. Relying on this type of treatment alone and avoiding or delaying conventional medical care for cancer may have serious health consequences.

This product is sold as a dietary supplement in the United States. Unlike companies that produce drugs (which must provide the FDA with results of detailed testing showing their product is safe and effective before the drug is approved for sale), the companies that make supplements do not have to show evidence of safety or health benefits to the FDA before selling their products. Supplement products without any reliable scientific evidence of health benefits may still be sold as long as the companies selling them do not claim the supplements can prevent, treat, or cure any specific disease. Some such products may not contain the amount of the herb or substance that is written on the label, and some may include other substances (contaminants). Though the FDA has written new rules to improve the quality of manufacturing processes for dietary supplements and the accurate listing of supplement ingredients, these rules do not take full effect until 2010. The new rules also do not address the safety of supplement ingredients or their effects on health when proper manufacturing techniques are used.

Most such supplements have not been tested to find out if they interact with medicines, foods, or other herbs and supplements. Even though some reports of interactions and harmful effects may be published, full studies of interactions and effects are not often available. Because of these limitations, any information on ill effects and interactions should be considered incomplete.

References

Anderson LA, Gross JB. Aromatherapy with peppermint, isopropyl alcohol, or placebo is equally effective in relieving postoperative nausea. *J Perianesth Nurs.* 2004;19:29-35.

Behrends M, Beiderlinden M, Peters J. Acute lung injury after peppermint oil injection. *Anesth Analg.* 2005;101:1160-1162.

Blumenthal M, ed. *The Complete German Commission E Monographs: Therapeutic Guide to Herbal Medicines.* Austin, TX: American Botanical Council; 1998.

dos Santos MA, Santos Galvão CE, Morato Castro F. Menthol-induced asthma: a case report. *J Investig Allergol Clin Immunol.* 2001;11:56-58.

Fetrow CW, Avila JR. *Professional's Handbook of Complementary & Alternative Medicines.* Philadelphia, PA: Lippincott Williams & Wilkins; 2004.

Gruenwald J. *PDR for Herbal Medicines.* 3rd ed. Montvale, NJ: Thomson PDR; 2004.

Hiki N, Kurosaka H, Tatsutomi Y, Shimoyama S, Tsuji E, Kojima J, Shimizu N, Ono H, Hirooka T, Noguchi C, Mafune K, Kaminishi M. Peppermint oil reduces gastric spasm during upper endoscopy: a randomized, double-blind, double-dummy controlled trial. *Gastrointest Endosc.* 2003;57:475-482.

Kingham JG. Peppermint oil and colon spasm. *Lancet.* 1995;346:986.

Madisch A, Heydenreich CJ, Wieland V, Hufnagel R, Hotz J. Treatment of functional dyspepsia with a fixed peppermint oil and caraway oil combination preparation as compared to cisapride. A multicenter, reference-controlled double-blind equivalence study. *Arzneimittelforschung.* 1999;49:925-932.

Madsen C, Würtzen G, Carstensen J. Short-term toxicity study in rats dosed with menthone. *Toxicol Lett.* 1986;32:147-152.

Manufacturer's product information: levo-Menthol. J.T. Baker Web site. http://www.jtbaker.com/msds/englishhtml/m1131.htm. Accessed January 24, 2006.

McKemy DD, Neuhausser WM, Julius D. Identification of a cold receptor reveals a general role for TRP channels in thermosensation. *Nature.* 2002;416:52-58.

Mizuno S, Kato K, Ono Y, Yano K, Kurosaka H, Takahashi A, Abeta H, Kushiro T, Miyamoto S, Kurihara R, Hiki N, Kaminishi M, Iwasaki A, Arakawa Y. Oral peppermint oil is a useful antispasmodic for double-contrast barium meal examination. *J Gastroenterol Hepatol.* 2006;21:1297-1301.

Nair B. Final report on the safety assessment of Mentha Piperita (Peppermint) Oil, Mentha Piperita (Peppermint)

Leaf Extract, Mentha Piperita (Peppermint) Leaf, and Mentha Piperita (Peppermint) Leaf Water. *Int J Toxicol.* 2001;20 Suppl 3:61-73.

Peppermint (Mentha x piperita L.). Medline Plus Web site. http://www.nlm.nih.gov/medlineplus/druginfo/natural/patient-peppermint.html. Updated January 1, 2008. Accessed June 6, 2008.

Pittler MH, Ernst E. Peppermint oil for irritable bowel syndrome: a critical review and metaanalysis. *Am J Gastroenterol.* 1998;93:1131-1135.

Tate S. Peppermint oil: a treatment for postoperative nausea. *J Adv Nurs.* 1997;26:543-549.

PHYTOCHEMICALS

Other common name(s): antioxidants, flavonoids, flavones, isoflavones, catechins, anthocyanidins, isothiocyanates, carotenoids, allyl sulfides, polyphenols
Scientific/medical name(s): various names

Description

The term "phytochemicals" refers to a wide variety of compounds produced by plants. They are found in fruits, vegetables, beans, grains, and other plants. Scientists have identified thousands of phytochemicals, although only a small fraction have been studied closely. Some of the more commonly known phytochemicals include beta carotene, ascorbic acid (vitamin C), folic acid, and vitamin E.

Overview

Some phytochemicals have either antioxidant or hormone-like actions. There is some evidence that a diet rich in fruits, vegetables, and whole grains reduces the risk for certain types of cancer and other diseases, and researchers are looking for specific compounds in these foods that may account for the beneficial effects in humans. Available scientific evidence does not support claims that taking phytochemical supplements is as helpful as consuming the fruits, vegetables, beans, and grains from which they are taken.

How are they promoted for use?

Phytochemicals are promoted for the prevention and treatment of many health conditions, including cancer, heart disease, diabetes, and high blood pressure. There is some evidence that certain phytochemicals may help prevent the formation of potential carcinogens (substances that cause cancer), block the action of carcinogens on their target organs or tissue, or act on cells to suppress cancer development. Many experts suggest that people can reduce their risk for cancer significantly by eating more fruits, vegetables, and other foods from plants that contain phytochemicals.

There are several major groups of phytochemicals. The polyphenols include a large subgroup of chemicals called flavonoids. Flavonoids are plant chemicals found in a broad range of fruits, grains, and vegetables. They are being studied to find out whether they can prevent chronic diseases such as cancer and heart disease. The isoflavones found in foods and supplements such as soy products, red clover, garbanzo beans and licorice, and the lignans found in flaxseed and whole grains, may mimic the actions of the female hormone estrogen (see "Licorice," page 410, and "Soybean," page 679). These estrogen-like substances from these plant sources are called phytoestrogens. They may play a role in the development of and protection against some hormone-dependent cancers such as some types of breast and prostate cancer.

Other polyphenols (including some flavonoids) act as antioxidants. These are thought to rid the body of harmful molecules known as free radicals, which can damage a cell's DNA and may trigger some forms of cancer and other diseases. These compounds are commonly found in vegetables such as broccoli, brussels sprouts, cabbage, and cauliflower and in teas. Grapes, eggplant, red cabbage, and radishes all contain anthocyanidins—flavonoids that act as antioxidants and may protect against some cancers and heart disease. Quercetin, another flavonoid with antioxidant properties, is found in apples, onions, teas, and red wine. Ellagic acid, found in raspberries, blackberries, cranberries, strawberries, and walnuts, also is said to have anticancer effects (see "Ellagic Acid," page 605).

Carotenoids, which give carrots, yams, cantaloupe, squash, and apricots their orange color, are also promoted as anticancer agents. Tomatoes, red peppers, and pink grapefruit contain lycopene, which proponents claim is a powerful antioxidant (see "Lycopene," page 633). The phytochemicals lutein and zeaxanthin, found in spinach, kale, and turnip greens, may reduce the risk for some cancers.

Another group of phytochemicals, called allyl sulfides, are found in garlic and onions (see "Garlic," page 611). These compounds may stimulate enzymes that help the body get rid of harmful chemicals. They may also help strengthen the immune system.

What does it involve?

Phytochemicals are present in virtually all of the fruits, vegetables, legumes (beans and peas), and grains we eat, so it is quite easy for most people to include them in their diet. For instance, a carrot contains more than a hundred phytochemicals. There are thousands of known phytochemicals, but only a few have been studied in detail.

Many of the better-known phytochemicals are now available as dietary supplements.

However, most available evidence suggests that these single supplements are not as beneficial as the foods from which they are derived.

What is the history behind it?

Only a few years ago, the term "phytochemical" was barely known. But doctors, nutritionists, and other health care practitioners have long advocated a low-fat diet that includes a variety of fruits, vegetables, legumes, and whole grains. Historically, cultures that consume such a diet have lower rates of certain cancers and heart disease.

Since the passage of the Dietary Supplement Health and Education Act (DSHEA) in the United States in 1994, a large number of phytochemicals are being sold as dietary supplements.

What is the evidence?

It has become a widely accepted notion that a diet rich in fruits, vegetables, legumes, and grains reduces the risk for cancer, heart disease, and other illnesses. But only recently have researchers begun to try to learn the effects of specific phytochemicals contained in those foods.

Much of the evidence so far has come from observations of cultures in which the diet consists mainly of plant sources, which seem to have lower rates of certain types of cancer and heart disease. For instance, the relatively low rates of breast and endometrial cancers in some Asian cultures are credited at least in part to dietary habits. These cancers are much more common in the United States, possibly because the typical American diet is higher in fat and lower in fruits, vegetables, legumes, and grains.

Because of the number of phytochemicals and the complexity of the chemical processes in which they are involved, it is difficult for researchers to determine which phytochemicals in foods may fight cancer and other diseases, which may have no effect, and which may even be harmful.

Many studies have looked at the relationship between cancer risk and eating fruits and vegetables, legumes, and whole grains. Most of the evidence indicates that eating a diet high in these foods seems to lower the risk for some cancers and other illnesses.

Some of the links between individual phytochemicals and cancer risk found in laboratory studies are compelling and make a strong case for further research. So far, however, none of the findings are conclusive. It is still uncertain which of the many phytochemicals in fruits and vegetables actively help the body fight disease.

Researchers have also shown much interest in phytochemical supplements. Some laboratory studies in cell cultures and animals have shown that certain phytochemicals have some activity against cancer cells or tumors. But at this time there have been no strong studies in humans showing that any phytochemical supplement can prevent or treat cancer.

Until conclusive research findings emerge, health care professionals advise a balanced diet with an emphasis on fruits, vegetables, legumes, and whole grains. The interaction between certain phytochemicals and the other compounds in foods is not well understood, but it is unlikely that any single compound offers the best protection against cancer. A balanced diet that includes five or more servings a day of fruits and vegetables, along with foods from a variety of other plant sources such as nuts, seeds, whole grain cereals, and beans, is likely to be more effective in reducing cancer risk than is consuming one particular phytochemical in large amounts.

Are there any possible problems or complications?

Phytochemicals, in the amounts consumed in a healthy diet, are likely to be helpful and are unlikely to cause any major problems. Some people assume that because phytochemical supplements come from "natural" sources, they must be safe and free from side effects, but this is not always true. Many phytochemical supplements, especially when taken in large amounts, have side effects and may interact with some drugs. Some of these interactions may be dangerous. Before taking a phytochemical in supplement form, always talk to your doctor and pharmacist to be sure it will not interact with other medicines or herbs you may be taking. Relying on the use of phytochemicals alone and avoiding or delaying conventional medical care for cancer may have serious health consequences.

This product is sold as a dietary supplement in the United States. Unlike companies that produce drugs (which must provide the FDA with results of detailed testing showing their product is safe and effective before the drug is approved for sale), the companies that make supplements do not have to show evidence of safety or health benefits to the FDA before selling their products. Supplement products without any reliable scientific evidence of health benefits may still be sold as long as the companies selling them do not claim the supplements can prevent, treat, or cure any specific disease. Some such products may not contain the amount of the herb or substance that is written on the label, and some may include other substances (contaminants). Though the FDA has written new rules to improve the quality of manufacturing processes for dietary supplements and the accurate listing of supplement ingredients, these rules do not take full effect until 2010. The new rules also do not address the safety of supplement ingredients or their effects on health when proper manufacturing techniques are used.

Most such supplements have not been tested to find out if they interact with medicines, foods, or other herbs and supplements. Even though some reports of interactions and harmful effects may be published, full studies of interactions and effects are not often available. Because of these limitations, any information on ill effects and interactions should be considered incomplete.

References

Craig WJ. Health-promoting properties of common herbs. *Am J Clin Nutr.* 1999;70:491S-499S.

Gruenwald J. *PDR for Herbal Medicines.* 3rd ed. Montvale, NJ: Thomson PDR; 2004.

Kushi LH, Byers T, Doyle C, Bandera EV, McCullough M, McTiernan A, Gansler T, Andrews KS, Thun MJ; American Cancer Society 2006 Nutrition and Physical Activity Guidelines Advisory Committee. American Cancer Society guidelines on nutrition and physical activity for cancer prevention: reducing the risk of cancer with healthy food choices and physical activity. *CA Cancer J Clin.* 2006;56:254-281.

Setchell KD, Cassidy A. Dietary isoflavones: biological effects and relevance to human health. *J Nutr.* 1999;129:758S-767S.

Wang YH, Chao PD, Hsiu SL, Wen KC, Hou YC. Lethal quercetin-digoxin interaction in pigs. *Life Sci.* 2004;74:1191-1197.

PINE BARK EXTRACT

Other common name(s): pygenol, Pycnogenol, Masquelier's Original OPCs (oligomeric proanthocyanidins)
Scientific/medical name(s): *Pinus pinaster*

Description

Pine bark extract is made from the bark of the maritime pine tree *(Pinus pinaster)*, which contains naturally occurring chemicals called proanthocyanidins. The maritime pine is native to the western Mediterranean, with a range extending over Portugal, Spain, France, Italy, and Morocco. Pine bark extract is commonly sold under the brand name Pycnogenol. Pycnogenol is also the name of a group of compounds that contain proanthocyanidins taken from a number of natural sources, such as grape seeds (see "Grapes," page 619) and other plants. In addition to the Pycnogenol brand, there are several other pine bark extract supplements available, which may use different types of pine bark and have different formulations. Pine bark extract is used for its antioxidant properties.

Overview

Although interest in pine bark extract is growing among medical researchers, only limited data from clinical trials support the claims made about its benefits for health. A few small early studies in humans have shown possible benefits in reducing swelling from a circulation disorder called chronic venous insufficiency. Some early studies have suggested it may help lower blood sugar in some diabetic patients. Laboratory studies have indicated pine bark extract may have some antioxidant properties.

How is it promoted for use?

Proponents claim that pine bark extract is a powerful antioxidant. Antioxidants are compounds that block the action of free radicals, activated oxygen molecules that can damage cells. Supporters believe pine bark extract protects against arthritis, complications from diabetes, cancer, heart disease, and problems with circulation such as swelling and varicose veins. Other reported benefits include improved memory, fewer effects from stress, better joint flexibility, and decreased inflammation. Some claim that pine bark extract supplements are much more effective in eliminating free radicals than vitamins C and E.

What does it involve?

Pine bark extract is available as a tablet and capsule in a range of strengths. Practitioners may recommend a dose ranging from 25 to 300 milligrams per day for up to three weeks. After that, some suggest a maintenance dose of 50 to 100 milligrams per day, while others recommend continuing a "saturation dose" of 20 to 30 milligrams per twenty pounds of body weight. Others recommend doses of 600 milligrams or more per day, depending on the reason for taking it.

What is the history behind it?

In the winter of 1535, a French explorer named Jacques Cartier found his ship ice-bound in the St. Lawrence River, in what is now Quebec. Having no fruits or vegetables, the crew became ill with scurvy, a disease resulting from vitamin C deficiency. Several had already died when a Native American told them how to prepare a tea made from tree bark. Many crew members recovered and attributed miraculous qualities to the tea. It is thought now that the tea was prepared from the bark of the Eastern White Cedar tree and that it contained large amounts of vitamin C.

In 1951, French researcher Dr. Jacques Masquelier reportedly read this account in Cartier's writings and began a search for the active ingredients in the tea. He was able to extract proanthocyanidins from the bark of the European coastal pine tree. He patented the process and named the compound Pycnogenol.

In 1970, proanthocyanidins were also extracted from grape seeds. The compound found in grape seeds and plants is referred to as either proanthocyanidins or pycnogenol. However, it differs somewhat from the Pycnogenol extracted by Dr. Masquelier.

What is the evidence?

There are not enough data from clinical trials to support most of the health claims made for any form of pine bark extract, although interest in proanthocyanidins among medical researchers is growing. There are reports from small human studies that pine bark extract may be helpful in treating circulation disorders. One clinical trial began in August 2003 to find out whether pycnogenol helps reduce lymphedema (swelling from fluid buildup that can occur after procedures in which lymph nodes are affected) after treatment for breast cancer. This study was still recruiting patients as of early 2007.

A small human study found that a single high dose of pine bark extract in the form of a bioflavonoid mixture was effective in reducing platelet clumping in smokers for more than three days, which would be expected to reduce blood clotting. This result may mean that pine bark extract could lower risk for stroke or heart attack, but clinical studies to find out whether this is true have not been done.

Some small brief studies have been done to look at pine bark extract's possible usefulness in treating asthma, menstrual pain, blood clots and leg swelling during long airplane flights, retinal disease in diabetics, high cholesterol, and other disorders. All of these studies need to be done on larger groups of people under carefully controlled conditions to find out whether pine bark extract actually helps any of these problems.

Studies also suggest pine bark extract has antioxidant properties, which are sometimes helpful in reducing cancer risk. Further research is needed to find out whether pine bark extract may have any benefit for preventing or treating cancer.

Are there any possible problems or complications?

Pine bark extract has been reported to be safe. Some people report mild problems such as headache, nausea, and upset stomach. Not much is known about possible interactions with other drugs and herbs. Always tell your doctor and pharmacist about any herbs or supplements you are taking.

Allergic reactions to pine are possible, although reactions to pine bark extract have not been reported in the available medical literature. Pine bark extract has not been studied in pregnant or breastfeeding women. Relying on this type of treatment alone and avoiding or delaying conventional medical care for cancer may have serious health consequences.

This product is sold as a dietary supplement in the United States. Unlike companies that produce drugs (which must provide the FDA with results of detailed testing showing their product is safe and effective before the drug is approved for sale), the companies that make supplements do not have to show evidence of safety or health benefits to the FDA before selling their products. Supplement products without any reliable scientific evidence of health benefits may still be sold as long as the companies selling them do not claim the supplements can prevent, treat, or cure any specific disease. Some such products may not contain the amount of the herb or substance that is written on the label, and some may include other substances (contaminants). Though the FDA has written new rules to improve the quality of manufacturing processes for dietary supplements and the accurate listing of supplement ingredients, these rules do not take full effect until 2010. The new rules also do not address the safety of supplement ingredients or their effects on health when proper manufacturing techniques are used.

Most such supplements have not been tested to find out if they interact with medicines, foods, or other herbs and supplements. Even though some reports of interactions and harmful effects may be published, full studies of interactions and effects are not often available. Because of these limitations, any information on ill effects and interactions should be considered incomplete.

References

Araghi-Niknam M, Hosseini S, Larson D, Rohdewald P, Watson RR. Pine bark extract reduces platelet aggregation. *Integr Med.* 2000;2:73-77.

Cesarone MR, Belcaro G, Rohdewald P, Pellegrini L, Ippolito E, Scoccianti M, Ricci A, Dugall M, Cacchio M, Ruffini I, Fano F, Acerbi G, Vinciguerra MG, Bavera P, Di Renzo A, Errichi BM, Mucci F. Prevention of edema in long flights with Pycnogenol. *Clin Appl Thromb Hemost.* 2005;11:289-294.

Devaraj S, Vega-López S, Kaul N, Schönlau F, Rohdewald P, Jialal I. Supplementation with a pine bark extract rich in polyphenols increases plasma antioxidant capacity and alters the plasma lipoprotein profile. *Lipids.* 2002;37:931-934.

Downs AM, Sansom JE. Colophony allergy: a review. *Contact Dermatitis.* 1999;41:305-310.

Fetrow CW, Avila JR. *Professional's Handbook of Complementary & Alternative Medicines.* Springhouse, PA: Springhouse Corp; 1999.

Huynh HT, Teel RW. Effects of intragastrically administered Pycnogenol on NNK metabolism in F344 rats. *Anticancer Res.* 1999;19:2095-2099.

Kohama T, Suzuki N, Ohno S, Inoue M. Analgesic efficacy of French maritime pine bark extract in dysmenorrhea: an open clinical trial. *J Reprod Med.* 2004;49:828-832.

Lau BH, Riesen SK, Truong KP, Lau EW, Rohdewald P, Barreta RA. Pycnogenol as an adjunct in the management of childhood asthma. *J Asthma.* 2004;41:825-832.

Petrassi C, Mastromarino A, Spartera C. PYCNOGENOL in chronic venous insufficiency. *Phytomedicine.* 2000;7:383-388.

Pine Bark. PDRhealth Web site. http://www.pdrhealth.com/drugs/altmed/altmed-mono.aspx?contentFileName=ame0425.xml&contentName=Pine+Bark+. Accessed June 6, 2008.

Pütter M, Grotemeyer KH, Würthwein G, Araghi-Niknam M, Watson RR, Hosseini S, Rohdewald P. Inhibition of smoking-induced platelet aggregation by aspirin and pycnogenol. *Thromb Res.* 1999;95:155-161.

Pycnogenol / polybioflavanoids. BC Cancer Agency Web site. http://www.bccancer.bc.ca/HPI/UnconventionalTherapies/PycnogenolPolybioflavanoids.htm. Updated February 2000. Accessed June 6, 2008.

Silliman K, Parry J, Kirk LL, Prior RL. Pycnogenol does not impact the antioxidant or vitamin C status of healthy young adults. *J Am Diet Assoc.* 2003;103:67-72.

Summary of data for chemical selection: oligomeric proanthocyanidins from grape seeds and pine bark. National Toxicology Program Web site. http://ntp.niehs.nih.gov/ntp/htdocs/Chem_Background/ExSumPdf/GrapeSeeds_PineBark.pdf. Accessed June 6, 2008.

Tyler VE. Pycnogenol fights cancer and the diseases of aging. *Prevention.* 1998;50:93.

US National Institutes of Health. Pycnogenol for the treatment of lymphedema. ClinicalTrials.gov Web site. http://www.clinicaltrials.gov/ct/show/NCT00214032. Accessed June 6, 2008.

POKEWEED

Other common name(s): common pokeweed, poke root, poke salad (or poke sallet), poke berry, poke, Virginia poke, inkberry, cancer root, American nightshade, pigeon berry
Scientific/medical name(s): *Phytolacca americana*

Description

Pokeweed is a perennial herb that is native to eastern North America and cultivated throughout the world. It can grow to a height of more than ten feet during the summer and dies back to the root each winter. The berries and dried roots are used in herbal remedies.

Overview

Some research has shown that a protein contained in pokeweed, called pokeweed antiviral protein (PAP), has antitumor effects in mice and in laboratory studies. In test tube studies, PAP has also shown action against viruses such as herpes and human immunodeficiency virus (HIV). Clinical trials have not yet determined whether these effects apply to humans. All parts of the mature pokeweed plant contain chemically active substances such as phytolaccine, formic acid, tannin, and resin acid. All parts of the plant are at least mildly poisonous when eaten, although the root is most toxic.

How is it promoted for use?

Proponents claim that pokeweed can be taken internally to treat a number of conditions, including rheumatoid arthritis, tonsillitis, mumps, swollen glands, chronic excess mucus, bronchitis, mastitis, and constipation. They also say that the herb is an effective treatment for fungal infections, joint inflammation, hemorrhoids, breast abscesses, ulcers, and bad breath. Herbalists also claim that external application of a preparation made from the plant relieves itching, inflammation, and skin diseases.

What does it involve?

Pokeweed supplements are available as liquid extracts, tinctures, powders, and poultices. There is no standard dose for pokeweed. Pokeweed berries are one of the ingredients in the Hoxsey formula (see "Hoxsey Herbal Treatment," page 390). Pokeweed antiviral protein, or PAP, is difficult to remove from the plant in its natural form. For research purposes, scientists have learned how to create PAP. The purified, laboratory-created version is also less toxic than that extracted from the plant.

What is the history behind it?

Young pokeweed shoots, which contain very low levels of toxins, were used as food by Native Americans and others. In the southeastern United States, some people still cook and eat "poke sallet." It is thoroughly boiled in water that is changed twice during cooking. Native Americans also used pokeweed in herbal remedies as a heart stimulant and to treat cancer, rheumatism, itching, and syphilis. The pokeweed root was also used as a laxative and to induce vomiting. European settlers adopted the use of pokeweed, which went on to become a common folk medicine.

Juice from the berries was once used to make ink and dye, and it is still used by the food industry to make red food coloring. Farmers and dairymen use an alcohol extract or tincture of pokeweed to reduce swelling of cows' udders. Followers of President James Polk wore pokeweed twigs during their candidate's election campaign, mistakenly believing that the plant was named for him.

What is the evidence?

Research has shown that pokeweed contains a compound that appears to enhance the immune system and has some anticancer effects in animals. According to one animal study, PAP demonstrated anticancer effects in rodents. Another study found that PAP, when combined with an immunotherapy drug called TP-3, holds promise as a potential treatment for advanced osteosarcomas and some soft tissue sarcomas. Laboratory studies have suggested that certain formulations of PAP may be turn out to be useful against cancer cells that depend on hormones for their growth, such as cells from prostate, breast, and ovarian cancer.

PAP also acts against some viruses such as herpes and HIV, and it is being studied as a possible antiviral agent. In laboratory studies, it seemed to help protect cells against HIV, and researchers are studying whether it might help protect people from HIV infection. However, even though animal and laboratory studies may show a certain compound looks promising, further research is necessary to find out whether the results hold true for humans.

Are there any possible problems or complications?

All parts of the pokeweed are poisonous, particularly the roots. The leaves and stems are next in toxicity, and the berries have the smallest amount of poison. However, children have been poisoned by eating raw pokeweed berries, and some have died. The practice of brewing pokeweed plant parts with hot water to make tea has caused poisoning. Thoroughly cooking the plant reduces its toxicity. The effects of eating the uncooked or improperly prepared plant can include nausea, vomiting, diarrhea, abdominal cramps, headaches, blurred vision, confusion, dermatitis, dizziness, and weakness. Convulsions, low blood pressure, rapid heartbeat, heart block (a blockage of the electrical impulses that stimulate the heart to contract), and death may occur. Animals can also die of toxic effects from eating pokeweed, although it does not happen often.

Pokeweed should not be used by people who are taking antidepressants, disulfiram (Antabuse), oral contraceptives, or fertility drugs. Other potential interactions between pokeweed and other drugs and herbs should be considered. Always tell your doctor and pharmacist about any herbs you are taking.

The plant may cause menstrual cycle irregularities and may also stimulate contractions of the uterus. Women who are pregnant or breastfeeding should not use pokeweed. Relying on this type of treatment alone and avoiding or delaying conventional medical care for cancer may have serious health consequences.

This product is sold as a dietary supplement in the United States. Unlike companies that produce drugs (which must provide the FDA with results of detailed testing showing their product is safe and effective before the drug is approved for sale), the companies that make supplements do not have to show evidence of safety or health benefits to the FDA before selling their products. Supplement products without any reliable scientific evidence of health benefits may still be sold as long as the companies selling them do not claim the supplements can prevent, treat, or cure any specific disease. Some such products may not contain the amount of the herb or substance that is written on the label, and some may include other substances (contaminants). Though the FDA has written new rules to improve the quality of manufacturing processes for dietary supplements and the accurate listing of supplement ingredients, these rules do not take full effect until 2010. The new rules also do not address the safety of supplement ingredients or their effects on health when proper manufacturing techniques are used.

Most such supplements have not been tested to find out if they interact with medicines, foods, or other herbs and supplements. Even though some reports of interactions and harmful effects may be published,

full studies of interactions and effects are not often available. Because of these limitations, any information on ill effects and interactions should be considered incomplete.

References

Allen GM, Bond MD, Main MB. 50 common native plants important in Florida's ethnobotanical history. University of Florida Web site. http://edis.ifas.ufl.edu/BODY_UW152. Accessed June 6, 2008.

Anderson PM, Meyers DE, Hasz DE, Covalcuic K, Saltzman D, Khanna C, Uckun FM. In vitro and in vivo cytotoxicity of an anti-osteosarcoma immunotoxin containing pokeweed antiviral protein. *Cancer Res.* 1995;55:1321-1327.

Bown D. *New Encyclopedia of Herbs & Their Uses.* New York: DK Publishing Inc; 2001.

Ek O, Waurzyniak B, Myers DE, Uckun FM. Antitumor activity of TP3(anti-p80)-pokeweed antiviral protein immunotoxin in hamster cheek pouch and severe combined immunodeficient mouse xenograft models of human osteosarcoma. *Clin Cancer Res.* 1998;4:1641-1647.

Fetrow CW, Avila JR. *Professional's Handbook of Complementary & Alternative Medicines.* Philadelphia, PA: Lippincott Williams & Wilkins; 2004.

Gruenwald J. *PDR for Herbal Medicines.* 3rd ed. Montvale, NJ: Thomson PDR; 2004.

Pokeweed. Memorial Sloan-Kettering Cancer Center Web site. http://www.mskcc.org/mskcc/html/69334.cfm. Updated September 17, 2007. Accessed June 6, 2008.

Pokeweed poisoning. Evanston Northwestern Healthcare Web site. http://www.enh.org/healthresources/encyclopedia/ency/article/002874.aspx. Accessed April 26, 2007. Content no longer available.

Qi L, Nett TM, Allen MC, Sha X, Harrison GS, Frederick BA, Crawford ED, Glode LM. Binding and cytotoxicity of conjugated and recombinant fusion proteins targeted to the gonadotropin-releasing hormone receptor. *Cancer Res.* 2004;64:2090-2095.

Urban herbs: medicinal plants at Georgetown University. Georgetown University Medical Center Web site. http://www8.georgetown.edu/departments/physiology/cam/urbanherbs/pokeweed.htm. Accessed June 6, 2008.

POTASSIUM

Other common name(s): none
Scientific/medical name(s): K, K+, potassium chloride (KCl), potassium citrate, potassium acetate, potassium carbonate, potassium gluconate, potassium bicarbonate

Description

Potassium is an essential mineral found in most foods. Along with sodium and calcium, potassium helps regulate major body functions, including normal heart rhythm, blood pressure, water balance in the body, digestion, nerve impulses, muscle contractions, and pH balance (the balance of acidity and alkalinity in the body). The body cannot manufacture potassium on its own and must obtain it from foods. Potassium is found in foods such as apricots, potatoes, bananas, oranges, pineapples, green leafy vegetables, whole grains, beans, nuts, and lean meat. Most salt substitutes also contain large amounts of potassium.

Overview

Potassium is a mineral that is required for normal body functioning. Most people get all the potassium they need in their diets. Available scientific evidence does not support claims that potassium supplements can prevent or treat cancer in humans. Excess potassium in the body can be toxic.

How is it promoted for use?

Some alternative medical practitioners maintain that low levels of potassium in the body may be linked to cancer, heart disease, high blood pressure, osteoporosis, depression, and schizophrenia. Some proponents claim that a diet high in sodium and low in potassium promotes tumor growth by changing the normal pH and water balance in human cells.

What does it involve?

Because most foods contain potassium, people usually get plenty of potassium from their normal food intake. Normally, the kidneys control the level of potassium in the blood and eliminate excess in the urine. The Food and Nutrition Board of the National Academies of Sciences has not set a Recommended Dietary Allowance for potassium, but has set Adequate Intake at 4.7 grams per day for most adults. There is no upper limit for potassium intake from food alone, but people with kidney disease, Addison's disease, or those taking certain blood pressure medicines may need to consume less than the Adequate Intake of potassium.

Potassium supplements are needed only by those who have low levels of potassium in their bloodstream, a condition known as hypokalemia. The causes of hypokalemia can include diarrhea and vomiting, diabetes, certain kidney diseases, excessive sweating, overuse of laxatives, and use of some types of diuretics (drugs that remove water from the body through urine). Use of potassium supplements can be dangerous unless monitored by health care providers.

What is the history behind it?

In the 1930s, Max Gerson began developing a controversial dietary treatment for cancer known as the Gerson Diet Therapy (see "Gerson Therapy," page 616). The cornerstone of his diet was the use of potassium supplements and low sodium intake. He claimed the diet could restore proper balance of salt and water within human cells and help stop tumor growth. However, this theory has not been supported by clinical or experimental data.

What is the evidence?

Some animal and human studies have indicated that eating foods high in potassium and low in sodium might help prevent high blood pressure, or hypertension. Dietary Approaches to Stop Hypertension, the so-called DASH diet, was designed to help control blood pressure. The DASH diet can reduce blood pressure and risk for heart disease through weight loss, reduced salt intake, moderation in drinking alcohol (for those who drink), and eating foods that are rich in potassium. These measures are especially helpful in older people and in African Americans, although the exact reasons are uncertain. For people who already have hypertension, these measures can be used along with medicines to gain better control over blood pressure. This can help reduce risk for stroke and heart attack.

Some observational epidemiologic studies have found that cancer rates are lower in a number of countries where there are high-potassium diets. In areas where there are low-potassium diets, these studies showed the cancer rates are higher. These types of studies, however, do not prove a direct connection, because there are many other factors involved. A few epidemiologic studies of individual potassium intake (rather than national averages) have found associations with cancer risk. However, the main sources of dietary potassium are fruits and vegetables, so people with a diet high in potassium may be at lower risk for cancer because of their intake of other beneficial phytochemicals. In addition, because these studies estimated potassium intake from food sources, the results are of uncertain relevance to potassium supplements.

One researcher has suggested a link between low potassium and high sodium levels in cells and an increased risk for cancer. However, available scientific evidence does not support the idea that changes in dietary potassium intake have any impact on potassium concentrations inside cancer cells. Further studies are needed to learn the effects of a high-potassium, low-sodium diet on the prevention or formation of cancer.

Are there any possible problems or complications?

Excessive use of potassium supplements or salt substitutes can cause potassium to build up in the blood, resulting in a condition known as hyperkalemia. The symptoms of hyperkalemia include muscle weakness, numbness and tingling, abnormal heart rhythm, muscle paralysis, trouble breathing, and even heart failure and death. Severe kidney failure and Addison's disease (a hormone deficiency) may also cause hyperkalemia. However, even people with normal kidneys can overdose on potassium if they take too many supplements at once.

People who are taking potassium-sparing diuretics (such as triamterene, amiloride, and spironolactone) or angiotensin-converting enzyme (ACE) inhibitors (such as lisinopril, enalapril, and captopril) can build up dangerously high potassium levels by using potassium supplements or salt substitutes. Those with kidney failure, diabetes, or Addison's disease should take potassium supplements only under the careful supervision of a doctor.

Other side effects of potassium supplements may include stomach or intestinal irritation, nausea, vomiting, abdominal pain, gas, and diarrhea. Talk with your doctor or pharmacist if you are thinking about potassium supplements. Relying on this type of treatment alone and avoiding or delaying conventional medical care for cancer may have serious health consequences.

This product is sold as a dietary supplement in the United States. Unlike companies that produce drugs (which must provide the FDA with results of detailed testing showing their product is safe and effective before the drug is approved for sale), the companies that make supplements do not have to show evidence of safety or health benefits to the FDA before selling their products. Supplement products without any reliable scientific evidence of health benefits may still be sold as long as the companies selling them do not claim the supplements can prevent, treat, or cure any specific disease. Some such products may not contain the amount of the herb or substance that is written on the label, and some may include other substances (contaminants). Though the FDA has written new rules to improve the quality of manufacturing processes for dietary supplements and the accurate listing of supplement ingredients, these rules do not take full effect until 2010. The new rules also do not address the safety of supplement ingredients or their effects on health when proper manufacturing techniques are used.

Most such supplements have not been tested to find out if they interact with medicines, foods, or other herbs and supplements. Even though some reports of interactions and harmful effects may be published, full studies of interactions and effects are not often available. Because of these limitations, any information on ill effects and interactions should be considered incomplete.

References

Appel LJ, Brands MW, Daniels SR, Karanja N, Elmer PJ, Sacks FM; American Heart Association. Dietary approaches to prevent and treat hypertension: a scientific statement from the American Heart Association. *Hypertension.* 2006;47:296-308.

Braunwald E, Fauci AS, Kasper DL, Hauser SL, Longo DL, Jameson JL, eds. *Harrison's Principles of Internal Medicine.* 15th ed. Washington DC: McGraw-Hill; 2001.

Cassileth B. *The Alternative Medicine Handbook: The Complete Reference Guide to Alternative and Complementary Therapies.* New York: W.W. Norton; 1998.

Food and Nutrition Board, Institute of Medicine, National Academies of Science. Dietary reference intakes (DRIs): recommended intakes for individuals, elements. Institute of Medicine Web site. http://www.iom.edu/Object.File/Master/21/372/DRI%20Tables%20after%20electrolytes%20plus%20micro-macroEAR_2.pdf. Accessed June 6, 2008.

Grimm RH Jr, Neaton JD, Elmer PJ, Svendsen KH, Levin J, Segal M, Holland L, Witte LJ, Clearman DR, Kofron, et al. The influence of oral potassium chloride on blood pressure in hypertensive men on a low-sodium diet. *N Engl J Med.* 1990;322:569-574.

Jacobs MM. Potassium inhibition of DMH-induced small intestinal tumors in rats. *Nutr Cancer.* 1990;14:95-101.

Jansson B. Potassium, sodium, and cancer: a review. *J Environ Pathol Toxicol Oncol.* 1996;15:65-73.

Levi F, Pasche C, Lucchini F, La Vecchia C. Dietary intake of selected micronutrients and breast-cancer risk. *Int J Cancer.* 2001;91:260-263.

Negri E, La Vecchia C, Franceschi S, D'Avanzo B, Talamini R, Parpinel M, Ferraroni M, Filiberti R, Montella M, Falcini F, Conti E, Decarli A. Intake of selected micronutrients and the risk of breast cancer. *Int J Cancer.* 1996;65:140-144.

Potassium. PDRhealth Web site. http://www.pdrhealth.com/drug_info/nmdrugprofiles/nutsupdrugs/pot_0208.shtml. Accessed June 6, 2008.

Tobian L. Dietary sodium chloride and potassium have effects on the pathophysiology of hypertension in humans and animals. *Am J Clin Nutr.* 1997;65:606S-611S.

Van Leer EM, Seidell JC, Kromhout D. Dietary calcium, potassium, magnesium and blood pressure in the Netherlands. *Int J Epidemiol.* 1995;24:1117-1123.

PSYLLIUM

Other common name(s): psyllium seed husk, isphagula, ispaghula, isabgol
Scientific/medical name(s): *Plantago psyllium, Plantago ovata, Plantago isphagula*

Description

Psyllium comes from the crushed seeds of the *Plantago ovata* plant, an herb native to parts of Asia, Mediterranean regions of Europe, and North Africa. It is now cultivated extensively in India and Pakistan as well as in the southwestern United States. The seed husks are used in herbal remedies and as laxatives. Although a member of the plantain family, it is not related to the banana-like fruit that is sometimes also called plantain.

Overview

Psyllium contains about 70 percent soluble fiber and 30 percent insoluble fiber and has been used for many years to treat constipation. It is also helpful in reducing cholesterol. It must be taken with plenty of water to avoid choking or blocking the esophagus, throat, or intestine. Some people are allergic to psyllium, with several types of reactions reported. Although fiber supplements are useful in treating constipation, fruits and vegetables are considered to be more effective in lowering cancer risk.

How is it promoted for use?

The psyllium seed husk is promoted mainly as a fiber supplement to ease bowel movements and lessen constipation. Fiber is the indigestible material in plant foods, also known as roughage. High-fiber diets help the digestive tract function properly. Psyllium absorbs water and expands as it travels through the digestive tract, which is why it is called a bulk-forming laxative. Psyllium is also sometimes promoted to treat side effects of cancer treatment such as diarrhea and constipation.

What does it involve?

Psyllium is available as a powder, tablet, capsule, and chewable wafer. It is also added to some cereals to increase fiber content. Most often, psyllium powder is mixed with water or juice, then stirred and drunk quickly before the liquid thickens. Doses range between 4 and 20 grams per day as needed (a level teaspoon is about 5 grams). In any form, it must be taken with plenty of water (one or two glasses per 3.5 grams). To avoid bloating and gas, it is recommended to start with a lower dose and increase it as the body adjusts. Psyllium is a common ingredient in laxatives. Laxatives are available over the counter and by prescription.

What is the history behind it?

Psyllium seed husk has been used as a laxative for generations. The leaves of the plant have also been used in many folk medicine traditions to treat a variety of conditions, such as blisters, bleeding, abrasions, sprains, insect bites, stings, burns, poison ivy, throat irritation, gout, inflammation of mucous membranes and skin, dysentery, urinary tract disorders, chronic diarrhea, and coughs and to make a wash for sore eyes.

What is the evidence?

Psyllium has been found to be effective in treating constipation, and it can also help reduce cholesterol. It is well known that a diet high in fiber helps the digestive tract work better. Too little fiber in the diet can lead to constipation, hemorrhoids, and diverticulitis, a common digestive disorder. Fiber supplements such as psyllium have been proven to be effective for easing constipation, but most nutritionists agree that the best source of fiber is from foods. Good sources of fiber are beans, vegetables, whole grains, and fruits.

Clinical trials have shown that psyllium, when taken with a low-fat diet, helps to lower LDL ("bad") cholesterol more than a low-fat diet alone. Because of this finding, the U.S. Food and Drug Administration (FDA) allows marketers to claim that using psyllium along with a low-fat diet may reduce risk for heart disease.

Psyllium and other fiber supplements have also been tested to see whether they help control symptoms of irritable bowel syndrome (IBS). Most reviews of this evidence have concluded that fiber supplements are not useful as the main treatment for IBS but that they may be helpful when used with other treatments, especially in IBS patients who also have constipation.

Studies clearly show that a diet high in fruits and vegetables can lower colorectal cancer risk, as well as the risk for several other diseases. However, conflicting results from studies of dietary fiber and colorectal cancer risk have created some confusion among the general public and even some health professionals. Recent studies have found that fiber may not be the ingredient in fruits and vegetables that lowers cancer risk. The studies confirm the benefits of eating fruits and vegetables, but suggest that other substances in these foods may be responsible for their protective effect.

Are there any possible problems or complications?

The use of psyllium is generally safe. However, when taken in excessive amounts, it can cause bloating, diarrhea, gas, and intestinal blockage. Not drinking enough water with psyllium can cause choking and blocking of the esophagus, throat, and intestines. A number of patients have had blockages from psyllium laxatives, especially people with a narrowing of the esophagus or intestine.

People with cancer who have severe constipation that is not helped by over-the-counter remedies should contact their doctors. Constipation can be a major side effect of certain pain medicines, such as morphine and similar drugs. It can become a serious problem if not addressed quickly and effectively.

Serious allergic reactions to psyllium have been reported, including breathing problems, skin rashes, hives, and anaphylaxis (shock). Some people with these allergies react to touching psyllium or breathing its dust. Allergic reactions are more likely in those who have had frequent exposure to psyllium dust.

Diabetics who are on medication for their condition may need to reduce their dosages while taking psyllium products. People who have problems swallowing, blocked or narrowed intestines, or fecal impaction should avoid psyllium.

Psyllium may influence absorption of medicines such as tetracycline, digoxin, lithium, tricyclic antidepressants, carbamazepine, some cholesterol-lowering drugs, and some drugs for diabetes (glyburide and metformin), if they are taken at the same time as psyllium. Such medicines should be taken an hour before or at least two hours after taking psyllium. Talk to your doctor or pharmacist about all the medicines you are taking, including herbs and supplements, to be sure there are no harmful interactions. Relying on this type of treatment alone and avoiding or delaying conventional medical care for cancer may have serious health consequences.

This product is sold as a dietary supplement in the United States. Unlike companies that produce drugs (which must provide the FDA with results of detailed testing showing their product is safe and effective before the drug is approved for sale), the companies that make supplements do not have to show evidence of safety or health benefits to the FDA before selling their products. Supplement products without any reliable scientific evidence of health benefits may still be sold as long as the companies selling them do not claim the supplements can prevent, treat, or cure any specific disease. Some such products may not contain the amount of the herb or substance that is written on the label, and some may include other substances (contaminants). Though the FDA has written new rules to improve the quality of manufacturing processes for dietary supplements and the accurate listing of supplement ingredients, these rules do not take full effect until 2010. The new rules also do not address the safety of supplement ingredients or their effects on health when proper manufacturing techniques are used.

Most such supplements have not been tested to find out if they interact with medicines, foods, or other herbs and supplements. Even though some reports of interactions and harmful effects may be published, full studies of interactions and effects are not often available. Because of these limitations, any information on ill effects and interactions should be considered incomplete.

References

Anderson JW, Allgood LD, Turner J, Oeltgen PR, Daggy BP. Effects of psyllium on glucose and serum lipid responses in men with type 2 diabetes and hypercholesterolemia. *Am J Clin Nutr.* 1999;70:466-473.

Blumenthal M, ed. *The Complete German Commission E Monographs: Therapeutic Guide to Herbal Medicines.* Austin, TX: American Botanical Council; 1998.

Fetrow CW, Avila JR. *Professional's Handbook of Complementary & Alternative Medicines.* Springhouse, PA: Springhouse Corp; 1999.

Gruenwald J. *PDR for Herbal Medicines.* 3rd ed. Montvale, NJ: Thomson PDR; 2004.

Lembo A, Camilleri M. Chronic constipation. *N Engl J Med.* 2003;349:1360-1368.

Petchetti L, Frishman WH, Petrillo R, Raju K. Nutriceuticals in cardiovascular disease: psyllium. *Cardiol Rev.* 2007;15:116-122.

Possible interactions with: psyllium. University of Maryland Medical Center Web site. http://www.umm.edu/altmed/articles/psyllium-000976.htm. Accessed July 31, 2008.

Psyllium. Drug Digest Web site. http://www.drugdigest.org/DD/DVH/Uses/0,3915,574|Psyllium,00.html#interactions. Accessed June 6, 2008.

Psyllium (plantago ovata, plantago isphagula). Medline Plus Web site. http://www.nlm.nih.gov/medlineplus/druginfo/natural/patient-psyllium.html. Updated February 1, 2008. Accessed June 6, 2008.

Psyllium. PDRhealth Web site. http://www.pdrhealth.com/drug_info/nmdrugprofiles/herbaldrugs/102270.shtml. Accessed June 6, 2008.

Roberts-Andersen J, Mehta T, Wilson RB. Reduction of DMH-induced colon tumors in rats fed psyllium husk or cellulose. *Nutr Cancer.* 1987;10:129-136.

Robertson DJ, Sandler RS, Haile R, Tosteson TD, Greenberg ER, Grau M, Baron JA. Fat, fiber, meat and the risk of colorectal adenomas. *Am J Gastroenterol.* 2005;100:2789-2795.

Rock CL. Primary dietary prevention: is the fiber story over? *Recent Results Cancer Res.* 2007;174:171-177.

RABDOSIA RUBESCENS

Other common name(s): dong ling cao, oridonin, ponicidin
Scientific/medical name(s): *Rabdosia rubescens, Isodon rubescens*

Description

Rabdosia rubescens is a Chinese herb promoted as a treatment for cancer of the esophagus. It was also one of the eight herbs used in PC-SPES, an herbal formula that was promoted as a treatment for prostate cancer prior to being removed from the market for irregularities in its manufacturing (see "PC-SPES, PC-HOPE, and PC-CARE," page 448). *Rabdosia rubescens* is an ingredient in the herbal products PC-HOPE and PC-CARE, which are similar to PC-SPES and are currently available.

Overview

There are some signs that extracts of this herb may have anticancer activity. Further research is needed to find out what role, if any, these substances may have in cancer treatment.

How is it promoted for use?

Rabdosia rubescens is promoted as a treatment for cancer of the esophagus. PC-HOPE and PC-CARE, two herbal products of which the herb is an ingredient, are promoted for the treatment of prostate cancer. Additional uses in Chinese herbal medicine include treatment of cancers of the stomach, breast, and liver and relief of insect bites, snake bites, and inflammation of the tonsils.

What does it involve?

The herbal products PC-HOPE and PC-CARE (of which *Rabdosia rubescens* is part) come in capsules and are taken daily, in varying dosages. PC-SPES is no longer produced. PC-HOPE and PC-CARE are available in health food stores, from some nutritionists, and directly from manufacturers. In one clinical trial of *Rabdosia rubescens* as a treatment for esophageal cancer, the herb was taken by mouth as a lozenge three times a day, once after each meal.

What is the history behind it?

Rabdosia rubescens has been used as a Chinese folk medicine to clear the body of toxins, nourish yin, relieve swelling, relieve pain and remove blood stasis (a condition described in traditional Chinese medicine as a pooling of the blood).

What is the evidence?

In the past few years, several laboratory studies have shown that two extracts of *Rabdosia rubescens*, called oridonin and ponicidin, have some activity against cancer cells. Oridonin has been tested against several types of human cancer cells in laboratory dishes and in mice. Most of these studies were done in China or Japan, and all showed activity against the cancer cells. Ponicidin was tested in the laboratory against human leukemia cells in China and found to help induce cell death, or apoptosis. Even though laboratory studies show promise, further studies are needed to find out whether the results apply to humans.

Other extracts from the herb are in earlier stages of study. No studies using the whole herb as a cancer treatment are available, although a few laboratory and animal studies report using an extract of the whole herb rather than isolated compounds. Extracted compounds are not the same as the herb, and study results are not likely to show the same effects. More research is needed to find out what role, if any, these substances may have in cancer treatment.

A clinical trial conducted in China compared *Rabdosia rubescens* with placebo for patients with localized esophageal cancer and compared chemotherapy with *Rabdosia rubescens* and chemotherapy without *Rabdosia rubescens* for advanced disease. In both situations, the researchers reported that the herbal lozenges improved survival.

Are there any possible problems or complications?

No serious side effects were reported in one Chinese study of patients with cancer of the esophagus; mild side effects included mild abdominal symptoms, diarrhea, and skin itching. Relying on this type of treatment alone and avoiding or delaying conventional medical care for cancer may have serious health consequences.

This product is sold as a dietary supplement in the United States. Unlike companies that produce drugs (which must provide the FDA with results of detailed testing showing their product is safe and effective before the drug is approved for sale), the companies that make supplements do not have to show evidence of safety or health benefits to the FDA before selling their products. Supplement products without any reliable scientific evidence of health benefits may still be sold as long as the companies selling them do not claim the supplements can prevent, treat, or cure any specific disease. Some such products may not contain the amount of the herb or substance that is written on the label, and some may include other substances (contaminants). Though the FDA has written new rules to improve the quality of manufacturing processes for dietary supplements and the accurate listing of supplement ingredients, these rules do not take full effect until 2010. The new rules also do not address the safety of supplement ingredients or their effects on health when proper manufacturing techniques are used.

Most such supplements have not been tested to find out if they interact with medicines, foods, or other herbs and supplements. Even though some reports of interactions and harmful effects may be published, full studies of interactions and effects are not often available. Because of these limitations, any information on ill effects and interactions should be considered incomplete.

References

Chen S, Gao J, Halicka HD, Huang X, Traganos F, Darzynkiewicz Z. The cytostatic and cytotoxic effects of oridonin (Rubescenin), a diterpenoid from *Rabdosia rubescens*, on tumor cells of different lineage. *Int J Oncol.* 2005;26:579-588.

Chu JHK. Dong ling cao. Complementary and Alternative Healing University Web site. http://alternativehealing.org/dong_ling_cao.htm. Accessed August 6, 2008.

Ikezoe T, Chen SS, Tong XJ, Heber D, Taguchi H, Koeffler HP. Oridonin induces growth inhibition and apoptosis of a variety of human cancer cells. *Int J Oncol.* 2003;23:1187-1193.

Ikezoe T, Yang Y, Bandobashi K, Saito T, Takemoto S, Machida H, Togitani K, Koeffler HP, Taguchi H. Oridonin, a diterpenoid purified from *Rabdosia rubescens*, inhibits the proliferation of cells from lymphoid malignancies in association with blockade of the NF-kappa B signal pathways. *Mol Cancer Ther.* 2005;4:578-586.

Liu JJ, Huang RW, Lin DJ, Wu XY, Lin Q, Peng J, Pan X, Song YQ, Zhang MH, Hou M, Chen F. Antiproliferation effects of ponicidin on human myeloid leukemia cells in vitro. *Oncol Rep.* 2005;13:653-657.

Liu JJ, Huang RW, Lin DJ, Wu XY, Peng J, Pan XL, Lin Q, Hou M, Zhang MH, Chen F. Antiproliferation effects of oridonin on HPB-ALL cells and its mechanisms of action. *Am J Hematol.* 2006;81:86-94.

Ren KK, Wang HZ, Xie LP, Chen DW, Liu X, Sun J, Nie YC, Zhang RQ. The effects of oridonin on cell growth, cell cycle, cell migration and differentiation in melanoma cells. *J Ethnopharmacol.* 2006;103:176-180.

Wang R, Cheng P, Fan Q, Wang R. Clinical efficacy for the treatment of esophageal cancer with rabdosia rubescens alone and combining with chemotherapy. *Life Sci J.* 2007;4(3)22-25.

RED CLOVER

Other common name(s): purple clover, trefoil, wild clover
Scientific/medical name(s): *Trifolium pratense*

Description

Red clover is a perennial plant that grows wild in the Americas, Europe, Australia, Asia, and northern Africa. The flower head, which ranges from pink to purple or red, is the part of the plant used in herbal remedies.

Overview

Available clinical evidence does not show that red clover is effective in treating or preventing cancer, menopausal symptoms, or any other medical conditions. It may also increase the risk for excessive bleeding in some people. Some of its extracts (isoflavones) are being tested to determine whether they help symptoms of menopause or reduce the level of bad cholesterol in the blood. So far, results are mixed. Studies looking at the extracts' effectiveness against prostate enlargement and prostate cancer have begun. Other researchers are looking at whether it will help blood pressure and insulin resistance in diabetics and osteoporosis in women. Early findings suggest it may merit further testing.

How is it promoted for use?

Proponents claim that red clover is useful for relieving menopausal symptoms because it contains chemicals that are similar to the hormone estrogen. They also claim that the herb suppresses coughs (particularly whooping cough) and slows blood clotting. According to some practitioners, people who take prescription blood-thinning medications, such as warfarin (Coumadin), may be able to reduce their dosage by taking red clover supplements.

Other supporters claim that red clover is effective for treating cancers of the breast, ovary, and lymphatic system, although available scientific evidence does not support this claim. A few claim that the herb acts as an antibiotic, an appetite suppressant, and a relaxant. Some believe that red clover preparations can be used to help speed wound healing and ease chronic skin conditions such as psoriasis.

What does it involve?

Red clover supplements are available as tablets, as capsules, or in liquid extract form. Dried red clover can be brewed into a tea. Practitioners generally use a daily dosage of about 4 grams of dried red clover or 1.5 to 3.0 milliliters of liquid extract. (Five milliliters is equal to one teaspoon, so this would be around ¼ to ½ teaspoon of the liquid.) The liquid extract can be rubbed directly on skin or applied with a compress. Dried red clover can also be made into a tea and either drunk or used as a wash. It also comes in cream, lotion, or ointment form for use on the skin and is sometimes used in cosmetics and soaps.

What is the history behind it?

For centuries, red clover has been grown in pastures to feed cattle and other grazing animals. The herb is an ingredient in the Hoxsey formula, Jason Winters' tea, and Essiac tea, which are common herbal remedies (see "Hoxsey Herbal Treatment," page 390, and "Essiac Tea," page 342).

What is the evidence?

Scientists have identified phytoestrogens (estrogen-like substances from plants) called isoflavones, mainly biochanin and formononetin, in red clover. These two are precursors of the isoflavones daidzein and genistein, which are found in smaller amounts in red clover and also in soy. Low levels of anticoagulant, or blood-thinning, chemicals called coumarins are also present in red clover. While these substances have been identified in the plant, however, most of the claims made for the herb have not been verified in humans through randomized clinical trials.

One group of Australian researchers gave red clover isoflavonoids to twenty men with prostate cancer before they had prostatectomies (surgery to remove the prostate). The men who had received flavonoids appeared to have more dying cancer cells in their surgically removed prostate tissue. This was a very small study, without a placebo group, and it did not compare survival, quality of life, or symptoms. How this result might affect treatment is not yet known. Further studies are needed.

Most studies suggest that long-term use (ten years or more) of estrogen replacement therapy after menopause may increase the risk for heart disease and breast and endometrial cancer. Scientists are looking for estrogen alternatives that do not increase these risks, and phytoestrogens from red clover have been targeted for research. In a small clinical study, researchers concluded that a diet supplemented with red clover sprouts and other plants that contain phytoestrogens may reduce the severity of menopausal symptoms. However, this conclusion needs to be confirmed in other studies before red clover can be routinely recommended. Studies of commercial red clover isoflavone supplements for relief of menopausal symptoms have shown conflicting results, although most (including the largest study) found no reduction of hot flashes and no improvement in relevant quality of life measures.

Several studies of isoflavone extracts from red clover have since shown mixed results on heart disease risk factors such as cholesterol and triglycerides. For example, in a 2005 study, sixty postmenopausal women taking red clover isoflavones had slightly lower triglyceride levels and fewer menopausal symptoms than those on placebo. No significant difference in LDL, or "bad," cholesterol was noted.

An Australian study looked at both men and women taking enriched red clover isoflavones. One supplement was enriched with the phytoestrogens formononetin and the other with biochanin. These were compared with placebo for six weeks. The men receiving the biochanin-enriched supplement had somewhat lower levels of LDL cholesterol, but the other study participants did not.

Preliminary studies have looked at the use of isoflavones from red clover to control blood pressure in diabetic patients and to treat insulin resistance, osteoporosis, and benign prostatic hypertrophy (enlarged prostate). Most of these studies were small and did not last very long, and no conclusions can be reached about red clover isoflavones' possible effectiveness for these conditions. Further studies are needed. It is also important to note that the extracts are not the same as the whole herb, and study results would not be likely to show the same effects.

Are there any possible problems or complications?

Red clover is categorized as "generally recognized as safe" by the U.S. Food and Drug Administration (FDA), and small amounts are included in some teas and "health drinks." Patients with bleeding problems or who take anticoagulant medications, including aspirin, may want to avoid red clover because of the slight chance it could increase the risk for serious bleeding. In addition, since the amount of the blood-thinning chemical coumarin in red clover varies, it cannot be relied upon to produce the same effect even when the same dose is taken. Additional potential interactions between red clover and other drugs and herbs should be considered. Always tell your doctor and pharmacist about any herbs you are taking.

Women who have had estrogen receptor–positive cancers or who are pregnant or breastfeeding should not use this herb. No reports of toxicity or overdose from red clover were found in the available medical literature, although those who are allergic to clover should avoid it. Relying on this type of treatment alone and avoiding or delaying conventional medical care for cancer may have serious health consequences.

This product is sold as a dietary supplement in the United States. Unlike companies that produce drugs (which must provide the FDA with results of detailed testing showing their product is safe and effective before the drug is approved for sale), the companies that make supplements do not have to show evidence of safety or health benefits to the FDA before selling their products. Supplement products without any reliable scientific evidence of health benefits may still be sold as long as the companies selling them do not claim the supplements can prevent, treat, or cure any specific disease. Some such products may not contain the amount of the herb or substance that is written on the label, and some may include other substances (contaminants). Though the FDA has written new rules to improve the quality of manufacturing processes for dietary supplements and the accurate listing of supplement ingredients, these rules do not take full effect until 2010. The new rules also do not address the safety of supplement ingredients or their effects on health when proper manufacturing techniques are used.

Most such supplements have not been tested to find out if they interact with medicines, foods, or other herbs and supplements. Even though some reports of interactions and harmful effects may be published, full studies of interactions and effects are not often available. Because of these limitations, any information on ill effects and interactions should be considered incomplete.

References

Bown D. *New Encyclopedia of Herbs & Their Uses.* New York: DK Publishing Inc; 2001.

Fetrow CW, Avila JR. *Professional's Handbook of Complementary & Alternative Medicines.* Philadelphia, PA: Lippincott Williams & Wilkins; 2004.

Gruenwald J. *PDR for Herbal Medicines.* 3rd ed. Montvale, NJ: Thomson PDR; 2004.

Howes JB, Bray K, Lorenz L, Smerdely P, Howes LG. The effects of dietary supplementation with isoflavones from red clover on cognitive function in postmenopausal women. *Climacteric.* 2004;7:70-77.

Howes JB, Tran D, Brillante D, Howes LG. Effects of dietary supplementation with isoflavones from red clover on ambulatory blood pressure and endothelial function in postmenopausal type 2 diabetes. *Diabetes Obes Metab.* 2003;5:325-332.

Jarred RA, Keikha M, Dowling C, McPherson SJ, Clare AM, Husband AJ, Pedersen JS, Frydenberg M, Risbridger GP. Induction of apoptosis in low to moderate-grade human prostate carcinoma by red clover-derived dietary isoflavones. *Cancer Epidemiol Biomarkers Prev.* 2002;11:1689-1696.

Knight DC, Howes JB, Eden JA. The effect of Promensil, an isoflavone extract, on menopausal symptoms. *Climacteric.* 1999;2:79-84.

Nestel P, Cehun M, Chronopoulos A, DaSilva L, Teede H, McGrath B. A biochanin-enriched isoflavone from red clover lowers LDL cholesterol in men. *Eur J Clin Nutr.* 2004;58:403-408.

Red clover. Drug Digest Web site. http://www.drugdigest.org/DD/DVH/HerbsWho/0,3923,552774|Red%2BClover,00.html. Accessed June 6, 2008.

Red clover. Memorial Sloan-Kettering Cancer Center Web site. http://www.mskcc.org/mskcc/html/69350.cfm. Updated November 21, 2007. Accessed June 6, 2008.

Tice JA, Ettinger B, Ensrud K, Wallace R, Blackwell T, Cummings SR. Phytoestrogen supplements for the treatment of hot flashes: the Isoflavone Clover Extract (ICE) study: a randomized controlled trial. *JAMA.* 2003;290:207-214.
Comment in:
ACP J Club. 2004;140:47.
J Fam Pract. 2003;52:846-847.

US Department of Health and Human Services. Substances generally recognized as safe. 21 CFR §182.10. http://www.accessdata.fda.gov/scripts/cdrh/cfdocs/cfcfr/CFRSearch.cfm?CFRPart=182&showFR=1&subpartNode=21:3.0.1.1.13.1. Revised April 1, 2008. Accessed November 18, 2008.

van de Weijer PH, Barentsen R. Isoflavones from red clover (Promensil) significantly reduce menopausal hot flush symptoms compared with placebo. *Maturitas.* 2002;42:187-193.

Wilcox G, Wahlqvist ML, Burger HG, Medley G. Oestrogenic effects of plant foods in postmenopausal women. *BMJ.* 1990;301:905-906.

SAW PALMETTO

Other common name(s): saw palmetto berry extract, shrub palmetto, dwarf palm
Scientific/medical name(s): *Serenoa repens*

Description

Saw palmetto is a low-growing palm tree found in the West Indies and in coastal regions of the southeastern United States. The tree grows to between six and ten feet in height and has a crown of large leaves. The berries are used in herbal remedies.

Overview

How is it promoted for use?

Saw palmetto is promoted for relieving some of the symptoms of BPH, which include difficult and frequent urination. Chemicals in saw palmetto berries called sterols are said to interfere with the ability of hormones such as testosterone to cause prostate cells to grow.

Saw palmetto is sometimes promoted by itself or with other herbs as a treatment for prostate cancer. Saw palmetto is also promoted as a treatment for prostatitis (inflamed prostate gland). Some proponents claim it increases sex drive and fertility and that it can be used to treat low thyroid function.

What does it involve?

Saw palmetto supplements are available as capsules, tablets, and extracts and as a tea. There is no standard dosage. In some clinical studies for the treatment of BPH, patients received 320 milligrams per day as a single dose or divided into two doses. A recent study showed wide variation in the contents of different brands of saw palmetto supplements.

What is the history behind it?

Native Americans ate the berries of the saw palmetto believing they served as a tonic that nourished the body, stimulated appetite, and promoted weight gain. They also used the herb to treat problems of the urinary tract, such as trouble urinating or frequent nighttime urination.

Saw palmetto supplements are very popular in Europe, especially in Germany, where doctors often prescribe them for patients with BPH. Saw palmetto is approved by Commission E (Germany's regulatory agency for herbs) for prostate complaints or irritable bladder. Saw palmetto supplements have become popular in the United States in recent years as well and are often marketed "for prostate health."

What is the evidence?

Some research has found that saw palmetto extract may reduce symptoms of BPH. A review published in 2002 looked at twenty-one clinical studies of saw palmetto conducted over the last thirty years and involving more than three thousand patients. The report concluded that saw palmetto provided mild to moderate improvement in urinary symptoms such as frequent nighttime urination and problems with urine flow. The improvements were similar to those seen in men who took the prescription drug finasteride (Proscar) for BPH. Saw palmetto also caused fewer and milder side effects than finasteride. Whether side effects are long-lasting is unclear. However, a 2006 study of 225 men that carefully evaluated symptoms, maximal urine flow rate, prostate size, and quality of life for one year found that saw palmetto had no effect on any of these outcomes. A recent review concluded that although most studies have suggested improvement in BPH, the precise clinical use of saw palmetto remains undefined. Saw palmetto is not currently recommended in major U.S. or European urology society guidelines for treatment of BPH.

It is important to note, however, that benign prostatic hyperplasia is not cancer. Some laboratory studies in cell cultures and animal studies have hinted that saw palmetto may affect prostate cancer cells (and therefore have potential for prevention or treatment), but others have found no effect. Available scientific studies do not support claims that saw palmetto can prevent or treat prostate cancer in humans. One epidemiologic study of more than thirty thousand men, published in 2006, concluded that saw palmetto had no detectable influence on prostate cancer risk. Further research in this area is needed.

Are there any possible problems or complications?

Side effects from saw palmetto are not common but may include headache, nausea, vomiting, upset stomach, dizziness, constipation or diarrhea, trouble sleeping, and fatigue. Its long-term effects and safety have not been studied.

Men who have symptoms that might be caused by BPH, such as difficult, frequent, or urgent urination, should see a doctor as soon as possible rather than treating themselves with saw palmetto. These symptoms can also result from prostate cancer or other serious conditions, and self-treatment with saw palmetto could delay diagnosis and treatment.

Saw palmetto does not seem to interfere with the measurement of prostate-specific antigen (PSA), a protein made by prostate cells that is used in testing for prostate cancer, although this has not been studied extensively. Since saw palmetto affects testosterone metabolism in the same way as finasteride (which does affect PSA levels), some doctors recommend that men have a baseline PSA test and digital rectal exam before starting treatment with saw palmetto, just to be safe.

Relying on the use of saw palmetto alone and avoiding or delaying conventional medical care for cancer may have serious health consequences.

This product is sold as a dietary supplement in the United States. Unlike companies that produce drugs (which must provide the FDA with results of detailed testing showing their product is safe and effective before the drug is approved for sale), the companies that make supplements do not have to show evidence of safety or health benefits to the FDA before selling their products. Supplement products without any reliable scientific evidence of health benefits may still be sold as long as the companies selling them do not claim the supplements can prevent, treat, or cure any specific disease. Some such products may not contain the amount of the herb or substance that is written on the label, and some may include other substances (contaminants). Though the FDA has written new rules to improve the quality of manufacturing processes for dietary supplements and the accurate listing of supplement ingredients, these rules do not take full effect until 2010. The new rules also do not address the safety of supplement ingredients or their effects on health when proper manufacturing techniques are used.

Most such supplements have not been tested to find out if they interact with medicines, foods, or other herbs and supplements. Even though some reports of interactions and harmful effects may be published,

full studies of interactions and effects are not often available. Because of these limitations, any information on ill effects and interactions should be considered incomplete.

References

Avins AL, Bent S. Saw palmetto and lower urinary tract symptoms: what is the latest evidence? *Curr Urol Rep.* 2006;7:260-265.

Bent S, Kane C, Shinohara K, Neuhaus J, Hudes ES, Goldberg H, Avins AL. Saw palmetto for benign prostatic hyperplasia. *N Engl J Med.* 2006;354:557-566.

Bonnar-Pizzorno RM, Littman AJ, Kestin M, White E. Saw palmetto supplement use and prostate cancer risk. *Nutr Cancer.* 2006;55:21-27.

Feifer AH, Fleshner NE, Klotz L. Analytical accuracy and reliability of commonly used nutritional supplements in prostate disease. *J Urol.* 2002;168:150-154.

Gruenwald J. *PDR for Herbal Medicines.* 3rd ed. Montvale, NJ: Thomson PDR; 2004.

Habib FK, Ross M, Ho CK, Lyons V, Chapman K. Serenoa repens (Permixon) inhibits the 5alpha-reductase activity of human prostate cancer cell lines without interfering with PSA expression. *Int J Cancer.* 2005;114:190-194.

Hill B, Kyprianou N. Effect of permixon on human prostate cell growth: lack of apoptotic action. *Prostate.* 2004;61:73-80.

Madersbacher S, Berger I, Ponholzer A, Marszalek M. Plant extracts: sense or nonsense? *Curr Opin Urol.* 2008;18:16-20.

Saw palmetto. Memorial Sloan-Kettering Cancer Center Web site. http://www.mskcc.org/mskcc/html/69364.cfm. Updated August 7, 2007. Accessed June 6, 2008.

Saw palmetto (Serenoa repens [Bartram] small). Mayo Clinic Web site. http://www.mayoclinic.com/health/saw-palmetto/NS_patient-sawpalmetto. Updated February 1, 2008. Accessed June 6, 2008.

Sinclair RD, Mallari RS, Tate B. Sensitization to saw palmetto and minoxidil in separate topical extemporaneous treatments for androgenetic alopecia. *Australas J Dermatol.* 2002;43:311-312.

Wadsworth TL, Worstell TR, Greenberg NM, Roselli CE. Effects of dietary saw palmetto on the prostate of transgenic adenocarcinoma of the mouse prostate model (TRAMP). *Prostate.* 2007;67:661-673.

Wilt T, Ishani A, Mac Donald R. Serenoa repens for benign prostatic hyperplasia. *Cochrane Database Syst Rev.* 2002;(3):CD001423.

SELENIUM

Other common name(s): high-selenium yeast, selenized yeast, chelated selenium
Scientific/medical name(s): Se, selenium dioxide, sodium selenate, sodium selenite, selenocysteine, selenomethionine

Description

Selenium is an essential mineral for both humans and animals. It is found in soil all over the world in varying amounts. Plants and small living organisms convert selenium to organic compounds, including selenomethione, the form selenium takes in foods. Selenomethione, which is sometimes called "chelated selenium," binds to proteins and can be used in body processes without further metabolic changes.

Overview

Selenium shows promise as a nutrient that may help prevent the development and progression of cancer; however, more research is needed. A small amount of selenium is all the human body needs. Large amounts in supplement form can be toxic.

How is it promoted for use?

Selenium is said to help preserve elasticity in body tissues, slow the aging process, improve the flow of oxygen to the heart, and help prevent abnormal blood clotting. Selenium may stimulate the formation of antibodies (proteins that help fight invading microorganisms) in response to vaccines. Selenium may also play a role in normal growth, development, and fertility.

Supporters claim selenium protects the body against cancer by causing cancer cells to die before they have a chance to grow and spread. Available scientific evidence does not support this claim.

What does it involve?

The best dietary sources of selenium are Brazil nuts, seafood, liver, kidney, poultry, meats, whole grains, and cereals. The amount of selenium in plants depends on the soil in which they are grown. Some regions have small amounts of selenium in their drinking water. Selenium in food and water is easily absorbed by the human body and used where needed.

A very small amount of selenium is good for the body, but too much can be toxic. The recommended intake of selenium is 40 to 70 micrograms per day for adults (1 milligram is equal to 1,000 micrograms). The amount of selenium supplement taken should not be more than 200 micrograms per day, especially if taken on a regular basis. Supplements are available in drugstores, health food stores, and on the Internet.

Selenium deficiency is rare in the United States, and supplements are usually not needed. The typical American diet provides about 50 to 150 micrograms per day. Those who are on long-term intravenous feeding must receive supplements. Deficiency can also develop in people who have had part of the stomach or intestine removed or who have severe intestinal problems such as Crohn's disease. A person with low selenium can develop a form of heart disease, poor thyroid function, and a weakened immune system. Selenium deficiency is common in some parts of China and Russia because of low selenium levels in the soil.

What is the history behind it?

Selenium was first discovered as an element in 1817 by Jons Berzelius and was recognized as an essential nutrient in the late 1950s. It was not until the 1960s that selenium began to be suggested as a possible cancer preventive. Researchers wondered if selenium's antioxidant properties could inhibit tumor growth and boost the immune system. Animal research into the relationship between selenium and cancer began in the 1960s, and a human trial followed in the 1980s.

What is the evidence?

Researchers have found that selenium activates an antioxidant enzyme in the body. Antioxidants are compounds that block the action of free radicals—activated oxygen molecules that can damage cells.

Large observational studies have shown that death rates from cancer are significantly lower in areas of the world where selenium levels in the soil are high. This finding held true for deaths caused by cancers of the lung, esophagus, bladder, breast, colon, rectum, pancreas, ovary, and cervix, as well as for total cancer deaths. However, observational studies are difficult to interpret because of the many factors that can affect outcome. In part because of this, observational studies cannot prove what caused differences in outcomes.

One long-term controlled study of people who had had skin cancer was started in 1983. The selenium supplement had no effect on the patients' skin cancer; however, it was found that patients given a supplement of 200 micrograms of selenium per day had significantly fewer cancers of the lung, colon, rectum, and prostate and had fewer deaths from lung cancer than those who did not take selenium. Since the impact on prostate cancer was especially notable, researchers started another large study in 2001, called the SELECT study. Researchers give the men either selenium or a combination of selenium and vitamin E to learn whether either will lower the risk of prostate cancer. The study includes more than thirty-two thousand men and was expected to conclude in 2013. However, a preliminary analysis in 2008 showed no difference in prostate cancer risk between the group taking the selenium supplement and the group taking the placebo. The results suggested that the selenium group might have a higher risk for developing diabetes. The vitamin E supplement did not appear to be beneficial either, and early results suggested that it might slightly increase prostate cancer risk. Because of these possible risks, the researchers advised participants to stop taking the supplements.

Another study looked at more than five thousand men, giving some of them a placebo and others a supplement containing vitamin E, vitamin C, beta carotene, zinc, and selenium every day for eight years. There was a reduction in prostate cancer in men who took the supplement, but only in those who had a normal level of prostate-specific antigen (a protein made by the prostate gland) at the beginning of the study.

A study published in 2004 (called SU.VI.MAX) reported on more than thirteen thousand French adults who had taken either a placebo or a combination of vitamin E, vitamin C, beta carotene, selenium, and zinc. After a median of more than seven years of follow-up, there were no major differences in cancer rates between the people who got real supplements and those who took the placebo. However, when researchers looked at men and women separately, the men who had taken the antioxidant supplement had lower risk for cancer and death from all causes than the men who had not. This was not true for the women in the study. However, the men had lower levels of antioxidants, especially beta carotene and vitamins C and E, in their bodies when the study began. This may partly explain why they benefited more. It is unclear whether and how much selenium contributed to this effect.

In another analysis of the SU.VI.MAX study, those who took antioxidants ended up with no better levels of heart disease risk factors, such as cholesterol and other fats in the blood, than those on placebo. In fact, the women who had received the supplement had slightly worse risk factors than those who did not. Since this study looked at several antioxidants all together, it is difficult to say what selenium's role might have been.

Very little is known about the potential benefits or harm of selenium supplements for people living with cancer. A 2006 review of this issue concluded that there is not enough evidence to say whether selenium might reduce side effects of surgery, radiation therapy, or chemotherapy.

A 2007 reanalysis of data from 385 studies found that people who took selenium supplements tended to live slightly longer than those who did not, whereas other antioxidant supplements (vitamins A, C, and E) either had no effect or shortened life span slightly.

Selenium has been tested in many small clinical trials to see whether it affects other health problems, such as pancreatitis, thyroid conditions, human immunodeficiency virus, asthma, hepatitis, and more. There is not enough evidence from any of these studies to prove that selenium supplements are helpful. Large, well-controlled clinical trials are necessary to learn more.

At this time, it is hard to say how each nutrient or nutrient combination affects a person's risk for cancer. On the other hand, studies of large groups of people have shown that those whose diets are high in vegetables and low in animal fat, meat, and/or calories have lower risk for some of the most common types of cancer. Until more is known about this relationship, the American

Cancer Society recommends eating a variety of healthful foods—with most of them coming from plant sources—rather than relying on supplements.

Are there any possible problems or complications?

Selenium supplements can be toxic to the human body if they raise selenium levels beyond what the body can tolerate. Massive overdoses taken all at once can result in kidney failure, breathing problems, and death. Too much selenium taken over a period of weeks or months can cause more gradual toxic effects. Early signs of selenium poisoning include vomiting, diarrhea, fatigue, irritability, garlicky-smelling breath, and numbness and loss of control in the arms and legs. Long-term effects can include hair loss, discolored nails, skin rash, and loss of nails.

In one clinical trial originally intended to study whether a 200-microgram selenium supplement reduced skin cancer risk, the researchers noticed that people receiving the supplement were 55 percent more likely to develop type 2 diabetes. A recent epidemiologic study in which researchers measured serum selenium levels of more than thirteen thousand people found that people with low selenium levels were at higher risk for dying of cancer and all causes combined, but also noticed there was an increased risk among people with the highest selenium levels. The researchers interpreted this finding as reason to be cautious about selenium supplements.

Selenium has antioxidant properties, and antioxidant supplements may interfere with the effectiveness of chemotherapy or radiation treatment. Patients who are undergoing cancer treatment should talk to their doctors before taking vitamins, minerals, or other supplements.

According to the U.S. Department of Health and Human Services, one compound of selenium, selenium sulfide (a chemical compound used in antidandruff shampoos, but not in supplements), might cause cancer if taken internally and therefore should not be ingested. Using these shampoos is considered safe because skin does not absorb selenium sulfide.

Relying on this type of treatment alone and avoiding or delaying conventional medical care for cancer may have serious health consequences.

This product is sold as a dietary supplement in the United States. Unlike companies that produce drugs (which must provide the FDA with results of detailed testing showing their product is safe and effective before the drug is approved for sale), the companies that make supplements do not have to show evidence of safety or health benefits to the FDA before selling their products. Supplement products without any reliable scientific evidence of health benefits may still be sold as long as the companies selling them do not claim the supplements can prevent, treat, or cure any specific disease. Some such products may not contain the amount of the herb or substance that is written on the label, and some may include other substances (contaminants). Though the FDA has written new rules to improve the quality of manufacturing processes for dietary supplements and the accurate listing of supplement ingredients, these rules do not take full effect until 2010. The new rules also do not address the safety of supplement ingredients or their effects on health when proper manufacturing techniques are used.

Most such supplements have not been tested to find out if they interact with medicines, foods, or other herbs and supplements. Even though some reports of interactions and harmful effects may be published, full studies of interactions and effects are not often available. Because of these limitations, any information on ill effects and interactions should be considered incomplete.

References

Bjelakovic G, Nikolova D, Gluud LL, Simonetti RG, Gluud C. Mortality in randomized trials of antioxidant supplements for primary and secondary prevention: systematic review and meta-analysis. *JAMA.* 2007;297:842-857.

Bleys J, Navas-Acien A, Guallar E. Serum selenium levels and all-cause, cancer, and cardiovascular mortality among US adults. *Arch Intern Med.* 2008;168:404-410.

Clark LC, Combs GF Jr, Turnbull BW, Slate EH, Chalker DK, Chow J, Davis LS, Glover RA, Grahm GF, Gross EG, Krongrad A, Lesher JL Jr, Park HK, Sanders BB Jr, Smith CL, Taylor JR. Effects of selenium supplementation for cancer prevention in patients with carcinoma of the skin. *JAMA.* 1996;276:1957-1963.
Erratum in:
JAMA. 1997;277:1520.

Clark RF, Strukle E, Williams SR, Manoguerra AS. Selenium poisoning from a nutritional supplement. *JAMA.* 1996;275:1087-1088.

Dennert G, Horneber M. Selenium for alleviating the side effects of chemotherapy, radiotherapy and surgery in cancer patients. *Cochrane Database Syst Rev.* 2006;(3):CD005037.

Duffield-Lillico AJ, Dalkin BL, Reid ME, Turnbull BW, Slate EH, Jacobs ET, Marshall JR, Clark LC; Nutritional Prevention of Cancer Study Group. Selenium supplementation, baseline plasma selenium status and incidence of prostate cancer: an analysis of the complete treatment period of the Nutritional Prevention of Cancer Trial. *BJU Int.* 2003;91:608-612.

Food and Nutrition Board. Dietary reference intakes: elements. Institute of Medicine Web site. http://www.iom.edu/Object.File/Master/7/294/0.pdf. Accessed June 6, 2008.

Galan P, Briançon S, Favier A, Bertrais S, Preziosi P, Faure H, Arnaud J, Arnault N, Czernichow S, Mennen L, Hercberg S. Antioxidant status and risk of cancer in the SU.VI.MAX study: is the effect of supplementation dependent on baseline levels? *Br J Nutr.* 2005;94:125-132.

Hercberg S, Bertrais S, Czernichow S, Noisette N, Galan P, Jaouen A, Tichet J, Briancon S, Favier A, Mennen L, Roussel AM. Alterations of the lipid profile after 7.5 years of low-dose antioxidant supplementation in the SU.VI.MAX Study. *Lipids.* 2005;40:335-342.

Hercberg S, Galan P, Preziosi P, Bertrais S, Mennen L, Malvy D, Roussel AM, Favier A, Briançon S. The SU.VI.MAX study: a randomized, placebo-controlled trial of the health effects of antioxidant vitamins and minerals. *Arch Intern Med.* 2004;164:2335-2342.

Klein EA. Selenium and vitamin E cancer prevention trial. *Ann N Y Acad Sci.* 2004;1031:234-241.

Kushi LH, Byers T, Doyle C, Bandera EV, McCullough M, McTiernan A, Gansler T, Andrews KS, Thun MJ; American Cancer Society 2006 Nutrition and Physical Activity Guidelines Advisory Committee. American Cancer Society guidelines on nutrition and physical activity for cancer prevention: reducing the risk of cancer with healthy food choices and physical activity. *CA Cancer J Clin.* 2006;56:254-281.

Lawenda BD, Kelly KM, Ladas EJ, Sagar SM, Vickers A, Blumberg JB. Should supplemental antioxidant administration be avoided during chemotherapy and radiation therapy? *J Natl Cancer Inst.* 2008;100:773-783.

Meyer F, Galan P, Douville P, Bairati I, Kegle P, Bertrais S, Estaquio C, Hercberg S. Antioxidant vitamin and mineral supplementation and prostate cancer prevention in the SU.VI.MAX trial. *Int J Cancer.* 2005;116:182-186.

Dietary supplement fact sheet: selenium. Office of Dietary Supplements Web site. http://ods.od.nih.gov/factsheets/selenium.asp. Accessed June 6, 2008.

Patterson BH, Levander OA. Naturally occurring selenium compounds in cancer chemoprevention trials: a workshop summary. *Cancer Epidemiol Biomarkers Prev.* 1997;6:63-69.

Review of prostate cancer prevention study shows no benefit for use of selenium and vitamin E supplements [press release]. Bethesda, MD: National Cancer Institute Office of Media Relations; October 27, 2008. http://www.cancer.gov/newscenter/pressrelease/SELECTresults2008. Accessed December 4, 2008.

Selenium. Memorial Sloan-Kettering Cancer Center Web site. http://www.mskcc.org/mskcc/html/69373.cfm. Updated August 7, 2007. Accessed June 6, 2008.

Selenium. PDRhealth Web site. http://www.pdrhealth.com/drug_info/nmdrugprofiles/nutsupdrugs/sel_0232.shtml. Accessed June 6, 2008.

Selenium (Se). Medline Plus Web site. http://www.nlm.nih.gov/medlineplus/druginfo/natural/patient-selenium.html. Updated March 1, 2008. Accessed June 6, 2008.

Stranges S, Marshall JR, Natarajan R, Donahue RP, Trevisan M, Combs GF, Cappuccio FP, Ceriello A, Reid ME. Effects of long-term selenium supplementation on the incidence of type 2 diabetes. A randomized trial. *Ann Intern Med.* 2007;147:217-223.

SIX FLAVOR TEA

Other common name(s): liu wei di huang wan, six flavor rehmanni, rehmannia six
Scientific/medical name(s): none

Description

Six Flavor Tea is a Chinese herbal combination that is promoted to enhance conventional treatment of small cell lung cancer.

Overview

Available scientific evidence does not support claims about Six Flavor Tea's health benefits.

How is it promoted for use?

Six Flavor Tea pills are mainly sold as a treatment for kidney deficiencies, which practitioners claim can cause a buildup of disease-causing toxins. They contend Six Flavor Tea can also treat weakness or pain in the lower back, insomnia, night sweats, dizziness, tinnitus, impotence, sore throat, headache, burning of the palms of the hands or soles of the feet, and high blood pressure. This product is also promoted as a cure for diabetes. In Chinese medicine, this herbal remedy is reportedly used for deficient liver or spleen qi or yin.

What does it involve?

Six Flavor Tea is sold in pill form.

What is the history behind it?

Some say that Six Flavor Tea is a traditional Chinese formula and that it has been used in Asia for thousands of years.

What is the evidence?

Available scientific evidence does not convincingly support any of these claims. Although a few Chinese studies have been reported, the studies contain insufficient information to evaluate their reliability. Most of the claims of proponents are not addressed in any studies published in peer-reviewed medical journals.

Are there any possible problems or complications?

Most Web sites recommending Six Flavor Tea claim that this product causes no side effects. Relying on this type of treatment alone and avoiding or delaying conventional medical care for cancer may have serious health consequences.

This product is sold as a dietary supplement in the United States. Unlike companies that produce drugs (which must provide the FDA with results of detailed testing showing their product is safe and effective before the drug is approved for sale), the companies that make supplements do not have to show evidence of safety or health benefits to the FDA before selling their products. Supplement products without any reliable scientific evidence of health benefits may still be sold as long as the companies selling them do not claim the supplements can prevent, treat, or cure any specific disease. Some such products may not contain the amount of the herb or substance that is written on the label, and some

may include other substances (contaminants). Though the FDA has written new rules to improve the quality of manufacturing processes for dietary supplements and the accurate listing of supplement ingredients, these rules do not take full effect until 2010. The new rules also do not address the safety of supplement ingredients or their effects on health when proper manufacturing techniques are used.

Most such supplements have not been tested to find out if they interact with medicines, foods, or other herbs and supplements. Even though some reports of interactions and harmful effects may be published, full studies of interactions and effects are not often available. Because of these limitations, any information on ill effects and interactions should be considered incomplete.

References

Hu SJ, Fang Q, Liu JS, Zhang L, Cao EZ. Clinical study on intervention of liuwei dihuang pill on hormonotherapy in treating nephrotic syndrome [in Chinese] [Abstract]. *Zhongguo Zhong Xi Yi Jie He Za Zhi.* 2005;25:107-110.

Shen JJ, Lin CJ, Huang JL, Hsieh KH, Kuo ML. The effect of liu-wei-di-huang wan on cytokine gene expression from human peripheral blood lymphocytes. *Am J Chin Med.* 2003;31:247-257.

Vickers A, Goyal N, Harland R, Rees R. Do certain countries produce only positive results? A systematic review of controlled trials. *Control Clin Trials.* 1998;19:159-166.

Zheng WC, Hu SJ, Fang Q. Intervention of liuwei dihuang pill on lupus nephropathy treated with cyclophosphamide and glucocorticoids [in Chinese] [Abstract]. *Zhongguo Zhong Xi Yi Jie He Za Zhi.* 2005;25:983-985.

SODIUM BICARBONATE

Other common name(s): Simoncini Cancer Therapy, baking soda
Scientific/medical name(s): NaHC03

Description

Sodium bicarbonate, also known as baking soda, is promoted by some alternative practitioners as cancer treatment. This treatment is based on the theory that cancer is caused by a form of yeast infection and that sodium bicarbonate can kill the yeast.

Sodium bicarbonate is used as a conventional treatment for disorders in which the blood is too acidic. It is also used as an over-the-counter remedy for heartburn.

Overview

Available scientific evidence does not support claims that cancer is caused by infection with a type of yeast known as *Candida albicans.* Available scientific evidence also does not support the idea that sodium bicarbonate works as a treatment for any form of cancer or that it cures yeast or fungal infections. There is substantial evidence, however, that these claims are false. Although sodium bicarbonate is safe when used in proper doses and as directed as a conventional treatment, high doses can cause serious problems or even death.

How is it promoted for use?

Sodium bicarbonate is promoted by some alternative practitioners, especially Dr. Tullio Simoncini, as a cure for all types of cancer. This claim is made on several Web sites, in videos of Dr. Simoncini posted on the Internet, and in a book written by Dr. Simoncini.

What does it involve?

Sodium bicarbonate is given by some alternative practitioners by mouth or intravenously. It is also given intra-arterially (into an artery supplying blood to the tumor) and is sometimes given as a solution directly through the trachea (windpipe) into the lungs to treat lung cancer.

What is the history behind it?

The main proponent of sodium bicarbonate as an alternative cancer treatment is Tullio Simoncini, MD. Information on the Internet describes how Dr. Simoncini concluded that cancer is caused by *Candida albicans* and can be cured with baking soda. The sequence of events and timeline are not described in detail.

According to the Cancer Treatment Watch Web site, "[Dr. Simoncini] has been using unsubstantiated cancer treatments for 15 years… in 2003, his [Italian] license to practice medicine was withdrawn, and in 2006 he was convicted by an Italian judge for wrongful death and swindling… This has not stopped him from continuing to provide his controversial treatments, not only in Italy, but apparently also in foreign countries, such as the Netherlands" (Koene and Jitta, 2008).

What is the evidence?

No peer-reviewed articles in medical journals were found supporting the theory that cancer is caused by a fungus infection or a yeast infection. Available peer-reviewed medical journals do not support claims that sodium bicarbonate works as a cancer treatment.

Scientists require certain kinds of evidence to support claims that a kind of germ causes a certain disease. The first requirement is that the germ should be present in all cases of the disease. Simoncini claims that all tumors contain fungi. But these fungi have not been found in tumors when biopsies are examined by methods capable of revealing fungi in infected tissue. Another requirement is that infecting laboratory animals with the germ should cause the disease. Infections can develop in animals that are exposed to *Candida albicans*, but there are no credible reports that this exposure or infection causes cancer. Finally, when researchers remove diseased tissue from infected laboratory animals, they should be able to recover the germs and grow them in laboratory dishes. There are no reports in scientific journals that this has been observed for *Candida albicans* and cancer of experimental animals.

A number of Web sites propose various reasons people believe there is a connection between fungus and cancer (for example, that *Candida albicans* can cause serious infections and that cancer is a serious disease). However, none of these Web sites show scientific evidence supported by credible experiments or clinical trials.

Fungal infection deep in the body is a serious health problem that can be fatal. Although a number of antifungal drugs are available to treat these infections, there is no evidence that sodium bicarbonate can. There is no evidence that most people with cancer have any deep tissue yeast or fungal infections. People whose immune systems are weakened by high doses of chemotherapy can sometimes contract these kinds of infections. While antifungal drugs can often cure the infection, there is no evidence that antifungal treatment causes the patients' tumors to shrink. If this had happened, the doctors caring for these patients would have been likely to report it in medical journals.

Some people with cancer have other health conditions for which sodium bicarbonate is used. But, again, there is no evidence that sodium bicarbonate has caused their tumors to shrink. Chewable sodium bicarbonate tablets and powder are common over-the-counter treatments that are used to neutralize stomach acid that causes heartburn. Intravenous sodium bicarbonate is used as a conventional treatment to reduce acidity of blood in serious conditions like shock, severe dehydration, and uncontrolled kidney failure or diabetes.

Are there any possible problems or complications?

In general, oral and intravenous treatment with sodium bicarbonate that is given for the right reasons and in proper doses is considered safe. Concern has been raised that the same substance can be dangerous in other medical situations. The Cancer Treatment Watch Web site quotes the Netherlands Health Inspectorate:

> … there are no scientific data that justify the administration of sodium bicarbonate to patients with cancer… [T]he administration of sodium bicarbonate even has risks for patients with high blood pressure, patients with diseases of lungs, heart, or kidneys and for patients with cancer. This is certainly the case if a number of specific blood levels are not monitored daily before, during and after the treatment. The balance of the body can become completely disturbed when large amounts are administered. In severely ill patients, this may lead to organ damage. In sick people, there is in fact

irresponsible health care if this product is administered without monitoring. (2008)

Relying on this type of treatment alone and avoiding or delaying conventional medical care for cancer may have serious health consequences.

This substance has not been thoroughly tested to find out how it interacts with medicines, foods, or dietary supplements. Even though some reports of interactions and harmful effects may be published, full studies of interactions and effects are not often available. Because of these limitations, any information on ill effects and interactions should be considered incomplete.

References

Cancer therapy Web site. http://www.curenaturalicancro.com/. Accessed October 16, 2008.

A fungus among us in oncology? Respectful insolence Web site. http://scienceblogs.com/insolence/2008/08/a_fungus_among_us_in_oncology.php. Posted August 7, 2008. Accessed October 16, 2008.

Koch's postulates. Wikipedia Web site. http://en.wikipedia.org/wiki/Henle_Koch_postulates. Accessed October 16, 2008.

Koene R, Jitta SJ. Be wary of Simoncini cancer therapy. Cancer Treatment Watch Web site. http://www.cancertreatmentwatch.org/reports/simoncini.shtml. Posted August 7, 2008. Accessed October 16, 2008.

Sodium bicarbonate. Drugs Web site. http://www.drugs.com/mtm/sodium-bicarbonate.html. Revised July 13, 2005. Accessed October 16, 2008.

Sodium bicarbonate. RxList Web site. http://www.rxlist.com/cgi/generic/sodbic_ids.htm. Accessed October 16, 2008.

ST. JOHN'S WORT

Other common name(s): goatweed, amber, klamath weed, tipton weed
Scientific/medical name(s): *Hypericum perforatum*

Description

St. John's wort is a shrub-like perennial herb with bright yellow flowers that is native to Europe, western Asia, and northern Africa. Colonists brought it to the United States, where it now grows widely. The parts of the plant used in herbal remedies are taken from the flowering tops.

Overview

St. John's wort has been shown to be effective in treating mild to moderate depression and causes fewer side effects than older types of antidepressants (tricyclics or TCAs). Data suggest it may be less effective in treating severe depression. More research is needed to compare it with newer antidepressants. St. John's wort is known to interfere with many prescription drugs, including some used for anesthesia and cancer treatment.

How is it promoted for use?

St. John's wort is widely used in Europe to treat depression, anxiety, and sleep disorders. In Germany, doctors prescribe it more often than the popular antidepressant drug Prozac. Hypericin is the most commonly studied active ingredient in St. John's wort, and the amount of this compound is often used to standardize extracts.

The herb is also promoted to treat bronchial inflammation, bed-wetting, stomach problems, hemorrhoids, hypothyroidism, insomnia, migraines, kidney disorders, and malaria. A balm made from St. John's wort can be used on the skin for burns, wounds, insect bites and stings, and other skin diseases. Although there is some evidence for using St. John's wort in some emotional conditions besides depression, available scientific evidence does not support claims that it works for these other diseases.

What does it involve?

Commission E (Germany's regulatory agency for herbs) has approved St. John's wort for the treatment of depression and anxiety, as well as for burns and skin lesions. It is available by prescription only in Germany. However, it can be purchased in drug stores and health food stores in the United States as a capsule, tablet, and liquid extract and as a tea. An average dose is 300 milligrams, taken three times a day for four to six weeks.

Unfortunately, the potency and purity of different extracts sold in the United States varies widely. The U.S. Food and Drug Administration does not regulate herbs as tightly as it does prescription and over-the-counter medicines and cannot guarantee strength or purity.

A 2003 study using a new type of test found that most brands of St. John's wort contained a different amount of hypericin (or pseudohypericin), one of the active ingredients in St. John's wort, from what was listed on the label, ranging from 0 percent to 109 percent of the amount listed for capsules, and 31 percent to 80 percent of the amount listed for tablets. On average, the labels stated that the product contained about twice as much hypericin and pseudohypericin as it actually contained. Some products contained no detectable St. John's wort, and others contained less than a third of what the label stated. Very few contained the amount stated on the label. This variability can affect the results people might get when they try to follow a standard dose. Standardized products are supposed to contain 0.3 percent hypericin. The variability in strength may also affect the outcomes of research on the herb, unless researchers confirm the contents of the brand before testing it.

What is the history behind it?

Use of St. John's wort dates back many centuries and is surrounded with folklore. Greeks used it to fight fevers and evil spirits. Its scientific name comes from the Greek words *hyper* (meaning "over") and *eikon* (meaning "ghost"). In pre-Christian rituals in England, the plant was used to protect a house from evil spirits and to banish witches. It was thought that a person could be protected from death during the following year by putting a piece of the plant under a pillow on St. John's Eve, after which the saint would appear in a dream and give his blessing. The plant's common name reflects the fact that the flowers typically bloom around the birthday of St. John the Baptist, June 24.

St. John's wort has been used as a folk remedy for centuries to treat everything from wounds, headaches, gout, and kidney problems to nervous disorders. After it was brought to this continent, Native Americans used several species of St. John's wort to treat diarrhea, wounds, and snakebites.

In the United States, the plant was not well known until after the 1900s. In 1959, the plant was first studied for its ability to fight bacteria. Extracts of St. John's wort have become extremely popular in the United States. Since its interactions with other drugs have been discovered, there are more concerns about its potential dangers (see the section on problems and complications on page 501 for more information). Ireland, for instance, banned over-the-counter sales of the herb in 2000, though it is still available by prescription there.

What is the evidence?

Clinical trials have shown that St. John's wort is effective in treating mild to moderate depression and causes fewer side effects than older standard antidepressants (tricyclics or TCAs). Researchers are uncertain about how St. John's wort works to relieve depression. Hypericin was first recognized as its active ingredient, but newer information indicates that hyperforin, another compound in the herb, also plays an important role.

One review that analyzed twenty-three randomized clinical trials concluded that St. John's wort was more effective than a placebo for the treatment of mild to moderate depression and was found to be as effective as standard antidepressants. A more recent review of controlled, double-blinded studies reached a similar conclusion. However, the review authors reported that there were problems with the way the studies were designed and analyzed.

In 2004, a German group analyzed thirty studies that looked at St. John's wort for mild to moderate depression and found that the herb compared well to newer antidepressants. In the studies looking at mild depression, patients taking St. John's wort sometimes had better results than with standard treatment.

Studies are mixed with regard to its effectiveness in treating severe depression, but recent clinical trials suggest that it does not work as well. The U.S. National Institutes of Health—in cooperation with the Office of Alternative Medicine, the National Institute of Mental Health, and the Office of Dietary Supplements—launched a double-blind, controlled clinical trial using St. John's wort in the treatment of patients with major depression. A total of 340 adult patients were followed over a period of two to six months. The study compared the effects of St. John's wort, a placebo, and a newer antidepressant called sertraline. The study showed that neither the St. John's wort nor the sertraline was more effective than the placebo. This and similar studies suggest that St. John's wort may not be effective for moderate to severe depression, although this study was criticized because the approved antidepressant also showed no benefit.

St. John's wort has also been studied as a treatment for attention-deficit/hyperactivity disorder. A recent clinical trial for this condition found St. John's wort to be no different from placebo.

New studies are looking more closely at the interaction of St. John's wort with birth control pills and strong pain medicines called opioids. St. John's wort is also being studied to find out whether it helps in the treatment of minor depression, social phobia, and obsessive-compulsive disorder.

One nonrandomized clinical trial suggested that St. John's wort may have potential in helping people to stop smoking. This is an interesting idea, as other antidepressants have been useful in smoking cessation. However, additional study is needed before St. John's wort can be considered to be effective in this situation.

A few laboratory studies are testing some substances from St. John's wort as a cancer treatment. However, this research is quite preliminary, and no clinical studies have been reported.

Are there any possible problems or complications?

Side effects are not common but include upset stomach, constipation, fatigue, dry mouth, dizziness, headache, drowsiness, sleep disturbances, skin rash, and extreme sensitivity to sunlight. People taking St. John's wort should use sunscreen and eye protection when exposed to sunlight and should avoid tanning beds. It can also lower the sex drive. Allergic reactions are rare, but rashes have been reported. Information on the long-term effects of St. John's wort is not currently known. In some patients, when the herb has been taken for more than a month, stopping it suddenly can cause withdrawal symptoms such as nausea, vomiting, dizziness, dry mouth, and extreme fatigue.

St. John's wort interferes with several important medicines, such as human immunodeficiency virus drugs (antiretrovirals), blood thinners, birth control pills, and heart medicines such as digoxin. The herb can reduce the effectiveness of some anticancer drugs such as irinotecan and imatinib. It may also interact with drugs such as cyclosporine that keep the body from rejecting transplanted organs. St. John's wort may increase sleepiness if used with alcohol, narcotics, sedatives, sleeping medicines, and anticonvulsants (drugs to prevent seizures). Other medicines that may interact badly with St. John's wort include an antidiarrhea medicine called loperamide, an asthma medicine called theophylline, and some blood pressure medicines.

St. John's wort should not be used with other antidepressants because it could cause serotonin syndrome. This is a potentially fatal complication of the brain chemistry involving confusion, fever, hallucinations, poor coordination, nausea, vomiting, shakiness, restlessness, sweating, and other symptoms caused by an increase in serotonin activity.

People taking any prescription medicines or other herbs should talk to their doctors or pharmacists about possible interactions before taking St. John's wort. Because of its potential to interfere with anesthetics, it should be discontinued at least a week before surgery.

People with severe depression or manic depression (bipolar disorder) should not use St. John's wort. The herb may also increase muscle contractions of the uterus and is known to pass into breast milk. It should not be used by pregnant or breastfeeding women. Relying on this type of treatment alone and avoiding or delaying conventional medical care for cancer may have serious health consequences.

This product is sold as a dietary supplement in the United States. Unlike companies that produce drugs (which must provide the FDA with results of detailed testing showing their product is safe and effective before the drug is approved for sale), the companies that make supplements do not have to show evidence of safety or health benefits to the FDA before selling their products. Supplement products without any reliable scientific evidence of health benefits may still be sold as long as the companies selling them do not claim the supplements can prevent, treat, or cure any specific disease. Some such products may not contain the amount of the herb or substance that is written on the label, and some may include other substances (contaminants). Though the FDA has written new rules to improve the quality of manufacturing processes for dietary supplements and the accurate listing of supplement ingredients, these rules do not take full effect until 2010. The new rules also do not address the safety of supplement ingredients or their effects on health when proper manufacturing techniques are used.

Most such supplements have not been tested to find out if they interact with medicines, foods, or other herbs and supplements. Even though some reports of interactions and harmful effects may be published, full studies of interactions and effects are not often available. Because of these limitations, any information on ill effects and interactions should be considered incomplete.

References

Barrett S. St. John's wort. Quackwatch Web site. http://www.quackwatch.org/01QuackeryRelatedTopics/DSH/stjohn.html. Updated April 16, 2000. Accessed June 6, 2008.

Blumenthal M, ed. *The Complete German Commission E Monographs: Therapeutic Guide to Herbal Medicines.* Austin, TX: American Botanical Council; 1998.

Brennan C. St John's wort-a natural remedy for depression? Net Doctor.co.uk Web site. http://www.netdoctor.co.uk/special_reports/depression/stjwort.htm. Updated January 2, 2000. Accessed June 6, 2008.

Center for Drug Evaluation and Research. Risk of drug interactions with St. John's wort and Indinavir and other drugs. FDA Public Health Advisory. US Food and Drug Administration Web site. http://www.fda.gov/cder/drug/advisory/stjwort.htm.Published February 10, 2000. Accessed June 6, 2008.

Draves AH, Walter SE. Analysis of the hypericin and pseudohypericin content of commercially available St. John's Wort preparations. *Can J Clin Pharmacol.* 2003;10:114-118.

Fetrow CW, Avila JR. *Professional's Handbook of Complementary & Alternative Medicines.* Philadelphia, PA: Lippincott Williams & Wilkins; 2004.

Frye RF, Fitzgerald SM, Lagattuta TF, Hruska MW, Egorin MJ. Effect of St. John's wort on imatinib mesylate pharmacotherapeutics. *Clin Pharmacol Ther.* 2004;76:323-329.

Kim HL, Streltzer J, Goebert D. St. John's wort for depression: a meta-analysis of well-defined clinical trials. *J Nerv Ment Dis.* 1999;187:532-538.

Lawvere S, Mahoney MC, Cummings KM, Kepner JL, Hyland A, Lawrence DD, Murphy JM. A phase II study of St. John's Wort for smoking cessation. *Complement Ther Med.* 2006;14:175-184.

Linde K, Ramirez G, Mulrow CD, Egger M. St John's wort for depression. *Cochrane Database of Syst Rev.* 2005;(2):CD00448.

Meijerman I, Beijnen JH, Schellens JH. Herb-drug interactions in oncology: focus on mechanisms of induction. *Oncologist.* 2006;11:742-752.

National Center for Complementary and Alternative Medicine, National Institutes of Health. St. John's wort and the treatment of depression. National Center for Complementary and Alternative Medicine Web site. http://nccam.nih.gov/health/stjohnswort/sjw.pdf. Updated March 2004. Accessed June 6, 2008.

St. John's wort. Drug Digest Web site. http://www.drugdigest.org/DD/DVH/HerbsWho/0,3923,4049|St%2E+John%27s+Wort,00.html. Accessed June 6, 2008.

St. John's wort. Memorial Sloan-Kettering Cancer Center Web site. http://www.mskcc.org/mskcc/html/69385.cfm. Updated August 6, 2007. Accessed June 6, 2008.

Piscitelli SC, Burstein AH, Chaitt D, Alfaro RM, Falloon J. Indinavir concentrations and St. John's wort. *Lancet.* 2000;355:547-548.

Quiney C, Billard C, Salanoubat C, Fourneron JD, Kolb JP. Hyperforin, a new lead compound against the progression of cancer and leukemia? *Leukemia.* 2006;20:1519-1525.

Röder C, Schaefer M, Leucht S. Meta-analysis of effectiveness and tolerability of treatment of mild to moderate depression with St. John's Wort [in German] [Abstract]. *Fortsch Neurol Psychiatr.* 2004;72:330-343.

Ruschitzka F, Meier PJ, Turina M, Lüscher TF, Noll G. Acute heart transplant rejection due to Saint John's wort. *Lancet.* 2000;355:548-549.

Stavropoulos NE, Kim A, Nseyo UU, Tsimaris I, Chung TD, Miller TA, Redlak M, Nseyo UO, Skalkos D. *Hypericum perforatum* L. extract - novel photosensitizer against human bladder cancer cells. *J Photochem Photobiol B.* 2006;84:64-69.

Vorbach EU, Arnoldt KH, Hübner WD. Efficacy and tolerability of St. John's wort extract LI 160 versus imipramine in patients with severe depressive episodes according to ICD-10. *Pharmacopsychiatry.* 1997;30:81-85.

Weber W, Vander Stoep A, McCarty RL, Weiss NS, Biederman J, McClellan J. *Hypericum perforatum* (St John's wort) for attention-deficit/hyperactivity disorder in children and adolescents: a randomized controlled trial. *JAMA.* 2008;299:2633-2641.

Zanoli P. Role of hyperforin in the pharmacological activities of St. John's wort. *CNS Drug Rev.* 2004;10:203-218.

STRYCHNOS NUX-VOMICA

Other common name(s): nux vomica, poison nut, Quaker buttons, strychnine tree, ma qian zi (also written maqianzi)

Scientific/medical name(s): *Strychnos nux-vomica*

Description

Strychnos nux-vomica is the name of an evergreen tree that is native to southeast Asia, especially India and Myanmar, and cultivated elsewhere. Its dried seeds or beans, and sometimes its bark (called nux vomica), are used in herbal remedies. The seeds contain organic substances, strychnine and brucine, that are used in herbal remedies.

Overview

Available scientific evidence does not support claims that *Strychnos nux-vomica* is effective in treating cancer, relieving the side effects of conventional cancer treatment, or in treating any other conditions. The chemicals in the seeds are poisonous and may cause convulsions and death.

How is it promoted for use?

In herbal medicine, *Strychnos nux-vomica* is recommended for liver cancer, upset stomach, vomiting, abdominal pain, constipation, intestinal irritation, hangovers, heartburn, insomnia, certain heart diseases, circulatory problems, eye diseases, depression, migraine headaches, nervous conditions, problems related to menopause, and respiratory diseases in the elderly. In folk medicine, it is used as a healing tonic and appetite stimulant. *Strychnos nux-vomica* is used in Chinese herbal medicine to unblock channels and obstructions, reduce swelling, alleviate pain, and to treat abscesses and yin-type ulcers. In traditional Chinese treatment of cancer, it can be used in combination with other herbs.

What does it involve?

The seeds of the *Strychnos nux-vomica* tree are removed from the ripened berries of the tree and dried in the sun. Sometimes they are heated or further processed, which may reduce the amount of poison in the seeds. Various herbal preparations are made from the dried seeds, including tablets, liquid extracts, and tinctures. Some practitioners use single dosages that range from 20 milligrams to 1 gram. Homeopathic dilutions are also made (see "Homeopathy," page 753), which contain little, if any, of the actual seeds.

What is the history behind it?

Strychnos nux-vomica is one of the ingredients used, in small amounts, in traditional Chinese herbal treatments for liver cancer and numerous other health problems. Native tribes in Central and South America have also used extracts from this plant for centuries as a medicine to inhibit muscle contractions and as a poison for the tips of arrows. Some physicians used *Strychnos nux-vomica* in the treatment of stomach cancer in the late nineteenth century. It was given to patients to induce vomiting, which was felt to help relieve the patient's discomfort.

Strychnos nux-vomica is still used as an active ingredient in pest control products, in gopher bait, and in some rat poisons. Today, it is rare to find any form other than the homeopathic preparation recommended for human treatment.

What is the evidence?

Strychnos nux-vomica has not been proven effective for the treatment of any illness. Since the seeds contain strychnine, which is poisonous to humans, conventional medical practitioners do not recommend it as a medicine. Some research has shown that the level of poison in nux vomica preparations may depend greatly on how the seeds are processed.

The herbal remedy is on the Commission E (Germany's regulatory agency for herbs) list of unapproved herbs, meaning it is not recommended for use because it has not been proven to be safe or effective.

There is no clinical trial evidence of effectiveness as a cancer treatment reported in peer-reviewed English-language journals. Some Chinese studies have reported that *Strychnos nux-vomica* can kill cancer cells grown in laboratory dishes.

Are there any possible problems or complications?

The seeds of the nux vomica tree contain strychnine, a poison that in doses as small as 5 milligrams (as little as one seed) can cause anxiety, restlessness, painful convulsions of the body, breathing difficulties, and even death from suffocation or exhaustion. Long-term intake of even small amounts of strychnine can cause liver damage. This herb should be avoided, especially by women who are pregnant or breastfeeding. Relying on this type of treatment alone and avoiding or delaying conventional medical care for cancer may have serious health consequences.

This product is sold as a dietary supplement in the United States. Unlike companies that produce drugs (which must provide the FDA with results of detailed testing showing their product is safe and effective before the drug is approved for sale), the companies that make supplements do not have to show evidence of safety or health benefits to the FDA before selling their products. Supplement products without any reliable scientific evidence of health benefits may still be sold as long as the companies selling them do not claim the supplements can prevent, treat, or cure any specific disease. Some such products may not contain the amount of the herb or substance that is written on the label, and some may include other substances (contaminants). Though the FDA has written new rules to improve the quality of manufacturing processes for dietary supplements and the accurate listing of supplement ingredients, these rules do not take full effect until 2010. The new rules also do not address the safety of supplement ingredients or their effects on health when proper manufacturing techniques are used.

Most such supplements have not been tested to find out if they interact with medicines, foods, or other herbs and supplements. Even though some reports of interactions and harmful effects may be published, full studies of interactions and effects are not often available. Because of these limitations, any information on ill effects and interactions should be considered incomplete.

References

Blumenthal M, ed. *The Complete German Commission E Monographs: Therapeutic Guide to Herbal Medicines.* Austin, TX: American Botanical Council; 1998.

Cai BC, Hattori M, Namba T. Processing of nux vomica. II. Changes in alkaloid composition of the seeds of Strychnos nux-vomica on traditional drug-processing. *Chem Pharm Bull (Tokyo).* 1990;38:1295-1298.

Cai BC, Wang TS, Kurokawa M, Shiraki K, Hattori M. Cytotoxicities of alkaloids from processed and unprocessed seeds of Strychnos nux-vomica. *Zhongguo Yao Li Xue Bao* 1998;19:425-428.

Chan TY. Herbal medicine causing likely strychnine poisoning. *Hum Exp Toxicol.* 2002;21:467-468.

Chu JHK. Ma qian zi, fan mu bie. Complementary and Alternative Healing University Web site. http://alternative healing.org/ma_qian_zi.htm. Accessed August 6, 2008.

Deng X, Yin F, Lu X, Cai B, Yin W. The apoptotic effect of brucine from the seed of Strychnos nux-vomica on human hepatoma cells is mediated via Bcl-2 and Ca2+ involved mitochondrial pathway. *Toxicol Sci.* 2006;91:59-69.

Gruenwald J. *PDR for Herbal Medicines.* 3rd ed. Montvale, NJ: Thomson PDR; 2004.

Ma qian zi. Chinese Medicine Tools Web site. http://www.chinesemedicinetools.com/ma-qian-zi. Accessed August 6, 2008.

Wang Z, Zhao J, Xing J, He Y, Guo D. Analysis of strychnine and brucine in postmortem specimens by RP-HPLC: a case report of fatal intoxication. *J Anal Toxicol.* 2004;28:141-144.

TEA TREE OIL

Other common name(s): Australian tea tree oil, melaleuca oil
Scientific/medical name(s): *Melaleuca alternifolia*

Description

Tea tree oil is a concentrated plant oil from the leaves of a tree native to Australian coastal areas. The tree is known as *Melaleuca alternifolia* (or tea tree) and is a member of the myrtle family. The oil is distilled into the air through a steam process and is also used on the skin as an herbal remedy.

Overview

Tea tree oil has been used in Australia for many years to treat skin infections. It holds some potential as a treatment for bacterial and fungal infections of the skin and nails. Available scientific evidence does not support claims that it boosts the immune system. Tea tree oil is toxic when swallowed and should never be taken internally.

How is it promoted for use?

Proponents believe tea tree oil is an antiseptic and use it to fight germs. It has been used to treat cuts, minor burns, athlete's foot, and insect bites. Some claim it can treat bacterial and fungal skin infections, wound infections, gum infections, acne, head lice, eczema, vaginal yeast infections, colds, pneumonia, and other respiratory illnesses.

While no one claims tea tree oil can prevent or treat cancer, some proponents claim the oil can boost the immune system. Some herbalists claim that tea tree oil can be used as a "lymphatic recharge" for a "sluggish" lymphatic system.

Household cleaners that contain tea tree oil have also been promoted as alternatives to products that contain cancer-causing chemicals, such as formaldehyde.

What does it involve?

Tea tree oil can be dissolved in water or used at full strength. It is also available in the form of ointments, creams, lotions, and soap. Tea tree oil is often sold in dark glass bottles to prevent light from affecting its potency. When used to treat infections and skin conditions, the oil can be applied directly to the skin in full strength or diluted form using cotton swabs. The oil can also be found in deodorants, shampoos, soaps, antiseptic first-aid creams, cosmetics, and household cleaning products.

Tea tree oil should never be taken internally. For colds and other respiratory illnesses, the oil is added to a vaporizer so that the mist can be inhaled. Drops of the oil can be added to bath water. The oil is sometimes mixed in water as a mouthwash.

What is the history behind it?

The aborigines of Australia were the first to discover the healing properties of tea tree oil thousands of years ago. They treated cuts, burns, and skin infections by crushing the leaves of the tree and applying them to cuts and injuries. In the 1770s, the British explorer Captain Cook observed the native Australians brewing tea from the leaves. He then brewed tea of his own to give to his crew to prevent scurvy. He coined the name tea tree.

In the 1920s, Australian physicians began to use the oil to clean wounds and prevent infections after surgery. They believed it to be more effective than carbolic acid, the antiseptic most used at that time. Average Australians then began to use the oil as a household remedy for skin conditions and fungus infections. During World War II, tea tree oil was included in the first-aid kits given to all Australian soldiers and sailors.

After the discovery of penicillin and other antibiotics in the late 1940s, tea tree oil went out of favor as an antiseptic until the 1980s, when it was discovered that some bacteria were resistant to certain antibiotics, such as methicillin and vancomycin. Today, there is renewed interest in tea tree oil as an alternative to these antibiotics for skin infections.

What is the evidence?

Recent laboratory experiments suggest that tea tree oil holds promise as an antiseptic when used on the skin to kill germs, including those that are resistant to methicillin, vancomycin, and other antibiotics. Other laboratory studies suggest that tea tree oil might be helpful against scabies (skin mites) and some types of fungus. A laboratory study published in 2006 showed that tea tree oil can kill yeasts that cause mouth infections in cancer patients with weakened immune systems. However, the safety and effectiveness of tea tree oil has not been tested in clinical studies of cancer patients with mouth infections, and the fact that tea tree oil is toxic when swallowed seems likely to limit its use to treat mouth infections. Even though laboratory studies may show promise, further studies are needed to find out whether the results apply to humans.

A few human studies have been done on tea tree oil's effectiveness in treating various conditions. In studies to determine whether tea tree oil helped fungal toenail infections, it compared well to clotrimazole cream, an older treatment. However, the testing procedure was scientifically somewhat weak. Tests to find out whether tea tree oil helped prevent cold sores showed no benefit, but the tests also had some design flaws that could have affected the results. Tea tree oil has also been tested to see whether it helped mild acne. It was compared with benzoyl peroxide for three months, and both groups showed similar improvement by the end of the study. Tests to see whether it cured athlete's foot showed mixed results. Despite years of use, available clinical evidence does not support the effectiveness of tea tree oil for treating skin problems and infections in humans.

Are there any possible problems or complications?

In rare cases, allergic reactions (such as rashes) to tea tree oil can occur. The rashes may be mild and itchy, but severe blistering has been reported as well. The rashes usually improve when the person stops using the oil. Serious allergic reactions are possible—one medical report described a man who had immediate dizziness and swelling in his throat when tea tree oil was applied to his skin. People who are allergic to other members of the myrtle family (*Myrtaceae*), such as eucalyptus, guava, clove, or allspice, may be more likely to have an allergic reaction. Those who are sensitive to pine or turpentine may also react to tea tree oil because of chemical similarities between the plants. As tea tree oil ages, it breaks down into substances that are more likely to cause reactions. Using fresher products that have not been exposed to air, light, and heat may cause fewer problems with allergies.

Full-strength tea tree oil may cause skin irritation even in people who are not allergic to the oil. These people may have less of a problem with more diluted oils. Some tea tree oil preparations contain other ingredients as well, some of which may cause irritation, allergic reaction, or rash on their own.

There is some evidence that the oil should not be used on burns. Tea tree oil is not recommended for children. Women who are pregnant or breastfeeding should not use this oil.

Tea tree oil is toxic when swallowed. It has been reported to cause drowsiness, confusion, hallucinations, coma, unsteadiness, weakness, vomiting, diarrhea, stomach upset, blood cell abnormalities, and severe rashes. It should be kept away from pets and children. Relying on this type of treatment alone and avoiding or delaying conventional medical care for cancer may have serious health consequences.

This substance has not been thoroughly tested to find out how it interacts with medicines, foods, or dietary supplements. Even though some reports of interactions and harmful effects may be published, full studies of interactions and effects are not often available. Because of these limitations, any information on ill effects and interactions should be considered incomplete.

References

Bagg J, Jackson MS, Petrina Sweeney M, Ramage G, Davies AN. Susceptibility to Melaleuca alternifolia (tea tree) oil of yeasts isolated from the mouths of patients with advanced cancer. *Oral Oncol.* 2006;42:487-492.

Carson CF, Ashton L, Dry L, Smith DW, Riley TV. Melaleuca alternifolia (tea tree) oil gel (6%) for the treatment of recurrent herpes labialis. *J Antimicrob Chemother.* 2001;48:450-451.

Carson CF, Riley TV. Antimicrobial activity of the major components of the essential oil of Melaleuca alternifolia. *J Appl Bacteriol.* 1995;78:264-269.

Faoagali J, George N, Leditschke JF. Does tea tree oil have a place in the topical treatment of burns? *Burns.* 1997;23:349-351.

Fetrow CW, Avila JR. *Professional's Handbook of Complementary & Alternative Medicines.* Philadelphia, PA: Lippincott Williams & Wilkins; 2004.

Gruenwald J. *PDR for Herbal Medicines.* 3rd ed. Montvale, NJ: Thomson PDR; 2004.

Hammer KA, Carson CF, Riley TV. In vitro activity of *Melaleuca alternifolia* (tea tree) oil against dermatophytes and other filamentous fungi. *J Antimicrob Chemother.* 2002;50:195-199.

Hausen BM, Reichling J, Harkenthal M. Degradation products of monoterpenes are the sensitizing agents in tea tree oil. *Am J Contact Dermat.* 1999;10:68-77.

Khanna M, Qasem K, Sasseville D. Allergic contact dermatitis to tea tree oil with erythema multiforme-like id reaction. *Am J Contact Dermat.* 2000;11:238-242.

Mozelsio NB, Harris KE, McGrath KG, Grammer LC. Immediate systemic hypersensitivity reaction associated with topical application of Australian tea tree oil. *Allergy Asthma Proc.* 2003;24:73-75.

Rubel DM, Freeman S, Southwell IA. Tea tree allergy: what is the offending agent? Report of three cases of tea tree allergy and review of the literature. *Australas J Dermatol.* 1998;39:244-247.

Tea tree oil. Drug Digest Web site. http://www.drugdigest.org/DD/DVH/HerbsWho/0,3923,551982|Tea+Tree+Oil,00.html. Accessed June 6, 2008.

Tea tree oil. Memorial Sloan-Kettering Cancer Center Web site. http://www.mskcc.org/mskcc/html/69396.cfm. Updated August 6, 2007. Accessed June 6, 2008.

Walton SF, McKinnon M, Pizzutto S, Dougall A, Williams E, Currie BJ. Acaricidal activity of *Melaleuca alternifolia* (tea tree) oil: in vitro sensitivity of *Sarcoptes scabiei* var *hominis* to terpinen-4-ol. *Arch Dermatol.* 2004;140:563-566.

THUJA

Other common name(s): Eastern white cedar, Northern white cedar, yellow cedar, tree of life, arborvitae, swamp cedar

Scientific/medical name(s): *Thuja occidentalis*

Description

Thuja (pronounced THOO-ya) is an evergreen in the cypress family, native to eastern North America. The tree is also grown in Europe as an ornamental plant. The parts used in herbal remedies are the branches and the tiny, flat, scale-like leaves, which contain the oil thujone.

Overview

Available scientific evidence does not support claims that thuja or its extract is safe or effective. Taken internally, the herb can cause serious side effects, and it may be toxic in large doses. The essential oil contained in the tree, also known as cedar leaf oil, is not generally sold for internal use. It is poisonous and can also irritate or burn the skin and eyes.

How is it promoted for use?

Thuja is promoted as a treatment for many medical conditions, including cancer. Some proponents claim that thuja decreases the toxic effects of chemotherapy and radiation therapy. Herbalists prescribe thuja to treat viral and bacterial infections and coughs and other respiratory ailments, including strep throat and respiratory distress related to congestive heart failure. Herbalists also use it as a diuretic to increase urination and as an astringent to "purify the blood," reduce inflammation, and cleanse the body of "toxins." Thuja is sometimes used with antibiotics to treat bacterial skin infections and herpes sores. It has even been used by some practitioners to induce abortions. Thuja ointment is applied to the skin for ailments such as psoriasis, eczema, vaginal infections, warts, muscle aches, and rheumatism.

Some practitioners of homeopathy (see "Homeopathy," page 753) recommend use of very dilute thuja, in pill or liquid form, for treating irritability, depression, sadness, impaired thinking, headache, warts, growths, rashes, runny nose, sores in the nose, mouth pain, toothache, gas, hemorrhoids, watery stool, enlarged prostate, gonorrhea, back pain, joint pain, bad dreams, tiredness, insomnia, fevers, shaking chills, muscle pain, and cancer.

What does it involve?

Leaves from the tree are harvested and dried. Liquid extracts, tinctures, and tea made from thuja are taken internally. There is no standard dose of the herb. Thuja ointment is applied directly to the skin. Thuja oil and capsules are available in health food stores and over the Internet. When properly prepared and dosed as dietary supplements, the thujone levels are reportedly below the toxic range. However, because dietary supplements are not considered drugs, the U.S. Food and Drug Administration (FDA) does not hold them to the same strict safety requirements that prescription or over-the-counter drugs must meet.

Homeopathic dilutions of thuja are available to take by mouth or in pill or liquid form. Thuja is also made into homeopathic creams or ointments to be applied to the skin. These contain very tiny or even undetectable amounts of thuja.

What is the history behind it?

Native Americans of the eastern United States and Canada used thuja for generations to treat menstrual problems, headaches, and heart ailments (see "Native American Healing," page 112). Loggers drank tea made from white cedar twigs to relieve rheumatism. During the seventeenth century, some people called the eastern white cedar the "tree of life," because they believed that its sap had healing powers. In the late 1800s, the U.S. Pharmacopoeia (the U.S. compendium of quality control tests and information on drugs) listed thuja as a treatment to stimulate the uterus and as a diuretic to increase urine flow.

Thujone (a major component of thuja oil) is banned as a food or drink additive in the United States, but small amounts are used in some alcoholic drinks in Europe. It is used in shoe polish and as a pest repellant. Cedar leaf oil, which is distilled from the leaves of *Thuja occidentalis*, is used in some furniture polishes and fragrances.

What is the evidence?

Human clinical trials of thuja by itself have not been reported. A 2005 German study looked at a mixture of extracts that included echinacea, baptisia, and thuja in the treatment of ninety-one adults with colds and runny noses. Those who received the extracts used fewer facial tissues than those who got placebo. However, it is impossible to say how much of this effect was related to thuja.

Available scientific evidence does not support claims that thuja is effective in treating cancer or any other disease. The medical literature contains no studies on the effects of thuja as an herbal remedy in humans, and there is very little scientific data to verify that the herb has any therapeutic value. Many supporters base their claims on limited laboratory experiments or individual reports. One laboratory study done in Germany found that a polysaccharide (a type of complex sugar) in thuja enhanced the immune system's ability to fight off invading germs. However, even though laboratory studies may show the substance holds promise, further studies are needed to find out whether the results apply to humans.

Are there any possible problems or complications?

Because so little is known about thuja, it is not recommended for any medicinal use. Taken internally, thuja can be toxic in large doses, although the exact amount that causes problems is uncertain. Some people who have consumed thuja reportedly experienced asthma attacks, intestinal irritation, excess stimulation of the nervous system, and spontaneous abortion (miscarriage). The essential oil causes spasms if taken internally, and in high doses it can cause seizures as well as damage to the liver and the kidneys. The fresh leaves and shoots can also cause poisoning. Deaths have been reported. Skin or eye contact with cedar leaf oil can cause severe irritation or burns. Asthma and rashes have occurred in people who work with the wood of this tree.

Thujone, a component of thuja, is known to cause muscle spasms, seizures, and hallucinations if taken internally. These neurologic toxicities are the results of thujone interfering with the action of gamma amino butyric acid, often known as GABA, on nerve cells in the brain. In high doses thujone is known to damage the liver and the kidneys. Thujone occurs in a number of other plants, most notably wormwood and mugwort (see pages 571 and 432 for more information on wormwood and mugwort).

People with seizure disorders or gastrointestinal problems (such as ulcers or gastritis) should avoid thuja. Women who are pregnant or breastfeeding should not use this herb. Relying on this type of treatment alone and avoiding or delaying conventional medical care for cancer may have serious health consequences.

This substance has not been thoroughly tested to find out how it interacts with medicines, foods, or dietary supplements. Even though some reports of interactions and harmful effects may be published, full studies of interactions and effects are not often available. Because of these limitations, any information on ill effects and interactions should be considered incomplete.

References

Alpha-thujone (546-80-5). National Toxicology Program Web site. http://ntp.niehs.nih.gov/index.cfm?objectid=03DB8C36-E7A1-9889-3BDF8436F2A8C51F. Updated May 2, 2006. Accessed June 6, 2008.

Cartier A, Chan H, Malo JL, Pineau L, Tse KS, Chan-Yeung M. Occupational asthma caused by eastern white cedar (*Thuja occidentalis*) with demonstration that plicatic acid is present in this wood dust and is the causal agent. *J Allergy Clin Immunol.* 1986;77:639-645.

Deane PM. Conifer pollen sensitivity in western New York: cedar pollens. *Allergy Asthma Proc.* 2005;26:352-355.

Fetrow CW, Avila JR. *Professional's Handbook of Complementary & Alternative Medicines.* Philadelphia, PA: Lippincott Williams & Wilkins; 2004.

Gruenwald J. *PDR for Herbal Medicines.* 3rd ed. Montvale, NJ: Thomson PDR; 2004.

Material safety data sheet: cedar leaf oil. ScienceLab Web site. http://www.sciencelab.com/xMSDS-Cedar_leaf_oil-9923339. Updated October 9, 2005. Accessed June 6, 2008.

Naser B, Lund B, Henneicke-von Zepelin HH, Köhler G, Lehmacher W, Scaglione F. A randomized, double-blind, placebo-controlled, clinical dose-response trial of an extract of Baptisia, Echinacea and Thuja for the treatment of patients with common cold. *Phytomedicine.* 2005;12:715-722.

Offergeld R, Reinecker C, Gumz E, Schrum S, Treiber R, Neth RD, Gohla SH. Mitogenic activity of high molecular polysaccharide fractions isolated from the cuppressaceae Thuja occidentalis L. enhanced cytokine-production by thyapolysaccharide, g-fraction (TPSg). *Leukemia.* 1992;3:189S-191S.

TURMERIC

Other common name(s): jiang huang, haridra, Indian saffron
Scientific/medical name(s): *Curcuma longa, Curcuma domestica*

Description

Turmeric is a spice grown in India and other tropical regions of Asia. It has a long history of use in herbal remedies, particularly in China, India, and Indonesia. The root and rootstock, or rhizome, of the plant contain the active ingredient, curcumin. Curcumin is not related to cumin, which is a spice made from the seeds of a different plant.

Overview

Turmeric is a common food flavoring and coloring in Asian cooking. Animal and laboratory studies have found that curcumin, an antioxidant that is an active ingredient in turmeric, demonstrated some anticancer effects. However, clinical research is needed to determine curcumin's role in cancer prevention and treatment in humans. Several types of cancer cells are inhibited by curcumin in the laboratory, and curcumin slows the spread of some cancers in some animal studies.

Curcumin is being studied to find out whether it helps other diseases such as arthritis, Alzheimer's disease, and stomach ulcers. It is also being studied to see whether it can help lower "bad cholesterol" and improve outcome in kidney transplants. A few early studies have been done in humans, but more human research is still needed to find out whether curcumin can be effective in these uses.

How is it promoted for use?

Some researchers believe turmeric may prevent and slow the growth of a number of types of cancer, particularly tumors of the esophagus, mouth, intestines, stomach, breast, and skin. One researcher reported that curcumin, the active ingredient in turmeric, inhibited the formation of cancer-causing enzymes in rodents.

Turmeric is promoted mainly as an anti-inflammatory herbal remedy and is said to produce fewer side effects than commonly used pain relievers. Some practitioners prescribe turmeric to relieve inflammation caused by arthritis, muscle sprains, swelling, and pain caused by injuries or surgical incisions. It is also promoted as a treatment for rheumatism and as an antiseptic for cleaning wounds. Some proponents claim turmeric interferes with the actions of some viruses, including hepatitis and human immunodeficiency virus (HIV).

Supporters also claim that turmeric protects against liver diseases, stimulates the gall bladder and circulatory system, reduces cholesterol levels, dissolves blood clots, helps stop external and internal bleeding, and relieves painful menstruation and angina, which are the chest pains that often occur with heart disease. It is also used as a remedy for digestive problems such as irritable bowel syndrome, colitis, Crohn's disease, and illnesses caused by toxins from parasites and bacteria.

What does it involve?

Turmeric root is on the Commission E (Germany's regulatory agency for herbs) list of approved herbs, and it is available in powdered form as a spice in most grocery stores. It can also be made into a tea or purchased as a tincture, capsule, or tablet. Ointments or pastes made from turmeric can be applied to the skin. Although there is no standardized dose for turmeric, some practitioners recommend taking a teaspoon with each meal. The dried root of turmeric normally contains from 3 percent to 5 percent curcumin. Today, many sellers market supplements that claim to be standardized to contain 95 percent curcumin compounds.

What is the history behind it?

The use of turmeric was described in traditional Chinese and Indian medicine as early as the seventh century AD. In various Asian folk medicine traditions, turmeric has been used to treat a long list of conditions, including diarrhea, fever, bronchitis, colds, parasitic worms, leprosy, and bladder and kidney inflammation. Herbalists have applied turmeric salve to bruises, leech bites, festering eye infections, mouth inflammations, skin conditions, and infected wounds. Some people inhale smoke from burning turmeric to relieve chronic coughs. Turmeric mixed with hot water and sugar is considered by some herbalists to be a remedy for colds.

In India and Malaysia, there is a custom of making turmeric paste to apply directly onto the skin, a practice now under study for the possibility that it may prevent skin cancer. The bright red forehead mark worn by some Hindu women is created by mixing turmeric with lime juice. Chefs frequently add turmeric to their creations because of its rich flavor and deep yellow-orange color. The seasoning is an important ingredient in Indian curries. It is also used to add color to foods such as butter, margarine, cheese, and mustard; to tint cotton, silk, paper, wood, and cosmetics; as a food preservative; and to make pickles.

What is the evidence?

Curcumin, an active ingredient in turmeric, is an antioxidant. Antioxidants are compounds that can protect the body's cells from damage caused by activated oxygen molecules called free radicals. Laboratory studies have also shown that curcumin interferes with several important molecular pathways involved in cancer development, growth, and spread.

Recently, curcumin has received a great deal more attention in studies than turmeric as a whole herb. Researchers are studying curcumin to learn whether it is an effective anti-inflammatory agent and whether it holds any promise for cancer prevention or treatment. A number of studies of curcumin have shown promising results. Curcumin can kill cancer cells in laboratory dishes and also reduces growth of surviving cells. Curcumin also has been found to reduce development of several forms of cancer in laboratory animals and to shrink animal tumors.

Human studies of curcumin in cancer prevention and treatment are in the very early stages. One study of fifteen patients with colorectal cancer was done to find out how much curcumin they could safely take and whether they could take a dose large enough to be detected in the blood. The patients were able to take 3.6 grams of curcumin without noting ill effects. At this high dose, some curcumin and its products were found in the blood. Lower doses may work for the stomach and intestine. Even though it does not absorb well into the body, it has been shown to absorb into the colon lining and into any cancerous tissue in the colon. The researchers recommended that the high dose be used when curcumin is tested for effects outside the intestine. Other small studies have found people were able to take up to 10 grams per day for a period of a few weeks without noting problems. Some researchers are currently working on ways to increase absorption of curcumin by combining it with other substances. Further clinical trials are needed to find out what role, if any, turmeric and curcumin may play in the prevention or treatment of cancer.

Curcumin is being studied to see whether it helps other diseases as well. One small study of curcumin and another antioxidant called quercetin was done in adults who had kidney transplants. Those who took the combination in high doses had fewer transplant rejections than those who received lower doses or placebo. More studies are needed to find out whether this will hold true. Curcumin may also promote the emptying of the gallbladder, but again, more studies are needed.

Early studies showed promise that curcumin could correct the problem of cystic fibrosis, but later studies have been inconsistent and often shown no effect. Curcumin also seemed to help prevent stomach ulcers in rodents, although there are not good studies in humans to recommend it for this use.

Early research has suggested that curcumin may help lower "bad" cholesterol, reduce inflammation, and help with arthritis symptoms, although more reliable human studies are still needed. Tests of curcumin and HIV have been mixed and have generally not shown it to be helpful. In studies of mice, curcumin appeared to help with blocking the plaque and proteins that cause problems in the brain during Alzheimer's disease.

Although laboratory and animal tests look very promising, careful study is needed to find out whether curcumin will be useful for treating these conditions in humans. It is important to remember that extracted compounds such as curcumin are not the same as the whole herb, and study results would not be likely to show the same effects.

Are there any possible problems or complications?

When used as a spice in foods, turmeric is considered safe. More research is needed to establish the safety of turmeric when used in herbal remedies. Little is known about the potential risks of taking the larger amounts used to treat illnesses. Taking large amounts may result in stomach pain, gas, indigestion, and nausea. Skin rash and stomach ulcers have been reported after long-term use, and allergic reactions are possible. People who are allergic to ginger or yellow food colorings are more likely to be allergic to turmeric.

A recent safety study in humans suggested that curcumin changes metabolism of oxalate, a substance that can form kidney stones. The researchers urged caution in use of this supplement by people with conditions that make them susceptible to kidney stones.

People taking blood-thinning medications, drugs that suppress the immune system, or nonsteroidal pain relievers (such as ibuprofen) should avoid turmeric because of the risk for harmful drug interactions. In animal and laboratory studies, turmeric made certain anticancer drugs less effective. Antioxidant supplements can interfere with the effectiveness of chemotherapy or radiation treatment. Patients who are in cancer treatment should talk to their doctors before taking vitamins, minerals, or other supplements.

In addition, other potential interactions between turmeric and other drugs and herbs should be considered. Always tell your doctor and pharmacist about any herbs or supplements you are taking.

People with bleeding disorders, obstructions of the bile duct, or a history of ulcers also should avoid turmeric. Women who are pregnant or breastfeeding should not use this herb. The amount of turmeric found in foods is thought to be safe for those who are not allergic to it. Applying turmeric to the skin for long periods of time can cause a yellow discoloration that may be difficult to remove.

Relying on this type of treatment alone and avoiding or delaying conventional medical care for cancer may have serious health consequences.

This product is sold as a dietary supplement in the United States. Unlike companies that produce drugs (which must provide the FDA with results of detailed testing showing their product is safe and effective before the drug is approved for sale), the companies that make supplements do not have to show evidence of safety or health benefits to the FDA before selling their products. Supplement products without any reliable scientific evidence of health benefits may still be sold as long as the companies selling them do not claim the supplements can prevent, treat, or cure any specific disease. Some such products may not contain the amount of the herb or substance that is written on the label, and some may include other substances (contaminants). Though the FDA has written new rules to improve the quality of manufacturing processes for dietary supplements and the accurate listing of supplement ingredients, these rules do not take full effect until 2010. The new rules also do not address the safety of supplement ingredients or their effects on health when proper manufacturing techniques are used.

Most such supplements have not been tested to find out if they interact with medicines, foods, or other herbs and supplements. Even though some reports of interactions and harmful effects may be published, full studies of interactions and effects are not often available. Because of these limitations, any information on ill effects and interactions should be considered incomplete.

References

Aggarwal BB, Kumar A, Bharti AC. Anticancer potential of curcumin: preclinical and clinical studies. *Anticancer Res.* 2003;23:363-398.

Aggarwal BB, Shishodia S, Takada Y, Banjerjee S, Newman RA, Bueso-Ramos CE, Price JE. Curcumin suppresses the paclitaxel-induced nuclear factor-kappaB pathway in breast cancer cells and inhibits lung metastasis of human breast cancer in nude mice. *Clin Cancer Res.* 2005;11:7490-7498.

Anand P, Kunnumakkara AB, Newman RA, Aggarwal BB. Bioavailability of curcumin: problems and promises. *Mol Pharm.* 2007;4:807-818.

Blumenthal M, ed. *The Complete German Commission E Monographs: Therapeutic Guide to Herbal Medicines.* Austin, TX: American Botanical Council; 1998.

Deshpande SS, Ingle AD, Maru GB. Inhibitory effects of curcumin-free aqueous turmeric extract on benzo[a]pyrene-induced forestomach papillomas in mice. *Cancer Lett.* 1997;118:79-85.

Egan ME, Pearson M, Weiner SA, Pearson M, Weiner SA, Rajendran V, Rubin D, Glöckner-Pagel J, Canny S, Du K, Lukacs GL, Caplan MJ. Curcumin, a major constituent of turmeric, corrects cystic fibrosis defects. *Science.* 2004;304:600-602.

Fetrow CW, Avila JR. *Professional's Handbook of Complementary & Alternative Medicines.* Springhouse, PA: Springhouse Corp; 1999.

Garcea G, Berry DP, Jones DJ, Singh R, Dennison AR, Farmer PB, Sharma RA, Steward WP, Gescher AJ. Consumption of the putative chemopreventive agent curcumin by cancer patients: assessment of curcumin levels in the colorectum and their pharmacodynamic consequences. *Cancer Epidemiol Biomarkers Prev.* 2005;14:120-125.

Goel A, Kunnumakkara AB, Aggarwal BB. Curcumin as "Curecumin": from kitchen to clinic. *Biochem Pharmacol.* 2008;75:787-809.

Grubb BR, Gabriel SE, Mengos A, Gentzsch M, Randell SH, Van Heeckeren AM, Knowles MR, Drumm ML, Riordan JR, Boucher RC. SERCA pump inhibitors do not correct biosynthetic arrest of deltaF508 CFTR in cystic fibrosis. *Am J Respir Cell Mol Biol.* 2006;34:355-363.

Gruenwald J. *PDR for Herbal Medicines.* 3rd ed. Montvale, NJ: Thomson PDR; 2004.

Hastak K, Lubri N, Jakhi SD, More C, John A, Ghaisas SD, Bhide SV. Effect of turmeric oil and turmeric oleoresin on cytogenetic damage in patients suffering from oral submucous fibrosis. *Cancer Lett.* 1997:116:265-269.

Kim DC, Kim SH, Choi BH, Baek NI, Kim D, Kim MJ, Kim KT. *Curcuma longa* extract protects against gastric ulcers by blocking H2 histamine receptors. *Biol Pharm Bull.* 2005;28:2220-2224.

Kunnumakkara AB, Diagaradjane P, Guha S, Deorukhkar A, Shentu S, Aggarwal BB, Krishnan S. Curcumin sensitizes human colorectal cancer xenografts in nude mice to gamma-radiation by targeting nuclear factor-kappaB-regulated gene products. *Clin Cancer Res.* 2008;14:2128-2136.

Lawenda BD, Kelly KM, Ladas EJ, Sagar SM, Vickers A, Blumberg JB. Should supplemental antioxidant administration be avoided during chemotherapy and radiation therapy? *J Natl Cancer Inst.* 2008;100:773-783.

Lin YG, Kunnumakkara AB, Nair A, Merritt WM, Han LY, Armaiz-Pena GN, Kamat AA, Spannuth WA, Gershenson DM, Lutgendorf SK, Aggarwal BB, Sood AK. Curcumin inhibits tumor growth and angiogenesis in ovarian carcinoma by targeting the nuclear factor-kappaB pathway. *Clin Cancer Res.* 2007;13:3423-3430.

Mall M, Kunzelmann K. Correction of the CF defect by curcumin: hypes and disappointments. *Bioessays.* 2005;27:9-13.

Rafatullah S, Tariq M, Al-Yahya MA, Mossa JS, Ageel AM. Evaluation of turmeric (Curcuma longa) for gastric and duodenal antiulcer activity in rats. *J Ethnopharmacol.* 1990;29:25-34.

Sharma RA, Euden SA, Platton SL, Cooke DN, Shafayat A, Hewitt HR, Marczylo TH, Morgan B, Hemingway D, Plummer SM, Pirmohamed M, Gescher AJ, Steward WP. Phase I clinical trial of oral curcumin: biomarkers of systemic activity and compliance. *Clin Cancer Res.* 2004;10:6847-6854.

Shoskes D, Lapierre C, Cruz-Corerra M, Muruve N, Rosario R, Fromkin B, Braun M, Copley J. Beneficial effects of the bioflavonoids curcumin and quercetin on early function in cadaveric renal transplantation: a randomized placebo controlled trial. *Transplantation.* 2005;80:1556-1559.

Tunstall RG, Sharma RA, Perkins S, Sale S, Singh R, Farmer PB, Steward WP, Gescher AJ. Cyclooxygenase-2 expression and oxidative DNA adducts in murine intestinal adenomas: modification by dietary curcumin and implications for clinical trials. *Eur J Cancer.* 2006;42:415-421.

Turmeric (*Curcuma longa*). Aetna Intelihealth Web site. http://www.intelihealth.com/IH/ihtIH/WSIHW000/8513/31402/348510.html. Updated June 17, 2005. Accessed June 6, 2008.

Turmeric (Curcuma longa linn.) and curcumin. Medline Plus Web site. http://www.nlm.nih.gov/medlineplus/druginfo/natural/patient-turmeric.html. Updated March 1, 2008. Accessed June 6, 2008.

Turmeric. Drug Digest Web site. http://www.drugdigest.org/DD/DVH/HerbsWho/0,3923,4046|Turmeric,00.html. Accessed June 6, 2008.

Turmeric. Memorial Sloan-Kettering Cancer Center Web site. http://www.mskcc.org/mskcc/html/69401.cfm. Updated December 11, 2007. Accessed June 6, 2008.

Yang F, Lim GP, Begum AN, Ubeda OJ, Simmons MR, Ambegaokar SS, Chen PP, Kayed R, Glabe CG, Frautschy SA, Cole GM. Curcumin inhibits formation of amyloid beta oligomers and fibrils, binds plaques, and reduces amyloid in vivo. *J Biol Chem.* 2005;280:5892-5901.

VALERIAN

Other common name(s): valerian tea, valerian root, valerian extract
Scientific/medical name(s): *Valeriana officinalis*

Description

Valerian is a flowering plant native to Europe, Asia, and the Americas. In herbal remedies, the plant's root is chopped and made into a tea or extract to be used primarily as a sedative. Although the fresh root has little odor, the dried root has an odor that is often described as being similar to dirty socks.

Overview

Valerian is an herb used for anxiety and sleeplessness. Although some research suggests that it is effective, the results have been inconsistent and, in many cases, the study methods have been flawed. More research is needed to make definite conclusions about its effectiveness. There are some side effects linked with long-term valerian use, and it has the potential to interfere with anesthesia and other medicines.

How is it promoted for use?

Herbal practitioners claim that valerian root or extract can lessen anxiety and nervous tension, promote sleep, help people quit smoking, ease congestion, and relieve muscle spasms. Generally, no one claims that valerian is useful for treating or preventing cancer.

What does it involve?

Valerian root is on the Commission E (Germany's regulatory agency for herbs) list of approved herbs. Supplements are available as tablets, capsules, or tinctures, and it can also be brewed as a tea. When taken as a sleep aid, the usual dosage of valerian extract in tablet form is 300 to 900 milligrams to be taken an hour or two before bedtime. For stress and anxiety, the usual dose is 50 to 100 milligrams taken two to three times a day, although some recommend doses of 200 milligrams or even 400 milligrams.

What is the history behind it?

For thousands of years, the Chinese, Greeks, Romans, and Indians have used valerian as a mild sedative. The origin of the word "pew" is said to come from the foul odor of the valerian root, which a first century AD Roman physician, Dioscorides, called "phu." In the mid-1800s in the United States, the Shakers began growing valerian and other herbs to market to doctors and pharmacists in America and Europe. Valerian is sometimes used to flavor foods and drinks such as root beer.

What is the evidence?

Several controlled human studies have been conducted comparing valerian with a placebo. Some studies showed that those who took valerian had less insomnia and better sleep quality, while other studies showed no difference between valerian and placebo.

A German study compared valerian extract to oxazepam (a prescription anti-anxiety drug) in 202 adults over a six-week period. The people taking valerian reported equal improvement in sleep quality, feeling rested, and how long they slept as those taking the prescription drug.

A randomized clinical trial reported in 2005 of nearly four hundred people compared valerian with kava (a plant commonly used as a sleep aid) or placebo. Neither valerian nor kava was significantly better than placebo in reducing anxiety or improving sleep. A number of other studies have found that valerian shortens the time it takes to fall asleep, although most of the studies had small sample sizes and short follow-up periods. In addition, the study used valerian from more than one source and used different doses, making results difficult to interpret.

Of interest, studies that have looked at only a single dose of the herb have tended to show no improvement in sleep at all. Longer studies suggested that improvement increased over a period of two to four weeks.

On the basis of animal studies and several clinical trials in Europe, German health officials have approved valerian as a sleep aid and mild sedative. While some experts trust in valerian's safety and effectiveness as a mild sedative, others are uncertain because of conflicting evidence. More research is needed to be sure of valerian's effectiveness as a sleep aid.

A 2006 evidence review of valerian and anxiety found only one study that used reliable research methods and concluded that there is not enough evidence to know whether valerian might be useful as a treatment for anxiety disorders.

A Norwegian clinical trial of 405 patients with insomnia suggested that valerian might be slightly better than placebo and concluded that "...valerian appears to be safe, but with modest beneficial effects at most on insomnia compared to placebo" (*PLoS ONE.* 2007;2:e1040,1).

Are there any possible problems or complications?

Valerian is considered to be relatively safe when used in recommended doses during four- to six-week periods. However, some people may notice restlessness and heart palpitations, especially with long-term use of valerian. Long-term or excessive use is not advised because of possible side effects, which include headaches, blurred vision, heart palpitations, and nausea. A few people become excitable and unable to sleep when they take valerian. Rarely, liver damage has been linked to valerian, although it is uncertain whether valerian, contaminants, or other herbs caused the damage. Those who take valerian should tell their doctors so that their liver function can be monitored. Allergic reactions may also be possible.

Valerian should not be taken with alcohol, antihistamines, muscle relaxants, sedatives, anti-seizure drugs, narcotics, or any drugs used in treatment of mental illnesses. People on cancer treatment medicines, antifungal drugs, allergy drugs, or medicines for high cholesterol should talk with their doctors or pharmacists about possible drug interactions before taking valerian. Because valerian may interact with anesthetics, people who are going to have surgery should not use valerian. However, suddenly stopping the herb has caused withdrawal symptoms in some people, so the dose of valerian should be tapered slowly, starting several weeks before surgery. Always tell your doctor and pharmacist about any herbs you are taking.

People with liver or kidney disease should talk to their doctors before taking valerian. In very high doses, the herb may weaken the heartbeat and cause paralysis. Women who are pregnant or breastfeeding should not take valerian. Relying on this type of treatment alone and avoiding or delaying conventional medical care for cancer may have serious health consequences.

This product is sold as a dietary supplement in the United States. Unlike companies that produce drugs (which must provide the FDA with results of detailed testing showing their product is safe and effective before the drug is approved for sale), the companies that make supplements do not have to show evidence of safety or health benefits to the FDA before selling their products. Supplement products without any reliable scientific evidence of health benefits may still be sold as long as the companies selling them do not claim the supplements can prevent, treat, or cure any specific disease. Some such products may not contain the amount of the herb or substance that is written on the label, and some may include other substances (contaminants). Though the FDA has written new rules to improve the quality of manufacturing processes for dietary supplements and the accurate listing of supplement ingredients, these rules do not take full effect until 2010. The new rules also do not address the safety of supplement ingredients or their effects on health when proper manufacturing techniques are used.

Most such supplements have not been tested to find out if they interact with medicines, foods, or other herbs and supplements. Even though some reports of interactions and harmful effects may be published, full studies of interactions and effects are not often available. Because of these limitations, any information on ill effects and interactions should be considered incomplete.

References

Barrett B, Kiefer D, Rabago D. Assessing the risks and benefits of herbal medicine: an overview of scientific evidence. *Altern Ther Health Med.* 1999;5:40-49.

Bent S, Padula A, Moore D, Patterson M, Mehling W. Valerian for sleep: a systematic review and meta-analysis. *Am J Med.* 2006;119:1005-1012.

Blumenthal M, ed. *The Complete German Commission E Monographs: Therapeutic Guide to Herbal Medicines.* Austin, TX: American Botanical Council; 1998.

Dietary supplement fact sheet: valerian. Office of Dietary Supplements Web site. http://ods.od.nih.gov/factsheets/Valerian_pf.asp. Accessed June 6, 2008.

Ernst E, ed. *The Desktop Guide to Complementary and Alternative Medicine: An Evidence-Based Approach.* New York: Mosby; 2001.

Fetrow CW, Avila JR. *Professional's Handbook of Complementary & Alternative Medicines.* Philadelphia, PA: Lippincott Williams & Wilkins; 2004.

Garges HP, Varia I, Doraiswamy PM. Cardiac complications and delirium associated with valerian root withdrawal. *JAMA.* 1998;280:1566-1567.

Hadley S, Petry JJ. Valerian. *Am Fam Physician.* 2003;67:1755-1758.

Jacobs BP, Bent S, Tice JA, Blackwell T, Cummings SR. An internet-based randomized, placebo-controlled trial of kava and valerian for anxiety and insomnia. *Medicine (Baltimore).* 2005;84:197-207.

Miller L. Herbal medicinals: selected clinical considerations focusing on know or potential drug-herb interactions. *Arch Intern Med.* 1998;158:2200-2211.

Miyasaka LS, Atallah AN, Soares BG. Valerian for anxiety disorders. *Cochrane Database Syst Rev.* 2006;(4):CD004515.

O'Hara M, Kiefer D, Farrell K, Kemper K. A review of 12 commonly used medicinal herbs. *Arch Fam Med.* 1998;7:523-536.

Oxman AD, Flottorp S, Håvelsrud K, Fretheim A, Odgaard-Jensen J, Austvoll-Dahlgren A, Carling C, Pallesen S, Bjorvatn B. A televised, web-based randomised trial of an herbal remedy (valerian) for insomnia. *PLoS ONE.* 2007;2:e1040.

Valerian. Drug Digest Web site. http://www.drugdigest.org/DD/PrintablePages/herbMonograph/0,11475,4047,00.html. Accessed June 6, 2008.

Ziegler G, Ploch M, Miettinen-Baumann A, Collet W. Efficacy and tolerability of valerian extract LI 156 compared with oxazepam in the treatment of non-organic insomnia—a randomized, double-blind, comparative clinical study. *Eur J Med Res.* 2002;7:480-486.

VENUS FLYTRAP

Other common name(s): Carnivora, plumbagin
Scientific/medical name(s): *Dionaea muscipula*

Description

The Venus flytrap is a perennial plant that traps and eats insects. It is native to the low-lying wetlands of the southeastern United States. After being harvested, the whole fresh plant is pressed to remove the liquid extract, which is used as an herbal remedy. It is also used in mixtures like Carnivora, a patented formula that includes many ingredients in addition to Venus flytrap extract. Venus flytrap extract is sold in capsule and liquid form to be taken by mouth and as an injectable liquid.

Overview

Available scientific evidence does not support claims that extract from the Venus flytrap plant is effective in treating skin cancer or any other type of cancer. Some side effects have been reported with its use.

How is it promoted for use?

Most sellers of Venus flytrap extract base information about their products on claims about Carnivora. Proponents claim that Carnivora and Venus flytrap extract have immune stimulant and anticancer properties. Some even claim that the extract can be applied directly to some skin cancer lesions to substitute for radiation therapy and chemotherapy. Some claim that Carnivora can lead to the total reversal of skin and other forms of cancer. Supporters also claim that Carnivora is effective for treating colitis, Crohn's disease, rheumatoid arthritis, multiple sclerosis, neurodermatitis, chronic fatigue syndrome, human immunodeficiency virus (HIV), and certain types of herpes.

What does it involve?

Proponents suggest that full-strength or diluted Venus flytrap liquid extracts can be placed under the tongue or mixed with water to make a drink. One form of Carnivora can be injected into the skin, a vein, or muscle. Carnivora can also be inhaled through a vaporizer or applied directly to the skin. Liquid Venus flytrap extracts for oral use, including Carnivora, contain about 25 percent to 30 percent alcohol.

There is no standard dose for the extracts, and instructions vary. One product, for example, recommends mixing 15 to 30 drops of the extract in warm water and drinking it one to three times a day. Another advises against swallowing the extract, since it may be inactivated by stomach acids. Instead, the seller suggests taking one half teaspoon and holding it under the tongue until absorbed, three to five times a day. The recommendation for Carnivora liquid is to take 30 drops mixed with water or tea three to five times per day. Carnivora capsules are said to contain 125 micrograms of Venus flytrap along with its other listed ingredients (1,000 micrograms is equal to 1 milligram). The manufacturer suggests taking 6 to 9 capsules per day. If the injectable form of Carnivora is obtained from Germany, a doctor or other health care professional is needed to inject it.

What is the history behind it?

In the 1970s, a German physician began testing liquids pressed from the Venus flytrap to determine whether they could digest abnormal proteins found in cancer cells. Several years later he patented Carnivora. In a 1985 study, he claimed that out of 210 people with various types of cancer, 56 percent experienced either remission or stabilization of their tumors. He published the findings in a little-known German medical journal, and the results were never verified. Carnivora is not approved by the U.S. Food and Drug Administration (FDA), and physicians in this country cannot legally prescribe the drug. The FDA prohibits its import into the United States except for personal use.

What is the evidence?

Available scientific evidence does not support the health claims made for Venus flytrap extract. Plumbagin, a substance found in many plants, is thought to be the active ingredient in the Venus flytrap. The plant also contains other compounds such as flavonoids, acids, and enzymes (digestive proteins).

Most of the studies done on the herbal extract were conducted by the physician who patented the drug Carnivora, who also has a large financial stake in a clinic that administers the drug and in the company that manufactures the drug.

An animal study conducted in India to study the effects of plumbagin (taken from the Indian medicinal plant *Plumbago rosea*) combined with radiation therapy was inconclusive.

A second animal study in India found that plumbagin demonstrated a small degree of antitumor activity. The results of several other studies from India were positive but inconclusive. A laboratory study in Japan indicated that plumbagin had some effect against intestinal tumors, and other laboratory studies show that plumbagin can induce cell death. While animal and laboratory studies show promise, further studies are necessary to determine whether the results apply to humans. It is important to remember that purified compounds such as plumbagin are not the same as the fresh plant extract, and study results would not be likely to show the same effects.

Are there any possible problems or complications?

Liquid extracts of Venus flytrap, including Carnivora, do not appear to be toxic when taken by mouth, but not enough is known about the active ingredients for scientists to ensure that they are safe. When liquid extracts have been injected into the skin, muscle, or veins, side effects have included nausea, vomiting, fever, chills, and collapse of the circulatory system. Skin contact with the fresh plant can cause irritation, and allergic reactions are possible.

Plumbagin is known to cause toxic side effects such as diarrhea, skin rash, liver damage, and abnormal blood counts. In animal studies, female rats given plumbagin failed to conceive, while those not given plumbagin conceived easily. In addition, pregnant rats given the drug were more likely to abort. It also affected sperm in male animals. Plumbagin appears to act as an oxidant, which can damage DNA, enzymes, and cell membranes. The extent of plumbagin's toxic effects is not yet known.

Most of the liquid extracts of Venus flytrap contain between 25 percent and 30 percent alcohol, which may cause harmful interactions with medicines such as disulfiram and metronidazole. Consult with your doctor or pharmacist before taking alcohol-containing medications. None of these preparations or extracts should be used by pregnant or breastfeeding women. Relying on these treatments alone and avoiding or delaying conventional medical care for cancer may have serious health consequences.

This product is sold as a dietary supplement in the United States. Unlike companies that produce drugs (which must provide the FDA with results of detailed testing showing their product is safe and effective before the drug is approved for sale), the companies that make supplements do not have to show evidence of safety or health benefits to the FDA before selling their products. Supplement products without any reliable scientific evidence of health benefits may still be sold as long as the companies selling them do not claim the supplements can prevent, treat, or cure any specific disease. Some such products may not contain the amount of the herb or substance that is written on the label, and some may include other substances (contaminants). Though the FDA has written new rules to improve the quality of manufacturing processes for dietary supplements and the accurate listing of supplement ingredients, these rules do not take full effect until 2010. The new rules also do not address the safety of supplement ingredients or their effects on health when proper manufacturing techniques are used.

Most such supplements have not been tested to find out if they interact with medicines, foods, or other herbs and supplements. Even though some reports of interactions and harmful effects may be published, full studies of interactions and effects are not often available. Because of these limitations, any information on ill effects and interactions should be considered incomplete.

References

Devi PU, Rao BS, Solomon FE. Effect of plumbagin on the radiation-induced cytogenetic and cell cycle changes in mouse Ehrlich ascites carcinoma in vivo. *Indian J Exp Biol.* 1998;36:891-895.

Gruenwald J. *PDR for Herbal Medicines.* 3rd ed. Montvale, NJ: Thomson PDR; 2004.

Kini DP, Pandey S, Shenoy BD, Singh UV, Udupa N, Umadevi P, Kamath R, Nagarajkumari, Ramanarayan K. Antitumor and antifertility activities of plumbagin-controlled release formulations. *Indian J Exp Biol.* 1997;35:374-379.

Srinivas G, Annab LA, Gopinath G, Banerji A, Srinivas P. Antisense blocking of BRCA1 enhances sensitivity to plumbagin but not tamoxifen in BG-1 ovarian cancer cells. *Mol Carcinog.* 2004;39:15-25.

Srinivas P, Gopinath G, Banerji A, Dinakar A, Srinivas G. Plumbagin induces reactive oxygen species, which mediate apoptosis in human cervical cancer cells. *Mol Carcinog.* 2004;40:201-211.

Sugie S, Okamoto K, Rahman KM, Tanaka T, Kawai K, Yamahara J, Mori H. Inhibitory effects of plumbagin and juglone on azoxymethane-induced intestinal carcinogenesis in rats. *Cancer Lett.* 1998;127:177-183.

Summary of data for chemical selection: plumbagin 481-42-5. 2000. National Toxicology Program Web site. http://ntp.niehs.nih.gov/ntp/htdocs/Chem_Background/ExSumPdf/Plumbagin.pdf. Accessed June 6, 2008.

VITAE ELIXXIR

Other common name(s): none
Scientific/medical name(s): none

Description

Vitae Elixxir is an herb and mineral mixture that is promoted as a treatment for arthritis, multiple sclerosis, lymphomas, leukemias, multiple myeloma, internal parasites, and other illnesses.

Overview

Available scientific evidence does not support claims that Vitae Elixxir can treat cancer or other illnesses.

How is it promoted for use?

Vitae Elixxir is promoted as a treatment for arthritis, multiple sclerosis, lymphomas, leukemias, multiple myeloma, internal parasites, and other illnesses.

What does it involve?

The ingredients of the formula are not well documented, although it reportedly contains St. John's wort (see page 498), as well as eleven main ingredients and seven trace minerals. People have reported that it has an unpleasant taste. It is taken by mouth after being mixed with water, juice, or food. Proponents also recommend mixing Vitae Elixxir with dimethyl sulfoxide (DMSO) to make a foot bath for people with advanced cancer who cannot tolerate taking the preparation orally; however, it has not been proven to be effective (see "DMSO," page 737).

What is the history behind it?

Vitae Elixxir was developed by a Wyoming businessman, Ralph Schauss, with no formal medical or scientific training. More precise information on the origins of Vitae Elixxir is not available.

What is the evidence?

Available scientific evidence does not support claims of Vitae Elixxir's health benefits. No published studies of Vitae Elixxir could be found in the peer-reviewed medical journals.

Are there any possible problems or complications?

Although proponents claim there is no toxicity, allergies to the herbs are possible. The reported side effects include diarrhea, gas, pain, and a general worsening of symptoms after the mixture is started. Relying on this type of treatment alone and avoiding or delaying conventional medical care for cancer may have serious health consequences.

This product is sold as a dietary supplement in the United States. Unlike companies that produce drugs (which must provide the FDA with results of detailed testing showing their product is safe and effective before the drug is approved for sale), the companies that make supplements do not have to show evidence of safety or health benefits to the FDA before selling their products. Supplement products without any reliable scientific evidence of health benefits may still be sold as long as the companies

selling them do not claim the supplements can prevent, treat, or cure any specific disease. Some such products may not contain the amount of the herb or substance that is written on the label, and some may include other substances (contaminants). Though the FDA has written new rules to improve the quality of manufacturing processes for dietary supplements and the accurate listing of supplement ingredients, these rules do not take full effect until 2010. The new rules also do not address the safety of supplement ingredients or their effects on health when proper manufacturing techniques are used.

Most such supplements have not been tested to find out if they interact with medicines, foods, or other herbs and supplements. Even though some reports of interactions and harmful effects may be published, full studies of interactions and effects are not often available. Because of these limitations, any information on ill effects and interactions should be considered incomplete.

References

Dunn S. Elixir vitae. CancerGuide Web site. http://cancerguide.org/elixir_vitae.html. Updated May 24, 1995. Accessed June 6, 2008.

Vitae Elixxir. Annieappleseedproject Web site. http://www.annieappleseedproject.org/vitaeelixxir.html. Accessed August 6, 2008.

VITAMIN A AND BETA CAROTENE

Other common name(s): none
Scientific/medical name(s): Retinol, retinoic acid, retinoids

Description

Vitamin A is a nutrient that is vital to growth and development. It is obtained in the diet from animal sources and is also derived from beta carotene in plant foods. Beta carotene is changed into vitamin A in the small intestine. Vitamin A is stored in the liver until needed by the body. Vitamin A and closely related molecules are also known as retinoids.

Overview

Vitamin A supplements have not been proven to be effective in preventing cancer in humans. However, further clinical studies are being done to explore the role of vitamin A and other retinoids in cancer prevention and treatment. High doses of vitamin A are toxic, and long-term use of high-dose supplements may increase the risk for lung cancer among people at high risk, such as smokers.

How is it promoted for use?

Vitamin A is essential for normal growth, bone development, reproduction, vision, the maintenance of healthy skin and mucous membranes (which line the nose and mouth), and protection against infections in the respiratory, digestive, and urinary tracts. Vitamin A is obtained in two ways: as vitamin A from animal sources such as liver, fish oils, and dairy products, and as beta carotene, which the body converts to retinol (a type of vitamin A) from many fruits and vegetables, including carrots, broccoli, spinach, squash, peaches, and apricots.

Some research suggests that vitamin A and some other retinoids are able to cause changes in cancer cells and can also prevent normal cells from becoming cancerous. Retinoids are given as a conventional prescription medication for some rare types of cancer or precancerous conditions. Some proponents say that vitamin A supplements prevent cancer in general.

What does it involve?

Vitamin A is absorbed from dietary animal fats (especially liver, fish, egg yolks, and milk fat), from dietary supplements, and in the form of beta carotene, which is found in some fruits and vegetables and is converted to vitamin A by the body. Vitamin A is stored in the liver until needed by the body, so it does not need to be consumed every day. The best way to get this vitamin is to eat a well-balanced diet. People who eat a balanced diet of fruits, vegetables, dairy products, and animal fats usually obtain enough vitamin A and beta carotene for good health, although supplements are available. The Recommended Dietary Allowance (RDA) of vitamin A is 2,310 IU (0.7 milligrams) per day for women (with larger doses for women who are pregnant or breastfeeding) and 3,000 IU (0.9 milligrams) per day for men.

What is the history behind it?

The discovery of vitamin A dates back to research from the early twentieth century. Over the past twenty years, vitamin A has been extensively studied as a cancer-fighting nutrient in laboratory, animal, and observational epidemiologic studies, and even in some clinical trials. In addition to studies of vitamin A and cancer prevention, related retinoids have also been evaluated in laboratory studies and in human clinical trials.

Several studies based on dietary surveys of large numbers of people have concluded that eating foods rich in vitamin A is associated with a lower risk for several forms of cancer. However, it is not clear whether the protective effect was due to vitamin A or to other helpful substances in these foods.

What is the evidence?

Vitamin A deficiency is rare in developed countries. It can cause a lowered resistance to infection, poor night vision or even blindness, poor growth in children, weak bones and teeth, inflamed eyes, diarrhea, and poor appetite.

Some animal studies have found that vitamin A and other retinoids may enhance the immune system, slow tumor growth, decrease the size of tumors, and increase the effectiveness of some cancer treatments. Some laboratory, animal, and human studies have found that certain retinoids may also inhibit cancer development.

Studies of vitamin A's possible role in cancer prevention have been generally disappointing. Clinical trials have found that vitamin A supplements do not lower the risk for lung cancer in smokers and actually increased their risk for dying of lung cancer and heart disease. Studies of overall health and longevity found no benefit to taking vitamin A supplements, and the U.S. Institute of Medicine does not recommend use of these supplements by the general public. Studies on vitamin A and other types of cancer have been mixed, but there have been no consistent findings showing a decreased risk for cancers of the stomach, intestines, skin, breast, cervix, bladder, or prostate due to vitamin A in the diet. The use of vitamin A supplements has also not been proven to be effective in reducing cancer risk in humans. It appears that the combination of micronutrients in fruits, vegetables, legumes, and grains is more likely to be helpful than individual vitamins. A 2007 review of sixty-eight studies of vitamin supplements concluded that people taking beta carotene or vitamin A supplements had a shorter life expectancy than those who did not take these supplements.

Synthetic retinoids that are more potent than natural vitamin A or beta carotene have shown some ability to reverse premalignancies in the cervix, mouth, throat, and skin. They also may help prevent new tumors in people who have already been treated for these forms of cancer. However, further clinical research is needed. Several clinical trials involving retinoids have been completed, and others are ongoing.

Retinoids are not currently used as a cancer treatment, with one notable exception. A relatively rare type of leukemia, promyelocytic leukemia, often responds to a combination of retinoic acid (a retinoid) and chemotherapy. Patients with this form of leukemia receive high doses of retinoic acid under the supervision of a hematologist and/or oncologist. Treatment of promyelocytic leukemia does not include use of nonprescription vitamin A supplements or dietary changes intended to increase intake of this vitamin.

Studies of other types of cancer, such as lung cancer, head and neck cancer, and melanoma, found that vitamin A supplements are not helpful. In addition, some oncologists are concerned that vitamin A and other vitamins that act as antioxidants may make chemotherapy and radiation therapy less effective when taken during treatment. For this reason, many oncologists recommend that their patients not take such antioxidant supplements until their treatment is complete.

Are there any possible problems or complications?

High doses of vitamin A supplements can cause nausea, vomiting, diarrhea, loss of appetite, tiredness, headaches, dizziness, blurred vision, poor muscle coordination, itchiness and scaling of the skin, bone pain, hair loss, irregular menstruation in women, and temporary or permanent liver damage and can cause birth defects if taken during pregnancy. Relying on this type of treatment alone and avoiding or delaying conventional medical care for cancer may have serious health consequences.

This product is sold as a dietary supplement in the United States. Unlike companies that produce drugs (which must provide the FDA with results of detailed testing showing their product is safe and effective before the drug is approved for sale), the companies that make supplements do not have to show evidence of safety or health benefits to the FDA before selling their products. Supplement products without any reliable scientific evidence of health benefits may still be sold as long as the companies selling them do not claim the supplements can prevent, treat, or cure any specific disease. Some such products may not contain the amount of the herb or substance that is written on the label, and some may include other substances (contaminants). Though the FDA has written new rules to improve the quality of manufacturing processes for dietary supplements and the accurate listing of supplement ingredients, these rules do not take full effect until 2010. The new rules also do not address the safety of supplement ingredients or their effects on health when proper manufacturing techniques are used.

Most such supplements have not been tested to find out if they interact with medicines, foods, or other herbs and supplements. Even though some reports of interactions and harmful effects may be published, full studies of interactions and effects are not often available. Because of these limitations, any information on ill effects and interactions should be considered incomplete.

References

Albanes D, Heinonen OP, Taylor PR, Virtamo J, Edwards BK, Rautalahti M, Hartman AM, Palmgren J, Freedman LS, Haapakoski J, Barrett MJ, Pietinen P, Malila N, Tala E, Liippo K, Salomaa ER, Tangrea JA, Teppo L, Askin FB, Taskinen E, Erozan Y, Greenwald P, Huttunen JK. Alpha-tocopherol and beta-carotene supplement and lung cancer incidence in the Alpha-Tocopherol, Beta-Carotene Cancer Prevention Study: effects of base-line characteristics and study compliance. *J Natl Cancer Inst.* 1996;88:1560-1570.

The Alpha-Tocopherol, Beta Carotene Cancer Prevention Study Group. The effect of vitamin E and beta carotene on the incidence of lung cancer and other cancers in male smokers. *N Engl J Med.* 1994;330:1029-1035.

Bjelakovic G, Nikolova D, Gluud LL, Simonetti RG, Gluud C. Mortality in randomized trials of antioxidant supplements for primary and secondary prevention: systematic review and meta-analysis. *JAMA.* 2007;297:842-857.

Bjelakovic G, Nikolova D, Simonetti RG, Gluud C. Antioxidant supplements for prevention of gastrointestinal cancers: a systematic review and meta-analysis. *Lancet.* 2004;364:1219-1228.

Clinical practice guidelines in oncology – v.1.2006. acute myeloid leukemia. National Comprehensive Cancer Network Web site. http://www.nccn.org/professionals/physician_gls/PDF/aml.pdf. Accessed May 2, 2007.

de Klerk NH, Musk AW, Ambrosini GL, Eccles JL, Hansen J, Olsen N, Watts VL, Lund HG, Pang SC, Beilby J, Hobbs MS. Vitamin A and cancer prevention II: comparison of the effects of retinol and beta-carotene. *Int J Cancer.* 1998;75:362-367.

Dietary supplement fact sheet: vitamin A and carotenoids. Office of Dietary Supplements Web site. http://ods.od.nih.gov/factsheets/vitamina.asp. Updated April 23, 2006. Accessed June 16, 2008.

Lawenda BD, Kelly KM, Ladas EJ, Sagar SM, Vickers A, Blumberg JB. Should supplemental antioxidant administration be avoided during chemotherapy and radiation therapy? *J Natl Cancer Inst.* 2008;100:773-783.

Meyskens FL Jr, Liu PY, Tuthill RJ, Sondak VK, Fletcher WS, Jewell WR, Samlowski W, Balcerzak SP, Rector DJ, Noyes RD, et al. Randomized trial of vitamin A versus observation as adjuvant therapy in high-risk primary malignant melanoma: a Southwest Oncology Group study. *J Clin Oncol.* 1994;12:2060-2065.

Omenn GS, Goodman GE, Thornquist MD, Balmes J, Cullen MR, Glass A, Keogh JP, Meyskens FL, Valanis B, Williams JH, Barnhart S, Hammar S. Effects of a combination of beta carotene and vitamin A on lung cancer and cardiovascular disease. *N Engl J Med.* 1996;334:1150-1155.

Pryor WA, Stahl W, Rock CL. Beta carotene: from biochemistry to clinical trials. *Nutr Rev.* 2000;58:39-53.

Redlich CA, Blaner WS, Van Bennekum AM, Chung JS, Clever SL, Holm CT, Cullen MR. Effect of supplementation with beta-carotene and vitamin A on lung nutrient levels. *Cancer Epidemiol Biomarkers Prev.* 1998;7:211-214.

Tsao AS, Kim ES, Hong WK. Chemoprevention of cancer. *CA Cancer J Clin.* 2004;54:150-180.

Van Zandwijk N, Dalesio O, Pastirino U, de Vries N, van Tinteren H. EUROSCAN, a randomized trial of vitamin A and N-acetylcysteine in patients with head and neck cancer or lung cancer. For the European Organization for Research and Treatment of Cancer Head and Neck and Lung Cancer Cooperative Groups. *J Natl Cancer Inst.* 2000;92:977-986.

Vitamin A. Memorial Sloan-Kettering Cancer Center Web site. http://www.mskcc.org/mskcc/html/69410.cfm. Updated September 24, 2007. Accessed June 16, 2008.

VITAMIN B COMPLEX

Other common name(s): B vitamins; vitamins B1, B2, B3, B5, B6, B7, B9, and B12
Scientific/medical name(s): thiamine (B1), riboflavin (B2), niacin (B3), pantothenic acid (B5), pyridoxine (B6), biotin (B7), folic acid or folate (B9), cobalamin (B12)

Description

B vitamins are essential nutrients for growth, development, and a variety of other bodily functions. They play a major role in the activities of enzymes, proteins that regulate chemical reactions in the body, which are important in turning food into energy and other needed substances. B vitamins are found in a variety of plant and animal food sources.

Overview

B vitamins are an important part of the diet and are needed to help avoid many health conditions. However, with the exception of vitamin B9 (folic acid), there is not enough scientific evidence to know whether B vitamins can reduce the risk for cancer. People with low intake of folic acid are at increased risk for certain types of cancer. A diet rich in vegetables containing this vitamin, and perhaps a daily multivitamin supplement containing the recommended daily value of vitamin B9 is recommended by some experts in cancer prevention (see "Folic Acid," page 356). Available scientific evidence does not support claims that any B vitamin is an effective treatment for people who already have cancer.

How is it promoted for use?

Scientists know that B vitamins influence several important bodily functions:

- Vitamin B1 (thiamin) and vitamin B2 (riboflavin) help the body produce energy and affect enzymes that influence the muscles, nerves, and heart.
- Vitamin B3 (niacin) has a role in energy production in cells and in maintaining the health of the skin, nervous system, and digestive system.
- Vitamin B5 (pantothenic acid) influences normal growth and development.
- Vitamin B6 (pyridoxine) helps the body break down protein and helps maintain the health of red blood cells, the nervous system, and parts of the immune system.
- Vitamin B7 (biotin) helps break down protein and carbohydrates and helps the body make hormones.
- Vitamin B9 (folic acid) helps the cells in the body make and maintain DNA and is important in the production of red blood cells.

- Vitamin B12 (cobalamin) plays a role in the body's growth and development. It also has a part in producing blood cells, the functions of the nervous system, and how the body uses folic acid and carbohydrates.

Deficiency of certain B vitamins can cause anemia, tiredness, loss of appetite, abdominal pain, depression, numbness and tingling in the arms and legs, muscle cramps, respiratory infections, hair loss, eczema, poor growth in children, and birth defects in the fetuses of pregnant women.

Women who are pregnant or breastfeeding require more folic acid than others. The Public Health Service recommends that women of childbearing age who can become pregnant should consume at least 400 micrograms of folic acid daily through dietary supplements and fortified foods, in addition to a diet containing folate-rich foods, to help prevent certain birth defects.

Some alternative medical practitioners claim that deficiencies in B vitamins weaken the immune system and make the body vulnerable to cancer. They recommend high doses of B vitamins as treatments for people with cancer. Many researchers are studying the relationships between vitamin intake and risk for developing certain cancers.

What does it involve?

Nutritionists maintain that a balanced diet that includes five daily servings of fruits and vegetables, as well as grains, is sufficient to provide most people with all the B vitamins they need. Only small amounts of these vitamins are needed to reach the recommended dietary intakes. Unfortunately, many people may not eat enough fruits, vegetables, or other healthy foods to get the recommended amounts. The National Academies of Science (NAS) recommends that adults over the age of fifty take B vitamin supplements, or eat foods enriched with these vitamins, in order to prevent deficiency, which is common in this age group.

Vitamins B1 and B2 are found in cereals and whole grains. B1 is also found in potatoes, pork, seafood, liver, and kidney beans. B2 is found in enriched bread, dairy products, liver, and green leafy vegetables. Vitamin B3 is found in liver, fish, chicken, lean red meat, nuts, whole grains, and dried beans. Vitamin B5 is found in almost all foods. Fish, liver, pork, chicken, potatoes, wheat germ, bananas, and dried beans are good sources of vitamin B6. Vitamin B7 is manufactured by intestinal bacteria and is also present in peanuts, liver, egg yolks, bananas, mushrooms, watermelon, and grapefruit. Green leafy vegetables, liver, citrus fruits, mushrooms, nuts, peas, dried beans, and wheat bread contain vitamin B9. Vitamin B12 is found in eggs, meat, poultry, shellfish, milk, and milk products.

Supplements that contain several B vitamins, usually in combination with other nutrients, are sold in grocery stores, health food stores, and over the Internet in pill form. Dosages vary by manufacturer.

What is the history behind it?

While diseases due to vitamin deficiencies have been known for centuries, just about all of the B vitamins were discovered in the early 1900s. Since then, B vitamins have been studied to determine how they affect the human body. As their importance and functions were clarified, the U.S. government began recommending daily intake levels to promote and maintain good health. Research on the possible role of some B vitamins in preventing cancer began in the last few decades.

What is the evidence?

The limited data concerning B vitamins and cancer come mainly from animal studies and from observational epidemiologic studies. These types of studies are not as strong as randomized controlled clinical trials and therefore must be interpreted with caution. There is some evidence from observational epidemiologic studies that increased intake of vitamin B9 (folic acid) is linked to a lower risk for colon cancer, especially in people who are vitamin-deficient, such as those who drink excessive amounts of alcohol. Evidence of effects on other types of cancer has been mixed.

Some (but not all) observational epidemiologic studies have also shown a possible link between intake of vitamin B6 and lower risks for colorectal and breast cancers in women. Possible links between other B vitamins and cancer risk have not been studied as extensively or have been studied with mixed results.

While the results of studies on vitamin B6 and folate are early and are not conclusive, they deserve further research. It is still unclear whether taking in more B vitamins will help protect against cancer or how much might be needed to reduce cancer risk.

Even if some B vitamins prove to be helpful in preventing certain cancers, it does not necessarily follow that B vitamins would be useful in treating cancers. In fact, some experts have cautioned that certain B vitamins, such as thiamine and folic acid, might actually make it easier for established tumors to grow. This is not well proven, but caution is advised when considering taking large doses of these vitamins.

At this time, it is hard to say how each nutrient or nutrient combination affects a person's risk for cancer. On the other hand, studies of large groups of people have shown that those whose diets are high in vegetables and low in animal fat, meat, and/or calories have lower risks for some of the most common types of cancer. Until more is known about this relationship, the American Cancer Society recommends eating a variety of healthful foods—with most of them coming from plant sources—rather than relying on supplements.

While it is best to get vitamins and minerals from foods, supplements may be helpful for some people. If a supplement is taken, the best choice for most people is a balanced multivitamin/mineral supplement that contains no more than 100 percent of the "Daily Value" of most nutrients. Pregnant women, women of childbearing age, and people with restricted food intakes should speak with their doctors about supplements containing higher levels of certain vitamins.

Are there any possible problems or complications?

B vitamins are water-soluble, meaning that any excess intake is largely excreted in the urine. Supplements containing B vitamins are generally thought to be safe but still should not be taken in very large doses. Possible side effects include gout, high blood sugar levels, and skin problems. Overdoses can lead to heart and liver problems. Rarely, large doses of vitamin B3 (niacin) supplements can cause blurred vision, nausea, vomiting, and can make stomach ulcers worse. High doses of folic acid supplements may interfere with at least one chemotherapy drug (methotrexate) and similar medicines. Always tell your doctor and pharmacist about any supplements and herbs you are taking.

Relying on the use of B vitamins alone and avoiding or delaying conventional medical care for cancer may have serious health consequences.

This product is sold as a dietary supplement in the United States. Unlike companies that produce drugs (which must provide the FDA with results of detailed testing showing their product is safe and effective before the drug is approved for sale), the companies that make supplements do not have to show evidence of safety or health benefits to the FDA before selling their products. Supplement products without any reliable scientific evidence of health benefits may still be sold as long as the companies selling them do not claim the supplements can prevent, treat, or cure any specific disease. Some such products may not contain the amount of the herb or substance that is written on the label, and some may include other substances (contaminants). Though the FDA has written new rules to improve the quality of manufacturing processes for dietary supplements and the accurate listing of supplement ingredients, these rules do not take full effect until 2010. The new rules also do not address the safety of supplement ingredients or their effects on health when proper manufacturing techniques are used.

Most such supplements have not been tested to find out if they interact with medicines, foods, or other herbs and supplements. Even though some reports of interactions and harmful effects may be published, full studies of interactions and effects are not often available. Because of these limitations, any information on ill effects and interactions should be considered incomplete.

References

Boros LG, Brandes JL, Lee WN, Cascante M, Puigjaner J, Revesz E, Bray TM, Schirmer WJ, Melvin WS. Thiamine supplementation to cancer patients: a double edged sword. *Anticancer Res.* 1998;18:595-602.

Centers for Disease Control and Prevention. Folate status in women of childbearing age, by race/ethnicity—United States, 1999-2000, 2001-2002, and 2003-2004. *MMWR Morb Mortal Wkly Rep.* 2007;55:1377-1380.

Food and Nutrition Board, Institute of Medicine. *Dietary Reference Intakes for Thiamin, Riboflavin, Niacin, Vitamin B6, Folate, Vitamin B12, Pantothenic Acid, Biotin, and Choline.* Washington, DC: National Academy Press; 1998.

Guyton JR, Bays HE. Safety considerations with niacin therapy. *Am J Cardiol.* 2007;99:22C-31C. Epub 2006 Nov 28.

Kushi LH, Byers T, Doyle C, Bandera EV, McCullough M, McTiernan A, Gansler T, Andrews KS, Thun MJ; American Cancer Society 2006 Nutrition and Physical Activity Guidelines Advisory Committee. American Cancer Society guidelines on nutrition and physical activity for cancer prevention: reducing the risk of cancer with healthy food choices and physical activity. *CA Cancer J Clin.* 2006;56:254-281.

Larsson SC, Giovannucci E, Wolk A. Vitamin B6 intake, alcohol consumption, and colorectal cancer: a longitudinal population-based cohort of women. *Gastroenterology.* 2005;128:1830-1837.

Lawenda BD, Kelly KM, Ladas EJ, Sagar SM, Vickers A, Blumberg JB. Should supplemental antioxidant administration be avoided during chemotherapy and radiation therapy? *J Natl Cancer Inst.* 2008;100:773-783.

Wu K, Helzlsouer KJ, Comstock GW, Hoffman SC, Nadeau MR, Selhub J. A prospective study on folate, B12, and pyridoxal 5'-phosphate (B6) and breast cancer. *Cancer Epidemiol Biomarkers Prev.* 1999;8:209-217.

Zhang SM, Willett WC, Selhub J, Hunter DJ, Giovannucci EL, Holmes MD, Colditz GA, Hankinson SE. Plasma folate, vitamin B6, vitamin B12, homocysteine, and risk of breast cancer. *J Natl Cancer Inst.* 2003;95:373-380.

VITAMIN C

Other common name(s): none
Scientific/medical name(s): ascorbic acid, ascorbate

Description

Vitamin C is an essential vitamin the human body needs to function well. It is a water-soluble vitamin that cannot be made by the body and must be obtained from foods or other sources. Vitamin C is found in abundance in citrus fruits, such as oranges, grapefruit, and lemons, and in green leafy vegetables, potatoes, strawberries, bell peppers, and cantaloupe.

Overview

Vitamin C is necessary for healthy skin, scar tissue, tendons, ligaments, bones, cartilage, and blood vessels and for the healing of wounds and injuries. A shortage of vitamin C causes scurvy.

Fortunately, vitamin C deficiency is very rare among people who eat a reasonably balanced diet.

Many studies have shown a connection between eating foods rich in vitamin C, such as fruits and vegetables, and a reduced risk for cancer. On the other hand, evidence indicates that vitamin C supplements do not reduce cancer risk. This suggests that the activity of fruits and vegetables in preventing cancer is due to a combination of many vitamins and other phytochemicals and not to vitamin C alone (see "Phytochemicals," page 458). Clinical trials of high doses of vitamin C taken by mouth as a treatment for cancer have not shown any benefit. Several studies of very high doses given intravenously are currently in progress. High doses of vitamin C can cause a number of side effects.

How is it promoted for use?

Vitamin C is an antioxidant, a compound that blocks the action of free radicals (activated oxygen molecules that can damage cells). Vitamin C is thought by some to enhance the immune system by stimulating the activities of anticancer agents and a type of white blood cell called natural killer cells. Some claim that the vitamin can prevent a variety of cancers from developing, including cancers of the lung, prostate, bladder, breast, cervix, intestine, esophagus, stomach, pancreas, and salivary gland, as well as leukemia and non-Hodgkin's lymphoma. Vitamin C is also said to prevent tumors from spreading, help the body heal after cancer surgery, enhance the effects of certain anticancer drugs, and reduce the toxic effects of other drugs used in chemotherapy. Some proponents recommend taking high doses of vitamin C by mouth or intravenously as a cancer treatment. Some practitioners recommend high doses of vitamin C supplements to protect against and treat colds.

What does it involve?

Vitamin C is water-soluble, which means that the body uses what it needs and excretes the rest. The Recommended Dietary Allowance (RDA) of vitamin C is 90 milligrams per day for men and 75 milligrams per day for women, with a larger dose recommended for those who are pregnant or breastfeeding. These recommendations were revised by the Food and Nutrition Board of the National Academy of Sciences (NAS) in April 2000. That NAS report set the upper limit for vitamin C from both food and supplements at 2,000 milligrams (2 grams) per day.

Vitamin C supplements are available in powder or chewable pill form at grocery stores, health food stores, drugstores, and over the Internet. Recommended dosages vary by manufacturer. Some of these supplements contain vitamin C only, whereas others are multivitamin supplements that contain variable amounts of vitamin C. Vitamin C is commonly added to foods and drinks. Some of these, such as breakfast cereals, typically contain no more than the RDA of vitamin C, but some other drinks and foods contain considerably more.

What is the history behind it?

First identified in 1928 by Nobel Prize winner Albert Szent-Gyorgyi, vitamin C has been studied ever since for its nutritional and disease-preventing role. In 1970, two-time Nobel Prize winner Linus Pauling advocated large doses of vitamin C (1,000 milligrams per day or more) to prevent colds and reduce their severity. In a 1979 book called *Vitamin C and Cancer*, Pauling claimed that high doses of vitamin C could also be effective against cancer. His claim was based on a 1976 study he did with a Scottish physician in which one hundred patients with advanced cancer were given 10,000 milligrams of vitamin C. The study concluded that the patients treated with vitamin C survived three to four times longer than patients not given the supplements. The Pauling study has been criticized by the National Cancer Institute as poorly designed, and later studies done at the Mayo Clinic found that advanced cancer patients given the same dose of vitamin C did not survive any longer than those not given the supplement. However, the Mayo Clinic trials have also been criticized for not fully addressing all the issues related to the effects of vitamin C. There are still questions about whether vitamin C is effective in treating cancer.

What is the evidence?

Many scientific studies have shown that eating a diet high in fruits and vegetables containing vitamin C significantly reduces the risk for cancers of the pancreas, esophagus, larynx, mouth, stomach, colon and rectum, breast, cervix, and lungs. Many of these studies show that a high intake of vitamin C from food sources has about a two-fold protective effect when compared with a low intake of the vitamin. Likewise, people with higher blood levels of vitamin C tend to have a lower risk for cancer than people with lower blood levels of vitamin C.

However, observational studies and clinical trials of vitamin C supplements have not shown the same strong protective effects against cancer. Apparently, vitamin C is most helpful when it is eaten naturally in fruits and vegetables. A 2007 review of sixty-eight clinical studies of antioxidant vitamin supplements concluded that taking vitamin C supplements had no detectable effect on life span.

The 2000 NAS report stated that there is not enough evidence to support claims that taking high doses of antioxidants (such as vitamins C and E, selenium, and beta carotene) can prevent chronic diseases. Some oncologists believe that taking high doses of antioxidant vitamins may actually interfere with the effectiveness of radiation therapy and some chemotherapy drugs. This conclusion is based on their understanding of the biochemical mechanisms through which these treatments kill cancer cells. However, no clinical trials have yet been done in humans to test this theory. More research is needed to evaluate this question.

Although high doses of vitamin C have been suggested as a cancer treatment, the available evidence from clinical trials has not shown any benefit. Some researchers have suggested that one reason for these results is that when vitamin C is taken by mouth, levels in the body are not high enough to kill cancer cells. Some laboratory studies support this idea, and there are a few case reports of long survival among people who received intravenous vitamin C. On the other hand, critics of this idea have noted that many of the patients in these reports received other conventional or alternative/complementary therapies and that the influence of vitamin C on their cancer is uncertain. In order to help resolve these questions, several clinical trials of high-dose intravenous vitamin C alone or in combination with conventional chemotherapy are currently in progress in patients with several types of cancer.

At this time, it is hard to say how each nutrient or nutrient combination affects a person's risk for cancer. On the other hand, studies of large groups of people have shown that those whose diets are high in vegetables and low in animal fat, meat, and/or calories have lower risks for some of the most common types of cancer. Until more is known about this relationship, the American Cancer Society recommends eating a variety of healthful foods—with most of them coming from plant sources—rather than relying on supplements.

While it is best to get vitamins and minerals from foods, supplements may be helpful for some people, such as pregnant women, women of childbearing age, and people with restricted food intakes. If a supplement is taken, the best choice for most people is a balanced multivitamin/mineral supplement that contains no more than 100 percent of the "Daily Value" of most nutrients.

Are there any possible problems or complications?

Vitamin C supplements are generally considered safe unless doses are higher than 2,000 milligrams per day. However, doses higher than 1,000 milligrams (1 gram) can cause headaches, diarrhea, nausea, heartburn, stomach cramps, and may cause kidney stones. Vitamin C can also increase the amount of iron the body absorbs, which is generally a problem only for those with too much iron in the body, a condition called hematochromatosis.

Most oncologists routinely recommend that people with cancer avoid gram-sized doses of vitamin C during treatment. People who have cancer should talk to their doctors before taking vitamin C or other vitamin supplements. Relying on this type of treatment alone and avoiding or delaying conventional medical care for cancer may have serious health consequences.

This product is sold as a dietary supplement in the United States. Unlike companies that produce drugs (which must provide the FDA with results of detailed testing showing their product is safe and effective before the drug is approved for sale), the companies that make supplements do not have to show evidence of safety or health benefits to the FDA before selling their products. Supplement products without any reliable scientific evidence of health benefits may still be sold as long as the companies

selling them do not claim the supplements can prevent, treat, or cure any specific disease. Some such products may not contain the amount of the herb or substance that is written on the label, and some may include other substances (contaminants). Though the FDA has written new rules to improve the quality of manufacturing processes for dietary supplements and the accurate listing of supplement ingredients, these rules do not take full effect until 2010. The new rules also do not address the safety of supplement ingredients or their effects on health when proper manufacturing techniques are used.

Most such supplements have not been tested to find out if they interact with medicines, foods, or other herbs and supplements. Even though some reports of interactions and harmful effects may be published, full studies of interactions and effects are not often available. Because of these limitations, any information on ill effects and interactions should be considered incomplete.

References

Assouline S, Miller WH. High-dose vitamin C therapy: renewed hope or false promise? *CMAJ.* 2006;174:956-957.

Bjelakovic G, Nikolova D, Gluud LL, Simonetti RG, Gluud C. Mortality in randomized trials of antioxidant supplements for primary and secondary prevention: systematic review and meta-analysis. *JAMA.* 2007;297:842-857.

Byers T, Guerrero N. Epidemiologic evidence for vitamin C and vitamin E in cancer prevention. *Am J Clin Nutr.* 1995;62:1385S-1392S.

Creagan ET, Moertel CG, O'Fallon JR, Schutt AJ, O'Connell MJ, Rubin J, Frytak S. Failure of high-dose vitamin C (ascorbic acid) therapy to benefit patients with advanced cancer. A controlled trial. *N Engl J Med.* 1979;301:687-690.

Hwang MY. How much vitamin C do you need? *JAMA.* 1999;281:1460.

Institute of Medicine (US). Panel on Dietary Antioxidants and Related Compounds. *Dietary Reference Intakes for Vitamin C, Vitamin E, Selenium, and Carotenoids : a Report of the Panel on Dietary Antioxidants and Related Compounds, Subcommittees on Upper Reference Levels of Nutrients and of Interpretation and Use of Dietary Reference Intakes, and the Standing Committee on the Scientific Evaluation of Dietary Reference Intakes, Food and Nutrition Board, Institute of Medicine.* Washington, DC: National Academy Press; 2000.

Kushi LH, Byers T, Doyle C, Bandera EV, McCullough M, McTiernan A, Gansler T, Andrews KS, Thun MJ; American Cancer Society 2006 Nutrition and Physical Activity Guidelines Advisory Committee. American Cancer Society guidelines on nutrition and physical activity for cancer prevention: reducing the risk of cancer with healthy food choices and physical activity. *CA Cancer J Clin.* 2006;56:254-281.

Lawenda BD, Kelly KM, Ladas EJ, Sagar SM, Vickers A, Blumberg JB. Should supplemental antioxidant administration be avoided during chemotherapy and radiation therapy? *J Natl Cancer Inst.* 2008;100:773-783.

Levine M, Rumsey SC, Daruwala R, Park JB, Wang Y. Criteria and recommendations for vitamin C intake. *JAMA.* 1999;281:1415-1423.

Moertel CG, Fleming TR, Creagan ET, Rubin J, O'Connell MJ, Ames MM. High-dose vitamin C versus placebo in the treatment of patients with advanced cancer who have had no prior chemotherapy. A randomized double-blind comparison. *N Engl J Med.* 1985;312:137-141.

Padayatty SJ, Riordan HD, Hewitt SM, Katz A, Hoffer LJ, Levine M. Intravenously administered vitamin C as cancer therapy: three cases. *CMAJ.* 2006;174:937-942.

Patterson RE, White E, Kristal AR, Neuhouser ML, Potter JD. Vitamin supplements and cancer risk: the epidemiologic evidence. *Cancer Causes Control.* 1997;8:786-802.

US National Institutes of Health. Pilot trial of intravenous vitamin C in refractory non-Hodgkin lymphoma (NHL). ClinicalTrials.gov Web site. http://clinicaltrials.gov/ct2/show/NCT00626444. Accessed September 4, 2008.

US National Institutes of Health. Study of high-dose intravenous (IV) vitamin C treatment in patients with solid tumors. ClinicalTrials.gov Web site. http://clinicaltrials.gov/ct2/show/NCT00441207. Accessed September 4, 2008.

US National Institutes of Health. Study of IV decitabine, arsenic trioxide and vitamin C in patients with MDS. ClinicalTrials.gov Web site. http://clinicaltrials.gov/ct2/show/NCT00671697. Accessed September 4, 2008.

US National Institutes of Health. Trisenox, ascorbic acid and bortezomib in patients with relapsed/refractory multiple myeloma (AAV). ClinicalTrials.gov Web site. http://clinicaltrials.gov/ct2/show/NCT00590603. Accessed September 4, 2008.

Vickers A. Alternative cancer cures: "unproven" or "disproven"? *CA Cancer J Clin.* 2004;54:110-118.

Vitamin C. Memorial Sloan-Kettering Cancer Center Web site. http://www.mskcc.org/mskcc/html/69413.cfm. Updated February 28, 2008. Accessed June 6, 2008.

Willett WC, Stampfer MJ. Clinical practice. What vitamins should I be taking, doctor? *N Engl J Med.* 2001;345:1819-1824.

VITAMIN D

Other common name(s): the sunshine vitamin, Calcitriol, calciferol, ergocalciferol (vitamin D2), cholecalciferol (vitamin D3), 1,25-D

Scientific/medical name(s): 1,25 dihydroxycholecalciferol; also called 1,25 dihydroxyvitamin D

Description

Vitamin D is an essential vitamin the body needs to regulate the amount of calcium and phosphorus in the body. It is best known for its role in using calcium to help build bones and keep them strong. Vitamin D affects many other tissues of the body, including the kidneys, intestines, and parathyroid glands. It is found in salmon, mackerel, tuna, and sardines, as well as in cod liver oil. Most of the milk supply in the United States has vitamin D added to it, as do some breakfast cereals, orange juices, and milk substitutes (such as soy milk). Some experts note that vitamin D acts more like a hormone than a vitamin, in part because the body can make its own vitamin D if the skin gets enough ultraviolet (UV) rays from sunlight.

Overview

Vitamin D is needed to keep a balance between calcium and phosphorus in the body by controlling how much of these nutrients are absorbed from foods or taking them from bones when needed. While known for its role in building bones and keeping them strong, the exact function of vitamin D in other cells and organs is not fully known.

After fairly brief exposure to sunlight, the body can make vitamin D for several hours afterward. However, the amount of sun it takes to make enough vitamin D depends on several factors (see "What does it involve?"). Because UV light exposure is linked to skin cancer and other diseases, safety is a concern when considering the use of sunlight to meet vitamin D requirements. Most people can meet their vitamin D requirements through dietary sources and supplements, if used properly. Food sources of vitamin D and vitamin D supplements have the added benefit of not causing cancer and other negative skin effects that can result from exposure to UV light.

Although some studies have found that cancer risk is lower for people who have higher levels of vitamin D in the body, more studies are needed to find out whether vitamin D is the reason for this decreased risk. If there is a link, researchers would still have to determine whether vitamin D deficiency raises a person's cancer risk and/or whether intake of vitamin D above the recommended daily value has a protective effect. The possible role of vitamin D in treating cancer is still being studied.

How is it promoted for use?

Vitamin D is promoted mainly for its role in balancing calcium and phosphorus and keeping bones healthy. Some practitioners claim that vitamin D is an immune system booster that can be used to prevent many problems, including autism, type 1 diabetes, schizophrenia, mood disorders, infectious diseases, cancer, and other illnesses. Others say it is helpful for weight loss. In orthomolecular medicine and some other forms of alternative medicine, large doses of vitamin D may be used along with other vitamins to treat cancer (see "Orthomolecular Medicine," page 439). Vitamin D is also being studied as a component of conventional treatment regimens together with chemotherapy.

What does it involve?

The body can make vitamin D after exposure to UV rays or it can be obtained through some foods or supplements. The amount of vitamin D made when the skin is exposed to sunlight depends on several factors, including skin color, age, how much skin is exposed, time of year, time of day, cloud cover, length of exposure, and geographic location. Latitudes farther away from the equator do not get much UV light through the earth's atmosphere in the winter months. This difference can be a problem for people who live in the northern United States and Canada and who do not take in much vitamin D in foods. In addition, darker-skinned people need somewhat longer UV exposures to trigger their bodies to make vitamin D, and older people do not make as much vitamin D as younger people in response to sunlight. Sunscreen also blocks UV rays, which reduces the body's ability to produce vitamin D.

Even in a sunny climate, sunlight's effects can be hard to predict. One study looked at ninety-three adults in Hawaii who reported several hours of sun exposure each week for at least three months. The researchers found that half of the study participants had low vitamin D levels in their blood. Closer analysis showed no link between vitamin D levels and age, lightest or darkest skin colors, or hours of sun exposure without sunscreen. Clearly, there is no "one size fits all" prescription for a reliable minimum amount of sun exposure to meet the vitamin D requirements of every person.

The body stores several forms of vitamin D. Vitamin D3 is the form that is made in the skin. Vitamin D2 (ergo calciferol) or D3 (cholecalciferol) can be absorbed from food. All must be changed into 25 hydroxyvitamin D (25 hydroxycholecalciferol), a form that can last for several weeks in the blood. This is the vitamin D level that doctors generally check.

The liver and kidneys change vitamin D into calcitrol (also called 1,25 dihydroxycholecalciferol or 1,25 dihydroxyvitamin D), which helps the intestine absorb more calcium and phosphorus.

After a review of evidence in the 1990s, the Institute of Medicine concluded that there was not enough scientific evidence to set a Recommended Dietary Allowance (RDA) for vitamin D. They were able to decide on an Adequate Intake (AI), which is a less definitive level. The AI of vitamin D for infants, children, and men and women up through age fifty is 200 International Units (IU) per day (equal to 5 micrograms). Adequate Intake is 400 IU per day (10 micrograms) for adults aged fifty-one to seventy and 600 IU a day (15 micrograms) for adults older than seventy. The safe upper limit for adults was set at 2,000 IU per day.

New evidence has some nutrition experts suggesting that the recommendations may be too low. Blood tests can now measure the body's stores of vitamin D, and many people have unexpectedly low levels. There is now serious discussion about how much vitamin D it takes to raise the body's stores of it to healthy levels.

Because it does not occur naturally in many foods, many adults may not get enough vitamin D from their everyday diet. The addition of vitamin D to milk and other breakfast foods has helped many people get more of it. For instance, one cup of fortified milk contains half of what is currently considered to be the AI of vitamin D for an adult between the ages of nineteen and fifty. That same cup supplies only one-quarter of the AI for an adult aged fifty-one to seventy, and about one-sixth of the AI for a person seventy-one or older.

Vitamin D supplements may be necessary for some people:

- People aged fifty and older, whose skin cannot make as much vitamin D and/or whose kidneys are less able to convert vitamin D to its active form
- People with limited sun exposure; for instance, those who are homebound, who live in northern areas such as New England and Alaska, women who wear robes and head coverings for religious reasons, and people whose work prevents sun exposure, if they are unable to consume enough vitamin D in foods
- Adults with darker skin. Some studies suggest that older adults with dark skin, especially women, are at even higher risk for vitamin D deficiency if they do not consume enough vitamin D in foods.
- People who do not absorb fat well. This is linked to several medical conditions:
    - deficiency of pancreatic enzymes
    - Crohn's disease
    - cystic fibrosis
    - sprue or celiac disease (gluten intolerance)
    - certain types of liver disease
    - surgical removal of all or part of the stomach or intestine
- Children and adolescents who are not exposed to sunlight and who do not drink at least two cups of fortified milk per day
- People who are lactose intolerant, allergic to milk, or who avoid milk products for any reason
- Infants who are breastfed only. Formula is fortified with vitamin D. An infant who consumes two cups of formula per day takes in adequate vitamin D.

Vitamin D supplements are most often taken in pill form, although cod liver oil is also still used. Supplements are available at drugstores, grocery stores, and health food stores and on the Internet.

What is the history behind it?

Rickets, a disease of weak bones and other deformities, was first described in the mid-1600s as a major problem among city children. Even though there were reports that rickets could be cured by sunbathing or cod liver oil, the disease was still widespread in northern Europe in the early twentieth century. After vitamin A was discovered in 1913 by Elmer McCollum as a cure for night blindness, a British doctor named Edward Mellanby induced rickets in dogs and then cured the condition using cod liver oil. He assumed that the vitamin A in the cod liver oil had cured the dogs. To test Mellanby's theory, McCollum devised a way to inactivate the vitamin A in cod liver oil. As expected, the oil no longer worked to treat night blindness. To the surprise of nearly everyone, however, it still cured rickets, which proved that another substance besides vitamin A was responsible. McCollum published these findings in 1922, calling this substance vitamin D. Soon after, a program to add vitamin D to milk was started in the United States, and rickets was nearly wiped out. Cod liver oil has remained a home remedy ever since.

Even though vitamin D was named and put to wide use, scientists in the early twentieth century knew almost nothing about what it was or how it worked. It took years of study and discoveries by a number of researchers to learn that there were several forms of vitamin D and to find out how they work in the body.

German researcher Adolf Windaus first discovered three forms of the vitamin, which he called D1, D2, and D3. (Because it was later learned that the product Windaus named vitamin D1 was a mixture of compounds rather than a pure vitamin D product, the term D1 is no longer used.) In the early 1950s, Arvid Carlsson found that vitamin D can remove calcium from the bones when the body needs it for other uses. Ragnar Nicolaysen, a dietary researcher, discovered that the amount of calcium absorbed from food is guided by an internal factor that tells the intestine how much the body needs. In 1975, another researcher named Mark Haussler confirmed that the intestines have a receptor protein that specifically binds to active vitamin D.

Today, vitamin D is still added to most milk sold in the United States, although it is not added to all milk products, such as cheese and ice cream. Some companies also add it to cereal, soy milk, and orange juice, usually along with calcium. It is now understood that rickets is the product of long-standing and severe vitamin D deficiency, and that milder cases of deficiency may have no symptoms.

Since a few studies in the early 2000s have suggested higher vitamin D intake may be related to lower cancer risk, more studies have begun to look at this possibility.

What is the evidence?

Laboratory and animal studies and observational epidemiologic studies suggest that higher intake of vitamin D may be linked to lower cancer risk. Observational studies suggest that the risk for cancer is lower in those who get more calcium and vitamin D (which may include vitamin D from foods as well as sunlight). Higher vitamin D levels in the blood have been linked in these studies to lower risk for some types of cancer, especially colorectal cancers. Vitamin D appeared to be a protective factor in a study of more than three thousand adults (mostly men) who had colonoscopies between 1994 and 1997 to look for polyps or cancer. Those with the highest vitamin D intake were less likely to have advanced cancer. Although this sounds promising, observational epidemiologic studies cannot rule out that other unknown factors may have caused the outcome.

Randomized clinical trials, which are considered much stronger evidence than observational studies, have since been started to more reliably study the role vitamin D may play in cancer prevention. A Women's Health Initiative study published in 2006 put more than thirty-six thousand menopausal women into two groups: half got vitamin D with calcium supplements and half got a placebo. After seven years, the researchers looked at colorectal cancer risk in the two groups. Cancer risk was not lower in the group that took vitamin D, but critics noted that the dose given (400 IU per day) may have been too low to make a difference, and that many women were not taking their pills at all. The average vitamin D and calcium intake of the women at the start of the study was also about twice as high as the national average, and close to the doses used in the study. This factor may have limited the ability of the study to find any differences. Interestingly, colorectal cancer risk was lower in women who had higher levels of vitamin D in their blood at the start of the study. This study is still going on, so a final conclusion has not been reached.

A four-year study published in 2007 looked at 1,179 healthy women over age fifty-five who were randomly selected from rural Nebraska. The researchers gave a third of the women 1,400 to 1,500 milligrams of calcium each day. Another third received calcium plus 1,100 IU of vitamin D3 each day, while the rest got a placebo. The women who took calcium and vitamin D had significantly less risk for all types of cancer, as did the women who had higher vitamin D levels when the study started. As this was only one study, it is difficult to be certain the vitamin D and calcium caused the difference. It is still possible that other differences between the groups may have accounted for the lower cancer rates. Before this information can be used to recommend increased supplements of vitamin D and calcium, it needs to be confirmed by other studies. It also needs to be shown that the findings hold true in other groups of people, that the supplements do not increase the risk for other problems, and that there are no unexpected side effects.

Additional well-designed clinical trials need to be done to confirm whether low levels of vitamin D raise cancer risk and to determine whether taking more vitamin D (with or without extra calcium) reduces cancer risk. Until such studies are completed, it is too early to advise people to take vitamin D supplements for cancer prevention.

Some researchers are interested in whether vitamin D can play a role in cancer treatment. Some small studies have looked at vitamin D along with standard treatment for prostate cancer.

In one study of sixteen men with metastatic prostate cancer, one in four had less bone pain and one in three had stronger muscles after taking 2,000 IU of vitamin D each day for twelve weeks. However, nearly half of the patients were deficient in vitamin D at the start of the study, which could have affected the results.

Another study looked at the effects of vitamin D3 on blood levels of prostate-specific antigen (PSA) in men whose prostate cancer had recurred after treatment. PSA is a substance produced by normal and cancerous prostate cells, and increased levels are considered to be an indicator of cancer growth. After treatment with radiation or surgery, the men took daily doses of vitamin D3 for a period of between six and fifteen months. The researchers observed that in six of seven patients, their PSA levels increased more slowly than their pretreatment rate. However, the men began to lose calcium in their urine, which limited the amount of vitamin D they could safely take. This was a small pilot study that called for further testing.

A 2003 study of twenty-two men with recurrent prostate cancer used larger weekly doses of vitamin D3. The researchers observed that the weekly dose was safe. However, while the rate of PSA increase in the men slowed to some extent, more studies are needed to determine whether vitamin D has a significant role in slowing the growth of prostate cancer.

Women who are vitamin D–deficient give birth to children with very little vitamin D in their bodies. In addition, past measurements have indicated that human breast milk contains very little vitamin D, leading to the recommendation that infants fed only breast milk be given vitamin D supplements. However, recent small early studies in breastfeeding women have found that women with high blood levels of vitamin D have adequate amounts in their breast milk. In order to reach these levels, though, researchers had to give the women very high doses of vitamin D each day. More research is needed to find out about safety and side effects, use of blood levels to determine vitamin D status, and optimum blood levels of the vitamin.

Results of an observational epidemiologic study presented at the 2008 annual meeting of the American Society of Clinical Oncology suggest that breast cancer patients with vitamin D deficiency do not live as long as those with adequate vitamin D status. Researchers are also testing whether vitamin D can increase the effectiveness of some chemotherapy drugs. Although preclinical studies and preliminary human studies in prostate cancer were encouraging, a 2008 report of a randomized, double-blinded clinical trial did not indicate that taxotere plus vitamin D was any more effective than the chemotherapy drug alone in prolonging the lives of men with advanced prostate cancer. Researchers are also testing deltanoids—compounds chemically related to vitamin D—for cancer prevention and for treatment, alone and in combination with other conventional drugs.

A vitamin D derivative was proven to be effective at reducing the symptoms of the skin condition psoriasis. Vitamin D can also prevent and treat some bone problems such as rickets in children and osteomalacia in adults. Vitamin D deficiency, which is often seen in older people, can lead to osteoporosis and is linked to an increased risk for broken hips. Studies of the effect of vitamin D supplements on hip fracture risk among older people have had conflicting results. More information is needed before any recommendations can be made for older people at risk for hip fracture.

Although low vitamin D levels seem to be linked to several diseases, further study is needed to learn whether the disease causes the low levels of vitamin D, the vitamin deficiency increases the risk for disease, or there is some other relationship between the two.

Are there any possible problems or complications?

Vitamin D is considered safe as part of a normal healthy diet. Too much vitamin D can cause nausea, vomiting, poor appetite, constipation, weakness, and weight loss. It can also raise blood calcium levels, causing changes in mental status such as confusion. High blood calcium can also cause abnormal heart rhythms. Too much vitamin D over a long time can cause depression, headaches, sleepiness, and weakness, as well as loss of calcium and bone. It can also cause the arteries and other soft tissues of the body (such as kidneys, heart, lungs) to become hardened and lined with layers of calcium, a condition known as calcinosis.

Getting vitamin D through sunlight may not work for some and may cause problems for others. In addition to the immediate danger of sunburn, exposure to ultraviolet light can cause skin cancer; wrinkled, sagging skin; damage to the eyes, including cataracts; and impairment of the immune system. Reflective surfaces make UV exposure more intense and can worsen these effects. Water, snow, and sand reflect the most. While sun exposure can cause other problems, it has never been reported to produce toxic levels of vitamin D. Vitamin D from foods is also unlikely to cause toxicity unless large amounts of cod liver oil are used. Vitamin D toxicity is much more likely to occur as a result of taking too many supplements. Vitamin D toxicity has also been caused by foods that were incorrectly fortified (foods or milk that had accidentally been mixed with far more vitamin D than intended).

Laxatives, steroids, and anti-cholesterol drugs like cholestyramine (Questran, Locholest) and colestipol (Colestid) may lower the amount of vitamin D you can absorb. Vitamin D should be taken several hours before or after these drugs. Anti-seizure drugs and rifampin (an anti-tuberculosis drug) can lower your vitamin D levels. Too much vitamin D may raise calcium levels, which can cause abnormal heart rhythms if you are taking digoxin.

If you take vitamin D with calcium, note that calcium can keep certain drugs from being absorbed. Always talk with your doctor and pharmacist about all the herbs, supplements, and medicines you are taking. Relying on this type of treatment alone and avoiding or delaying conventional medical care for cancer may have serious health consequences.

This product is sold as a dietary supplement in the United States. Unlike companies that produce drugs (which must provide the FDA with results of detailed testing showing their product is safe and effective before the drug is approved for sale), the companies that make supplements do not have to show evidence of safety or health benefits to the FDA before selling their products. Supplement products without any reliable scientific evidence of health benefits may still be sold as long as the companies selling them do not claim the supplements can prevent, treat, or cure any specific disease. Some such products may not contain the amount of the herb or substance that is written on the label, and some may include other substances (contaminants). Though the FDA has written new rules to improve the quality of manufacturing processes for dietary supplements and the accurate listing of supplement ingredients, these rules do not take full effect until 2010. The new rules also do not address the safety of supplement ingredients or their effects on health when proper manufacturing techniques are used.

Most such supplements have not been tested to find out if they interact with medicines, foods, or other herbs and supplements. Even though some reports of interactions and harmful effects may be published, full studies of interactions and effects are not often available. Because of these limitations, any information on ill effects and interactions should be considered incomplete.

References

Attia S, Eickhoff J, Wilding G, McNeel D, Blank J, Ahuja H, Jumonville A, Eastman M, Shevrin D, Glode M, Alberti D, Staab MJ, Horvath D, Straus J, Marnocha R, Liu G. Randomized, double-blinded phase II evaluation of docetaxel with or without doxercalciferol in patients with metastatic, androgen-independent prostate cancer. *Clin Cancer Res.* 2008;14:2437-2443.

Beer TM, Lemmon D, Lowe BA, Henner WD. High-dose weekly oral calcitriol in patients with a rising PSA after prostatectomy or radiation for prostate carcinoma. *Cancer.* 2003;97:1217-1224.

Binkley N, Novotny R, Krueger D, Kawahara T, Daida YG, Lensmeyer G, Hollis BW, Drezner MK. Low vitamin D status despite abundant sun exposure. *J Clin Endocrinol Metab.* 2007;92:2130-2135.

Chapuy MC, Pamphile R, Paris E, Kempf C, Schlichting M, Arnaud S, Garnero P, Meunier PJ. Combined calcium and vitamin D3 supplementation in elderly women: confirmation of reversal of secondary hyperparathyroidism and hip fracture risk: the Decalyos II study. *Osteoporos Int.* 2002;13:257-264.

de Sevaux RGL, Hoitsma AJ, Corstens FHM, Wetzels JFM. Treatment with vitamin D and calcium reduces bone loss after renal transplantation: a randomized study. *J Am Soc Nephrol.* 2002;13:1608-1614.

Dietary supplement fact sheet: vitamin D. Office of Dietary Supplements Web site. http://ods.od.nih.gov/factsheets/vitamind.asp. Accessed July 16, 2007.

Duthie MS, Kimber I, Norval M. The effects of ultraviolet radiation on the human immune system. *Br J Dermatol.* 1999;140:995-1009.

EXCITE: skin cancer module: practice exercises. Centers for Disease Control and Prevention Web site. http://www.cdc.gov/excite/skincancer/mod06.htm. Updated August 27, 2004. Accessed August 6, 2007.

Goodwin PJ, Ennis M, Pritchard KI, Koo J, Hood N. Frequency of vitamin D (Vit D) deficiency at breast cancer (BC) diagnosis and association with risk of distant recurrence and death in a prospective cohort study of T1-3, N0-1, M0 BC. *J Clin Oncol.* 2008;26 (May 20 supplement; abstract 511).

Grant AM, Avenell A, Campbell MK, McDonald AM, MacLennan GS, McPherson GC, Anderson FH, Cooper C, Francis RM, Donaldson C, Gillespie WJ, Robinson CM, Torgerson DJ, Wallace WA; RECORD Trial Group. Oral vitamin D3 and calcium for secondary prevention of low-trauma fractures in elderly people (Randomised Evaluation of Calcium Or vitamin D, RECORD): a randomised placebo-controlled trial. *Lancet.* 2005;365:1621-1628.

Gross C, Stamey T, Hancock S, Feldman D. Treatment of early recurrent prostate cancer with 1,25-dihydroxyvitamin D3 (calcitriol). *J Urol.* 1998;159:2035-2039.

Holick MF. *Vitamin D: Physiology, Molecular Biology, and Clinical Applications.* Totowa, NJ: Humana Press; 1999.

Holick MF, Krane SM. Introduction to bone and mineral metabolism. In: Braunwald E, Fauci AS, Kasper DL, Hauser SL, Longo DL, Jameson JL, eds. *Harrison's Principles of Internal Medicine.* 15th ed. New York: McGraw Hill; 2001: 2192-2205.

Hollis BW, Wagner CL. Assessment of dietary vitamin D requirements during pregnancy and lactation. *Am J Clin Nutr.* 2004:79: 717-726.

Jackson RD, LaCroix AZ, Gass M, Wallace RB, Robbins J, Lewis CE, Bassford T, Beresford SA, Black HR, Blanchette P, Bonds DE, Brunner RL, Brzyski RG, Caan B, Cauley JA, Chlebowski RT, Cummings SR, Granek I, Hays J, Heiss G, Hendrix SL, Howard BV, Hsia J, Hubbell FA, Johnson KC, Judd H, Kotchen JM, Kuller LH, Langer RD, Lasser NL, Limacher MC, Ludlam S, Manson JE, Margolis KL, McGowan J, Ockene JK, O'Sullivan MJ, Phillips L, Prentice RL, Sarto GE, Stefanick ML, Van Horn L, Wactawski-Wende J, Whitlock E, Anderson GL, Assaf AR, Barad D; Women's Health Initiative Investigators. Calcium plus vitamin D supplementation and the risk of fractures. *N Engl J Med.* 2006;354:669-683.

Lappe JM, Travers-Gustafson D, Davies KM, Recker RR, Heaney RP. Vitamin D and calcium supplementation reduces cancer risk: results of a randomized trial. *Am J Clin Nutr.* 2007;85:1586-1591.

Porthouse J, Cockayne S, King C, Saxon L, Steele E, Aspray T, Baverstock M, Birks Y, Dumville J, Francis R, Iglesias C, Puffer S, Sutcliffe A, Watt I, Torgerson DJ. Randomised controlled trial of calcium and supplementation with cholecalciferol (vitamin D3) for prevention of fractures in primary care. *BMJ.* 2005;330:1003.

Unraveling the enigma of vitamin D. National Academy of Sciences, Beyond Discovery Web site. http://www.beyonddiscovery.org/content/view.article.asp?a=414. Accessed August 2, 2007.

Van Veldhuizen PJ, Taylor SA, Williamson S, Drees BM. Treatment of vitamin D deficiency in patients with metastatic prostate cancer may improve bone pain and muscle strength. *J Urol.* 2000;163:187-190.

Vitamin D. Medline Plus Web site. http://www.nlm.nih.gov/medlineplus/druginfo/natural/patient-vitamind.html. Accessed August 9, 2007.

Vitamin D. Memorial Sloan-Kettering Cancer Center Web site. http://www.mskcc.org/mskcc/html/69414.cfm. Accessed July 16, 2007.

Vitamin D. New Zealand Dermatological Society Web site. http://dermnetnz.org/systemic/vitamin-d.html. Accessed August 6, 2007.

Wactawski-Wende J, Kotchen JM, Anderson GL, Assaf AR, Brunner RL, O'Sullivan MJ, Margolis KL, Ockene JK, Phillips L, Pottern L, Prentice RL, Robbins J, Rohan TE, Sarto GE, Sharma S, Stefanick ML, Van Horn L, Wallace RB, Whitlock E, Bassford T, Beresford SA, Black HR, Bonds DE, Brzyski RG, Caan B, Chlebowski RT, Cochrane B, Garland C, Gass M, Hays J, Heiss G, Hendrix SL, Howard BV, Hsia J, Hubbell FA, Jackson RD, Johnson KC, Judd H, Kooperberg CL, Kuller LH, LaCroix AZ, Lane DS, Langer RD, Lasser NL, Lewis CE, Limacher MC, Manson JE; Women's Health Initiative Investigators. Calcium plus vitamin D supplementation and the risk of colorectal cancer. *N Engl J Med.* 2006;354:684-696.

Wagner CL, Hulsey TC, Fanning D, Ebeling M, Hollis BW. High-dose vitamin D3 supplementation in a cohort of breastfeeding mothers and their infants: a 6-month follow-up pilot study. *Breastfeed Med.* 2006;1:59-70.

Weaver CM, Fleet JC. Vitamin D requirements: current and future. *Am J Clin Nutr.* 2004;80:1735S-1739S.

VITAMIN E

Other common name(s): none
Scientific/medical name(s): alpha-tocopherol, tocopherols, tocotrienols

Description

Vitamin E is an essential nutrient the human body needs to function normally. The term vitamin E actually represents a group of substances, the most important (to the human body) being alpha-tocopherol. The main sources of vitamin E in the diet are vegetable oils (especially safflower oil, sunflower oil, and cottonseed oil), green leafy vegetables, nuts, cereals, meats, egg yolks, wheat germ, and whole wheat products. Vitamin E deficiency is rare and occurs almost exclusively in people with an inherited or acquired condition that impairs their ability to absorb this vitamin. Symptoms of vitamin E deficiency include muscle weakness, visual problems (especially at night), and a poor sense of balance. Over a long period, vitamin E deficiency may progress to blindness, heart disease, and impaired thinking. Supplements are usually necessary or recommended only for people with vitamin E deficiency or a condition that puts them at risk for this deficiency.

Overview

There is some evidence of the protective effects of vitamin E against prostate, bladder, and colorectal cancer; however, more research is needed. The consensus of most clinical studies is that vitamin E supplements do not have any overall health benefit or any beneficial effect on heart disease and cancer in general, and may even lead to increased risk for heart failure. Available scientific evidence does not support claims that vitamin E significantly affects the growth of cancers that have already formed.

How is it promoted for use?

Some proponents claim vitamin E plays a role in protecting the body against cancer by bolstering the immune system. Some also believe the vitamin can increase the effectiveness of some chemotherapy drugs and may reduce some side effects of chemotherapy and radiation therapy. However, others believe high doses of vitamin E might interfere with the effectiveness of radiation therapy and chemotherapy.

Proponents also claim that vitamin E supplements protect against heart attacks by preventing a buildup of harmful cholesterol in the blood. There are also claims that vitamin E eases the inflammation associated with arthritis, speeds the healing of wounds in people who have suffered burns or have had surgery, and slows the progression of Parkinson's disease and Alzheimer's disease. Vitamin E is also used to protect against the effects of pollution and overexposure to the sun and to lessen the risk for cataracts.

What does it involve?

A balanced diet normally provides adequate amounts of vitamin E for the body's needs, especially a diet low in fat and high in green leafy vegetables and fiber from grains and cereals. The Recommended Dietary Allowance (RDA) of vitamin E for adults is 15 milligrams per day from food, with 19 milligrams per day recommended for women who are breastfeeding. Vitamin E is often measured as International Units (IU); 1 milligram is equal to 1.5 IU. This recommendation was revised by the National Academy of Science (NAS) in April 2000. It also set the upper limit of intake from supplements at 1,000 milligrams per day (1,500 IU).

Vitamin E supplements are taken as capsules, with a typical dose being 400 IU per day.

What is the history behind it?

Since the 1940s, researchers and others have thought that vitamin E might prevent heart disease. Researchers have observed that people who have cancer often also have low levels of vitamin E in their blood. More recently, several clinical trials have been completed (and others are still in progress) comparing the risk for cancer among volunteers randomly assigned to receive either vitamin E supplements or a placebo.

What is the evidence?

Vitamin E is an antioxidant, a compound that blocks the action of free radicals (activated oxygen molecules that can damage cells). Most of the evidence for the preventive effects of antioxidants such as vitamin E comes from animal studies and from observational epidemiologic studies using surveys estimating how much vitamin E a person consumes from food and supplements. However, the most reliable studies on this issue are controlled clinical trials, such as a large 1994 study of antioxidant vitamins and cancer conducted by the National Cancer Institute (NCI) and the National Public Health Institute of Finland. The study was designed to find out whether antioxidant vitamins in higher doses than the RDA could reduce the incidence of lung cancer, other types of cancer, and other illnesses among twenty-nine thousand male smokers. The study found no beneficial effect of vitamin E supplements on lung cancer incidence. It found lower rates of prostate and colorectal cancer among those who received vitamin E, but higher rates of bladder, stomach, and other types of cancer.

The 2000 National Academy of Sciences report stated that there is not enough evidence to support claims that taking high doses of antioxidants (such as vitamins C and E, selenium, and beta carotene) can prevent chronic diseases.

Individual clinical trials can sometimes provide misleading results because of variation in research methods or random statistical variation. Because of this possibility, researchers often analyze the combined data from many studies. This approach is called meta-analysis. A meta-analysis published in 2005 combined data from nineteen clinical trials that looked at vitamin E supplements. The results showed that vitamin E supplements do not lower the risk for heart disease or of cancer overall, and that people who received the placebo actually lived slightly longer than those receiving the supplements.

Another large clinical trial published in 2005 also found no risk reduction for heart disease or cancer overall. It even suggested that heart failure was slightly more common among people taking vitamin E. A 2007 review of sixty-eight studies of antioxidant vitamin supplements found that people taking vitamin E supplements had a shorter life expectancy than those who did not take these supplements.

At least two more clinical trials of vitamin E for disease prevention are still in progress. The Women's Health Study began in 1991 and is expected to be completed in 2009. The SELECT (Selenium and Vitamin E Cancer Prevention Trial) is studying the effect of vitamin E alone or in combination with selenium (an antioxidant mineral; see also "Selenium," page 488) on prostate cancer risk. The SELECT study was expected to conclude in 2013. However, a preliminary analysis in 2008 showed no difference in prostate cancer risk between the group taking the vitamin E supplement and the group taking the placebo. The results suggested that vitamin E might even have slightly increased the risk for prostate cancer. The selenium supplement did not appear to be beneficial either, and early results suggested that it might slightly increase the risk of developing diabetes. Because of these possible risks, the researchers advised participants to stop taking the supplements. Follow-up tests will continue for several years to learn more about any long-term effects of the supplements.

Vitamin E has also been studied in clinical trials of people who have had one cancer in order to see whether it could prevent cancer recurrence or formation of a second cancer. Clinical trials of people with head and neck cancer found it did not reduce the risk for recurrence or the risk for a second cancer.

Some scientists believe that taking high doses of antioxidant vitamins may actually interfere with the effectiveness of radiation therapy and some chemotherapy drugs. No studies have yet been done in humans to test this theory. However, one animal study found that vitamin E actually increased the effectiveness of the chemotherapy drug 5-FU against colon cancer in mice. Further studies are necessary to find out whether the results apply to humans.

Are there any possible problems or complications?

Vitamin E supplements found in multivitamins are generally considered safe as long as the levels do not exceed the Recommended Dietary Allowance. However, doses of vitamin E supplements of more than 800 IU (533 milligrams) taken over a long time can cause nausea, vomiting, stomach pain, and diarrhea. High doses of supplements may also slow the way the body absorbs vitamins A, D, and K and can result in deficiencies of these vitamins. Megadoses of vitamin E supplements are not advised for people who are taking blood-thinning medications, such as warfarin, because the supplements might counteract the effects of the drugs. People with cancer should talk to their doctors before taking vitamin E or other vitamin supplements, especially while they are undergoing chemotherapy or radiation therapy. Relying on this type of treatment alone and avoiding or delaying conventional medical care for cancer may have serious health consequences.

This product is sold as a dietary supplement in the United States. Unlike companies that produce drugs (which must provide the FDA with results of detailed testing showing their product is safe and effective before the drug is approved for sale), the companies that make supplements do not have to show evidence of safety or health benefits to the FDA before selling their products. Supplement products without any reliable scientific evidence of health benefits may still be sold as long as the companies selling them do not claim the supplements can prevent, treat, or cure any specific disease. Some such products may not contain the amount of the herb or substance that is written on the label, and some may include other substances (contaminants). Though the FDA has written new rules to improve the quality of manufacturing processes for dietary supplements and the accurate listing of supplement ingredients, these rules do not take full effect until 2010. The new rules also do not address the safety

of supplement ingredients or their effects on health when proper manufacturing techniques are used.

Most such supplements have not been tested to find out if they interact with medicines, foods, or other herbs and supplements. Even though some reports of interactions and harmful effects may be published, full studies of interactions and effects are not often available. Because of these limitations, any information on ill effects and interactions should be considered incomplete.

References

Alpha-Tocopherol, Beta Carotene Cancer Prevention Study Group. The effect of vitamin E and beta carotene on the incidence of lung cancer and other cancers in male smokers. *N Eng J Med.* 1994;330:1029-1035.

Bairati I, Meyer F, Gélinas M, Fortin A, Nabid A, Brochet F, Mercier JP, Têtu B, Harel F, Mâsse B, Vigneault E, Vass S, del Vecchio P, Roy J. A randomized trial of antioxidant vitamins to prevent second primary cancers in head and neck cancer patients. *J Natl Cancer Inst.* 2005;97:481-488.

Bjelakovic G, Nikolova D, Gluud LL, Simonetti RG, Gluud C. Mortality in randomized trials of antioxidant supplements for primary and secondary prevention: systematic review and meta-analysis. *JAMA.* 2007;297:842-857.

Byers T, Guerrero N. Epidemiologic evidence for vitamin C and vitamin E in cancer prevention. *Am J Clin Nutr.* 1995;62:1385S-1392S.

Dietary supplement fact sheet: vitamin E. Office of Dietary Supplements Web site. http://ods.od.nih.gov/factsheets/vitamine.asp. Updated January 23, 2007. Accessed June 6, 2008.

HOPE-TOO: NCI comment on published results. National Cancer Institute Web site. http://www.cancer.gov/newscenter/pressreleases/Hope-Too. Posted March 15, 2005. Accessed June 6, 2008.

Institute of Medicine (US). Panel on Dietary Antioxidants and Related Compounds. *Dietary Reference Intakes for Vitamin C, Vitamin E, Selenium, and Carotenoids : a Report of the Panel on Dietary Antioxidants and Related Compounds, Subcommittees on Upper Reference Levels of Nutrients and of Interpretation and Use of Dietary Reference Intakes, and the Standing Committee on the Scientific Evaluation of Dietary Reference Intakes, Food and Nutrition Board, Institute of Medicine.* Washington, DC: National Academy Press; 2000.

Jacobs EJ, Henion AK, Briggs PJ, Connell CJ, McCullough ML, Jonas CR, Rodriguez C, Calle EE, Thun MJ. Vitamin C and vitamin E supplement use and bladder cancer mortality in a large cohort of US men and women. *Am J Epidemiol.* 2002;156:1002-1010.

Kaplan GE, Collins T. Vitamin E deficiency. E-medicine Web site. http://www.emedicine.com/med/topic2383.htm. Updated July 19, 2006. Accessed June 6, 2008.

Lawenda BD, Kelly KM, Ladas EJ, Sagar SM, Vickers A, Blumberg JB. Should supplemental antioxidant administration be avoided during chemotherapy and radiation therapy? *J Natl Cancer Inst.* 2008;100:773-783.

Lonn E, Bosch J, Yusef S, Sheridan P, Pogue J, Arnold JM, Ross C, Arnold A, Sleight P, Probstfield J, Dagenais GR; HOPE and HOPE-TOO Trial Investigators. Effects of long-term vitamin E supplementation on cardiovascular events and cancer: a randomized controlled trial. *JAMA.* 2005;293:1338-1347.

Miller ER III, Pastor-Barriuso R, Dalal D, Reimersma RA, Appel LJ. Meta-analysis: high-dosage vitamin E supplementation may increase all-cause mortality. *Ann Intern Med.* 2005;142:37-46. Epub 2004 Nov 10.

Review of prostate cancer prevention study shows no benefit for use of selenium and vitamin E supplements [press release]. Bethesda, MD: National Cancer Institute Office of Media Relations; October 27, 2008. http://www.cancer.gov/newscenter/pressreleases/pressreleases/SELECTresults2008. Accessed December 4, 2008.

Vitamin E. Memorial Sloan-Kettering Cancer Center Web site. http://www.mskcc.org/mskcc/html/69415.cfm. Updated March 4, 2008. Accessed June 6, 2008.

Willett WC, Stampfer MJ. Clinical practice. What vitamins should I be taking, doctor? *N Engl J Med.* 2001;345:1819-1824.

VITAMIN K

Other common name(s): the clotting vitamin, vitamin K1, vitamin K2, vitamin K3
Scientific/medical name(s): phylloquinone, phytonadione, menaquinone, menadione

Description

Vitamin K is an essential nutrient that is needed by the liver in order to form proteins that promote blood clotting and prevent abnormal bleeding. There are three forms of vitamin K: K1, K2, and K3. Vitamin K1 (phylloquinone or phytonadione) is a natural nutrient found in green leafy vegetables, such as lettuce, cabbage, collard greens, broccoli, and turnip greens. Some oils, such as soybean oil and canola oil, contain vitamin K. It is also found in beans, olives, cereals, dairy products, some fruits, liver, and pork. Cooking does not remove the vitamin. Vitamin K2 (menaquinone) is a natural product of bacteria that reside in the lower intestinal tract. Vitamin K3 (menadione) is a potent synthetic (manmade) form of vitamin K.

Overview

Vitamin K is necessary for normal blood clotting and may be necessary for other activities. The human body obtains vitamin K from certain foods and bacteria that normally live in the intestines. Available scientific evidence does not support the use of vitamin K supplements for cancer treatment or prevention. However, a small clinical trial found that a compound similar to vitamin K2 seemed to reduce the recurrence of liver cancer after surgery.

How is it promoted for use?

Vitamin K is known primarily as a blood-clotting nutrient. However, some alternative medical practitioners claim that vitamin K3 is also an anticancer agent. Others claim that high doses of vitamin K3 and vitamin C supplements can inhibit tumor growth when taken together.

Vitamin K is also promoted as an ingredient in some cosmetic or herbal creams to lighten redness caused by broken blood vessels and to treat skin irritation (burns and sunburns) and scarring. They are often called "clarifying" creams and are usually recommended to be applied to the skin every day for several weeks.

What does it involve?

Healthy adults who eat plenty of leafy green vegetables generally get all the vitamin K they need from natural sources. The Food and Nutrition Board considers 90 micrograms per day for women and 120 micrograms per day for men to be an Adequate Intake (1 milligram is equal to 1,000 micrograms). Foods usually provide the body with about half of the normal supply of the vitamin, while intestinal bacteria produce the rest.

Only those who have symptoms of a vitamin K deficiency may need to take supplements. The signs of a deficiency include abnormal or excessive bleeding, such as frequent nosebleeds, abnormally bleeding gums, heavy menstruation, or blood in the urine or stool. People with these symptoms should see a doctor because these signs may also signal other, more serious, problems. A deficiency may result from extended treatment with antibiotics, which can kill the bacteria that produce vitamin K; liver damage; or intestinal disorders such as celiac disease, cystic fibrosis, or removal of part of the intestine. Chronic malnutrition, including alcoholism, can also cause vitamin K deficiency.

Newborns lack the bacteria in their intestines to produce vitamin K and may be at risk for serious bleeding. Newborns are usually given vitamin K supplements, either by injection or by mouth, while in the hospital. Babies who receive the supplements in the hospital do not need more supplements after they leave.

Phytonadione or phylloquinone (vitamin K1) and menaquinone (vitamin K2) supplements are available in tablet and capsule form from health food stores and on the Internet. The U.S. Food and Drug Administration (FDA) does not allow menadione (vitamin K3) to be sold as a dietary supplement for humans, although it is allowed in some feeds for farm animals.

What is the history behind it?

In 1935, a Danish scientist discovered that vitamin K was essential to blood clotting and named it for the Danish word for clotting, *koagulations*. Since then, laboratory and animal studies have been conducted to see whether vitamin K plays a role in preventing the development or spread of cancer, but there is no convincing evidence available to suggest that it does. However, in the 1990s, researchers began to worry about a possible link between childhood cancers, especially leukemia, and injections of vitamin K supplements in newborns. Further study has found no link between cancer and vitamin K injections. The American Academy of Pediatrics' latest recommendations advise that all newborns should receive the injection to prevent serious bleeding.

What is the evidence?

There is overwhelming scientific evidence that vitamin K is necessary for blood clotting. The intestinal bacteria that produce vitamin K are not present at birth. To avoid a deficiency of this vitamin that can lead to serious bleeding, most pediatricians recommend that an injection of vitamin K be given to newborns.

Some studies have suggested a link between low vitamin K intake or low blood levels of this vitamin and increased risk for some types of cancer. A large European epidemiologic study published in 2008 found higher risk for prostate cancer in men with low intake of some forms of vitamin K. A small clinical trial from Japan suggested that vitamin K lowers the risk for developing liver cancer among women with cirrhosis.

An animal study done in 1998 found that a manmade form of vitamin K known as compound 5 might slow the growth of cancer cells. Since then, several additional studies have suggested that some forms of vitamin K might be active against cancer cells in laboratory dishes or mice. Laboratory studies are pinpointing how it works and what kinds of cancer it might help. However, clinical trials in humans will be needed to find out whether vitamin K compounds play a role in cancer treatment.

There have been some studies examining whether menadione (vitamin K3) can help overcome resistance to certain types of chemotherapy drugs. Results in laboratory animals and cell cultures are mixed, but there is no evidence available of significant effects in humans yet. A small phase I clinical trial in California recently tested different doses of intravenous vitamin K3 in people with advanced cancer. The patients showed no improvement. In that study, several patients also had allergic reactions, especially at higher doses.

A 2006 clinical trial suggested that menatetrenone, a compound very similar to vitamin K2, may be able to reduce recurrence of liver cancer after surgery. This was a small pilot study, and more research is needed to be sure of this effect.

Some small, early studies also suggest that vitamin K might have a role in keeping bones strong, especially in older people. Further research is needed to confirm this possibility and, if confirmed, to determine the best way to use the vitamin.

One small human study looked at vitamin K cream to see whether it helped bruises to disappear faster after laser treatments. Researchers had people apply vitamin K cream twice a day to one side of their body and a dummy cream, or placebo, to the other. Bruises seemed to go away more quickly on the side of the body on which vitamin K cream was used. More studies are needed to find out whether this holds true and what concentration of cream is most effective.

Are there any possible problems or complications?

Natural vitamin K is considered safe as a normal part of a daily diet. Supplements of the vitamin are not usually needed unless recommended by a physician.

Injectable formulas of vitamin K (vitamin K3) can cause allergic reactions and some toxic effects. During clinical trials of vitamin K3, some patients experienced flushing of the face, numbness in their arms and legs, chest pain, and shortness of breath. Immediate severe allergies can cause shock and even death. Sometimes a milder reaction happens in the form of an itchy bump that comes up where the injection was given. The bump can take over a month to go away and can sometimes cause scarring. Injectable vitamin K can also cause red blood cells to be destroyed in some people. Rarely, allergic rashes can develop after using vitamin K creams on the skin.

Those who are on the blood-thinning medication warfarin (Coumadin) should know that vitamin K can make warfarin less effective. Talk with your health care provider before taking vitamin K supplements or changing the amount of vitamin K you take in through your diet.

Pregnant women who are on antiseizure medicines should get vitamin K supplements for two to four weeks before giving birth because of increased risk for bleeding in the newborn. Otherwise, the safety of vitamin K supplements during pregnancy is not known, although the vitamin K in foods is thought to be safe.

Relying on this type of treatment alone and avoiding or delaying conventional medical care for cancer may have serious health consequences.

This product is sold as a dietary supplement in the United States. Unlike companies that produce drugs (which must provide the FDA with results of detailed testing showing their product is safe and effective before the drug is approved for sale), the companies that make supplements do not have to show evidence of safety or health benefits to the FDA before selling their products. Supplement products without any reliable scientific evidence of health benefits may still be sold as long as the companies selling them do not claim the supplements can prevent, treat, or cure any specific disease. Some such products may not contain the amount of the herb or substance that is written on the label, and some may include other substances (contaminants). Though the FDA has written new rules to improve the quality of manufacturing processes for dietary supplements and the accurate listing of supplement ingredients, these rules do not take full effect until 2010. The new rules also do not address the safety of supplement ingredients or their effects on health when proper manufacturing techniques are used.

Most such supplements have not been tested to find out if they interact with medicines, foods, or other herbs and supplements. Even though some reports of interactions and harmful effects may be published, full studies of interactions and effects are not often available. Because of these limitations, any information on ill effects and interactions should be considered incomplete.

References

American Academy of Pediatrics Committee on Fetus and Newborn. Controversies concerning vitamin K and the newborn. *Pediatrics.* 2003;112:191-192.

Ansell P, Bull D, Roman E. Childhood leukaemia and intramuscular vitamin K: findings from a case-control study. *BMJ.* 1996;313:204-205.

Center for Food Safety and Applied Nutrition. Food additive status list. US Food and Drug Administration Web site. http://www.cfsan.fda.gov/~acrobat/opa-appa.pdf. Accessed June 6, 2008.

Food and Nutrition Board. Dietary reference intakes: vitamins. Institute of Medicine Web site. http://www.iom.edu/Object.File/Master/7/296/webtablevitamins.pdf. Accessed June 6, 2008.

Ge L, Wang Z, Wang M, Kar S, Carr BI. Involvement of c-Myc in growth inhibition of Hep 3B human hepatoma cells by a vitamin K analog. *J Hepatol.* 2004;41:823-829.

Habu D, Shiomi S, Tamori A, Takeda T, Tanaka T, Kubo S, Nishiguchi S. Role of vitamin K2 in the development of hepatocellular carcinoma in women with viral cirrhosis of the liver. *JAMA.* 2004;292:358-361.

Kaneda M, Zhang D, Bhattacharjee R, Nakahama K, Arii S, Morita I. Vitamin K2 suppresses malignancy of HuH7 hepatoma cells via inhibition of connexin 43. *Cancer Lett.* 2008;263:53-60.

Lim D, Morgan RJ Jr, Akman S, Margolin K, Carr BI, Leong L, Odujinrin O, Doroshow JH. Phase I trial of menadiol diphosphate (vitamin K3) in advanced malignancy. *Invest New Drugs.* 2005;23:235-239.

McKinney PA, Juszczak E, Findlay E, Smith K. Case-control study of childhood leukaemia and cancer in Scotland: findings for neonatal intramuscular vitamin K. *BMJ.* 1998;316:173-177.

Mizuta T, Ozaki I, Eguchi Y, Yasutake T, Kawazoe S, Fujimoto K, Yamamoto K. The effect of menatetrenone, a vitamin K2 analog, on disease recurrence and survival in patients with hepatocellular carcinoma after curative treatment: a pilot study. *Cancer.* 2006;106:867-872.

Nimptsch K, Rohrmann S, Linseisen J. Dietary intake of vitamin K and risk of prostate cancer in the Heidelberg cohort of the European Prospective Investigation into Cancer and Nutrition (EPIC-Heidelberg). *Am J Clin Nutr.* 2008;87:985-992.

Ni R, Nishikawa Y, Carr BI. Cell growth inhibition by a novel vitamin K is associated with induction of protein tyrosine phosphorylation. *J Biol Chem.* 1998;273:9906-9911.

Parker L, Cole M, Craft AW, Hey EN. Neonatal vitamin K administration and childhood cancer in the north of England: retrospective case-control study. *BMJ.* 1998;316:189-193.

Passmore SJ, Draper G, Brownbill P, Kroll M. Case-control studies of relation between childhood cancer and neonatal vitamin K administration. *BMJ.* 1998;316:178-184.

Passmore SJ, Draper G, Brownbill P, Kroll M. Ecological studies of relation between hospital policies on neonatal vitamin K administration and subsequent occurrence of childhood cancer. *BMJ.* 1998;316:184-189.

Russell RM. Vitamin and trace mineral deficiency and excess. In: Braunwald E, Fauci AS, Kasper DL, Hauser SL, Longo DL, Jameson JL, eds. *Harrison's Principles of Internal Medicine.* 15th ed. New York: McGraw-Hill; 2001:467.

Serra-Baldrich E, Dalmau J, Pla C, Muntañola AA. Contact dermatitis due to clarifying cream. *Contact Dermatitis.* 2005;53:174-175.

Shah NS, Lazarus MC, Budgodel R, Hsia SL, He J, Duncan R, Baumann L. The effects of topical vitamin K on bruising after laser treatment. *J Am Acad Dermatol.* 2002;47:241-244.

Tetef M, Margolin K, Ahn C, Akman S, Chow W, Coluzzi P, Leong L, Morgan RJ Jr, Raschko J, Shibata S, et al. Mitomycin C and menadione for the treatment of advanced gastrointestinal cancers: a phase II trial. *J Cancer Res Clin Oncol.* 1995;121:103-106.

US Department of Agriculture. Vitamin K: another reason to eat your greens. Agricultural Research Service Web site. http://www.ars.usda.gov/is/AR/archive/jan00/green0100.htm. Updated August 13, 2004. Accessed June 6, 2008.

Vitamin K deficiency. Merck Manual of Diagnosis and Therapy Online Edition. Merck Web site. http://www.merck.com/mmpe/sec01/ch002/ch002a.html#tb002_1. Accessed June 23, 2008.

Vitamin K. Medline Plus Web site. http://www.nlm.nih.gov/medlineplus/druginfo/natural/patient-vitamink.html. Updated March 1, 2008. Accessed June 6, 2008.

von Kries R. Oral versus intramuscular phytomenadione: safety and efficacy compared. *Drug Saf.* 1999;21:1-6.

von Kries R, Hachmeister A, Göbel U. Can 3 oral 2 mg doses of vitamin K effectively prevent late vitamin K deficiency bleeding? *Eur J Pediatr.* 1999;158(suppl 3):S183-S186.

Xu CJ, Zhang Y, Wang J, Zhang TM. Menadione reduced doxorubicin resistance in Ehrlich ascites carcinoma cells in vitro. *Zhongguo Yao Li Xue Bao.* 1998;19:273-276.

WHITE BIRCH

Other common name(s): white birch, silver birch, butalin, betulinic acid
Scientific/medical name(s): *Betula pendula, Betula alba*

Description

White birch is a tree that grows in northern Europe and North America. The bark, leaves, and buds from this and related birch trees are used in herbal and folk medicines. One of the chemicals that has been isolated from birch bark is called betulin. Betulinic acid, which is made from betulin, is being studied as a possible cancer treatment. Betulin has also been found in many other plants.

Overview

Birch bark, buds, and leaves are used in folk medicine but have not been studied to find out whether they are safe or effective. However, betulinic acid may hold promise as an anticancer agent. Some laboratory and animal studies of betulinic acid have reported antitumor activity. Additional studies are under way to find out whether it has a role in treating several forms of cancer, including melanoma and certain brain cancers. Clinical trials are needed to determine what effect, if any, betulinic acid may have in treating cancer in humans.

How is it promoted for use?

Birch bark or white birch (which contains betulinic acid and other compounds) is used on the skin to treat warts, eczema, and other skin conditions. Promoters say that birch tea can be taken internally as a diuretic or a mild sedative and that it can be used as a treatment for rheumatism, gout, and kidney stones. The leaves are sometimes used on the scalp to help with hair loss and dandruff. Birch tar (an oil distilled from birch bark) is used on the skin for skin irritations and parasites. Other claims for birch bark include the treatment of diarrhea, dysentery, and cholera.

Some researchers believe that betulin, which can be extracted from birch bark and other sources, causes some types of tumor cells to start a process of self-destruction called apoptosis. They also believe that betulinic acid slows the growth of several types of tumor cells and the human immunodeficiency virus (HIV). Some researchers also think it has antibacterial properties.

What does it involve?

Pure betulinic acid is not directly available for public use, but birch bark flakes, powder, capsules, oil, sap, and liquid extracts are sold in herbal medicine shops and on the Internet. Birch bark, buds, or leaves are used internally or externally. Tea can be made by steeping a teaspoon of the birch bark in a cup of boiling water for fifteen minutes. Proponents recommend drinking from two to five cups of tea per day. Birch leaves or powder can also be used to make tea. For skin conditions, birch leaf tea may be used as a wash or added to bath water. Birch bark or leaves can be applied directly to the skin as well. Birch oil is sometimes used in ointments or liniments and is considered a substitute for wintergreen. Some people also drink small amounts of fresh or bottled birch sap as a tonic.

What is the history behind it?

White birch bark has been used by Native Americans as a folk remedy for some time. It was used in tea and other beverages to treat stomach and intestinal problems such as diarrhea and dysentery. In Russia, it has been used since 1834. In Europe, birch sap was fermented into beer, wine, and other spirits. Its inner bark was sometimes eaten as food.

In 1994, scientists at the University of North Carolina reported that chemicals found in white birch bark slowed the growth of HIV. The following year, a researcher at the University of

Illinois reported that betulinic acid killed melanoma cells in mice. Since then, a number of researchers have conducted laboratory tests on betulinic acid to determine its antitumor properties. Since that time, betulin has been found in several other plant sources.

What is the evidence?

There has not been enough scientific study of white birch in humans to draw conclusions about its usefulness in treating illness, although some birch extracts have been studied for safety. Xylitol, a type of sugar, can be made from birch and has been approved to flavor food. Several other compounds extracted from birch have also been approved by the U.S. Food and Drug Administration (FDA) for use as food additives.

Betulinic acid has not been studied in humans, but several laboratory studies have looked at its effects when it is added to cancer cells growing in laboratory dishes. These studies, using the pure chemical betulinic acid rather than birch bark, have been published in peer-reviewed medical journals and suggest that betulinic acid holds some promise for patients with melanoma, certain nervous system tumors, and other forms of cancer. Three German studies concluded that betulinic acid showed antitumor activity against cells from certain types of nervous system cancers in children. Two laboratory studies conducted at the University of Illinois indicated that betulinic acid may prove useful as an antitumor drug.

Several studies have found that betulinic acid increases sensitivity of cancer cells in laboratory dishes or in rodents to chemotherapy drugs such as vincristine, 5-fluorouracil, irinotecan, and oxaliplatin. Some researchers are testing synthetic chemicals related to betulinic acid to determine which are most effective at killing cancer cells or preventing their growth. Studies are still going on to find out whether these results can be applied to humans.

Results from a German nonrandomized clinical trial published in 2006 indicated that birch bark extract may be an effective treatment for actinic keratosis, a precancerous skin condition. However, birch bark extract cannot be recommended for actinic keratoses until further studies have compared it with conventional treatments already known to be safe and effective.

Are there any possible problems or complications?

Birch products that are sold as supplements have not been studied for safety. However, people who are sensitive to aspirin should not use birch products, because birch contains large amounts of aspirin-like compounds. Birch may also pose a hazard to people with poor heart or kidney function. The full range of effects is not well known. Pregnant women, breastfeeding women, and children should not use birch products. Birch has been reported to cause skin rashes and, like most plants, may cause allergic reactions.

Researchers are still studying betulinic acid. Further testing is needed to find out whether it is safe for humans. Relying on this type of treatment alone and avoiding or delaying conventional medical care for cancer may have serious health consequences.

This product is sold as a dietary supplement in the United States. Unlike companies that produce drugs (which must provide the FDA with results of detailed testing showing their product is safe and effective before the drug is approved for sale), the companies that make supplements do not have to show evidence of safety or health benefits to the FDA before selling their products. Supplement products without any reliable scientific evidence of health benefits may still be sold as long as the companies selling them do not claim the supplements can prevent, treat, or cure any specific disease. Some such products may not contain the amount of the herb or substance that is written on the label, and some may include other substances (contaminants). Though the FDA has written new rules to improve the quality of manufacturing processes for dietary supplements and the accurate listing of supplement ingredients, these rules do not take full effect until 2010. The new rules also do not address the safety of supplement ingredients or their effects on health when proper manufacturing techniques are used.

Most such supplements have not been tested to find out if they interact with medicines, foods, or other herbs and supplements. Even though some reports of interactions and harmful effects may be published, full studies of interactions and effects are not often available. Because of these limitations, any information on ill effects and interactions should be considered incomplete.

References

Beaulieu JE. Herbal therapy interactions with immunosuppressive agents. US Pharmacist Web site. http://www.uspharmacist.com/oldformat.asp?url=newlook/files/feat/herbals.htm. Accessed June 9, 2008.

Betulaceae (birch family). Botanical Dermatology Data Base Web site. http://bodd.cf.ac.uk/BotDermFolder/BotDermB/BETU.html. Accessed June 9, 2008.

Center for Food Safety and Applied Nutrition. EAFUS: a food additive database. US Food and Drug Administration Web site. http://vm.cfsan.fda.gov/~dms/eafus.html. Accessed June 9, 2008.

Chintharlapalli S, Papineni S, Ramaiah SK, Safe S. Betulinic acid inhibits prostate cancer growth through inhibition of specificity protein transcription factors. *Cancer Res.* 2007;67:2816-2823.

Eiznhamer DA, Xu ZQ. Betulinic acid: a promising anticancer candidate. *IDrugs.* 2004;7:359-373.

Gruenwald J. *PDR for Herbal Medicines.* 3rd ed. Montvale, NJ: Thomson PDR; 2004.

Huyke C, Laszczyk M, Scheffler A, Ernst R, Schempp CM. Treatment of actinic keratoses with birch bark extract: a pilot study [in German]. *J Dtsch Dermatol Ges.* 2006;4:132-136.

Jung GR, Kim KJ, Choi CH, Lee TB, Han SI, Han HK, Lim SC. Effect of betulinic acid on anticancer drug-resistant colon cancer cells. *Basic Clin Pharmacol Toxicol.* 2007;101:277-285.

Kasperczyk H, La Ferla-Brühl K, Westhoff MA, Behrend L, Zwacka RM, Debatin KM, Fulda S. Betulinic acid as new activator of NF-kappaB: molecular mechanisms and implications for cancer therapy. *Oncogene.* 2005;24:6945-6956.

Kessler JH, Mullauer FB, de Roo GM, Medema JP. Broad in vitro efficacy of plant-derived betulinic acid against cell lines derived from the most prevalent human cancer types. *Cancer Lett.* 2007;251:132-145.

Liby K, Honda T, Williams CR, Risingsong R, Royce DB, Suh N, Dinkova-Kostova AT, Stephenson KK, Talalay P, Sundararajan C, Gribble GW, Sporn MB. Novel semisynthetic analogues of betulinic acid with diverse cytoprotective, antiproliferative, and proapoptotic activities. *Mol Cancer Ther.* 2007;6:2113-2119.

Pisha E, Chai H, Lee IS, Chagwedera TE, Farnsworth NR, Cordell GA, Beecher CW, Fong HH, Kinghorn AD, Brown DM, et al. Discovery of betulinic acid as a selective inhibitor of human melanoma that functions by induction of apoptosis. *Nat Med.* 1995;1:1046-1051.

Sawada N, Kataoka K, Kondo K, Arimochi H, Fujino H, Takahashi Y, Miyoshi T, Kuwahara T, Monden Y, Ohnishi Y. Betulinic acid augments the inhibitory effects of vincristine on growth and lung metastasis of B16F10 melanoma cells in mice. *Br J Cancer.* 2004;90:1672-1678.

Schmidt ML, Kuzmanoff KL, Ling-Indeck L, Pezzuto JM. Betulinic acid induces apoptosis in human neuroblastoma cell lines. *Eur J Cancer.* 1997;33:2007-2010.

Thurnher D, Turhani D, Pelzmann M, Wannemacher B, Knerer B, Formanek M, Wacheck V, Selzer E. Betulinic acid: a new cytotoxic compound against malignant head and neck cancer cells. *Head Neck.* 2003;25:732-740.

WILD YAM

Other common name(s): wild Mexican yam, colic root, rheumatism root, Chinese yam, shan yao

Scientific/medical name(s): *Dioscorea villosa, Dioscorea oppositifolia, Dioscorea opposita, Dioscorea batatas*

Description

Wild yam is a perennial vine, also known as the wild Mexican yam or *Dioscorea villosa*, which is native to North America. A similar variety called the Chinese yam is an ornamental plant native to China that now grows in North America as well. It is known as *Dioscorea oppositifolia* and *Dioscorea batatas* but is called *shan yao* in Chinese herbal medicine. The roots and rootstock, or rhizomes, of both types of yam are used in herbal remedies. These plants are different from the yams and sweet potatoes commonly eaten in North America.

Overview

Although creams and oral supplements containing wild yam extracts are popular among women as an alternative to postmenopausal hormone therapy, available scientific evidence does not support claims that they are safe or effective. Neither estrogen nor progesterone can be found in wild yams, although these yams may contain compounds that have effects similar to, but milder than, estrogen. Some wild yam creams have synthetic (sometimes called "natural") progesterone added to them.

How is it promoted for use?

The wild Mexican yam and the Chinese yam are two types of yams that are promoted in similar ways. Proponents claim that a cream made from the wild Mexican yam contains natural progesterone (a hormone that plays a vital role in women's health) and is therefore effective in treating premenstrual syndrome (PMS) and menstrual irregularity, as well as hot flashes and other symptoms of menopause. Supporters say that using wild yam as an alternative to postmenopausal hormone therapy significantly lowers the risk for breast and endometrial cancer. Marketers also claim that their product helps women lose weight, increases energy and stamina, and enhances sex drive. A few marketers imply that wild yam can be used as herbal birth control. By contrast, some suggest that it improves fertility. It is also recommended to enlarge breasts and reduce wrinkles.

Supporters claim that the wild Mexican yam, when taken internally, helps arthritis pain, morning sickness, painful menstruation, bronchitis, asthma, whooping cough, cramps, and intestinal ailments such as Crohn's disease, colitis, and chronic diarrhea.

The Chinese yam is claimed to stimulate appetite and to be a remedy for chronic diarrhea, asthma, fatigue, uncontrollable or frequent urination, diabetes, and emotional instability. Proponents claim the Chinese yam can be used externally to speed the healing of boils and abscesses. Herbalists also use it to treat colic because it is thought to relieve intestinal spasms.

What does it involve?

Creams or gels made from wild yams are rubbed directly onto the skin and are available from health food stores and on the Internet. Some of these creams have synthetic, or manmade, progesterone added to them, although most don't advertise this addition; if they do, it is often mentioned as "natural" progesterone. Wild yam is also sold as a capsule, liquid, dried root, and tincture to be taken by mouth. Some sellers combine it with vitamins, minerals, or other herbs, such as black cohosh (see page 273). In homeopathic medicine, the wild yam from the *Dioscorea villosa* plant is used fresh or dried and put in liquid extracts (see "Homeopathy," page 753). The Chinese yam can also be used fresh or baked with flour or clay. Wild yam capsules and other forms are available in herbal shops and over the Internet. Dosages vary by manufacturer.

What is the history behind it?

In East Indian traditional medicine, the wild yam is used to treat sexual and hormonal problems. Chinese herbalists have long used the herb for rheumatism, asthma, and digestive and urinary complaints. Wild yam has also been used in American folk medicine to treat coughs and to induce sweating and vomiting. Some sources suggest that Native Americans and early settlers used it for its ability to relieve intestinal spasms, which is how it got the name "colic root."

In the 1960s, progesterone and other steroid hormones were chemically manufactured, in part using ingredients from the Mexican wild yam. This practice may be the reason for the misconception that the progesterone "precursors" in wild yam could be converted into progesterone in the body.

Some wild yam creams have been found to contain added synthetic progesterone.

What is the evidence?

Contrary to claims, wild yam cannot supply the body with progesterone. The plant contains the chemical diosgenin, which can be converted into a synthetic form of progesterone through a lengthy process in the laboratory. There is no available scientific evidence that suggests the body can convert diosgenin into progesterone. Some of the chemicals in the plant resemble a weak form of estrogen, another hormone that is important in female physiology, but estrogen's effects on the body are very different from those of progesterone. Drugs manufactured from diosgenin are used to treat asthma, arthritis, eczema, and to control fertility.

Available scientific evidence does not support claims that the wild yam can help the symptoms of menopause or premenstrual syndrome, reduce wrinkles, or enlarge breasts. However, since progesterone is absorbed through the skin and mucous membranes, a wild yam cream with added progesterone can have pharmacologic effects on the whole body.

Are there any possible problems or complications?

Large doses of wild yam can cause nausea, vomiting, and diarrhea. Women who are pregnant or breastfeeding should not use wild yam. Although rare, allergic reactions to wild yam can occur, including rashes, asthma, and other symptoms.

There are several problems with using wild yam creams with added progesterone. They are often not labeled as containing added progesterone, and the amount in the cream varies. Even if the amount of progesterone in the cream was consistent and declared, the body absorbs progesterone in different amounts at different times and from different places on the body, meaning that any effect on the body is unreliable. In addition, progesterone can have side effects such as headache, breast tenderness, upset stomach, constipation, tiredness, and irritability. In rare cases, there can be serious side effects, such as dizziness, faintness, shortness of breath, blurred vision, seizures, and swelling of the lips, mouth, or throat. Relying on this type of treatment alone and avoiding or delaying conventional medical care for cancer may have serious health consequences.

This product is sold as a dietary supplement in the United States. Unlike companies that produce drugs (which must provide the FDA with results of detailed testing showing their product is safe and effective before the drug is approved for sale), the companies that make supplements do not have to show evidence of safety or health benefits to the FDA before selling their products. Supplement products without any reliable scientific evidence of health benefits may still be sold as long as the companies selling them do not claim the supplements can prevent, treat, or cure any specific disease. Some such products may not contain the amount of the herb or substance that is written on the label, and some may include other substances (contaminants). Though the FDA has written new rules to improve the quality of manufacturing processes for dietary supplements and the accurate listing of supplement ingredients, these rules do not take full effect until 2010. The new rules also do not address the safety of supplement ingredients or their effects on health when proper manufacturing techniques are used.

Most such supplements have not been tested to find out if they interact with medicines, foods, or other herbs and supplements. Even though some reports of interactions and harmful effects may be published, full studies of interactions and effects are not often available. Because of these limitations, any information on ill effects and interactions should be considered incomplete.

References

Bown D. *New Encyclopedia of Herbs & Their Uses.* New York: DK Publishing Inc; 2001.

Burry KA, Patton PE, Hermsmeyer K. Percutaneous absorption of progesterone in postmenopausal women treated with transdermal estrogen. *Am J Obstet Gynecol.* 1999;180:1504-1511.

Carey BJ, Carey AH, Patel S, Carter G, Studd JW. A study to evaluate serum and urinary hormone levels following short and long term administration of two regimens of progesterone cream in postmenopausal women. *BJOG.* 2000;107:722-726.

Foster S, Duke JA. *A Field Guide to Medicinal Plants: Eastern and Central North America.* Boston, MA: Houghton Mifflin; 1990.

Fugh-Berman A. "Bust enhancing" herbal products. *Obstet Gynecol.* 2003;101:1345-1349.

Fugh-Berman A. Wild yam cream, diosgenin, and natural progesterone: what can they really do for you? National Women's Health Network. *The Network News.* January 1, 1999.

Gorski T. "Wild yam cream" threatens women's health. Quackwatch Web site. http://www.quackwatch.org/01QuackeryRelatedTopics/wildyam.html. Updated July 19, 2002. Accessed June 9, 2008.

Komesaroff PA, Black CV, Cable V, Sudhir K. Effects of wild yam extract on menopausal symptoms, lipids and sex hormones in healthy menopausal women. *Climacteric.* 2001;4:144-150.

Progesterone. Medline Plus Web site. http://www.nlm.nih.gov/medlineplus/druginfo/medmaster/a604017.html. Updated July 1, 2004. Accessed June 9, 2008.

Tu M. Element stewardship abstract for *Dioscorea oppositifolia* L. syn. *Dioscoria batatas* (Decne): Chinese yam, cinnamon vine. The Nature Conservatory Web site. http://tncinvasives.ucdavis.edu/esadocs/documnts/diosopp.rtf. Accessed June 9, 2008.

Wild Yam (Discorea villosa). Medline Plus Web site. http://www.nlm.nih.gov/medlineplus/druginfo/natural/patient-wildyam.html. Updated February 1, 2008. Accessed June 9, 2008.

Wild yam. Memorial Sloan-Kettering Cancer Center Web site. http://www.mskcc.org/mskcc/html/69420.cfm. Updated July 20, 2007. Accessed June 9, 2008.

Wild yam. WholeHealthMD Web site. http://www.wholehealthmd.com/ME2/dirmod.asp?sid=17E09E7CFFF640448FFB0B4FC1B7FEF0&nm=Reference+Library&type=AWHN_Supplements&mod=Supplements&mid=&id=8BD6A74701414C1C9131AC1DE48FC415&tier=2. Updated September 12, 2005. Accessed June 9, 2008.

WORMWOOD

Other common name(s): absinthium, absinth wormwood
Scientific/medical name(s): *Artemisia absinthium*

Description

Wormwood is a shrubby perennial plant whose upper shoots, flowers, and leaves are used in herbal remedies and as a bitter flavoring for alcoholic drinks. It is native to Europe, northern Africa, and western Asia, and now also grows in North America.

Overview

Available scientific evidence does not support claims that wormwood is effective in treating cancer, the side effects of cancer treatment, or any other conditions. The plant contains a volatile oil with a high level of thujone (see "Thuja," page 511). There are reports that taking large doses of wormwood internally can cause serious problems with the liver and kidneys. It can also cause nausea, vomiting, stomach pain, headache, dizziness, seizures, numbness of the legs and arms, delirium, and paralysis.

Wormwood, or *Artemisia absinthium*, should not be confused with sweet wormwood, or *Artemisia annua*. While wormwood is related to sweet wormwood, they are used in different ways. Extracts of sweet wormwood have been used in traditional herbal medicine, and an active ingredient, artemisinin, is now used in conventional medical treatment of malaria.

How is it promoted for use?

Wormwood is promoted as a sedative and anti-inflammatory. There are also claims that it can treat loss of appetite, stomach disorders, and liver and gallbladder complaints. In folk medicine it is used for a wide range of stomach disorders, fever, and irregular menstruation. It is also used to fight intestinal worms. Externally, it is applied to poorly healing wounds, ulcers, skin blotches, and insect bites. It is used in moxibustion treatments for cancer (see "Moxibustion," page 223).

What does it involve?

Wormwood is taken in small doses for a short period of time, usually a maximum of four weeks. It is available as a capsule and as a liquid that can be added to water to make a tincture. The whole herb is sometimes brewed as a tea. Wormwood oil, washes, or poultices can also be used on the skin. Although pure wormwood is not available, "thujone-free" wormwood extract has been approved by the U.S. Food and Drug Administration (FDA) for use in foods and as a flavoring in alcoholic drinks such as vermouth.

What is the history behind it?

Artemisia absinthium was used by Hippocrates, and the earliest references to wormwood in Western civilization can be found in the Bible. Extract of wormwood was also used in ancient Egypt. The herb is mentioned often in first-century Greek and Roman writings and reportedly was placed in the sandals of Roman soldiers to help soothe their sore feet. It was taken as a treatment for tapeworms as far back as the Middle Ages.

In 1797, Henri Pernod developed absinthe, an alcoholic drink containing distilled spirits of wormwood, fennel, anise and sometimes other herbs. Absinthe became very popular in Europe and the United States in the nineteenth century. It was eventually banned in several countries in the early twentieth century due to its purported ill effects and addictive qualities. More recent analysis has suggested that, when properly prepared and distilled, the thujone content in these drinks was very low. It appears more likely that the addictiveness and other ill effects of absinthe were due to its alcohol content, which is around 60 to 85 percent. Varying additives or impurities from different distillers may have also produced some of these effects. Even though absinthe is illegal in some countries, various types can be found in some European countries. However, their thujone content is strictly limited. Wormwood is also an ingredient in vermouth and other drinks.

What is the evidence?

Available scientific studies do not support the use of wormwood for the treatment of cancer or the side effects of conventional cancer treatment. There is not enough evidence available to support its use for other conditions. Wormwood oil has been tested in laboratory studies and appears to inhibit the growth of some fungi. However, human tests have not been completed.

Some derivatives of *Artemisia annua*, or sweet wormwood, a relative of wormwood, have been shown to be effective in the treatment of malaria. In fact, the World Health Organization approved artemisinin for use against malaria in Africa in 2004. These extracts also show some promise in laboratory studies as cancer treatment drugs. Further studies are required to find out whether the anticancer results apply to people. It is important to remember that extracted compounds are not the same as the whole herb, and study results are not likely to show the same effects.

Are there any possible problems or complications?

Wormwood should be avoided, especially by women who are pregnant or breastfeeding, by people who have had seizures, and by those with ulcers or stomach irritation. Thujone, a component of wormwood, is known to cause muscle spasms, seizures, and hallucinations if taken internally. In high doses it is known to damage the liver and the kidneys.

Because of its thujone content, large doses of wormwood taken internally can lead to vomiting, stomach and intestinal cramps, headaches, dizziness, nervous system problems, and seizures. Wormwood can also lead to liver failure. *The New England Journal of Medicine* reported that a man who ordered essential oil of wormwood over the Internet, thinking he had purchased absinthe, suffered liver failure shortly after drinking the oil. Wormwood may also make seizures more likely and may interfere with the anticonvulsant effects of medicines such as phenobarbital.

The plant is a relative of ragweed and daisies. Those with allergies to these types of plants may also be allergic to wormwood. Contact with wormwood can cause rashes. Relying on this type of treatment alone and avoiding or delaying conventional medical care for cancer may have serious health consequences.

This product is sold as a dietary supplement in the United States. Unlike companies that produce drugs (which must provide the FDA with results of detailed testing showing their product is safe and effective before the drug is approved for sale), the companies that make supplements do not have to show evidence of safety or health benefits to the FDA before selling their products. Supplement products without any reliable scientific evidence of health benefits may still be sold as long as the companies selling them do not claim the supplements can prevent, treat, or cure any specific disease. Some such products may not contain the amount of the herb or substance that is written on the label, and some may include other substances (contaminants). Though the FDA has written new rules to improve the quality of manufacturing processes for dietary supplements and the accurate listing of supplement ingredients, these rules do not take full effect until 2010. The new rules also do not address the safety of supplement ingredients or their effects on health when proper manufacturing techniques are used.

Most such supplements have not been tested to find out if they interact with medicines, foods, or other herbs and supplements. Even though some reports of interactions and harmful effects may be published, full studies of interactions and effects are not often available. Because of these limitations, any information on ill effects and interactions should be considered incomplete.

References

Alpha-thujone (546-80-5). National Toxicology Program Web site. http://ntp.niehs.nih.gov/index.cfm?objectid=03DB8C36-E7A1-9889-3BDF8436F2A8C51F. Updated May 2, 2006. Accessed June 9, 2008.

Arnold WN. Vincent van Gogh and the thujone connection. *JAMA.* 1998;260:3042-3044.

Baggot MJ. Absinthe: frequently asked questions and some attempted answers. The Vaults of Erowid Web site. http://www.erowid.org/chemicals/absinthe/absinthe_faq.shtml. Accessed June 10, 2008.

Blumenthal M, ed. *The Complete German Commission E Monographs: Therapeutic Guide to Herbal Medicines.* Austin, TX: American Botanical Council; 1998.

Bown D. *New Encyclopedia of Herbs & Their Uses.* New York: DK Publishing Inc; 2001.

Efferth T. Molecular pharmacology and pharmacogenomics of artemisinin and its derivatives in cancer cells. *Curr Drug Targets.* 2006;7:407-421.

Fetrow CW, Avila JR. *Professional's Handbook of Complementary & Alternative Medicines.* Philadelphia, PA: Lippincott Williams & Wilkins; 2004.

Gruenwald J. *PDR for Herbal Medicines.* 3rd ed. Montvale, NJ: Thomson PDR; 2004.

Hsu E. Reflections on the 'discovery' of the antimalarial qinghao. *Br J Clin Pharmacol.* 2006;61:666-670.

Kordali S, Cakir A, Mavi A, Kilic H, Yildirim A. Screening of chemical composition and antifungal and antioxidant activities of the essential oils from three Turkish artemisia species. *J Agric Food Chem.* 2005;53:1408-1416.

Lachenmeier DW, Emmert J, Kuballa T, Sartor G. Thujone—cause of absinthism? *Forensic Sci Int.* 2006;158:1-8.

Miller LG. Herbal medicinals: selected clinical considerations focusing on known or potential drug-herb interactions. *Arch Intern Med.* 1998;158:2200-2211.

Mutabingwa TK, Anthony D, Heller A, Hallett R, Ahmed J, Drakeley C, Greenwood BM, Whitty CJ. Amodiaquine alone, amodiaquine+sulfadoxine-pyrimethamine, amodiaquine+artesunate, and artemether-lumefantrine for outpatient treatment of malaria in Tanzanian children: a four-arm randomised effectiveness trial. *Lancet.* 2005;365:1474-1480.

Nam W, Tak J, Ryu JK, Jung M, Yook JI, Kim HJ, Cha IH. Effects of artemisinin and its derivatives on growth inhibition and apoptosis of oral cancer cells. *Head Neck.* 2007;29:335-340.

Rediscovering wormwood: qinghaosu for malaria. *Lancet.* 1992;339:649-651.

Singh NP, Lai HC. Artemisinin induces apoptosis in human cancer cells. *Anticancer Res.* 2004;24:2277-2280.

van Agtmael MA, Eggelte TA, van Boxtel CJ. Artemisinin drugs in the treatment of malaria: from medicinal herb to registered medication. *Trends Pharmacol Sci.* 1999;20:199-205.

Weisbord SD, Soule JB, Kimmel PL. Poison on line--acute renal failure caused by oil of wormwood purchased through the Internet. *N Engl J Med.* 1997;337(12):825-827.
Erratum in:
N Engl J Med. 1997;337(20):1483.

Wormwood. PDRhealth Web site. http://www.pdrhealth.com/drug_info/nmdrugprofiles/herbaldrugs/102980.shtml. Accessed June 9, 2008.

YOHIMBE

Other common name(s): yohimbe bark, yohimbine hydrochloride, johimbe, Actibine, Aphrodyne, Dayto Himbin, Yocon, Yohimex, Yomax
Scientific/medical name(s): *Pausinystalia yohimbe, Corynanthe yohimbe*

Description

Yohimbe is an evergreen tree native to western Africa, specifically the countries of Nigeria, Cameroon, Gabon, and the Congo. It can reach a height of ninety feet. The dried bark is used in folk and herbal remedies.

The drug yohimbine hydrochloride (called yohimbine) is derived from yohimbe bark and has been approved by the U.S. Food and Drug Administration (FDA) for prescription use only.

Overview

Yohimbe bark has been used as an aphrodisiac for many years. It has been declared an unsafe herb in Germany because of such complications as increased heart rate and blood pressure and even kidney failure. In the United States, supplements that are labeled as containing yohimbe bark often contain very little of it.

On the other hand, yohimbine hydrochloride, the substance in yohimbe bark thought to help with erections, is regulated as a prescription drug and is standardized to contain a precise amount of the labeled ingredient. It is mainly used as a treatment for erectile dysfunction (impotence), although there are concerns about its side effects and interactions with other medicines, alcohol, and even some foods. Yohimbine hydrochloride is often called simply yohimbine, although it is made under several brand names.

How is it promoted for use?

Yohimbe bark extract is promoted as an aphrodisiac and sexual enhancer for men and women. Proponents say that yohimbe extracts are powerful antioxidants that can prevent heart attacks. Some also tout it as a stimulant, antidepressant, and aid to weight loss.

Yohimbine hydrochloride, often simply called yohimbine, is thought to be the most vital active ingredient of yohimbe bark. The drug yohimbine is available by prescription for the treatment of erectile dysfunction and is supposed to improve blood flow to the penis. It has also been promoted to treat exhaustion, drug overdose (from clonidine), and a form of low blood pressure that occurs when standing, called postural hypotension. Yohimbine can also be used to enlarge the pupil of the eye to help doctors examine the inside of the eyes.

What does it involve?

Yohimbe bark and bark extracts are sold as capsules, tablets, liquids, and powders. Some people make the bark into a tea, while others place the powdered bark under the tongue or sniff it.

Extracts and supplements labeled as yohimbine that are sold in health food stores and over the Internet contain varying amounts of yohimbe and other ingredients. FDA researchers analyzed a number of commercial yohimbe bark products available over the counter. They found that the supplements contained less of the amount of yohimbine than would be found in actual yohimbe bark and also contained substances that do not occur in yohimbe bark.

The prescription form of yohimbine is strictly regulated by the FDA. It is approved only for the treatment of impotence and is available in tablets and capsules. The standard dosage is 5.4 milligrams taken three times a day for no longer than ten weeks.

What is the history behind it?

In Africa, yohimbe has been used for generations as an aphrodisiac and a treatment for erectile dysfunction. It was also used to treat fevers, leprosy, high blood pressure, and heart problems. In addition, it was used by warriors as a stimulant before battle. The powder was sometimes smoked to induce hallucinations, and yohimbe poultices were placed on the skin as an antiseptic and treatment for pain. In the 1890s, yohimbe began to be used medicinally in Europe. Yohimbe has been used to treat erectile dysfunction for more than one hundred years.

After manufacturers purified the substance called yohimbine hydrochloride from the tree's bark, it has been sold by prescription only in the United States. Yohimbe was in use by 1938, before new drugs were required to be reviewed and approved by the FDA. When stricter regulatory practices were introduced, sales of existing drugs were allowed to continue. Its popularity has decreased as sildenafil (Viagra) and similar drugs were approved starting in the late 1990s. Even with this decline in popularity, there is concern that the yohimbe trees of Africa are being killed by over-harvesting because of yohimbe's popularity as a drug and dietary supplement.

What is the evidence?

Most clinical trials have looked at yohimbine rather than yohimbe bark. Clinical trials have found contradictions regarding the effectiveness of yohimbine for treating erectile dysfunction. The American Urological Association guidelines on treatment of erectile dysfunction state that it could not draw conclusions about yohimbine's effectiveness and safety and that larger studies are needed to evaluate it.

A randomized clinical trial found that yohimbine may be a useful treatment for erectile dysfunction caused by psychological problems. Another randomized clinical study found that yohimbine was no better than a placebo as a first treatment for erectile dysfunction that had some physical basis. Other studies with yohimbine have shown it helps some with mild erectile problems, even those that have a physical basis. A review study concluded that yohimbine has a modest effect on erectile dysfunction caused by psychological factors, but not on erectile dysfunction due to physical causes. It appears that more research needs to be done to clarify the role of yohimbine in the treatment of erectile dysfunction. No studies to date have compared yohimbine with newer treatments for this problem.

It is important to note that these studies were done using the drug yohimbine. Extracted chemicals are not the same as yohimbe bark. Studies of yohimbine would be expected to produce different results from studies using the raw plant. The unpurified plant extract would have different amounts of active compounds, more compounds that may cause unexpected effects, and many other differences.

Yohimbine is now being used with other substances for the treatment of erectile dysfunction and may be helpful for men who cannot take the newer drugs for impotence. A 2002 study looked at yohimbine combined with L-arginine glutamate (a substance thought to affect erections), given to forty-five men as a one-time dose one to two hours before intended sexual intercourse. Results showed that it worked better than placebo, although men with mild to moderate erectile dysfunction had more improvement than those with more severe problems.

Yohimbine has also been tested in small studies with people who have low blood pressure and in those who faint after standing up. It appeared to be somewhat helpful, but more studies need to be done before it can be recommended for this use. Early studies have also suggested that it can dilate the pupil of the eye to help doctors examine the inside of the eye, but more information is needed. Several other drugs are available and widely used for that purpose by eye specialists.

Are there any possible problems or complications?

Yohimbine and yohimbe bark can increase heart rate and raise blood pressure. People who have high blood pressure; heart, kidney or liver disease; and anxiety or nervous disorders should not take yohimbe or yohimbine. Those who drink alcohol or take antidepressants, antipsychotic drugs, methadone, certain nausea medicines, or opioid pain medicines (such as morphine) should not use yohimbe or yohimbine. Other potential interactions between yohimbe and other drugs and herbs should be considered. Some of these combinations may be dangerous. Always tell your doctor and pharmacist about any herbs you are taking.

Side effects of yohimbe bark or yohimbine include difficulty breathing, chest pain, palpitations, anxiety, queasiness, sleeplessness, and vomiting. Normal doses of yohimbine can cause a rise in blood pressure. Large doses of yohimbine (40 milligrams per day or more) can cause a drop in blood pressure and have been blamed for heart attacks and even deaths. Yohimbine can make heart disease or blood pressure problems worse. Less common side effects that do not usually require medical attention include dizziness, headache, flushing, nausea, nervousness, sweating, and tremors.

People with emotional or psychiatric problems may have worsening of post-traumatic stress disorder, sleeplessness, and anxiety. New onset of panic attacks or manic episodes have been reported. Yohimbine has been linked to psychotic episodes.

Yohimbine can also act as a monoamine oxidase inhibitor (MAOI), a type of powerful antidepressant. Foods that contain tyramine, such as beer, red wine, liver, aged or smoked meats, and aged cheese can raise blood pressure to dangerous levels if you eat them while taking yohimbine.

Yohimbine or yohimbe bark should not be used by children, elderly people, or women who are pregnant or breastfeeding. Yohimbe bark is on the Commission E (Germany's regulatory agency for herbs) list of unapproved herbs. This means that it is not recommended for use because it has not been proven to be safe or effective. Relying on this type of treatment alone and avoiding or delaying conventional medical care for cancer may have serious health consequences.

This product is sold as a dietary supplement in the United States. Unlike companies that produce drugs (which must provide the FDA with results of detailed testing showing their product is safe and effective before the drug is approved for sale), the companies that make supplements do not have to show evidence of safety or health benefits to the FDA before selling their products. Supplement products

without any reliable scientific evidence of health benefits may still be sold as long as the companies selling them do not claim the supplements can prevent, treat, or cure any specific disease. Some such products may not contain the amount of the herb or substance that is written on the label, and some may include other substances (contaminants). Though the FDA has written new rules to improve the quality of manufacturing processes for dietary supplements and the accurate listing of supplement ingredients, these rules do not take full effect until 2010. The new rules also do not address the safety of supplement ingredients or their effects on health when proper manufacturing techniques are used.

Most such supplements have not been tested to find out if they interact with medicines, foods, or other herbs and supplements. Even though some reports of interactions and harmful effects may be published, full studies of interactions and effects are not often available. Because of these limitations, any information on ill effects and interactions should be considered incomplete.

References

Betz JM, White KD, der Marderosian AH. Gas chromatographic determination of yohimbine in commercial yohimbe products. *J AOAC Int.* 1995;78:1189-1194.

Blumenthal M, ed. *The Complete German Commission E Monographs: Therapeutic Guide to Herbal Medicines.* Austin, TX: American Botanical Council; 1998.

Brinker FJ. *Herb Contraindications and Drug Interactions: With Appendices Addressing Specific Conditions and Medicines.* 2nd ed. Sandy, OR: Eclectic Medical Publications; 1998.

Cassileth B. *The Alternative Medicine Handbook: The Complete Reference Guide to Alternative and Complementary Therapies.* New York: W.W. Norton; 1998.

Center for Drug Evaluation and Research. Personal communication. November 1, 2005.

Ernst E, Pittler MH. Yohimbine for erectile dysfunction: a systemic review and meta analysis of randomized clinical trials. *J Urol.* 1998;159:433-436.

Fetrow CW, Avila JR. *Professional's Handbook of Complementary & Alternative Medicines.* Philadelphia, PA: Lippincott Williams & Wilkins; 2004.

Gruenwald J. *PDR for Herbal Medicines.* 3rd ed. Montvale, NJ: Thomson PDR; 2004.

Kunelius P, Häkkinen J, Lukkarinen O. Is high-dose yohimbine hydrochloride effective in the treatment of mixed-type impotence? A prospective, randomized, controlled double-blind crossover study. *Urology.* 1997;49:441-444.

Lebret T, Hervé JM, Gorny P, Worcel M, Botto H. Efficacy and safety of a novel combination of L-arginine glutamate and yohimbine hydrochloride: a new oral therapy for erectile dysfunction. *Eur Urol.* 2002;41:608-613.

Management of erectile dysfunction ('05/updated '06). American Urological Association Web site. http://www.auanet.org/guidelines/edmgmt.cfm. Accessed June 9, 2008.

Morales A. Yohimbine in erectile dysfunction: the facts. *Int J Impot Res.* 2000;12 Suppl 1:S70-S74.

Pittler MH, Ernst E. Trials have shown yohimbine is effective for erectile dysfunction. *BMJ.* 1998;317:478.

Stine SM, Southwick SM, Petrakis IL, Kosten TR, Charney DS, Krystal JH. Yohimbine-induced withdrawal and anxiety symptoms in opioid-dependent patients. *Biol Psychiatry.* 2002;51:642-651.

Summary of data for chemical selection: Yohimbe bark extract / yohimbine. National Toxicology Program Web site. http://ntp.niehs.nih.gov/ntp/htdocs/Chem_Background/ExSumPdf/Yohimbe.pdf. Accessed June 9, 2008.

Telöken C, Rhoden EL, Sogari P, Dambros M, Souto CA. Therapeutic effects of high dose yohimbine hydrochloride on organic erectile dysfunction. *J Urol.* 1998;159:122-124.

Vogt HJ, Brandl P, Kockott G, Schmitz JR, Wiegand MH, Schadrack J, Gierend M. Double-blind, placebo-controlled safety and efficacy trial with yohimbine hydrochloride in the treatment of nonorganic erectile dysfunction. *Int J Impot Res.* 1997;9:155-161.

Wagner G, Saenz de Tejada I. Update on male erectile dysfunction. *BMJ.* 1998;316:678-682.

Yohimbe. Drug Digest Web site. Mayo Clinic Web site. http://www.drugdigest.org/DD/DVH/HerbsWho/0,3923,4048|Yohimbe,00.html. Accessed June 9, 2008.

Yohimbe. Memorial Sloan-Kettering Cancer Center Web site. http://www.mskcc.org/mskcc/html/69423.cfm. Updated July 19, 2007. Accessed June 9, 2008.

Yohimbine (oral route). Mayo Clinic Web site. http://www.mayoclinic.com/health/drug-information/DR601453. Updated November 1, 2007. Accessed June 9, 2008.

Yohimbe. PDRhealth Web site. http://www.pdrhealth.com/drug_info/nmdrugprofiles/herbaldrugs/103010.shtml. Accessed June 9, 2008.

ZINC

Other common name(s): zinc gluconate, zinc sulfate, zinc acetate, zinc carbonate, zinc picolinate

Scientific/medical name(s): Zn, Zn++

Description

Zinc is an essential trace mineral that plays a key role in many important body processes such as building DNA and RNA, producing energy, regulating the immune system, and cell metabolism. It is required for wound healing, tasting, and smelling. Zinc is found in seafood, meats, nuts, eggs, cheese, grains, and other foods.

Overview

Some studies have found that zinc supplements may help reduce cancer risk in animals, but research in humans has not been as promising. A few early studies have suggested that zinc might help fight some side effects of radiation therapy, such as loss of taste and mouth sores in people being treated for cancer of the head or neck.

Zinc supplements can help fight infections in those with zinc deficiency and may be useful in people with sickle cell disease. Although zinc is very popular as a cold remedy, studies are mixed on whether it actually helps cold symptoms. Zinc nasal spray has been blamed by some people for the loss of their ability to smell and taste. Too much zinc can lead to serious side effects.

How is it promoted for use?

Some people claim zinc protects against certain types of cancer, shrinks enlarged prostate glands, decreases asthma and allergy symptoms, and fortifies the skin. Marketers claim it helps everything from anthrax and gout to menopause and varicose veins.

Some supporters claim that zinc reduces the severity and duration of the common cold. It is also promoted as an antioxidant, a compound that blocks the action of free radicals, activated oxygen molecules that can damage cells.

What does it involve?

Zinc is in a number of foods, such as enriched breakfast cereals, lean beef and pork, oysters, poultry, soybeans, nuts, pumpkin and sunflower seeds, eggs, cheese, and wheat bran. The Recommended Dietary Allowance, or RDA, of zinc is 11 milligrams per day for men, 8 milligrams per day for women, 11 milligrams per day for pregnant women, and 12 milligrams per day for breastfeeding women. Zinc capsules, tablets, lozenges, and liquid "ionic zinc" are available in most drugstores and pharmacies. Zinc spray or ointment is sometimes applied to wounds, burns, or injuries to speed healing.

What is the history behind it?

Zinc has been found in metals that date back to 1400 BC. In the thirteenth century, metallic zinc was produced in India. In 1500, zinc was recognized as an element by Andreas Marggraf in Germany. In the 1700s, zinc factories were built in Europe. Medical researchers began serious investigations of zinc in the body in the early 1970s.

What is the evidence?

There have been a number of studies looking at the possible roles of zinc in the body. Some researchers have focused on zinc levels in the body in people with cancer and other diseases. A few studies found that zinc levels in serum and/or inside white blood cells were often lower in patients with head and neck cancer or childhood leukemia. Low zinc levels were also linked to larger head or neck tumors, more advanced stage of disease, and a greater number of unplanned hospitalizations. However, it is impossible to know whether the low zinc level was due to the effects of the cancer, to lower dietary intake of zinc, or to some other unknown factor.

Another study found a connection between zinc intake from food and supplements and a lower risk for melanoma (the most serious form of skin cancer) and precancerous lesions of the mouth. More recent studies in humans do not show a consistent link between zinc supplements and lower cancer risk.

A study published in 2004 (called SU.VI.MAX) reported on more than thirteen thousand French adults who had taken either a combination of low doses of vitamin E, vitamin C, beta carotene, selenium, and zinc, or a placebo. After a median of more than seven years of follow-up, there were no major differences in cancer rates between the people who took real supplements and those who received placebo supplements. However, when researchers looked at men and women separately, the men who took antioxidants had lower risks for cancer and death from all causes than the men who had not. This was not true for the women in the study. However, the men began the study with lower levels of antioxidants, especially beta carotene and vitamins C and E, in their bodies. This fact may partly explain why they benefited more. It is unclear whether or how much zinc contributed to this effect.

A subgroup of more than five thousand men from the SU.VI.MAX study were looked at specifically for prostate cancer. After about eight years, there appeared to be a slightly lower risk for prostate cancer in the men who had taken the antioxidant supplements than in those who had taken a placebo. However, the difference was not statistically significant (that is, the result could have occurred by chance). Of more interest, in the men who started the study with a normal level of prostate-specific antigen (PSA, a protein made by the prostate gland), the risk of getting prostate cancer was significantly lower for those who took the supplement than for those who took the placebo. In contrast, for the men who started with a higher PSA (3 or greater), the prostate cancer risk tended to be higher for those who got the supplements than for those who took the placebo. This increased risk was not considered statistically significant.

A very small randomized clinical trial in Italy involving patients with head and neck cancer found that zinc sulfate tablets helped reverse the loss of taste caused by radiation therapy. However, a large randomized clinical trial from the Mayo Clinic reported that loss of taste was the same in patients who received the placebo and those who were treated with zinc supplements. Another small study in Turkey looked at patients receiving radiation therapy for head and neck cancers to find out whether zinc helped with mouth sores. Those who took zinc had milder mouth sores and sores that developed later in the course of radiation than people who took a placebo.

In an analysis of the SU.VI.MAX study that focused on heart disease risk, those who took antioxidants ended up with no difference in risk factors such as cholesterol compared with those on placebo. In fact, the women who had received the supplement had slightly worse risk factors than those who did not. Since this study looked at several antioxidants all together, it is difficult to say what zinc's role might have been.

It is known that the immune system does not work as well when a person does not take in enough zinc. In people with zinc deficiency, supplements may help immune function. For example, studies that were done in malnourished children from developing countries found that zinc helped prevent pneumonia and diarrhea. It also helped to slow down and shorten the duration of diarrhea that was caused by infection. However, zinc supplements do not help people with normal zinc levels and may cause harm if too much is taken.

Zinc has also proven useful in helping people with sickle cell disease, apparently because the illness causes zinc deficiency. Studies in those with sickle cell disease report that children often grow faster if given zinc supplements. Studies also report that adults with sickle cell disease tend to have fewer serious infections and hospitalizations if they take zinc supplements.

Zinc has been proven to reduce the body's absorption of copper, which has been proven useful for one rare health problem. The U.S. Food and Drug Administration (FDA) has approved a form of zinc known as zinc acetate for people with Wilson's disease, an inborn condition in which copper builds up in the body. Unlike zinc supplements sold over the counter, the prescription drug is regulated by the FDA. This difference in regulatory status means that it must meet strict quality standards, including containing the labeled amount of zinc in each tablet.

Results of studies on zinc and its effects on cold symptoms have been mixed. Two randomized, double-blind placebo studies found that zinc gluconate in a glycine base reduced the length of cold symptoms. In a review of eight clinical trials, researchers concluded that zinc reduced the duration and severity of the common cold. A later study found that zinc gluconate lozenges were not effective in treating cold symptoms in children and adolescents. Later studies were mixed. The type of lozenge or spray, dose, timing, and other factors may affect zinc's effectiveness. Generally, zinc seemed to work best when used as soon as symptoms started and then every couple of hours for a few days. Further study is needed to determine what role zinc plays in affecting cold symptoms.

There is some evidence that zinc, with other antioxidants, may delay age-related macular degeneration in older people and the loss of vision that goes with it. One study of the effect of zinc supplements on macular degeneration observed that men taking high doses of zinc were more likely to be admitted to the hospital with urinary problems, including enlarged prostate, kidney stones, and infections, than those not taking zinc. Women taking high doses of zinc had more urinary tract infections, than those who were not taking zinc supplements. However, those who took zinc also seemed to live longer than those who did not. These findings deserve careful study to see whether they hold true in other groups and settings.

At this time, it is hard to say how each nutrient or nutrient combination affects a person's risk for cancer. On the other hand, studies of large groups of people have shown that those whose diets are high in vegetables and low in animal fat, meat, and/or calories have lower risks for some of the most common types of cancer. Until more is known about this relationship, the American Cancer Society recommends eating a variety of healthful foods—with most of them coming from plant sources—rather than relying on supplements.

While it is best to get vitamins and minerals from foods, supplements may be helpful for some people, such as pregnant women, women of childbearing age, and people with restricted food intakes. If a supplement is taken, the best choice for most people is a balanced multivitamin/mineral supplement that contains no more than 100 percent of the "Daily Value" of most nutrients.

Are there any possible problems or complications?

An overdose of zinc can lead to a weakened immune system, vomiting, headache, and fatigue. Very high exposure to zinc, which occurs in some industries, may contribute to the development of prostate cancer. High zinc doses over long periods may increase the risk for urinary tract problems, including infections.

Taking 150 milligrams to 450 milligrams of zinc per day is linked to low copper levels, anemia, poor immune function, low levels of "good" cholesterol, and changes in the way iron works in the body. Zinc can reduce the body's ability to absorb antibiotics, copper, and iron. Other potential interactions between zinc and other drugs and herbs should be considered. Always tell your doctor and pharmacist about any supplements or herbs you are taking.

The National Institute of Health says that an adult should not take in more than 40 milligrams of zinc per day from foods and supplements. Zinc overdose can occur with a single overdose or by taking too much zinc over a longer period of time. A zinc overdose can cause severe nausea and vomiting within half an hour, and at least one death has been reported due to kidney failure.

Manufacturers of zinc nasal spray have been sued by several hundred people who reported that they lost some or all of their ability to smell and taste because of zinc nasal spray, and most have not gotten it back. Typically, these users noted severe burning in their noses when using the spray and right away found their sense of smell and taste was lost or greatly reduced. Some companies have stopped making zinc nasal sprays.

Women who are pregnant or breastfeeding should take zinc supplements only if advised to do so by their doctors. If the mother has high zinc levels, it can be passed to the baby and cause copper deficiency. However, low zinc levels in the mother can also be harmful to the infant during pregnancy, and getting enough zinc is important. Pregnant women should speak to their doctor before taking any zinc supplement. Relying on this type of treatment alone and avoiding or delaying conventional medical care for cancer may have serious health consequences.

This product is sold as a dietary supplement in the United States. Unlike companies that produce drugs (which must provide the FDA with results of detailed testing showing their product is safe and effective before the drug is approved for sale), the companies that make supplements do not have to show evidence of safety or health benefits to the FDA before selling their products. Supplement products without any reliable scientific evidence of health benefits may still be sold as long as the companies selling them do not claim the supplements can prevent, treat, or cure any specific disease. Some such products may not contain the amount of the herb or substance that is written on the label, and some may include other substances (contaminants). Though the FDA has written new rules to improve the quality of manufacturing processes for dietary supplements and the accurate listing of supplement ingredients, these rules do not take full effect until 2010. The new rules also do not address the safety of supplement ingredients or their effects on health when proper manufacturing techniques are used.

Most such supplements have not been tested to find out if they interact with medicines, foods, or other herbs and supplements. Even though some reports of interactions and harmful effects may be published, full studies of interactions and effects are not often available. Because of these limitations, any information on ill effects and interactions should be considered incomplete.

References

Age-Related Eye Disease Study Research Group. A randomized, placebo-controlled, clinical trial of high-dose supplementation with vitamins C and E, beta carotene, and zinc for age-related macular degeneration and vision loss: AREDS report no. 8. *Arch Ophthalmol.* 2001;119:1417-1436.

Clemons TE, Kurinij N, Sperduto RD; AREDS Research Group. Associations of mortality with ocular disorders and an intervention of high-dose antioxidants and zinc in the Age-Related Eye Disease Study: AREDS Report No. 13. *Arch Ophthalmol.* 2004;122:716-726.

Ertekin MV, Koç M, Karslioglu I, Sezen O. Zinc sulfate in the prevention of radiation-induced oropharyngeal mucositis: a prospective, placebo-controlled, randomized study. *Int J Radiat Oncol Biol Phys.* 2004;58:167-174.

Facts about dietary supplements: zinc. Office of Dietary Supplements Web site. http://ods.od.nih.gov/factsheets/cc/zinc.html. Updated December 9, 2002. Accessed June 9, 2008.

Galan P, Briançon S, Favier A, Bertrais S, Preziosi P, Faure H, Arnaud J, Arnault N, Czernichow S, Mennen L, Hercberg S. Antioxidant status and risk of cancer in the SU.VI.MAX study: is the effect of supplementation dependent on baseline levels? *Br J Nutr.* 2005;94:125-132.

Godfrey JC, Godfrey NJ, Novick SG. Zinc for treating the common cold: review of all clinical trials since 1984. *Altern Ther Health Med.* 1996;2:63-72.

Gruenwald J. *PDR for Herbal Medicines.* 3rd ed. Montvale, NJ: Thomson PDR; 2004.

Gupta PC, Hebert JR, Bhonsle RB, Mutri PR, Mehta H, Mehta FS. Influence of dietary factors on oral precancerous lesions in a population-based case-control study in Kerala, India. *Cancer.* 1999;85:1885-1893.

Halyard MY, Jatoi A, Sloan JA, Bearden JD 3rd, Vora SA, Atherton PJ, Perez EA, Soori G, Zalduendo AC, Zhu A, Stella PJ, Loprinzi CL. Does zinc sulfate prevent therapy-induced taste alterations in head and neck cancer patients? Results of phase III double-blind, placebo-controlled trial from the North Central Cancer Treatment Group (N01C4). *Int J Radiat Oncol Biol Phys.* 2007;67:1318-1322.

Hercberg S, Bertrais S, Czernichow S, Noisette N, Galan P, Jaouen A, Tichet J, Briançon S, Favier A, Mennen L, Roussel AM. Alterations of the lipid profile after 7.5 years of low-dose antioxidant supplementation in the SU.VI.MAX Study. *Lipids.* 2005;40:335-342.

Hercberg S, Galan P, Preziosi P, Bertrais S, Mennen L, Malvy D, Roussel AM, Favier A, Briançon S. The SU.VI.MAX Study: a randomized, placebo-controlled trial of the health effects of antioxidant vitamins and minerals. *Arch Intern Med.* 2004;164:2335-2342.

Jackson JL, Lesho E, Peterson C. Zinc and the common cold: a meta-analysis revisited. *J Nutr.* 2000;130:1512S-1515S.

Jafek BW, Linschoten MR, Murrow BW. Anosmia after intranasal zinc gluconate use. *Am J Rhinol.* 2004;18:137-141.

Johnson AR, Munoz A, Gottlieb JL, Jarrard DF. High dose zinc increases hospital admissions due to genitourinary complications. *J Urol.* 2007;177:639-643.

Kirkpatrick CS, White E, Lee JA. Case-control study of malignant melanoma in Washington State. II. Diet, alcohol, and obesity. *Am J Epidemiol.* 1994;139:869-880.

Kristal AR, Stanford JL, Cohen JH, Wicklund K, Patterson RE. Vitamin and mineral supplement use is associated with reduced risk of prostate cancer. *Cancer Epidemiol Biomarkers Prev.* 1999;8:887-892.

Leitzmann MF, Stampfer MJ, Wu K, Colditz GA, Willett WC, Giovannucci EL. Zinc supplement use and risk of prostate cancer. *J Natl Cancer Inst.* 2003;95:1004-1007.

Macknin ML, Piedmonte M, Calendine C, Janosky J, Wald E. Zinc gluconate lozenges for treating the common cold in children: a randomized controlled trial. *JAMA.* 1998;279:1962-1967.

Meyer F, Galan P, Douville P, Bairati I, Kegle P, Bertrais S, Estaquio C, Hercberg S. Antioxidant vitamin and mineral supplementation and prostate cancer prevention in the SU.VI.MAX trial. *Int J Cancer.* 2005;116:182-186.

Mossad SB, Macknin ML, Medendorp SV, Mason P. Zinc gluconate lozenges for treating the common cold. A randomized, double-blind, placebo-controlled study. *Ann Intern Med.* 1996;125:81-88.

Mossad SB. Treatment of the common cold. *BMJ.* 1998;317:33-36.

Phillips MJ, Ackerley CA, Superina RA, Roberts EA, Filler RM, Levy GA. Excess zinc associated with severe progressive cholestasis in Cree and Ojibwa-Cree children. *Lancet.* 1996;347(9005):866-868.
Erratum in:
Lancet. 1996;347(9017):1776

Prasad AS, Beck FW, Doerr TD, Shamsa FH, Penny HS, Marks SC, Kaplan J, Kucuk O, Mathog RH. Nutritional and zinc status of head and neck cancer patients: an interpretive review. *J Amer Coll Nutr.* 1998;17:409-418.

Prasad AS, Beck FW, Kaplan J, Chandrasekar PH, Ortega J, Fitzgerald JT, Swerdlow P. Effect of zinc supplementation on incidence of infections and hospital admissions in sickle cell disease (SCD). *Am J Hematol.* 1999;61:194-202.

Ripamonti C, Zecca E, Brunelli C, Fulfaro F, Villa S, Balzarini A, Bombardieri E, De Conno F. A randomized, controlled clinical trial to evaluate the effects of zinc sulfate on cancer patients with taste alterations caused by head and neck irradiation. *Cancer.* 1998;15:1938-1945.

Zemel BS, Kawchak DA, Fung EB, Ohene-Frempong K, Stallings VA. Effect of zinc supplementation on growth and body composition in children with sickle cell disease. *Am J Clin Nutr.* 2002;75:300-307.

Zicam maker settles lawsuit over users' loss of smell. 7 News Denver Channel Web site. http://www.thedenverchannel.com/7newsinvestigates/6279576/detail.html. Accessed June 9, 2008.

Zinc. Memorial Sloan-Kettering Cancer Center Web site. http://www.mskcc.org/mskcc/html/69427.cfm. Updated February 18, 2008. Accessed June 9, 2008.

Zinc. PDRhealth Web site. http://www.pdrhealth.com/drug_info/nmdrugprofiles/nutsupdrugs/zin_0281.shtml. Accessed June 9, 2008.

Chapter Eight

Diet and Nutrition Therapies

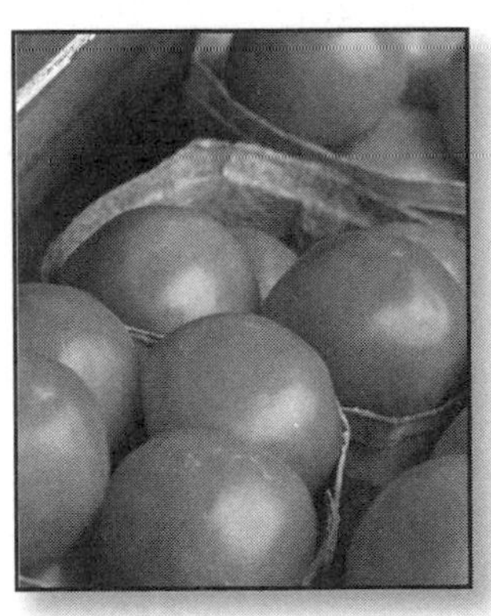

ACIDOPHILUS

Other common name(s): lactic acid bacteria
Scientific/medical name(s): *Lactobacillus acidophilus*

Description

Acidophilus is a type of germ, or bacterium, commonly found in the normal digestive tract of mammals, mainly in the small intestine. It is also found in many dairy products, especially yogurt. Acidophilus and some related bacteria are considered to be "probiotic" because they may help the body maintain or restore its normal balance of helpful bacteria.

Overview

Acidophilus has been promoted for a wide variety of conditions, including cancer. There have been no studies with humans on the role of *Lactobacillus acidophilus* (commonly referred to as *L. acidophilus*) in preventing or treating human cancers. Animal studies looking at the role of *L. acidophilus* in reducing the risk for cancer have shown varying results. Further research is needed.

How is it promoted for use?

Acidophilus is often promoted as a supplement to help "maintain a healthy bowel." It has also been suggested to prevent or treat diarrhea and vaginal infections, to lower cholesterol, to help with lactose digestion in lactose-sensitive people, and to help prevent the growth of disease-causing bacteria and yeast.

Some supporters claim acidophilus may lower the risk for cancer, especially colon cancer. It is supposed to lower risk by neutralizing cancer-causing agents, or carcinogens, in the diet and by directly killing tumor cells. Some also claim that acidophilus works against cancer by boosting the immune system by making B vitamins and vitamin K, and that it reduces levels of cholesterol, which proponents say tumor cells need in order to grow.

What does it involve?

When taking acidophilus, the dosage usually refers to the number of live bacteria. Most sources suggest one billion to ten billion bacteria as a recommended dose. This amount is available in tablets, capsules, and powder form. Average dosage suggestions vary from one to three times per day. However, some scientists warn that the concentration of the bacteria in the supplements varies widely from one manufacturer to another. Yogurt with "live cultures" and milk with *L. acidophilus* added to it are other sources.

What is the history behind it?

Interest in the health benefits of acidophilus began in the late 1800s, when it was proposed that the long life span of the Balkan people was due to their ingestion of fermented milk products. It was later found that these milk products were rich in *L. acidophilus*. Since then, the exact role of acidophilus in the digestive tract and in human health has been a controversial subject, with few clear results.

What is the evidence?

Laboratory and animal studies on the ability of acidophilus to prevent cancer have had mixed results, and there have been no large studies reported in humans. Acidophilus has been studied in the laboratory for possible antitumor properties. In some studies, milk that was fermented by acidophilus was able to slow or prevent the growth of breast and colon cancer cells grown in the laboratory.

In other studies, animals that were given *L. acidophilus* were found to be less prone to DNA damage in the colon after being given known carcinogens, suggesting acidophilus might have an effect on colon cancer. However, animal studies have shown that diets that include acidophilus do not seem to affect the formation of breast or skin cancers. In either case, randomized studies in people have not been done. Further studies are needed to determine whether the results apply to humans.

Researchers have also studied the effects of *L. acidophilus* and other probiotics on certain reproductive hormones known in high levels to increase risk for breast cancer. In studies of both pre- and postmenopausal women, acidophilus had no effect.

A Japanese study looked at the effect of a related bacterium *(Lactobacillus casei)* on the risk for colon tumors in about four hundred men and women who had had previous tumors removed. The risk for new tumor development was not significantly lower in those who took *L. casei*, although the tumors that did develop contained cells that were less abnormal.

A review of research on the effects of acidophilus and other closely related bacteria found that they lowered cholesterol in some, but not all, studies. It also found that a related bacterium *(Lactobacillus GG)* may shorten the duration of diarrhea due to viral or bacterial infections, but other health effects of these types of bacteria are not clear.

A few recent studies suggest that acidophilus or related *Lactobacillus* species may reduce the severity of diarrhea occurring with chemotherapy for colorectal cancer or with radiation therapy for colorectal or cervical cancer. On study suggest that adding *Lactobacillus* to chemotherapy instilled into the bladder might help prevent recurrence of bladder cancer after surgery.

Are there any possible problems or complications?

There appear to be few short-term problems with taking acidophilus. Some people have reported excess bloating or gas for the first few days while taking the supplement. In rare cases, acidophilus may cause serious infections that are hard to treat with antibiotics. People with weakened immune systems, such as those who are taking steroids or undergoing chemotherapy, who have received organ transplants, or who have AIDS, should use acidophilus with caution.

The lack of standardization makes it hard to be sure of the quality of acidophilus products. Because acidophilus must contain live cultures in order to be effective, proper packaging and storage is essential. Many products may contain other bacteria or may not contain enough of the active organisms, especially if the product has been sitting on a shelf for a while.

Relying on this type of treatment alone and avoiding or delaying conventional medical care for cancer may have serious health consequences.

This product is sold as a dietary supplement in the United States. Unlike companies that produce drugs (which must provide the FDA with results of detailed testing showing their product is safe and effective before the drug is approved for sale), the companies that make supplements do not have to show evidence of safety or health benefits to the FDA before selling their products. Supplement products without any reliable scientific evidence of health benefits may still be sold as long as the companies selling them do not claim the supplements can prevent, treat, or cure any specific disease. Some such products may not contain the amount of the herb or substance that is written on the label, and some may include other substances (contaminants). Though the FDA has written new rules to improve the quality of manufacturing processes for dietary supplements and the accurate listing of supplement ingredients, these rules do not take full effect until 2010. The new rules also do not address the safety of supplement ingredients or their effects on health when proper manufacturing techniques are used.

Most such supplements have not been tested to find out if they interact with medicines, foods, or other herbs and supplements. Even though some reports of interactions and harmful effects may be published, full studies of interactions and effects are not often available. Because of these limitations, any information on ill effects and interactions should be considered incomplete.

References

Baricault L, Denariaz G, Houri JJ, Bouley C, Sapin C, Trugnan G. Use of HT-29, a cultured human colon cancer cell line, to study the effect of fermented milks on colon cancer cell growth and differentiation. *Carcinogenesis.* 1995;16:245-252.

Biffi A, Coradini D, Larsen R, Riva L, Di Fronzo G. Antiproliferative effect of fermented milk on the growth of a human breast cancer cell line. *Nutr Cancer.* 1997;28:93-99.

Bolognani F, Rumney CJ, Pool-Zobel BL, Rowland IR. Effect of lactobacilli, bifidobacteria and inulin on the formation of aberrant crypt foci in rats. *Eur J Nutr.* 2001;40:293-300.

Bonorden MJ, Greany KA, Wangen KE, Phipps WR, Feirtag J, Adlercreutz H, Kurzer MS. Consumption of *Lactobacillus acidophilus* and *Bifidobacterium longum* do not alter urinary equol excretion and plasma reproductive hormones in premenopausal women. *Eur J Clin Nutr.* 2004;58:1635-1642.

Delia P, Sansotta G, Donato V, Frosina P, Messina G, De Renzis C, Famularo G. Use of probiotics for prevention of radiation-induced diarrhea. *World J Gastroenterol.* 2007;13:912-915.

de Roos NM, Katan MB. Effects of probiotic bacteria on diarrhea, lipid metabolism, and carcinogenesis: a review of papers published between 1988 and 1998. *Am J Clin Nutr.* 2000;71:405-411.

Hove H, Nørgaard H, Mortensen PB. Lactic acid bacteria and the human gastrointestinal tract. *Eur J Clin Nut.* 1999;53:339-350.

Ishikawa H, Akedo I, Otani T, Suzuki T, Nakamura T, Takeyama I, Ishiguro S, Miyaoka E, Sobue T, Kakizoe T. Randomized trial of dietary fiber and *Lactobacillus casei* administration for prevention of colorectal tumors. *Int J Cancer.* 2005;116:762-767.

Naito S, Koga H, Yamaguchi A, Fujimoto N, Hasui Y, Kuramoto H, Kinukawa N; Kyushu University Urological Oncology Group. Prevention of recurrence with epirubicin and lactobacillus casei after transurethral resection of bladder cancer. *J Urol.* 2008;179:485-490.

Natural Standard. Herbal/plant therapies: *Lactobacillus acidophilus*. Complementary/Integrative Medicine Education Resources, The University of Texas M. D. Anderson Cancer Center Web site. http://www.mdanderson.org/departments/cimer/display.cfm?id=28A0EE0D-11E2-4060-B5CEE2CE90A7295B&method=displayFull. Accessed June 10, 2008.

Nettleton JA, Greany KA, Thomas W, Wangen KE, Adlercreutz H, Kurzer MS. Short-term soy and probiotic supplementation does not markedly affect concentrations of reproductive hormones in postmenopausal women with and without histories of breast cancer. *J Altern Complement Med.* 2005;11:1067-1074.

Osterlund P, Ruotsalainen T, Korpela R, Saxelin M, Ollus A, Valta P, Kouri M, Elomaa I, Joensuu H. Lactobacillus supplementation for diarrhoea related to chemotherapy of colorectal cancer: a randomised study. *Br J Cancer.* 2007;97:1028-1034.

Pool-Zobel BL, Neudecker C, Domizlaff I, Ji S, Schillinger U, Rumney C, Moretti M, Vilarini I, Scassellati-Sforzolini R, Rowland I. Lactobacillus-and bifidobacterium-mediated antigenotoxicity in the colon of rats. *Nutr Cancer.* 1996;26:365-380.

Rao CV, Sanders ME, Indranie C, Simi B, Reddy BS. Prevention of colonic preneoplastic lesions by the probiotic Lactobacillus acidophilus NCFMTM in F344 rats. *Int J Oncol.* 1999;14:939-944.

Rice LJ, Chai YJ, Conti CJ, Willis RA, Locniskar MF. The effect of dietary fermented milk products and lactic acid bacteria on the initiation and promotion stages of mammary carcinogenesis. *Nutr Cancer.* 1995;24:99-109.

BROCCOLI

Other common name(s): none
Scientific/medical name(s): *Brassica oleracea italica*

Description

Broccoli is a cruciferous vegetable that belongs to the cabbage family, which also includes arugula, cauliflower, collard greens, bok choy, kale, mustard greens, radishes, turnips, watercress, rutabaga, and brussels sprouts. It is identified by its dense clusters of green flower buds.

Overview

Broccoli contains certain chemicals that may reduce the risk for colorectal or other cancers, although it is not clear which individual compounds may be responsible for the protective effects. While research in this area continues, the best advice at this time to reduce cancer risk is to eat a wide variety of vegetables. It is reasonable to include broccoli as part of a balanced diet.

How is it promoted for use?

Broccoli is considered a good source of nutrients because it is rich in vitamin C, carotenoids (vitamin A–like substances), fiber, calcium, and folate. Broccoli is also a source of many substances called phytochemicals, or plant chemicals, that may have anticancer properties. For example, broccoli contains several compounds called isothiocyanates, including sulforaphane and indole-3-carbinol (I3C), which have been touted as possible anticancer agents in recent years. Early studies have shown these substances may act as antioxidants and may boost detoxifying enzymes in the body. Some studies have also suggested they may alter the levels of estrogen in the body, which might affect breast cancer risk.

The chemical composition of broccoli and other cruciferous vegetables is complex, which makes it hard to determine which compound or combination of compounds may provide protection against cancer. Eating a wide variety of plant-based foods may be the best way to get the necessary components.

What does it involve?

Broccoli can be eaten raw or cooked in a variety of ways. It can be purchased fresh or frozen in most grocery and organic food stores. Broccoli retains the most nutrients when eaten raw. Cooking reduces some of the benefits of broccoli because the heating process seems to destroy some anticancer compounds. Some chemicals found in broccoli, such as indole-3-carbinol, are also available in pill form as dietary supplements.

What is the history behind it?

Broccoli has been around for more than two thousand years but has only been commercially grown in the United States since the 1920s. Today, more than 90 percent of the broccoli harvested in the United States comes from California, although it is also grown in other parts of the country.

About two decades ago, researchers first suggested a possible link between diets high in cruciferous vegetables (a group of plants including cauliflower, cabbage, broccoli, and brussels sprouts) and a lower risk for cancer. However, it was not until the 1990s that certain chemicals found in broccoli were identified as possible cancer-preventing compounds. In 1997, a study was published that noted broccoli sprouts had higher levels of one of these compounds than mature broccoli.

What is the evidence?

Diets high in cruciferous vegetables appear to be linked with a lower risk for certain types of cancer. An observational epidemiologic study found that those who ate diets high in lutein, a vitamin A–like chemical obtained from vegetables such as broccoli, spinach, and lettuce, had fewer cases of colon cancer. A similar study suggested that those who ate cruciferous vegetables seemed to have a lower risk for bladder cancer, but a similar study of smokers found no such benefit. Recent studies suggest that the effect of broccoli and related cruciferous vegetables on cancer risk may partly depend on an inherited variation in certain metabolic enzymes. For example, when people with certain glutathione S-transferase types eat a diet high in cruciferous vegetables, their risk for lung cancer is lower. Randomized clinical trials are needed to clarify these results.

Laboratory and animal studies have suggested that certain compounds in broccoli may have anticancer properties. These types of studies can suggest possible helpful effects, but they do not provide proof that such effects can be achieved in humans. Further studies are needed to find out whether possible anticancer properties could benefit humans. Some research has suggested that sulforaphane, a substance that is present at much higher levels in broccoli sprouts than in the mature vegetable, may be a powerful cancer-preventing agent. Some researchers have suggested that eating small amounts of broccoli sprouts may protect against the risk for cancer as effectively as much larger amounts of the mature vegetable. We are not aware of any clinical studies that have been done in humans to verify this claim. Sulforaphane is thought to prompt the body to make higher levels of enzymes that protect against cancer-causing chemicals. One study showed that breast tumor development was significantly reduced in laboratory animals that ate sulforaphane. Other laboratory studies have shown that sulforaphane may help protect against cancers of the prostate, colon, and pancreas as well as other types of cancer. Some studies have also suggested that the compound may help treat some types of cancer. More research in animals and humans will be needed to confirm these findings.

Another substance in broccoli, indole-3-carbinol (I3C), seems to alter estrogen levels and may also raise levels of protective enzymes in the body. Several studies of cancer cells growing in laboratory dishes or flasks have shown it may slow or stop the growth of breast, prostate, and other cancer cells. Some early studies in animals have shown similar results. Small studies in humans have found it may prevent the development of precancerous growths in the cervix, as well as growths called papillomas in the throat. Again, larger studies are needed to find out what benefits I3C may have against cancer.

Scientists caution that while broccoli appears promising as an excellent food for preventing cancer, the results of such studies cannot be considered by themselves. The anticancer effects of any single food cannot be completely understood without looking at it as part of a bigger dietary picture. It is still unclear, for example, whether the phytochemicals in broccoli have benefit on their own or whether it is the vitamin C, beta carotene, folate, and other compounds, working together and in the right quantities, that might protect people against cancer.

A balanced diet that includes five or more servings a day of fruits and vegetables, along with foods from a variety of other plant sources such as nuts, seeds, whole grain cereals, and beans, is likely to be more healthful than eating large amounts of one food.

Are there any possible problems or complications?

Broccoli and broccoli sprouts are generally safe to eat. Since broccoli is high in fiber, eating large amounts of it may cause gas. High-fiber foods should be reduced or avoided in people with diarrhea and some other colon problems. Raw broccoli may be more likely to cause irritation, especially in those with certain bowel conditions. Relying on this type of diet alone and avoiding or delaying conventional medical care may have serious health consequences.

This product is sold as a dietary supplement in the United States. Unlike companies that produce drugs (which must provide the FDA with results of detailed testing showing their product is safe and effective before the drug is approved for sale), the companies that make supplements do not have to show evidence of safety or health benefits to the FDA before selling their products. Supplement products without any reliable scientific evidence of health benefits may still be sold as long as the companies selling them do not claim the supplements can prevent, treat, or cure any specific disease. Some such products may not contain the amount of the herb or substance that is written on the label, and some may include other substances (contaminants). Though the FDA has written new rules to improve the quality of manufacturing processes for dietary supplements and the accurate listing of supplement ingredients, these rules do not take full effect until 2010. The new rules also do not address the safety

of supplement ingredients or their effects on health when proper manufacturing techniques are used.

Most such supplements have not been tested to find out if they interact with medicines, foods, or other herbs and supplements. Even though some reports of interactions and harmful effects may be published, full studies of interactions and effects are not often available. Because of these limitations, any information on ill effects and interactions should be considered incomplete.

References

Bell MC, Crowley-Nowick P, Bradlow HL, Sepkovic DW, Schmidt-Grimminger D, Howell P, Mayeaux EJ, Tucker A, Turbat-Herrera EA, Mathis JM. Placebo-controlled trial of indole-3-carbinol in the treatment of CIN. *Gynecol Oncol.* 2000;78:123-129.

Brennan P, Hsu CC, Moullan N, Szeszenia-Dabrowska N, Lissowska J, Zaridze D, Rudnai P, Fabianova E, Mates D, Bencko V, Foretova L, Janout V, Gemignani F, Chabrier A, Hall J, Hung RJ, Boffetta P, Canzian F. Effect of cruciferous vegetables on lung cancer in patients stratified by genetic status: a Mendelian randomisation approach. *Lancet.* 2005;366:1558-1560.

Cao G, Booth SL, Sadowski JA, Prior RL. Increases in human plasma antioxidant capacity after consumption of controlled diets high in fruit and vegetables. *Am J Clin Nutr.* 1998;68:1081-1087.

Cover CM, Hsieh SJ, Tran SH, Hallden G, Kim GS, Bjeldanes LF, Firestone GL. Indole-3-carbinol inhibits the expression of cyclin-dependent kinase-6 and induces a G1 cell cycle arrest of human breast cancer cells independent of estrogen receptor signaling. *J Biol Chem.* 1998;273:3838-3847.

Fahey JW, Zhang Y, Talalay P. Broccoli sprouts: an exceptionally rich source of inducers of enzymes that protect against chemical carcinogens. *Proc Natl Acad Sci U S A.* 1997;94:10367-10372.

Indole-3-Carbinol. PDRhealth Web site. http://www.pdrhealth.com/drug_info/nmdrugprofiles/nutsupdrugs/ind_0315.shtml. Accessed June 10, 2008.

Michaud DS, Pietinen P, Taylor PR, Virtanen M, Virtamo J, Albanes D. Intakes of fruits and vegetables, carotenoids and vitamins A, E, C in relation to the risk of bladder cancer in the ATBC cohort study. *Br J Cancer.* 2002;87:960-965.

Michaud DS, Spiegelman D, Clinton SK, Rimm EB, Willett WC, Giovannucci EL. Fruit and vegetable intake and incidence of bladder cancer in a male prospective cohort. *J Natl Cancer Inst.* 1999;91:605-613.

Nestle M. Broccoli sprouts in cancer prevention. *Nutr Rev.* 1998;56:127-130.

Parnaud G, Li P, Cassar G, Rouimi P, Tulliez J, Combaret L, Gamet-Payrastre L. Mechanism of sulforaphane-induced cell cycle arrest and apoptosis in human colon cancer cells. *Nutr Cancer.* 2004;48:198-206.

Shapiro TA, Fahey JW, Dinkova-Kostova AT, Holtzclaw WD, Stephenson KK, Wade KL, Ye L, Talalay P. Safety, tolerance, and metabolism of broccoli sprout glucosinolates and isothiocyanates: a clinical phase I study. *Nutr Cancer.* 2006;55:53-62.

Shapiro TA, Fahey JW, Wade KL, Stephenson KK, Talalay P. Human metabolism and excretion of cancer chemoprotective glucosinolates and isothiocyanates of cruciferous vegetables. *Cancer Epidemiol Biomarkers Prev.* 1998;7:1091-1100.

Singh SV, Srivastava SK, Choi S, Lew KL, Antosiewicz J, Xiao D, Zeng Y, Watkins SC, Johnson CS, Trump DL, Lee YJ, Xiao H, Herman-Antosiewicz A. Sulforaphane-induced cell death in human prostate cancer cells is initiated by reactive oxygen species. *J Biol Chem.* 2005;280:19911-19924. Epub 2005 Mar 11.

Slattery ML, Benson J, Curtin K, Ma KN, Schaeffer D, Potter JD. Carotenoids and colon cancer. *Am J Clin Nutr.* 2000;71:575-582.

Sulforaphane. PDRhealth Web site. http://www.pdrhealth.com/drug_info/nmdrugprofiles/nutsupdrugs/sul_0243.shtml. Accessed June 12, 2007. Content no longer available.

Tang L, Zhang Y, Jobson HE, Li J, Stephenson KK, Wade KL, Fahey JW. Potent activation of mitochondria-mediated apoptosis and arrest in S and M phases of cancer cells by a broccoli sprout extract. *Mol Cancer Ther.* 2006;5:935-944.

CASSAVA

Other common name(s): cassava plant, tapioca, tapioca plant, manioc
Scientific/medical name(s): *Manihot esculenta Crantz*

Description

The cassava plant is a staple crop in Africa, Asia, and South America. Tapioca is a starch found in the roots, or tubers, of the plant. Different parts of the plant, such as the root, leaves, and sometimes the whole plant, are used in herbal remedies.

Overview

There is no convincing scientific evidence that cassava or tapioca is effective in preventing or treating cancer. However, some researchers have proposed an idea that might eventually lead to treatments that use an enzyme from the cassava plant. This approach has not been scientifically tested.

How is it promoted for use?

In folk medicine, the cassava plant is promoted for the treatment of snakebites, boils, diarrhea, flu, hernia, inflammation, conjunctivitis, sores, and several other problems including cancer. Cassava plants can produce the poisonous substance cyanide as a way to fend off animals trying to eat them. Chewing the plant causes it to release an enzyme called linamarase, and linamarase, in turn, converts a compound in the plant called linamarin into cyanide. Researchers have suggested that this ability might be useful as a form of gene therapy. First, the gene for linamarase could be selectively put into cancer cells. If linamarin were then introduced into the body, cancer cells would break it down and release cyanide only in the area around the cancer cells, killing them. Since normal cells would not have the linamarase gene and would not be able to convert linamarin into cyanide, they would not be affected.

What does it involve?

In herbal remedies, the roots of the cassava are made into a poultice and applied directly to the skin as a treatment for sores. The leaf, root, and flour obtained from the plant can also be used in a wash that is applied to the skin. In some developing countries, tapioca starch made from the cassava plant is used to help restore body fluids. Cassava leaves are sold in health food stores and on the Internet in capsule or powder form. Cassava root starch may be used in vitamin C supplements. The parts of cassava used for food are the tubers, which are usually eaten raw, boiled, or fried. A form of flour is also made from the cassava plant. In Western countries, tapioca is found in baby foods and prepared as a dessert.

What is the history behind it?

Cassava has been used as a food source by many cultures for centuries. Today, it is consumed by millions of people in developing countries and is sometimes used as an herbal medicine. It has been theorized that the plant's ability to make cyanide may be useful as a type of gene therapy to treat cancer, but further research is needed to determine whether the technique will work in humans. This use would be quite different from the use of the cassava plant as an herbal remedy.

What is the evidence?

Available scientific evidence does not support claims that botanical products currently made from the cassava plant have anticancer properties. A British researcher identified the cassava genes involved in making hydrogen cyanide in the early 1990s. In collaboration with cancer specialists in Spain, she has conducted studies of the linamarase gene. They added this gene to a virus, which was then injected into rat brain tumors. These tumors were killed when the rats were infused with linamarin. Further research is needed to determine whether this technique will work in people.

Many scientists around the world are currently developing gene therapy methods for introducing DNA selectively into the tumor cells of cancer patients. More research is needed to determine whether linamarin and linamarase can be safely and effectively used to kill cancer cells in people with cancer.

Extracted chemicals or substances are different from the raw plant. Study results of extracts are not expected to have the same result as studies using the raw plant.

Are there any possible problems or complications?

The cassava plant produces cyanide, a poison that can be deadly to humans, and cassava can be a serious health hazard if it is not processed properly. Some of the signs of cyanide poisoning are headache, dizziness, agitation, confusion, coma, and convulsions. Some people in developing countries have been poisoned by eating parts of the cassava plant that were not prepared properly.

In regions of Africa and Latin America where cassava is a staple food, illnesses due to consuming smaller amounts of cyanide over a long period of time can occur if cassava leaves or roots are not processed properly. Effects can include paralysis of the legs, trouble walking, and poor vision and hearing. Malnutrition can also occur when cassava is a major part of the diet because the plant is low in protein and certain micronutrients.

Some people are allergic to cassava. Those with allergies to natural rubber latex may be more likely to have serious reactions. Relying on this type of treatment alone and avoiding or delaying conventional medical care for cancer may have serious health consequences.

References

Cardoso AP, Mirione E, Ernesto M, Massaza F, Cliff J, Haque MR, Bradbury JH. Processing of cassava roots to remove cyanogens. *J Food Comp Anal.* 2005;18:451-460.

Cortés ML, García-Escudero V, Hughes M, Izquierdo M. Cyanide bystander effect of the linamarase/linamarin killer-suicide gene therapy system. *J Gene Med.* 2002;4:407-414.

Gaspar A, Neto-Braga C, Pircs G, Murta R, Morais-Almcida M, Rosado-Pinto J. Anaphylactic reaction to manioc: cross-reactivity to latex. *Allergy*. 2003;58:683-684.

Hughes J, Keresztessy Z, Brown K, Suhandono S, Hughes MA. Genomic organization and structure of alpha-hydroxynitrile lyase in cassava (*Manihot esculenta* Crantz). *Arch Biochem Biophys.* 1998;356:107-116.

Manihot esculenta crantz. Purdue University Center for New Crops & Plants Products Web site. http://www.hort.purdue.edu/newcrop/duke_energy/Manihot_esculenta.html. Updated January 7, 1998. Accessed June 10, 2008.

Teles FF. Chronic poisoning by hydrogen cyanide in cassava and its prevention in Africa and Latin America. *Food Nutr Bull.* 2002;23:407-412.

Wapnir RA, Wingertzahn MA, Moyse J, Teichberg S. Proabsorptive effects of modified tapioca starch as an additive of oral rehydration solutions. *J Pediatr Gastroenterol Nutr.* 1998;27:17-22.

White WLB, Arias-Garzon DI, McMahon JM, Sayre RT. Cyanogenesis in cassava. The role of hydroxynitrile lyase in root cyanide production. *Plant Physiol.* 1998;116:1219-1225.

Wingertzahn MA, Teichberg S, Wapnir RA. Modified starch enhances absorption and accelerates recovery in experimental diarrhea in rats. *Pediatr Res.* 1999;45:397-402.

CORIOLUS VERSICOLOR

Other common name(s): "Turkey Tail" mushroom, Yun zhi, polysaccharide K (PSK), polysaccharide-peptide (PSP), versicolor polysaccharide (VPS)
Scientific/medical name(s): *Coriolus versicolor, Trametes versicolor*

Description

Coriolus versicolor is a mushroom used in traditional Asian herbal remedies. Two substances extracted from the mushroom, polysaccharide K (PSK) and polysaccharide-peptide (PSP), are being studied as possible complementary cancer treatments. Versicolor polysaccharide (VPS), another extract that is sold as a dietary supplement in the United States, is also being studied. A polysaccharide is a carbohydrate formed by many sugar molecules.

Overview

Available scientific evidence does not support claims that the raw mushroom itself is an effective anticancer agent in humans. But there is some scientific evidence that substances derived from parts of the mushroom may be useful against cancer. Clinical trials suggest that PSK may help people with certain types of cancer by increasing survival rates and lengthening periods of time without disease, without causing major side effects. PSK is commonly used with other cancer treatments in Japan. PSP and VPS have not been studied as thoroughly.

How is it promoted for use?

Herbalists claim *Coriolus versicolor* and its extracts are useful against a number of conditions, including cancer and certain infections. PSK, one of the substances that can be extracted from *Coriolus versicolor,* is believed to be a strong antioxidant, a compound that blocks the action of free radicals, activated oxygen molecules that can damage cells.

What does it involve?

Coriolus versicolor can be taken as a capsule, as an extract, or as a tea. The doses usually range from 1 to 9 grams per day, depending on the patient's condition. *Coriolus versicolor* can be obtained in herbal medicine shops, health food stores, and on the Internet. A variety of extracts of the mushroom, including PSP and VPS, are also sold as dietary supplements in the United States.

What is the history behind it?

Coriolus versicolor has been a component of traditional Asian medicine for centuries. In the 1980s, the Japanese government approved the use of PSK for treating several types of cancer. In Japan, PSK is a best-selling anticancer drug, where it is currently used as a cancer treatment along with surgery, chemotherapy, and radiation therapy. PSP was discovered more recently and has been studied mainly in China.

What is the evidence?

No reports of controlled clinical trials with the *Coriolus versicolor* mushroom itself could be found in the available peer-reviewed journals. However, there have been many studies looking at the usefulness of the extract PSK.

Researchers have found that PSK, one of the substances that can be extracted from *Coriolus versicolor*, has several anticancer properties. In some animal studies, it slows the spread of cancer cells. PSK also appears to have some immune system–boosting properties in people undergoing chemotherapy and may lessen some side effects of chemotherapy and radiation therapy. PSK is also believed to be a strong antioxidant, a compound that blocks the action of free radicals, activated oxygen molecules that can damage cells.

More than two dozen human studies of PSK have been reviewed by experts at the University of Texas M. D. Anderson Cancer Center. Almost all of these studies were done in Japan and focused on cancer of the esophagus, stomach, colon, or breast. Most of them found that people with cancer were helped by PSK. People who received PSK with other treatments, such as surgery, chemotherapy, or radiation therapy, generally had longer periods of time without disease and had increased survival rates compared with patients who received only standard treatment. Side effects from PSK in these studies were very mild. Smaller studies have suggested PSK may not be as effective against liver cancer or leukemia.

The effects of PSP are less well known. While some early Chinese studies of PSP have reportedly shown it may help protect the immune system from the effects of cancer treatment, most studies published in medical journals thus far have been in cell cultures or animals. These types of studies can suggest possible helpful effects, but they do not provide proof that such effects can be achieved in humans. Studies in animals have suggested that PSP may slow the growth of lung cancer and sarcoma and may help make radiation therapy more effective in treating certain brain tumors. One small study in humans found that lung cancer patients taking PSP seemed to maintain their levels of health longer than those who did not take PSP, although they did not get better and did not report improvement in cancer-related symptoms. Larger human studies will be needed to determine whether PSP can be helpful for people.

A 2005 study using mice treated with a chemical that causes colon cancer did not find any reduction in colon tumors in mice also given VPS. A 2006 study found that VPS may have actually increased the number of large colon tumors in mice.

Are there any possible problems or complications?

No serious risks have been reported as linked with the use of *Coriolus versicolor* or products derived from this mushroom. Rarely, side effects include nausea, vomiting, loss of appetite, and diarrhea. Even less common are darkening of the fingernails and low blood cell counts. Relying on this type of treatment alone and avoiding or delaying conventional medical care for cancer may have serious health consequences.

This product is sold as a dietary supplement in the United States. Unlike companies that produce drugs (which must provide the FDA with results of detailed testing showing their product is safe and effective before the drug is approved for sale), the companies that make supplements do not have to show evidence of safety or health benefits to the FDA before selling their products. Supplement products without any reliable scientific evidence of health benefits may still be sold as long as the companies selling them do not claim the supplements can prevent, treat, or cure any specific disease. Some such products may not contain the amount of the herb or substance that is written on the label, and some may include other substances (contaminants). Though the FDA has written new rules to improve the quality of manufacturing processes for dietary supplements and the accurate listing of supplement ingredients, these rules do not take full effect until 2010. The new rules also do not address the safety of supplement ingredients or their effects on health when proper manufacturing techniques are used.

Most such supplements have not been tested to find out if they interact with medicines, foods, or other herbs and supplements. Even though some reports of interactions and harmful effects may be published, full studies of interactions and effects are not often available. Because of these limitations, any information on ill effects and interactions should be considered incomplete.

References

Coles M, Toth B. Lack of prevention of large intestinal cancer by VPS, an extract of Coriolus versicolor mushroom. *In Vivo.* 2005;19:867-871.

Coriolus versicolor. Memorial Sloan-Kettering Cancer Center Web site. http://www.mskcc.org/mskcc/html/69194.cfm. Accessed June 10, 2008.

Fisher M, Yang LX. Anticancer effects and mechanisms of polysaccharide-K (PSK): implications of cancer immunotherapy. *Anticancer Res.* 2002;22:1737-1754.

Herbal/plant therapies: *Coriolus versicolor* detailed scientific review. Complementary/Integrative Medicine Education Resources, The University of Texas M. D. Anderson Cancer Center Web site. http://www.mdanderson.org/departments/CIMER/display.cfm?id=BF40CDD9-ED6B-11D4-810200508B603A14&method=displayFull. Accessed June 10, 2008.

Nakazato H, Koike A, Saji S, Ogawa N, Sakamoto J; Study Group of Immunochemotherapy with PSK for Gastric

Cancer. Efficacy of immunochemotherapy as adjuvant treatment after curative resection of gastric cancer. *Lancet.* 1994;343:1122-1126.

Ng TB. A review of research on the protein-bound polysaccharide (polysaccharopeptide, PSP) from the mushroom *Coriolus versicolor* (basidomycetes: Polyporacae). *Gen Pharmacol.* 1998;30:1-4.

Torisu M, Hayashi Y, Ishimitsu T, Fujimura T, Iwasaki K, Katano M, Yamamoto H, Kimura Y, Takesue M, Kondo M, Nomoto K. Significant prolongation of disease-free period gained by oral polysaccharide K (PSK) administration after curative surgical operation of colorectal cancer. *Cancer Immunol Immunother.* 1990;31:261-268.

Toth B, Coles M, Lynch J. Effects of VPS extract of Coriolus versicolor on cancer of the large intestine using a serial sacrifice technique. *In Vivo.* 2006;20:341-346.

Tsang KW, Lam CL, Yan C, Mak JC, Ooi GC, Ho JC, Lam B, Man R, Sham JS, Lam WK. Coriolus versicolor polysaccharide peptide slows progression of advanced non-small cell lung cancer. *Respir Med.* 2003;97:618-624.

ELLAGIC ACID

Other common name(s): none
Scientific/medical name(s): none

Description

Ellagic acid is a phytochemical, or plant chemical, found in raspberries, strawberries, cranberries, walnuts, pecans, pomegranates, and other plant foods.

Overview

Research in cell cultures and laboratory animals has found that ellagic acid may slow the growth of some tumors caused by certain carcinogens. While this finding is promising, at this time there is no reliable evidence available from human clinical studies showing that ellagic acid can prevent or treat cancer. Further research is needed to determine what benefits it may have.

How is it promoted for use?

Ellagic acid seems to have some anticancer properties. It can act as an antioxidant and has been found to cause cell death in cancer cells in the laboratory. In other laboratory studies, ellagic acid seems to reduce the effect of estrogen in promoting growth of breast cancer cells in tissue cultures. There are also reports that it may help the liver to break down or remove some cancer-causing substances from the blood.

Some supporters have claimed these results mean that ellagic acid can prevent or treat cancer in humans. This claim has not been proven. Unfortunately, many substances that show promise against cancer in laboratory and animal studies are not found to be useful in people.

Ellagic acid has also been said to reduce heart disease, birth defects, liver problems, and to promote wound healing.

What does it involve?

The highest levels of ellagic acid are found in raspberries, strawberries, and pomegranates, especially when they are freeze-dried. Extracts from red raspberry leaves or seeds, pomegranates, or other sources are said to contain high levels of ellagic acid and are available as dietary supplements in capsule, powder, or liquid form. The best dose of these preparations is not known.

What is the history behind it?

Ellagic acid was studied in the 1960s mainly for its effects on blood clotting. Early published research on ellagic acid and cancer first appeared in the 1970s and 1980s. With the publication of several small laboratory studies in the mid-1990s, ellagic acid began to be promoted on the Internet and elsewhere as a means of preventing and treating cancer.

What is the evidence?

Almost all studies conducted on ellagic acid have been done in cell cultures or laboratory animals. Several animal studies have found that ellagic acid can inhibit the growth of tumors of the skin, esophagus, and lungs, as well as other tumors caused by carcinogens. A recent study in cell cultures found that ellagic acid may act against substances that help tumors to form new blood vessels. Further studies are needed to determine whether these results apply to humans.

In the only study reported thus far in humans, Italian researchers found that ellagic acid seemed to reduce the side effects of chemotherapy in men with advanced prostate cancer, although it did not slow disease progression or improve survival. The researchers cautioned that more research would be needed to confirm these results.

The interaction between phytochemicals like ellagic acid and other compounds in foods is not well understood, but it is unlikely that any single compound offers the best protection against cancer. A balanced diet that includes five or more servings a day of fruits and vegetables along with foods from a variety of other plant sources such as nuts, seeds, whole grain cereals, and beans is likely to be more effective in reducing cancer risk than eating one particular food in large amounts. However, some studies suggest that foods high in ellagic acid might be useful additions to a balanced diet. For example, one nonrandomized clinical study of men with prostate cancer reported that pomegranate juice slowed the increase in blood levels of prostate-specific antigen, a substance that is routinely measured to estimate growth of prostate cancer.

Are there any possible problems or complications?

Eating berries or other natural sources of ellagic acid is generally considered safe. These foods should be part of a balanced diet that includes several servings of fruits and vegetables each day.

Ellagic acid is available in supplement form. Some reports indicate it may affect certain enzymes in the liver, which could alter the way in which some drugs are absorbed in the body. For this reason, people taking medicines or other dietary supplements should talk with their doctors or pharmacists about all their medicines and supplements before taking ellagic acid. The raspberry leaf, or preparations made from it, should be used with caution during pregnancy because it may initiate labor. Relying on this type of treatment alone and avoiding or delaying conventional medical care for cancer may have serious health consequences.

This product is sold as a dietary supplement in the United States. Unlike companies that produce drugs (which must provide the FDA with results of detailed testing showing their product is safe and effective before the drug is approved for sale), the companies that make supplements do not have to show evidence of safety or health benefits to the FDA before selling their products. Supplement products without any reliable scientific evidence of health benefits may still be sold as long as the companies selling them do not claim the supplements can prevent, treat, or cure any specific disease. Some such products may not contain the amount of the herb or substance that is written on the label, and some may include other substances (contaminants). Though the FDA has written new rules to improve the quality of manufacturing processes for dietary supplements and the accurate listing of supplement ingredients, these rules do not take full effect until 2010. The new rules also do not address the safety of supplement ingredients or their effects on health when proper manufacturing techniques are used.

Most such supplements have not been tested to find out if they interact with medicines, foods, or other herbs and supplements. Even though some reports of interactions and harmful effects may be published, full studies of interactions and effects are not often available. Because of these limitations, any information on ill effects and interactions should be considered incomplete.

References

Ahn D, Putt D, Kresty L, Stoner GD, Fromm D, Hollenberg PF. The effects of dietary ellagic acid on rat hepatic and esophageal mucosal cytochromes P450 and phase II enzymes. *Carcinogenesis.* 1996;17:821-828.

Ellagic acid. Memorial Sloan-Kettering Cancer Center Web site. http://www.mskcc.org/mskcc/html/11571.cfm?RecordID=644&tab=HC. Accessed June 10, 2008.

Falsaperla M, Morgia G, Tartarone A, Ardito R, Romano G. Support ellagic acid therapy in patients with hormone refractory prostate cancer (HRPC) on standard chemotherapy using vinorelbine and estramustine phosphate. *Eur Urol.* 2005;47:449-454; discussion 454-455. Epub 2005 Jan 19.

Harttig U, Hendricks JD, Stoner GD, Bailey GS. Organ specific, protocol dependent modulation of 7,12-dimethylbenz-[a]anthracene carcinogenesis in rainbow trout (*Oncorhyncus mykiss*) by dietary ellagic acid. *Carcinogenesis.* 1996;17:2403-2409.

Kresty LA, Morse MA, Morgan C, Carlton PS, Lu J, Gupta A, Blackwood M, Stoner GD. Chemoprevention of esophageal tumorigenesis by dietary administration of lyophilized black raspberries. *Cancer Res.* 2001;61:6112-6119.

Labrecque L, Lamy S, Chapus A, Mihoubi S, Durocher Y, Cass B, Bojanowski MW, Gingras D, Béliveau R. Combined inhibition of PDGF and VEGF receptors by ellagic acid, a dietary-derived phenolic compound. *Carcinogenesis.* 2005;26:821-826.

Mandal S, Stoner GD. Inhibition of N-nitrosobenzylmethylamine-induced esophageal tumorigenesis in rats by ellagic acid. *Carcinogenesis.* 1990;11:55-61.

Mertens-Talcott SU, Lee JH, Percival SS, Talcott ST. Induction of cell death in Caco-2 human colon carcinoma cells by ellagic acid rich fractions from muscadine grapes (*Vitis rotundifolia*). *J Agric Food Chem.* 2006;54:5336-5343.

Mukhtar H, Del Tito BJ Jr, Marcelo CL, Das M, Bickers DR. Ellagic acid: a potent naturally occurring inhibitor of benzo[a]pyrene metabolism and its subsequent glucuronidation, sulfation and covalent binding to DNA in cultured BALB/C mouse keratinocytes. *Carcinogenesis.* 1984;5:1565-1571.

Narayanan BA, Re GG. IGF-II down regulation associated cell cycle arrest in colon cancer cells exposed to phenolic antioxidant ellagic acid. *Anticancer Res.* 2001;21:359-364.

Pantuck AJ, Leppert JT, Zomorodian N, Aronson W, Hong J, Barnard RJ, Seeram N, Liker H, Wang H, Elashoff R, Heber D, Aviram M, Ignarro L, Belldegrun A. Phase II study of pomegranate juice for men with rising prostate-specific antigen following surgery or radiation for prostate cancer. *Clin Cancer Res.* 2006;12:4018-4026.

Papoutsi Z, Kassi E, Tsiapara A, Fokialakis N, Chrousos GP, Moutsatsou P. Evaluation of estrogenic/antiestrogenic activity of ellagic acid via the estrogen receptor subtypes ERalpha and ERbeta. *J Agric Food Chem.* 2005;53:7715-7720.

Thresiamma KC, George J, Kuttan R. Protective effect of curcumin, ellagic acid and bixin on radiation induced genotoxicity. *J Exp Clin Cancer Res.* 1998;17:431-434.

FASTING

Other common name(s): none
Scientific/medical name(s): none

Description

Fasting involves eating no food and drinking only water or juice for a period of one to five days or longer. Tea or broth may sometimes be part of the fasting process. Fasting is often promoted as part of a "detoxification" process in some types of metabolic therapies for cancer or other conditions.

Overview

Available scientific evidence does not support claims that fasting is effective for preventing or treating cancer. Even a short-term fast can have negative health effects, while fasting for a longer time could cause serious health problems.

How is it promoted for use?

Practitioners of a type of alternative therapy called metabolic therapy (see page 646) believe the body contains environmental toxins and other harmful substances that can be removed by fasting or detoxifying the body. They claim that fasting allows the body to focus energy on cleansing and healing itself. According to these practitioners, fasting helps the immune system work more efficiently, allows more oxygen and white blood cells to flow through the body, helps the body to burn more fat, helps increase energy, and allows other healing functions to improve. Some supporters claim that fasting by a person who has cancer can "starve" a tumor, leading to cell death.

Other illnesses and conditions proponents claim can be treated by fasting include acne, allergies, arthritis, asthma, noncancerous tumors, digestive disorders, fever, glaucoma, headaches, heart disease, high blood pressure, inflammatory diseases, pain, polyps, and ulcers. Fasting is also promoted to rejuvenate the body, help maintain normal body weight, increase longevity and sex drive, and to improve mental clarity, self-awareness, and self-esteem. It is also said to be helpful in quitting or cutting back on use of tobacco, alcohol, caffeine, or nonprescription drugs. Some practitioners claim it can heighten spiritual awareness.

What does it involve?

Short fasts, lasting from one to five days, are often done at home. Other than drinking only water or juice, fasting involves a lot of rest. Sometimes other methods of detoxification, such as liver flushes or enemas, are recommended as part of the regimen. (See also "Juicing," page 628, "Liver Flush," page 784, and "Colon Therapy," page 184.) Longer fasts require professional supervision and often take place at a spa, resort, or similar facility.

What is the history behind it?

Ancient cultures believed fasting could purify the soul. The belief that fasting could also purify or cleanse the body is a fairly modern idea, gaining popularity in the second half of the twentieth century.

What is the evidence?

Available scientific evidence does not support fasting as a treatment for cancer. Some studies in animals have suggested that long-term calorie restriction—consuming less than one's normal amount of calories each day—may slow the growth of certain tumors, but this is not the same as fasting. In fact, some animal studies have found that actual fasting, in which no food is eaten for several days, could actually promote the growth of some tumors. No human studies on the effects of fasting on cancer have been published in the available medical literature.

A brief fast (usually eight to twelve hours) is often advised by medical professionals in preparation for certain diagnostic tests. In this case, the fast helps to produce more accurate test results. Fasting may also be advised for a period of time before and after surgery, especially if digestive system organs are involved. This recommendation is mainly to ensure the stomach and bowels are empty during surgery. Such preparations are important in order to avoid getting stomach contents into the lungs, since anesthesia disables the usual protections, such as swallowing and coughing, that keep a person from inhaling foreign matter into the lungs when he or she is awake. It also allows the intestines time to recover from anesthesia before reintroducing food.

As for reaching and maintaining proper weight, most experts recommend a combination of limiting portion sizes, choosing healthful foods, and being physically active instead of fasting.

Some research has suggested that short-term fasts may briefly improve the symptoms of rheumatoid arthritis. However, the benefits do not last longer than ten days, and fasting is not a recommended component of arthritis care.

Are there any possible problems or complications?

Fasting can have short-term side effects such as headaches, dizziness, fatigue, abnormal heart rhythms, and a fruity taste in the mouth. It can also raise the risk for an attack in people with gout. Longer-term fasting can interfere with the immune system and vital bodily functions and can damage the liver, kidneys, and other organs. Fasting can be especially dangerous in people who are already malnourished, such as those with some forms of advanced cancer. Women who are pregnant or breastfeeding should not fast. Relying on this type of treatment alone and avoiding or delaying conventional medical care for cancer may have serious health consequences.

References

Caderni G, Perrelli MG, Cecchini F, Tessitore L. Enhanced growth of colorectal aberrant crypt foci in fasted/refed rats involves changes in TGFbeta1 and p21CIP expressions. *Carcinogenesis.* 2002;23:323-327.

Cassileth B. *The Alternative Medicine Handbook: The Complete Reference Guide to Alternative and Complementary Therapies.* New York: W.W. Norton; 1998.

Detoxification therapy. PDRhealth Web site. http://www.pdrhealth.com/content/natural_medicine/chapters/201160.shtml. Accessed August 4, 2005. Content no longer available.

Fasting. PDRhealth Web site. http://www.pdrhealth.com/content/natural_medicine/chapters/201200.shtml. Accessed August 4, 2005. Content no longer available.

Hikita H, Nuwaysir EF, Vaughan J, Babcock K, Haas MJ, Dragan YP, Pitot HC. The effect of short-term fasting, phenobarbital and refeeding on apoptotic loss, cell replication and gene expression in rat liver during the promotion stage. *Carcinogenesis.* 1998;19:1417-1425.

Hikita H, Vaughan J, Pitot HC. The effect of two periods of short-term fasting during the promotion stage of hepatocarcinogenesis in rats: the role of apoptosis and cell proliferation. *Carcinogenesis.* 1997;18:159-166.

Legro RS, Finegood D, Dunaif A. A fasting glucose to insulin ratio is a useful measure of insulin sensitivity in women with polycystic ovary syndrome. *J Clin Endocrinol Metab.* 1998;83:2694-2698.

Sesca E, Premoselli F, Binasco V, Bollito E, Tessitore L. Fasting-refeeding stimulates the development of mammary tumors induced by 7,12-dimethylbenz[a]anthracene. *Nutr Cancer.* 1998;30:25-30.

GARLIC

Other common name(s): garlic clove, garlic powder, garlic oil, allium, allyl sulfides, ajoene
Scientific/medical name(s): *Allium sativum*

Description

Garlic is a member of the lily family and is closely related to onions, leeks, and chives. Extracts and oils made from garlic are sometimes used as herbal remedies.

Overview

Garlic is currently under study for its ability to reduce cancer risk. However, there is not enough evidence at this time to support eating large amounts of garlic or taking garlic supplements for cancer prevention. Garlic may have the potential to interfere with anesthesia or other medicines. It is reasonable to include garlic as part of a balanced diet, unless one has a particular health problem or is taking medication that has been shown to be adversely affected by garlic.

How is it promoted for use?

Garlic and garlic supplements are sometimes promoted to prevent or treat cancer. Several compounds in garlic may have anticancer properties, but compounds of one type in particular—the allyl sulfur compounds—are said to play a major role. These compounds reportedly help the body get rid of cancer-causing chemicals and help cause cancer cells to die naturally, a process called apoptosis. There have also been claims that garlic has immune-boosting properties that may reduce cancer cell growth and help the body fight off diseases such as colds or the flu.

Proponents claim garlic can be used to treat bacterial, yeast, fungal, and parasitic infections and can be used to treat high blood sugar levels. They also say it has properties that may help stomach and abdominal problems. Garlic has also been claimed to reduce risk for heart disease, lower cholesterol, and reduce blood pressure.

What does it involve?

Garlic is a vegetable commonly used to enhance the flavor of foods. Extracts of garlic are also sold as dietary supplements in health food stores, drug stores, and over the Internet.

There is much debate about what form and amount of garlic to use to influence health. Proponents disagree as to whether garlic is more helpful when eaten, either raw or cooked, or whether garlic extracts, powders, and oils available in tablet form are more or less effective.

Garlic is on the Commission E (Germany's regulatory agency for herbs) list of approved herbs. They suggest a dosage of fresh garlic equal to 4 grams per day (or about one large clove per day) to help reduce heart disease risk.

What is the history behind it?

Garlic has been used in cooking throughout recorded history in many cultures around the world, especially those in the Orient, Middle East, and the Mediterranean. Garlic is believed to be one of the first cultivated plants, with cultivation thought to have begun about five thousand years ago in the Middle East. Garlic has also been used medicinally for thousands of years and continues to be popular today.

What is the evidence?

Several studies from around the world have found that people who eat more garlic seem to have a lower risk for certain types of cancer. In particular, observational epidemiologic studies that looked at diet and cancer have suggested that people who eat more garlic have a lower risk for stomach, prostate, mouth and throat, kidney, and colorectal cancer. The effect on risk for breast, bladder, ovarian, and lung cancers is less clear. As always in observational studies, it is possible that other factors may account for the differences in cancer risk. The few human studies that have looked at garlic supplements have not found them to be helpful against cancer.

Many laboratory studies done in cell cultures and animals suggest garlic may help reduce tumor growth. Cell culture studies have shown garlic can help cancer cells die off naturally. Other studies in cell cultures have found that substances in garlic seem to be able to act as antioxidants. Some studies have also suggested that garlic can act against *Helicobacter pylori*, a bacterium thought to be a major cause of stomach cancer. Studies in laboratory animals have found garlic may help protect against cancer of the colon, skin, liver, and breast, among others.

Although results of some observational studies are encouraging, randomized clinical trials in which people receive either garlic or an inactive control substance provide more reliable information. Very few studies of this type have studied garlic and cancer risk. In one recent study conducted in China, where stomach cancer is quite common, aged garlic extract and steam-distilled garlic oil did not prevent this disease.

Some studies suggest that garlic can lower blood cholesterol levels, although a recent clinical study funded by the National Center of Complementary and Alternative Medicine did not confirm any effect. This California study compared raw garlic with aged garlic extract, powdered garlic, and a placebo in nearly two hundred randomly assigned volunteers. The garlic was given in doses of 4 grams per day over six months. At the end of the study, there was no significant difference in LDL ("bad") cholesterol levels among the four groups. Other studies suggest that garlic makes blood less likely to form clots, which might help prevent heart disease and stroke. However, there is no reliable direct clinical evidence that garlic can actually prevent heart attacks or strokes. Evidence on garlic and blood pressure is mixed.

While some research on garlic is promising, it is very hard to determine the exact role a particular food may have in the treatment or prevention of cancer. It is even more difficult when the food in question is often used in small amounts, as is garlic. A balanced diet that includes five or more servings a day of fruits and vegetables, along with foods from a variety of other plant sources such as nuts, seeds, whole grain cereals, and beans, is likely to be more healthful than eating one particular food in large amounts.

Are there any possible problems or complications?

Eating large amounts of garlic may lead to irritation of the digestive tract, causing stomach pain, gas, and vomiting. Some research suggests that garlic may increase the risk for bleeding because of its anti-clotting properties. It should not be used by people who will be having surgery soon, especially if they are given blood thinners or if bleeding after surgery is a concern. People on blood-thinning medications, such as warfarin (Coumadin) or aspirin, should consult with their doctor before taking garlic supplements.

Garlic seems to affect enzymes in the liver that help remove certain drugs from the body. This effect may result in reduced levels of some drugs in the body, which could be especially important in people undergoing chemotherapy. This issue is currently under study, but people thinking about taking garlic supplements should speak with their doctors first.

Relying on this type of treatment alone and avoiding or delaying conventional medical care for cancer may have serious health consequences.

This product is sold as a dietary supplement in the United States. Unlike companies that produce drugs (which must provide the FDA with results of detailed testing showing their product is safe and effective before the drug is approved for sale), the companies that make supplements do not have to show evidence of safety or health benefits to the FDA before selling their products. Supplement products without any reliable scientific evidence of health benefits may still be sold as long as the companies selling them do not claim the supplements can prevent, treat, or cure any specific disease. Some such products may not contain the amount of the herb or substance that is written on the label, and some may include other substances (contaminants). Though the FDA has written new rules to improve the quality of manufacturing processes for dietary supplements and the accurate listing of supplement ingredients, these rules do not take full effect until 2010. The new rules also do not address the safety of supplement ingredients or their effects on health when proper manufacturing techniques are used.

Most such supplements have not been tested to find out if they interact with medicines, foods, or other herbs and supplements. Even though some reports of interactions and harmful effects may be published, full studies of interactions and effects are not often available. Because of these limitations, any information on ill effects and interactions should be considered incomplete.

References

Blumenthal M, ed. *The Complete German Commission E Monographs: Therapeutic Guide to Herbal Medicines.* Austin, TX: American Botanical Council; 1998.

Dorant E, van den Brandt PA, Goldbohm RA. Allium vegetable consumption, garlic supplement intake, and female breast carcinoma incidence. *Breast Cancer Res Treat.* 1995;33:163-170.

Fleischauer AT, Arab L. Garlic and cancer: a critical review of the epidemiologic literature. *J Nutr.* 2001;131:1032S-1040S.

Galeone C, Pelucchi C, Levi F, Negri E, Franceschi S, Talamini R, Giacosa A, La Vecchia C. Onion and garlic use and human cancer. *Am J Clin Nutr.* 2006;84:1027-1032.

Gardner CD, Lawson LD, Block E, Chatterjee LM, Kiazand A, Balise RR, Kraemer HC. Effect of raw garlic vs commercial garlic supplements on plasma lipid concentrations in adults with moderate hypercholesterolemia: a randomized clinical trial. *Arch Intern Med.* 2007;167:346-353.

Garlic. Memorial Sloan-Kettering Cancer Center Web site. http://www.mskcc.org/mskcc/html/69230.cfm. Accessed June 10, 2008.

Garlic. National Center for Complementary and Alternative Medicine Web site. http://nccam.nih.gov/health/garlic/. Accessed June 10, 2008.

Garlic. PDRhealth Web site. http://www.pdrhealth.com/drug_info/nmdrugprofiles/herbaldrugs/101190.shtml. Accessed June 10, 2008.

González CA, Pera G, Agudo A, Bueno-de-Mesquita HB, Ceroti M, Boeing H, Schultz M, Del Giudice G, Plebani M, Carneiro F, Berrino F, Sacerdote C, Tumino R, Panico S, Berglund G, Simán H, Hallmans G, Stenling R, Martinez C, Dorronsoro M, Barricarte A, Navarro C, Quiros JR, Allen N, Key TJ, Bingham S, Day NE, Linseisen J, Nagel G, Overad K, Jensen MK, Olsen A, Tjønneland A, Büchner FL, Peeters PH, Numans ME, Clavel-Chapelon F, Boutron-Ruault MC, Roukos D, Trichopoulou A, Psaltopoulou T, Lund E, Casagrande C, Slimani N, Jenab M, Riboli E. Fruit and vegetable intake and the risk of stomach and oesophagus adenocarcinoma in the European Prospective Investigation into Cancer and Nutrition (EPIC-EURGAST). *Int J Cancer.* 2006;118:2559-2566.

Hsing AW, Chokkalingam AP, Gao YT, Madigan MP, Deng J, Gridley G, Fraumeni JF Jr. Allium vegetables and risk of prostate cancer: a population-based study. *J Natl Cancer Inst.* 2002;94:1648-1651.

Meijerman I, Beijen JH, Schellens JH. Herb-drug interactions in oncology: focus on mechanisms of induction. *Oncologist.* 2006;11:742-752.

Ngo SN, Williams DB, Cobiac L, Head RJ. Does garlic reduce risk of colorectal cancer? A systematic review. *J Nutr.* 2007;137:2264-2269.

Phytochemicals and cardiovascular disease. American Heart Association Web site. http://www.americanheart.org/presenter.jhtml?identifier=4722. Accessed June 10, 2008.

Riggs DR, DeHaven JI, Lamm DL. *Allium sativum* (garlic) treatment for murine transitional cell carcinoma. *Cancer.* 1997;79:1987-1994.

Schulz M, Lahmann PH, Boeing H, Hoffmann K, Allen N, Key TJ, Bingham S, Wirfält E, Berglund G, Lundin E, Hallmans G, Lukanova A, Martínez Garcia C, González CA, Tormo MJ, Quirøs JR, Ardanaz E, Larrañaga N, Lund E, Gram IT, Skeie G, Peeters PH, van Gils CH, Bueno-de-Mesquita HB, Büchner FL, Pasanisi P, Galasso R, Palli D, Tumino R, Vineis P, Trichopoulou A, Kalapothaki V, Trichopoulos D, Chang-Claude J, Linseisen J, Boutron-Ruault MC, Touillaud M, Clavel-Chapelon F, Olsen A, Tjønneland A, Overvad K, Tetsche M, Jenab M, Norat T, Kaaks R, Riboli E. Fruit and vegetable consumption and risk of epithelial ovarian cancer: the European Prospective Investigation into Cancer and Nutrition. *Cancer Epidemiol Biomarkers Prev.* 2005;14:2531-2535.

Sundaram SG, Milner JA. Diallyl disulfide induces apoptosis of human colon tumor cells. *Carcinogenesis.* 1996;17:669-673.

Steinmetz KA, Kushi LH, Bostick RM, Folsom AR, Potter JD. Vegetables, fruit, and colon cancer in the Iowa Women's Health Study. *Am J Epidemiol.* 1994;139:1-15.

Tanaka S, Haruma K, Yoshihara M, Kajiyama G, Kira K, Amagase H, Chayama K. Aged garlic extract has potential suppressive effect on colorectal adenomas in humans. *J Nut.* 2006;136:821S-826S.

You WC, Brown LM, Zhang L, Li JY, Jin ML, Chang YS, Ma JL, Pan KF, Liu WD, Hu Y, Crystal-Mansour S, Pee D, Blot WJ, Fraumeni JF Jr, Xu GW, Gail MH. Randomized double-blind factorial trial of three treatments to reduce the prevalence of precancerous gastric lesions. *J Natl Cancer Inst.* 2006;98:974-983.

GERSON THERAPY

Other common name(s): Gerson diet, Gerson method, Gerson treatment, Gerson program
Scientific/medical name(s): none

Description

Gerson therapy is a form of alternative cancer treatment involving coffee enemas, supplements, and a special diet that is claimed to cleanse the body, boost the immune system, and stimulate metabolism.

Overview

Available scientific evidence does not support claims that Gerson therapy is effective in treating cancer, and the principles behind it are not widely accepted by the medical community. It is not approved for use in the United States. Gerson therapy can be dangerous. Coffee enemas have been associated with serious infections, dehydration, constipation, colitis (inflammation of the colon), electrolyte imbalances, and even death.

How is it promoted for use?

Gerson therapy is considered a metabolic therapy (see "Metabolic Therapy," page 646), and it is based on the theory that disease is caused by the body's accumulation of toxic substances. Practitioners believe that fertilizers, insecticides, herbicides, and other chemicals contaminate food by lowering its potassium content and raising its sodium content. Food processing and cooking adds more sodium, which they believe changes the metabolism of cells in the body and eventually causes cancer.

According to practitioners of Gerson therapy, people who have cancer have too much sodium and not enough potassium in their cells. The fruit and vegetable diet that is part of Gerson therapy is used to correct this imbalance and revitalize the liver so it can rid the body of malignant cells. Coffee enemas, also part of Gerson therapy, are claimed to relieve pain and eliminate liver toxins in a process called detoxification.

The goal of metabolic therapies is to eliminate toxins from the body and enhance immune function so that the body can "fight off" cancer. Liver extract injections, pancreatic enzymes, and various supplements are said to stimulate metabolism. Proponents of metabolic therapy claim that it addresses the underlying cause of disease rather than treating the symptoms.

What does it involve?

Gerson therapy requires following a strict low-salt, low-fat, vegetarian diet and drinking juice from about twenty pounds of fresh fruits and vegetables each day. One glass of juice is consumed each hour, thirteen times a day. In addition, patients are given several coffee enemas each day. Various supplements, such as potassium, vitamin B12, pancreatic enzymes, thyroid hormone, and liver extracts, are used to stimulate organ function, particularly of the liver and thyroid. Sometimes other treatments such as laetrile may also be recommended (see "Laetrile," page 776).

Treatment is usually begun at an inpatient clinic over several weeks. The Gerson Institute does not own or operate any medical facilities and instead refers patients to clinics it licenses. Currently the only licensed clinic is in Tijuana, Mexico. Clinic fees often exceed $4,000 per week. Treatment may last from a few months to ten years or more. It is generally recommended for at least two years in cancer patients. The Gerson Institute also offers a home therapy package.

What is the history behind it?

One of the oldest nutritional approaches to cancer treatment, the Gerson therapy was developed by Max Gerson, MD, a German doctor who immigrated to the United States in the late 1930s. He designed the dietary program to treat his own migraine headaches. He later expanded his method to treat other conditions such as arthritis, tuberculosis, and cancer. In 1945, Gerson published a preliminary report of his results in treating cancer in the *Review of Gastroenterology*. The National Cancer Institute and New York County Medical Society examined records of his patients and found no evidence that the method was effective against cancer. After his death in 1959, his work was carried on by his daughter, Charlotte Gerson, who established the Gerson Institute in the late 1970s.

What is the evidence?

There have been no well-controlled studies published in the available medical literature that show the Gerson therapy is effective in treating cancer. In a recent review of the medical literature, researchers from The University of Texas M. D. Anderson Cancer Center identified seven human studies of Gerson therapy that have been published or presented at medical conferences. None of them were randomized controlled studies. One study was a retrospective review conducted by the Gerson Research Organization. They reported that survival rates were higher than would normally be expected for patients with melanoma, colorectal cancer, and ovarian cancer who were treated with surgery and Gerson therapy, but they did not provide statistics to support the results. Other studies have been small, had inconclusive results, or have been plagued by other problems (such as a large percentage of patients not completing the study), making it impossible to draw firm conclusions about the effectiveness of treatment.

Some ideas put forth as part of the Gerson regimen, such as eating large amounts of fruits and vegetables and limiting fat intake, can be part of a healthy diet if not taken to an extreme. Researchers are continuing to study the potential anticancer properties of different substances in fruits and vegetables, but their actual effects are not well understood at this time. Because of this, the best advice may be to eat a balanced diet that includes five or more servings a day of vegetables and fruit, choosing whole grains over processed and refined foods, and limiting red meats and animal fats. Choosing foods from a variety of fruits, vegetables and other plant sources such as nuts, seeds, whole grain cereals, and beans is likely to be healthier than consuming large amounts of one particular food. Based on currently available evidence, diet is likely to play a greater role in preventing cancer than in treating it.

There is very little scientific evidence to support the use of other components of the Gerson regimen, such as consuming only fresh, raw juices prepared in a certain way, eliminating salt from the diet, and "detoxifying" the liver through coffee enemas and injected liver extracts.

Are there any possible problems or complications?

Use of the Gerson therapy can lead to a number of significant problems. Serious illness and death have occurred from some of the components of the treatment, such as the coffee enemas, which remove potassium from the body and can lead to electrolyte imbalances. Continued home use of enemas may cause the colon's normal function to weaken, worsening constipation problems and colitis. Some metabolic diets used in combination with enemas cause dehydration.

Serious infections may result from poorly administered liver extracts. Thyroid supplements may cause severe bleeding in patients with cancer that has spread to the liver.

Gerson therapy may be especially hazardous to women who are pregnant or breastfeeding. Relying on this treatment alone and avoiding or delaying conventional medical care for cancer may have serious health consequences.

These substances may have not been thoroughly tested to find out how they interact with medicines, foods, or dietary supplements. Even though some reports of interactions and harmful effects may be published, full studies of interactions and effects are not often available. Because of these limitations, any information on ill effects and interactions should be considered incomplete.

References

American Cancer Society. Questionable methods of cancer management: 'nutritional' therapies. *CA Cancer J Clin.* 1993;43:309-319.

Gerson regimen. Memorial Sloan-Kettering Cancer Center Web site. http://www.mskcc.org/mskcc/html/69233.cfm. Updated August 14, 2007. Accessed June 10, 2008.

Green S. A critique of the rationale for cancer treatment with coffee enemas and diet. *JAMA.* 1992;268:3224-3227.

Hildenbrand G, Hildenbrand L. Defining the role of diet therapy in complementary cancer management: prevention of recurrence vs. regression of disease. Proceedings of the 1996 Alternative Therapies Symposium: Creating Integrated Healthcare. San Diego, CA: January 18-21, 1996.

Hildenbrand GL, Hildenbrand LC, Bradford K, Cavin SW. Five-year survival rates of melanoma patients treated by diet therapy after the manner of Gerson: a retrospective review. *Altern Ther Health Med.* 1995;1:29-37.

National Institutes of Health. *Alternative Medicine: Expanding Medical Horizons: A Report to the National Institutes of Health on Alternative Medical Systems and Practices in the United States.* Washington, DC: US Government Printing Office; 1994. NIH publication 94-066.

Nutrition & special diets: Gerson detailed scientific review. Complementary/Integrative Medicine Education Resources, The University of Texas M. D. Anderson Cancer Center Web site. http://www.mdanderson.org/departments/cimer/display.cfm?id=17508EEC-F2C5-11D4-810400508B603A14&method=displayFull. Accessed June 10, 2008.

US Congress, Office of Technology Assessment. *Unconventional Cancer Treatments: OTA-H-405.* Washington, DC: US Government Printing Office; 1990.

GRAPES

Other common name(s): grape diet, grape cure, grape seed extract (GSE), grape seed proanthocyanidin extract (GSPE), grape seed oil, grape skins, proanthocyanidins, oligomeric proanthocyanidins (OPCs), resveratrol

Scientific/medical name(s): *Vitis vinifera, Vitis coignetiae*

Description

Grapes grow wild on vines or are cultivated. They are believed to be native to northwest Asia, although they have been grown throughout Europe and the United States for centuries. The seeds, skin, leaves, stems, and grape itself are used in herbal remedies. At times in the past, diets consisting solely of grapes have been touted as an alternative means of treating cancer. Some chemicals found in grape extracts (called proanthocyanidins) and in grape skins (called resveratrol) are currently being studied for possible use in the prevention and treatment of cancer and other illnesses.

Overview

Available scientific evidence does not support claims that a diet of grapes alone is effective for treating cancer or any other disease. Some laboratory evidence suggests that certain chemicals in grapes and their seeds and skins may help prevent heart disease and cancer, but more research is needed in people to understand the possible long-term benefits.

How is it promoted for use?

Alternative practitioners recommend the use of grapes and parts of the grape plant for high blood pressure, menopause, varicose veins, high cholesterol, skin rashes, and urination problems. They also claim it works for inflammation of the gums, throat, eyes, and mouth. Although used rarely today, the grape diet was promoted at different times in the twentieth century as a treatment to flush toxins from the body and protect the body against cancer and virtually all other diseases. Some supporters believed that the diet cured cancer.

Evidence suggests that proanthocyanidins, the chemicals found in grape seed extract, are powerful antioxidants. Antioxidants are compounds that block the action of free radicals, activated oxygen molecules that can damage cells. Proponents claim that antioxidants inhibit the development of some types of cancer, protect against heart disease, and are useful for treating a variety of medical conditions such as arthritis, allergies, circulatory problems, diabetes, water retention, and vision problems.

A compound called resveratrol, which is found in the skins of red grapes, is being studied to see how it affects the development and progression of heart disease and cancer.

What does it involve?

Fresh, preserved, and dried grapes are used as is or in the form of liquid extracts, tinctures, gargles, enemas, douches, and compresses. Grape skins are also used in making red wine. Grape seed extract and resveratrol are available as dietary supplements in tablet and capsule form. The amount of these substances in different supplements varies by manufacturer.

The complete grape diet begins with fasting and daily enemas for a few days and is followed by a diet of grapes and water for one to two weeks. Then, fresh fruits and sour milk can also be consumed. The next stage of the diet includes raw vegetables, salads, nuts, dairy products, honey, and olive oil. During the final stage of the diet, if a person is doing well, he or she may be allowed to add one cooked meal per day.

What is the history behind it?

Grapes have been associated with health for many centuries. Evidence of fossilized grape leaves, stems, and seeds dating back ten to twelve million years has been found in the Northern hemisphere. Grapes from the *Vitis vinifera* species were grown for thousands of years in the Old World before they were brought to the United States.

Johanna Brandt, a South African dietitian, proposed the grape diet in 1925. Brandt claimed to have cured herself of stomach cancer by following the diet. After immigrating to the United States in 1927, she opened the Harmony Healing Centre in New York City and began promoting the treatment. She wrote a book that was first published in 1928 and was republished several times throughout the twentieth century. Because no scientific evidence supported their claims that the treatment improved health or cured disease, Brandt and some of her followers who prescribed or promoted the grape diet as a cure for cancer eventually became the targets of intense criticism and even legal action.

During the past few decades, interest in understanding the role of antioxidants in health has begun to grow. Proanthocyanidins were extracted from grape seeds in 1970. In the mid-1990s, a compound called resveratrol, found mostly in the skins of red grapes, was first suggested to be responsible for the "French paradox," the low occurrence of heart disease among the French, who tend to eat a high-fat diet.

What is the evidence?

While some substances in grapes may hold promise against cancer, there is very little reliable scientific evidence available at this time that drinking red wine, eating grapes, or following the grape diet can prevent or treat cancer in people.

Several laboratory studies in cell cultures have shown that proanthocyanidins, the chemicals found in grape seed extract, have antioxidant properties. A small randomized clinical trial of grape seed extract in healthy volunteers supported this finding. Some laboratory studies have also found that proanthocyanidins may reduce the body's production of estrogen, which could possibly affect hormone-sensitive tumors such as some types of breast cancer. It is not yet clear whether these properties will translate into anticancer benefits in people. Early clinical trials are currently in progress to find the best dose of grape seed extract for suppressing estrogen levels for breast cancer prevention.

Studies in laboratory animals have suggested that grape seed extract may act against prostate, colon, and breast cancer. One laboratory study found that grape seed extract seemed to make the chemotherapy drug doxorubicin more effective against breast cancer cells. Randomized clinical trials are needed to determine whether grape seed extract can be helpful in cancer treatment.

Laboratory and animal studies have shown that resveratrol may help prevent heart disease and cancer. It appears to have antioxidant, anti-inflammatory, and possibly antiestrogenic properties. It also seems to activate liver enzymes that are responsible for ridding the body of unwanted chemicals. These properties may mean it will be active against cancer in people, but randomized clinical trials are needed to confirm this effect. Early clinical trials are now under way in healthy volunteers to determine the amount of resveratrol that can be given safely. This dose will then be used in studies of resveratrol for cancer prevention. Note, however, that a study of extracted chemicals would not be expected to have the same result as a study using the raw plant.

Some observational epidemiologic studies have found that people who drink red wine may have lower incidences of lung and prostate cancer. As always in these types of studies, many other factors could account for the difference in cancer risk. In addition, several studies have found that high intake of alcohol, regardless of the type, is linked to an increase in breast cancer and some other types of cancer.

While the early research on some substances in grapes is promising, it is very hard to determine the exact role a particular food may have against cancer. A balanced diet that includes five or more servings a day of fruits and vegetables, along with foods from a variety of other plant sources such as nuts, seeds, whole grain cereals, and beans, is likely to be more effective than eating one particular food in large amounts.

Are there any possible problems or complications?

An exclusive grape diet is unhealthy and does not supply the body with adequate amounts of protein and important nutrients. Grape seed extract is believed to be safe, but additional research is needed for confirmation.

The amount of resveratrol in red wine varies greatly, and increased consumption of wine to raise resveratrol intake may pose certain health risks. Alcohol is linked with a higher risk for cancer of the mouth, esophagus, pharynx, larynx, and liver in both men and women and a higher risk for breast cancer in women. Cancer risk also increases with the amount of alcohol consumed. However, the cardiovascular benefits of moderate drinking (two drinks a day for men, one drink a day for women) may outweigh the risk for cancer in men over age fifty and in women over age sixty.

Some substances in grapes may affect how quickly enzymes in the body get rid of certain chemicals, which could possibly affect the blood levels of certain drugs. If you are thinking about taking a grape-derived supplement, talk to your doctor.

The possible effects on pregnancy or breastfeeding have not been well studied. Relying on this treatment alone and avoiding or delaying conventional medical care for cancer may have serious health consequences.

This product is sold as a dietary supplement in the United States. Unlike companies that produce drugs (which must provide the FDA with results of detailed testing showing their product is safe and effective before the drug is approved for sale), the companies that make supplements do not have to show evidence of safety or health benefits to the FDA before selling their products. Supplement products without any reliable scientific evidence of health benefits may still be sold as long as the companies selling them do not claim the supplements can prevent, treat, or cure any specific disease. Some such products may not contain the amount of the herb or substance that is written on the label, and some

may include other substances (contaminants). Though the FDA has written new rules to improve the quality of manufacturing processes for dietary supplements and the accurate listing of supplement ingredients, these rules do not take full effect until 2010. The new rules also do not address the safety of supplement ingredients or their effects on health when proper manufacturing techniques are used.

Most such supplements have not been tested to find out if they interact with medicines, foods, or other herbs and supplements. Even though some reports of interactions and harmful effects may be published, full studies of interactions and effects are not often available. Because of these limitations, any information on ill effects and interactions should be considered incomplete.

References

American Cancer Society. Unproven methods of cancer management. Grape diet. *CA Cancer J Clin.* 1974;24: 144-146.

Athar M, Back JH, Tang X, Kim KH, Kopelovich L, Bickers DR, Kim AL. Resveratrol: a review of preclinical studies for human cancer prevention. *Toxicol Appl Pharmacol.* 2007;224:274-283.

Barrett S. The grape cure. Quackwatch Web site. http://www.quackwatch.org/01QuackeryRelatedTopics/Cancer/grape.html. Updated September 18, 2001. Accessed June 10, 2008.

Eng ET, Ye J, Williams D, Phung S, Moore RE, Young MK, Gruntmanis U, Braunstein G, Chen S. Suppression of estrogen biosynthesis by procyanidin dimers in red wine and grape seeds. *Cancer Res.* 2003;63:8516-8522.

Grape seed. Memorial Sloan-Kettering Cancer Center Web site. http://www.mskcc.org/mskcc/html/69243.cfm. Accessed June 10, 2008.

Grape seed proanthocyanidins. PDRhealth Web site. http://www.pdrhealth.com/drugs/altmed/altmedmono.aspx?contentFileName=ame0089.xml&contentName=Grape+Seed+Extract. Accessed June 10, 2008.

IH636 grape seed extract in preventing breast cancer in postmenopausal women at risk of developing breast cancer. ClinicalTrials.gov Web site. http://clinicaltrials.gov/show/NCT00100893. Accessed June 10, 2008.

Kaur M, Singh RP, Gu M, Agarwal R, Agarwal C. Grape seed extract inhibits in vitro and in vivo growth of human colorectal carcinoma cells. *Clin Cancer Res.* 2006;12:6194-6202.

Kijima I, Phung S, Hur G, Kwok SL, Chen S. Grape seed extract is an aromatase inhibitor and a suppressor of aromatase expression. *Cancer Res.* 2006;66:5960-5967.

Kim H, Hall P, Smith M, Kirk M, Prasain JK, Barnes S, Grubbs C. Chemoprevention by grape seed extract and genistein in carcinogen-induced mammary cancer in rats is diet dependent. *J Nutr.* 2004;134:3445S-3452S.

Kushi LH, Byers T, Doyle C, Bandera EV, McCullough M, McTiernan A, Gansler T, Andrews KS, Thun MJ; American Cancer Society 2006 nutrition and physical activity Guidelines Advisory Committee. American Cancer Society guidelines on nutrition and physical activity for cancer prevention: reducing the risk of cancer with healthy food choices and physical activity. *CA Cancer J Clin.* 2006;56:254-281.

Mantena SK, Baliga MS, Katiyar SK. Grape seed proanthocyanidins induce apoptosis and inhibit metastasis of highly metastatic breast carcinoma cells. *Carcinogenesis.* 2006;27:1682-1691. Epub 2006 Apr 5.

Mitchell SH, Zhu W, Young CY. Resveratrol inhibits the expression and function of the androgen receptor in LNCaP prostate cancer cells. *Cancer Res.* 1999;59:5892-5895.

Mohan J, Gandhi AA, Bhavya BC, Rashmi R, Karunagaran D, Indu R, Santhoshkumar TR. Caspase-2 triggers Bax-Bak-dependent and -independent cell death in colon cancer cells treated with resveratrol. *J Biol Chem.* 2006;281:17599-17611.

Moss R. *Herbs Against Cancer: History and Controversy.* New York: Equinox Press; 1998.

Nuttall SL, Kendall MJ, Bombardelli E, Morazzoni P. An evaluation of the antioxidant activity of a standardized grape seed extract, Leucoselect. *J Clin Pharm Ther.* 1998;23:385-389.

Resveratrol. PDRhealth Web site. http://www.pdrhealth.com/drug_info/nmdrugprofiles/nutsupdrugs/res_0224.shtml. Accessed June 10, 2008.

Ruano-Ravina A, Figueiras A, Barros-Dios JM. Type of wine and risk of lung cancer: a case-control study in Spain. *Thorax.* 2004;59:981-985.

Sharma G, Tyagi AK, Singh RP, Chan DC, Agarwal R. Synergistic anti-cancer effects of grape seed extract and conventional cytotoxic agent doxorubicin against human breast carcinoma cells. *Breast Cancer Res Treat.* 2004;85:1-12.

Veluri R, Singh RP, Liu Z, Thompson JA, Agarwal R, Agarwal C. Fractionation of grape seed extract and identification of gallic acid as one of the major active constituents causing growth inhibition and apoptotic death of DU145 human prostate carcinoma cells. *Carcinogenesis.* 2006;27:1445-1453.

INOSITOL HEXAPHOSPHATE

Other common name(s): IP6, IP-6, InsP-6, inositol, phytic acid, phytate, myo-inositol hexaphosphate

Scientific/medical name(s): inositol-1,2,3,4,5,6-hexakisphosphate

Description

Inositol hexaphosphate (IP6) is a chemical found in beans, brown rice, corn, sesame seeds, wheat bran, and other high-fiber foods. It is converted into compounds in the body that are used by cells to relay messages to the cell nucleus. IP6 also aids the body in its metabolism of calcium and other minerals.

Overview

Animal and laboratory research has found that IP6 may be effective in lowering tumor incidence and slowing tumor growth. However, studies of IP6 have not yet been done in people. Clinical trials are needed to find out how it might work in preventing or treating cancer in humans.

How is it promoted for use?

Proponents call IP6 a "natural cancer fighter" and claim it slows or reverses the growth of various forms of cancer, including breast, colon, and prostate cancer. It is thought to be an antioxidant, a compound that blocks the action of free radicals, which can damage cells. It may help to prevent the transmission of abnormal signals that tell a cancer cell to keep growing. Some research shows IP6 slows abnormal cell division and may transform tumor cells into normal cells. Supporters also claim it prevents kidney stones, high cholesterol, heart disease, and liver disease.

IP6 is one form of inositol. Inositol is a kind of sugar formed by six carbon atoms, six oxygen atoms, and twelve hydrogen atoms. This combination of atoms can also form glucose, but the atoms are arranged differently in inositol and glucose. There are actually several forms of inositol, each with subtle differences in the arrangement of atoms, with myo-inositol being the most common form. IP6 is formed by substituting phosphate groups (each with a phosphorous and three oxygens) for each of the six hydroxyl (an oxygen and hydrogen) groups of inositol. Thus, IP6 is related, yet chemically distinct, from myo-inositol, which is being studied for its possible role in illnesses such as depression and anxiety.

What does it involve?

Many high-fiber food sources contain IP6, and it is also available in pill form as a dietary supplement combining inositol and IP6. Scientists do not know enough about the chemical to recommend a standard supplement dose. It is not known whether taking a supplement provides the same effect as getting IP6 from food sources.

What is the history behind it?

The existence of IP6 has been known for several decades. Interest in its potential anticancer properties emerged in the mid-1980s when Dr. Abulkalam Shamsuddin, a pathologist at the University of Maryland, began to conduct research on inositol in the laboratory. He published a book on the subject in 1998. He and other researchers continue to study the effects of IP6.

What is the evidence?

All of the evidence regarding the anticancer effects of IP6 has come from laboratory cell cultures and animal studies. Laboratory studies of cell cultures have shown that IP6 may help put cancer cells on a path to normal cell death and may help prevent metastasis. It may also affect the growth of blood vessels that supply the tumor and the immune system in general. IP6 may have activity against cancer of the pancreas, breast, prostate, colon, and other types of cancer. Results of some cell studies have suggested that IP6 may help certain chemotherapy or hormone therapy drugs work better.

Studies in animals have found that supplementing the animals' diets with IP6 may help prevent tumors in the prostate, lung, colon, skin, and other areas. Further studies are needed to find out whether the results apply to humans. One preliminary human study suggested that IP6 may cause regression of precancerous lung changes in smokers. IP6 has not yet been studied in humans as a treatment for cancer.

Inositol hexaphosphate and similar chemicals have also been studied for treatment of polycystic ovary syndrome, panic disorders, autism, obsessive-compulsive disorders, Alzheimer's disease, post-traumatic stress disorder, and depression. Researchers have reached no firm conclusions about its impact on these conditions.

Are there any possible problems or complications?

When taken in moderate amounts, IP6 appears to be safe. However, no studies have been done to determine its safety. Some experts advise those who wish to increase their intake of IP6 to add beans, whole grains, and other foods rich in IP6 to their diets before resorting to supplements.

Inositol hexaphosphate may reduce the body's ability to absorb some minerals such as zinc, calcium, and iron. This concern has been raised mainly in regard to infants. IP6 can also reduce the amounts absorbed from mineral supplements. No studies have tested the safety of IP6 in women who are pregnant or breastfeeding. Relying on this treatment alone and avoiding or delaying conventional medical care for cancer may have serious health consequences.

This product is sold as a dietary supplement in the United States. Unlike companies that produce drugs (which must provide the FDA with results of detailed testing showing their product is safe and effective before the drug is approved for sale), the companies that make supplements do not have to show evidence of safety or health benefits to the FDA before selling their products. Supplement products without any reliable scientific evidence of health benefits may still be sold as long as the companies selling them do not claim the supplements can prevent, treat, or cure any specific disease. Some such products may not contain the amount of the herb or substance that is written on the label, and some may include other substances (contaminants). Though the FDA has written new rules to improve the quality of manufacturing processes for dietary supplements and the accurate listing of supplement ingredients, these rules do not take full effect until 2010. The new rules also do not address the safety of supplement ingredients or their effects on health when proper manufacturing techniques are used.

Most such supplements have not been tested to find out if they interact with medicines, foods, or other herbs and supplements. Even though some reports of interactions and harmful effects may be published, full studies of interactions and effects are not often available. Because of these limitations, any information on ill effects and interactions should be considered incomplete.

References

Inositol hexaphosphate. Memorial Sloan-Kettering Cancer Center Web site. http://www.mskcc.org/mskcc/html/69264.cfm. Updated December 19, 2007. Accessed June 18, 2008.

Inositol hexaphosphate. PDRhealth Web site. http://www.pdrhealth.com/drug_info/nmdrugprofiles/nutsupdrugs/ino_0333.shtml. Accessed June 13, 2007. Content no longer available.

Janus SC, Weurtz B, Ondrey FG. Inositol hexaphosphate and paclitaxel: symbiotic treatment of oral cavity squamous cell carcinoma. *Laryngoscope.* 2007;117:1381-1388.

Jariwalla RJ. Inositol hexaphosphate (IP6) as an anti-neoplastic and lipid-lowering agent. *Anticancer Res.* 1999;19:3699-3702.

Jenab M, Thompson LU. The influence of phytic acid in wheat bran on early biomarkers of colon carcinogenesis. *Carcinogenesis.* 1998;19:1087-1092.

Myo-Inositol. PDRhealth Web site. http://www.pdrhealth.com/drug_info/nmdrugprofiles/nutsupdrugs/myo_0145.shtml. Accessed June 10, 2008.

Nestler JE, Jakubowicz DJ, Reamer P, Gunn RD, Allan G. Ovulatory and metabolic effects of D-chiro-inositol in the polycystic ovary syndrome. *N Engl J Med.* 1999;340:1314-1320.

Singh RP, Agarwal C, Agarwal R. Inositol hexaphosphate inhibits growth, and induces G1 arrest and apoptotic death of prostate carcinoma DU145 cells: modulation of CDKI-CDK-cyclin and pRb-related protein-E2F complexes. *Carcinogenesis.* 2003;24:555-563.

Singh RP, Sharma G, Mallikarjuna GU, Dhanalakshmi S, Agarwal C, Agarwal R. In vivo suppression of hormone-refractory prostate cancer growth by inositol hexaphosphate: induction of insulin-like growth factor binding protein-3 and inhibition of vascular endothelial growth factor. *Clin Cancer Res.* 2004;10:244-250.

Somasundar P, Riggs DR, Jackson BJ, Cunningham C, Vona-Davis L, McFadden DW. Inositol hexaphosphate (IP6): a novel treatment for pancreatic cancer. *J Surg Res.* 2005;126:199-203.

Tantivejkul K, Vucenik I, Eiseman J, Shamsuddin AM. Inositol hexaphosphate (IP6) enhances the anti-proliferative effects of adriamycin and tamoxifen in breast cancer. *Breast Cancer Res Treat.* 2003;79:301-312.

Vucenik I, Shamsuddin AM. Cancer inhibition by inositol hexaphosphate (IP6) and inositol: from laboratory to clinic. *J Nutr.* 2003;133:3778S-3784S.

JUICING

Other common name(s): juice therapy
Scientific/medical name(s): none

Description

Juicing involves the consumption of freshly extracted juices from fresh fruits and uncooked vegetables as the main part of the diet.

Overview

There is no convincing scientific evidence that extracted juices are healthier than whole foods.

How is it promoted for use?

Juicing is promoted to enhance the immune system and prevent and treat a wide variety of conditions. The Internet abounds with promises of "glowing good health" from juicing. According to practitioners, "unnatural" foods cause imbalances in the body's cell composition, imbalances that are corrected and rebalanced with the juices' nutrients. This treatment method is frequently used to sustain the body during long fasts or as part of the Gerson regimen (see "Gerson Therapy," page 616). Some other proponents suggest juicing as a way to add more plant-derived nutrients to a person's usual diet.

What does it involve?

Juice extractors grind food into small pieces that are spun to extract juice from the pulp.

What is the history behind it?

Juicing first became popular in the early 1990s, when proponents claimed that it could reverse everything from the natural aging process to chronic diseases such as cancer.

What is the evidence?

There is no convincing scientific evidence that extracted juices are healthier than whole foods. Juice extractors remove the fiber-containing pulp from the fruits and vegetables, which results in less fiber intake. Some proponents suggest eating the pulp from the juiced vegetables and fruits, which helps to keep enough fiber in the diet. Some vitamins that are present in the raw food are destroyed by heat. And a diet high in vegetables and fruits has been shown to reduce cancer risk and to improve overall health. On the other hand, available scientific evidence does not support claims that the enzymes from raw foods have special, health-giving properties, since they are broken down during digestion anyway.

Are there any possible problems or complications?

Overuse of juicing or consuming too much of certain juices can cause severe diarrhea, sometimes claimed to be "cleansing" by proponents who believe that "toxins" are removed from the body during this process. The juices from fruits and starchy vegetables such as carrots or beets can contain a lot of sugar, which may be harmful for diabetics and can contribute to weight gain. Overall, however, juicing is considered safe when it is used as part of a healthy diet. Commercially juiced products should be pasteurized to kill harmful germs, which can cause serious infections in some people whose immune systems have been weakened by cancer. Relying on this type of treatment alone and avoiding or delaying conventional medical care for cancer may have serious health consequences.

References

Barrett S. Juicing. Quackwatch Web site. http://www.quackwatch.org/01QuackeryRelatedTopics/juicing.html. Updated September 7, 1999. Accessed June 10, 2008.

Doyle C, Kushi LH, Byers T, Courneya KS, Demark-Wahnefried W, Grant B, McTiernan A, Rock CL, Thompson C, Gansler T, Andrews KS, The 2006 Nutrition, Physical Activity and Cancer Survivorship Advisory Committee; American Cancer Society. Nutrition and physical activity during and after cancer treatment: an American Cancer Society guide for informed choices. *CA Cancer J Clin.* 2006;56:323-353.

Kushi LH, Byers T, Doyle C, Bandera EV, McCullough M, McTiernan A, Gansler T, Andrews KS, Thun MJ; American Cancer Society 2006 Nutrition and Physical Activity Guidelines Advisory Committee. American Cancer Society guidelines on nutrition and physical activity for cancer prevention: reducing the risk of cancer with healthy food choices and physical activity. *CA Cancer J Clin.* 2006;56:254-281.

KOMBUCHA TEA

Other common name(s): Manchurian tea, Kargasok tea, tea fungus
Scientific/medical name(s): none

Description

Kombucha tea is made by fermenting sweetened black tea with a flat, pancake-like culture of yeasts and bacteria known as the Kombucha mushroom. It is not actually a mushroom, but is called one because of the shape and color of the sac that forms on top of the tea after it ferments.

Overview

Available scientific evidence does not support claims that Kombucha tea promotes good health, prevents any ailments, or is effective in treating cancer or any other disease. Serious side effects and occasional deaths have been associated with drinking Kombucha tea.

How is it promoted for use?

Kombucha tea is promoted as a cure-all for a wide variety of conditions, including baldness, insomnia, intestinal disorders, arthritis, chronic fatigue syndrome, multiple sclerosis, AIDS, and cancer. Supporters assert that Kombucha tea can boost the immune system and reverse the aging process. Kombucha tea is said to contain antioxidants, compounds that block the action of free radicals, activated oxygen molecules that can damage cells. For people who have cancer, proponents claim the tea can improve the body's defenses (especially in the early stages of cancer) by detoxifying the body and enhancing the immune system. After the body has been detoxified, the tea is said to help repair and balance the body and fight off disease.

What does it involve?

The culture used in Kombucha tea varies but consists of several species of yeast and bacteria. It may include *Saccharomycodes ludwigii*, *Schizosaccharomyces pombe*, *Brettanomyces bruxellensis*, *Bacterium xylinum*, *Bacterium gluconicum*, *Bacterium xylinoides*, *Bacterium katogenum*, *Pichia fermentans*, *Candida stellata*, and *Torula* species, among others.

Kombucha tea is made by steeping the "mushroom" culture in tea and sugar for about a week. During this process, the original mushroom floats in the tea and produces a "baby mushroom" on its surface. These new mushrooms can be passed along to other people for starting their own cultures or can be kept to make new batches of the tea when the original mushroom "goes bad" (indicated when it turns dark brown). Proponents often recommend drinking very small daily doses of the tea (one to two ounces) to start and slowly increasing it over a few days or weeks.

Some proponents also encourage people to remove all chemicals from their diets and eat only fresh fruits and vegetables in order to help the "detoxification" process. They may also be told to quit smoking and to avoid caffeine, soft drinks, alcohol, hormone-fed meat, fertilized or sprayed foods, preservatives, and artificial colorings and flavorings.

Kombucha mushroom cultures can be obtained from commercial manufacturers in the United States; however, most people obtain Kombucha mushrooms from friends. Because of increased demand, some companies now sell bottles of brewed Kombucha tea. Other products include capsules made from the dried tea and Kombucha liquid extract, drops of which are put under the tongue.

What is the history behind it?

Kombucha tea originated in East Asia and was introduced into Germany at the turn of the century. Since the early nineteenth century, Kombucha tea has been promoted as an immunity-boosting tea that can strengthen the body against many ailments. It has become prevalent in the United States because it can be grown and harvested at home. It is especially popular among people with human immunodeficiency virus (HIV) and the elderly because of claims of its immunity-boosting and anti-aging powers.

What is the evidence?

No human studies have been published in the available scientific literature that support any of the health claims made for Kombucha tea. There have, however, been reports of serious complications associated with the tea. In April 1995, two women who had been drinking the tea daily for two months were hospitalized with severe acidosis—an abnormal increase of acid levels in body fluids. Both had high levels of lactic acid upon hospitalization. One woman died of cardiac arrest two days after admission. The second woman's heart also stopped, but she stabilized and was able to recover. The mushrooms used by both women came from the same "parent" mushroom. While no direct link to Kombucha tea was proven in this case, the U.S. Food and Drug Administration (FDA) has warned consumers to use caution when making and drinking the tea.

Are there any possible problems or complications?

Because several types of yeast and bacteria can grow under Kombucha tea's brewing conditions, different Kombucha teas may contain different varieties. Since cultures and preparation methods vary, Kombucha tea may contain contaminants such as molds and fungi, some of which can cause illness. After the tea is fermented, it is usually highly acidic and contains alcohol, ethyl acetate, acetic acid, and lactate.

Deaths from acidosis have been linked with the tea. Drinking excessive amounts of the tea is not recommended. Several experts warn that since home-brewing facilities vary significantly, the tea could become contaminated with harmful germs, which could be especially dangerous to people with HIV, cancer, or other immune problems. Allergic reactions, possibly to molds in the tea, have been reported, as have anthrax of the skin and jaundice, a yellowing of the skin and eyes that is usually caused by liver damage.

Kombucha tea should not be brewed in ceramic, lead crystal, or painted containers, as the acidity of the tea can cause it to absorb harmful elements from its container. Lead poisoning has been reported in at least two people who brewed Kombucha tea in a ceramic pot.

Since the potential health risks of Kombucha tea are unknown, anyone with an immune deficiency or any other medical condition should consult a physician before drinking the tea. Women who are pregnant or breastfeeding should not use this tea. Relying on this type of treatment alone and avoiding or delaying conventional medical care for cancer may have serious health consequences.

This product is sold as a dietary supplement in the United States. Unlike companies that produce drugs (which must provide the FDA with results of detailed testing showing their product is safe and effective before the drug is approved for sale), the companies that make supplements do not have to show evidence of safety or health benefits to the FDA before selling their products. Supplement products without any reliable scientific evidence of health benefits may still be sold as long as the companies selling them do not claim the supplements can prevent, treat, or cure any specific disease. Some such products may not contain the amount of the herb or substance that is written on the label, and some may include other substances (contaminants). Though the FDA has written new rules to improve the quality of manufacturing processes for dietary supplements and the accurate listing of supplement ingredients, these rules do not take full effect until 2010. The new rules also do not address the safety of supplement ingredients or their effects on health when proper manufacturing techniques are used.

Most such supplements have not been tested to find out if they interact with medicines, foods, or other herbs and supplements. Even though some reports of interactions and harmful effects may be published, full studies of interactions and effects are not often available. Because of these limitations, any information on ill effects and interactions should be considered incomplete.

References

Boik J. *Cancer and Natural Medicine: A Textbook of Basic Science and Clinical Research.* Princeton, MN: Oregon Medical Press; 1995.

Cassileth B. *The Alternative Medicine Handbook: The Complete Reference Guide to Alternative and Complementary Therapies.* New York: W.W. Norton; 1998.

Centers for Disease Control and Prevention. Unexplained severe illness possibly associated with consumption of Kombucha tea—Iowa, 1995. *JAMA.* 1996;275:96-98.

Derk CT, Sandorfi N, Curtis MT. A case of anti-Jo1 myositis with pleural effusions and pericardial tamponade developing after exposure to a fermented Kombucha beverage. *Clin Rheumatol.* 2004;23:355-357. Epub 2004 Apr 16.

Kombucha. Memorial Sloan-Kettering Cancer Center Web site. http://www.mskcc.org/mskcc/html/69274.cfm. Accessed June 10, 2008.

Mayser P, Fromme S, Leitzmann C, Gründer K. The yeast spectrum of the 'tea fungus Kombucha.' *Mycoses.* 1995;38:289-295.

Phan TG, Estell J, Duggin G, Beer I, Smith D, Ferson MJ. Lead poisoning from drinking Kombucha tea brewed in a ceramic pot. *Med J Aust.* 1998;169:644-646.

Spaulding-Albright N. A review of some herbal and related products commonly used in cancer patients. *J Am Diet Assoc.* 1997;97:S208-S215.

Teoh AL, Heard G, Cox J. Yeast ecology of Kombucha fermentation. *Int J Food Microbiol.* 2004;95:119-126.

US Food and Drug Administration. FDA Talk Paper: FDA cautions consumers on "Kombucha mushroom tea." Rockville, MD: National Press Office; March 23,1995. Talk Paper T95-15.

LYCOPENE

Other common name(s): Rhodopurpurin
Scientific/medical name(s): none

Description

Lycopene is an antioxidant compound that gives tomatoes and certain other fruits and vegetables their color. It is one of the major carotenoids in the diet of North Americans and Europeans. Carotenoids are pigments that give yellow, red, and orange vegetables and fruits their color. The body uses some types of carotenoids (but not lycopene) to make vitamin A.

Overview

People who have diets rich in tomatoes, which contain lycopene, appear to have a lower risk for certain types of cancer, especially cancers of the prostate, lung, and stomach. Further research is needed to find out what role, if any, lycopene has in the prevention or treatment of cancer. It is likely that the preventive effect of diets high in fruits and vegetables cannot be explained by just one single part of the diet.

How is it promoted for use?

Proponents claim that lycopene may lower the risk for heart disease; macular degenerative disease, an age-related illness that can lead to blindness; and lipid oxidation, damage to normal fat molecules that can cause inflammation and disease. It is also said to lower LDL, or "bad," cholesterol, enhance the body's defenses, and protect enzymes, DNA, and cellular fats.

A major claim for lycopene's benefits is in the prevention and treatment of cancers of the lung, prostate, stomach, bladder, cervix, skin, and, especially, prostate. In support of these claims regarding cancer, proponents note that lycopene is a powerful antioxidant, a compound that blocks the action of free radicals, activated oxygen molecules that can damage cells, and that several scientific studies have found lower risk for cancer among people who eat lycopene-rich foods.

What does it involve?

Tomatoes are the most concentrated food source of lycopene, although apricots, guava, watermelon, papaya, and pink grapefruit are also significant sources. Studies that looked at lycopene levels in the blood found that levels were higher after people ate cooked tomatoes than after they ate raw tomatoes or drank tomato juice. This finding suggests that lycopene in cooked tomato products such as tomato sauce or paste may be more readily absorbed by the body than lycopene in raw tomatoes. Eating lycopene-rich vegetables and fruits together with a small amount of oil or fat (for example, salad oil or cheese on pizza) increases the amount of lycopene absorbed by the intestines. Lycopene is also available in soft-gel capsule supplements. Dosages vary according to manufacturer.

What is the history behind it?

In recent years, the role of the diet in preventing cancer has been a popular and important area of research. The examination of the role of carotenoids, specifically beta carotene, in preventing cancer began in the 1920s. However, interest in lycopene did not really begin until the late 1980s, when it was found that the antioxidant activity of lycopene was twice that of beta carotene.

What is the evidence?

Observational epidemiologic studies in many countries have shown that the risk for some types of cancer is lower in people who have diets high in tomato products or who have higher levels of lycopene in their blood. Studies suggest that diets rich in tomatoes may account for this reduction in risk. Evidence is strongest for lycopene's protective effect against cancer of the lung, stomach, and prostate. It may also help to protect against cancer of the cervix, breast, mouth, pancreas, esophagus, and colon and rectum.

Some observational epidemiologic studies have found that a diet high in lycopene from tomato-based foods was linked with a lower risk for prostate cancer. Other studies, however, found no link between tomato products or other lycopene-rich foods and prostate cancer. A recent study suggested that variation in a particular gene (known as XRCC1) that helps repair damaged DNA influences whether lycopene intake will affect a man's prostate cancer risk.

Since tomatoes also contain vitamins, potassium, and other carotenoids and antioxidants, it is possible that other compounds in tomatoes, either alone or in combination with lycopene, may be responsible for some of the protective effects attributed to lycopene in some studies. When researchers look at large groups with different lifestyles and habits, it is also possible that their findings can be explained by other factors that were not examined.

A 2004 review that analyzed twenty-one observational studies concluded that tomato products appear to have a weak protective effect against prostate cancer. This review did not include lycopene supplements, only tomato and tomato-based foods. Some of the individual studies, however, did consider lycopene levels in the blood. The analysis noted that the protective effect was slightly stronger for cooked tomato products and that small amounts of added fat improved lycopene absorption. On the other hand, two studies from 2007, one of about 1,500 men and the second of more than twenty-eight thousand men, found no difference in blood lycopene levels between those in whom prostate cancer later developed and those in whom it did not.

There have been several experimental studies on the role of lycopene in preventing or treating cancer. One animal study found that lycopene treatment reduced the growth of brain tumors. Another animal study showed that frequent intake of lycopene over a long period of time considerably suppressed breast tumor growth in mice. However, breast cancer in humans is very different from breast cancer in mice, and those results may not apply to the disease in humans. In laboratory studies, lycopene has also been shown to interfere with the growth of many different types of human cancer cells growing in test tubes or Petri dishes, especially those that grow in response to insulin-like growth factor I. Laboratory and animal studies can suggest possible helpful effects, but they do not provide proof that such effects can be achieved in humans. Further studies are needed to find out whether possible anticancer properties could benefit humans.

To test whether lycopene is the main cancer-fighting substance in tomatoes, one animal study compared lycopene supplements to powdered tomatoes. Groups of rats that were fed tomato powder were compared with rats given lycopene. The rats that received tomato powder had much lower cancer risk, whereas the rats receiving lycopene supplements did not differ significantly from the group that received no special supplements.

Results from a few controlled studies on the effects of lycopene in humans have been published recently, but more clinical information (including results of several studies already under way) will be needed to determine whether lycopene-rich foods can be helpful in preventing or treating cancer. All of the clinical trials completed so far have reported relatively short-term effects on the level of prostate-specific antigen (PSA) in the blood, which is generally considered a good indicator of prostate cancer growth. Although these studies are an important step, they are not as valuable as long-term studies that determine whether a treatment actually helps patients live longer or relieves their symptoms.

One study assigned men at high risk for prostate cancer to take an ordinary multivitamin either with or without a lycopene supplement and found no difference in PSA levels between the two groups. A controlled study in a small group of men with prostate cancer found that lycopene supplements appeared to reduce the rapid growth of prostate cancer cells. However, a more recent study with men whose prostate cancer had stopped responding to hormone therapy found that lycopene did not have a significant effect. One short-term study from 2006 reported that lycopene supplements were safe but that they did not lower the levels of PSA in men with recurrent prostate cancer. Another reported that the combination of lycopene and soy supplements prevented PSA levels from increasing in some men with prostate cancer.

The American Cancer Society's nutrition guidelines recommend eating a balanced diet that includes five or more servings a day of vegetables and fruit, choosing whole grains over processed and refined foods, and limiting red meats and animal fats. Choosing foods from a variety of fruits, vegetables, and other plant sources such as nuts, seeds, whole grain cereals, and beans is likely to be healthier than consuming large amounts of one particular food. Based on currently available evidence, diet is likely to play a greater role in preventing cancer than in treating it.

Are there any possible problems or complications?

Lycopene obtained from eating fruits and vegetables has no known side effects and is thought to be safe for humans. The potential side effects of lycopene supplements are not fully known. Patients in one study who took a lycopene-rich tomato supplement of 15 milligrams twice a day had some intestinal side effects such as nausea, vomiting, diarrhea, indigestion, gas, and bloating. When consumed over a long period of time, very large amounts of tomato products can give the skin an orange color.

Supplements containing antioxidants such as lycopene may interfere with radiation therapy and chemotherapy if taken during cancer treatment. Even though studies have not been done in humans, antioxidants are known to destroy free radicals, which could interfere with one of the methods by which chemotherapy and radiation destroy cancer cells. Eating fruits and vegetables high in antioxidants is still considered safe during cancer treatment.

Relying on this type of treatment alone and avoiding or delaying conventional medical care for cancer may have serious health consequences.

This product is sold as a dietary supplement in the United States. Unlike companies that produce drugs (which must provide the FDA with results of detailed testing showing their product is safe and effective before the drug is approved for sale), the companies that make supplements do not have to show evidence of safety or health benefits to the FDA before selling their products. Supplement products without any reliable scientific evidence of health benefits may still be sold as long as the companies selling them do not claim the supplements can prevent, treat, or cure any specific disease. Some such products may not contain the amount of the herb or substance that is written on the label, and some may include other substances (contaminants). Though the FDA has written new rules to improve the quality of manufacturing processes for dietary supplements and the accurate listing of supplement ingredients, these rules do not take full effect until 2010. The new rules also do not address the safety

of supplement ingredients or their effects on health when proper manufacturing techniques are used.

Most such supplements have not been tested to find out if they interact with medicines, foods, or other herbs and supplements. Even though some reports of interactions and harmful effects may be published, full studies of interactions and effects are not often available. Because of these limitations, any information on ill effects and interactions should be considered incomplete.

References

Boileau TW, Liao Z, Kim S, Lemeshow S, Erdman JW Jr, Clinton SK. Prostate carcinogenesis in N-methyl-N-nitrosourea (NMU)-testosterone-treated rats fed tomato powder, lycopene, or energy-restricted diets. *J Natl Cancer Inst.* 2003;95:1578-1586.

Bunker CH, McDonald AC, Evans RW, de la Rosa N, Boumosleh JM, Patrick AL. A randomized trial of lycopene supplementation in Tobago men with high prostate cancer risk. *Nutr Cancer.* 2007;57:130-137.

Campbell JK, Canene-Adams K, Lindshield BL, Boileau TW, Clinton SK, Erdman JW Jr. Tomato phytochemicals and prostate cancer risk. *J Nutr.* 2004;134:3486S-3492S.

Clark PE, Hall MC, Borden LS Jr, Miller AA, Hu JJ, Lee WR, Stindt D, D'Agostino R Jr, Lovato J, Harmon M, Torti FM. Phase I-II prospective dose-escalating trial of lycopene in patients with biochemical relapse of prostate cancer after definitive local therapy. *Urology.* 2006;67:1257-1261.

Davis CD, Swanson CA, Ziegler RG, Clevidence B, Dwyer JT, Milner JA. Executive Summary Report: Promises and Perils of Lycopene/Tomato Supplementation and Cancer Prevention. Conference proceedings. Division of Cancer Epidemiology and Genetics. National Cancer Institute Web site. http://dceg.cancer.gov/pdfs/davis1352014s2005.pdf. Accessed June 10, 2008.

Doyle C, Kushi LH, Byers T, Courneya KS, Demark-Wahnefried W, Grant B, McTiernan A, Rock CL, Thompson C, Gansler T, Andrews KS, The 2006 Nutrition, Physical Activity and Cancer Survivorship Advisory Committee; American Cancer Society. Nutrition and physical activity during and after cancer treatment: an American Cancer Society guide for informed choices. *CA Cancer J Clin.* 2006;56:323-353.

Etminan M, Takkouche B, Caamaño-Isorna F. The role of tomato products and lycopene in the prevention of prostate cancer: a meta-analysis of observational studies. *Cancer Epidemiol Biomarkers Prev.* 2004;13:340-345.

Gerster H. The potential role of lycopene for human health. *J Am Coll Nutr.* 1997;16:109-126.

Giovannucci E. Tomatoes, tomato-based products, lycopene, and cancer: review of the epidemiologic literature. *J Natl Cancer Inst.* 1999;91:317-331.

Goodman M, Bostick RM, Ward KC, Terry PD, van Gils CH, Taylor JA, Mandel JS. Lycopene intake and prostate cancer risk: effect modification by plasma antioxidants and the XRCC1 genotype. *Nutr Cancer.* 2006;55:13-20.

Jatoi A, Burch P, Hillman D, Vanyo JM, Dakhil S, Nikcevich D, Rowland K, Morton R, Flynn PJ, Young C, Tan W; North Central Cancer Treatment Group. A tomato-based, lycopene-containing intervention for androgen-independent prostate cancer: results of a Phase II study from the North Central Cancer Treatment Group. *Urology.* 2007;69:289-294.

Kirsh VA, Mayne ST, Peters U, Chatterjee N, Leitzmann MF, Dixon LB, Urban DA, Crawford ED, Hayes RB. A prospective study of lycopene and tomato product intake and risk of prostate cancer. *Cancer Epidemiol Biomarkers Prev.* 2006;15:92-98.

Kushi LH, Byers T, Doyle C, Bandera EV, McCullough M, McTiernan A, Gansler T, Andrews KS, Thun MJ; American Cancer Society 2006 Nutrition and Physical Activity Guidelines Advisory Committee. American Cancer Society guidelines on nutrition and physical activity for cancer prevention: reducing the risk of cancer with healthy food choices and physical activity. *CA Cancer J Clin.* 2006;56:254-281.

Lawenda BD, Kelly KM, Ladas EJ, Sagar SM, Vickers A, Blumberg JB. Should supplemental antioxidant administration be avoided during chemotherapy and radiation therapy? *J Natl Cancer Inst.* 2008;100:773-783.

Lycopene: an antioxidant for good health. American Dietetic Association Web site. http://www.eatright.org/cps/rde/xchg/ada/hs.xsl/nutrition_5328_ENU_HTML.htm. Accessed June 10, 2008.

Norrish AE, Jackson RT, Sharpe SJ, Skeaff CM. Prostate cancer and dietary carotenoids. *Am J Epidemiol.* 2000;151:119-123.

Paiva SA, Russell RM. Beta-carotene and other carotenoids as antioxidants. *J Am Coll Nutr.* 1999;18:426-433.

Peters U, Leitzmann MF, Chatterjee N, Wang Y, Albanes D, Gelmann EP, Friesen MD, Riboli E, Hayes RB. Serum lycopene, other carotenoids, and prostate cancer risk: a nested case-control study in the Prostate, Lung, Colorectal, and Ovarian Cancer Screening Trial. *Cancer Epidemiol Biomarkers Prev.* 2007;16:962-968.

Vaishampayan U, Hussain M, Banerjee M, Seren S, Sarkar FH, Fontana J, Forman JD, Cher ML, Powell I, Pontes JE, Kucuk O. Lycopene and soy isoflavones in the treatment of prostate cancer. *Nutr Cancer.* 2007;59:1-7.

MACROBIOTIC DIET

Other common name(s): macrobiotics
Scientific/medical name(s): none

Description

A macrobiotic diet is generally vegetarian and consists largely of whole grains, cereals, and cooked vegetables. More extreme versions of the diet that consist solely of cooked whole grains are no longer promoted.

Overview

Available scientific evidence does not support claims that a macrobiotic diet is effective in treating cancer. A diet consisting mostly of vegetables, fruits, and whole grains is associated with general health benefits and lower risk for several diseases, and a macrobiotic diet, by virtue of its main components, can also achieve these benefits. However, macrobiotic diets can lead to poor nutrition if not properly planned. Some earlier, more limited, versions of the diet may actually pose a danger to health. Research is under way to find out whether a macrobiotic diet may play a role in preventing cancer.

How is it promoted for use?

Some proponents of the macrobiotic diet claim that it can prevent and cure disease, including cancer, and that it can enhance spiritual and physical well-being. An important goal of a macrobiotic diet is to balance the yin and yang—the two elementary and complementary energy forms that, according to ancient Asian spiritual traditions, are present within all people, foods, and objects. These two forces must be balanced in order to achieve health and vitality. A macrobiotic diet is considered to be a way of life, not just a diet.

What does it involve?

A macrobiotic diet combines elements of Buddhism with dietary principles based on simplicity and avoidance of "toxins" that come from eating dairy products, meats, and oily foods. Older versions of the macrobiotic diet were quite restrictive. One variation allowed only the consumption of whole grains. Current proponents of the diet advocate flexibility but still discourage dairy products, meats, and refined sugars.

The standard macrobiotic diet of today consists of 50 to 60 percent organically grown whole grains, 20 to 25 percent locally and organically grown fruits and vegetables, and 5 to 10 percent soups made with vegetables, seaweed, grains, beans, and miso (a fermented soy product). Other elements may include occasional helpings of fresh white fish, nuts, seeds, pickles, Asian condiments, and nonstimulating and nonaromatic teas. Early versions of the diet excluded all animal products. Proponents still discourage dairy products, eggs, coffee, sugar, stimulant and aromatic herbs, red meat, poultry, and processed foods. Some vegetables, such as potatoes, tomatoes, eggplant, peppers, asparagus, spinach, beets, zucchini, and avocados, are discouraged. The diet also advises against eating fruit that does not grow locally (for example, in most of the United States and Europe, bananas, pineapples, and other tropical fruits).

The macrobiotic diet also prescribes specific ways of cooking food. Pots, pans, and utensils should be made only from certain materials, such as wood, glass, ceramic, stainless steel, and enameled pieces. People who practice the diet do not usually cook with microwaves or electricity, nor do they consume vitamin or mineral supplements or heavily processed foods. Food is chewed until it is fluid in order to help with digestion. Since food is thought to be sacred, it is prepared in a peaceful setting.

The macrobiotic diet can vary slightly according to a person's age, sex, level of physical activity, and native climate. Although macrobiotic dietary guidelines are only one aspect of a larger philosophical and spiritual system, the diet has drawn the most attention in the West.

What is the history behind it?

The word "macrobiotic" comes from Greek roots and means "long life," reflecting the view toward long-term health and spirituality embodied by the macrobiotic philosophy. The macrobiotic philosophy and diet were developed by George Ohsawa, a Japanese philosopher who sought to integrate Zen Buddhism, Asian medicine, Christian teachings, and some aspects of Western medicine. Ohsawa believed simplicity in diet was the key to good health and that a diet based on simplicity and abstention from certain foods could cure cancer and other serious illnesses. In the 1930s, he began advocating his philosophy of health and healing through proper diet and natural medicine. Ohsawa brought his teachings to the United States in the 1960s. His diet involved ten stages that were progressively more restrictive. The last stage consisted only of brown rice and water. This restrictive diet was found to be unhealthy and is no longer promoted by macrobiotic counselors.

An early disciple, Michio Kushi, adopted and expanded Ohsawa's ideas and became a leader of the macrobiotic lifestyle. He opened the Kushi Institute in Boston in 1978 to promote the philosophy and its practices. According to Kushi, a macrobiotic diet is a common-sense approach to daily living, not just a type of therapy. Although macrobiotic diets were not developed primarily as cancer treatments, they have been widely promoted for that purpose. During the 1980s, interest in the diet grew through a book written by a physician and president of Philadelphia Hospital, Anthony Sattilaro, who felt that his prostate cancer went into remission because of the diet.

What is the evidence?

There have been no randomized clinical studies published in the available medical literature to show the macrobiotic diet can be used to prevent or cure cancer. One of the earlier versions of the macrobiotic diet that involved eating only brown rice and water has been linked to severe nutritional deficiencies and even death. However, low-fat, high-fiber diets that consist mainly of plant products are believed to reduce the risk for cardiovascular disease and some forms of cancer. The National Institutes of Health's National Center for Complementary and Alternative Medicine has funded a study to determine whether a macrobiotic diet may prevent cancer.

The American Cancer Society's nutrition guidelines recommend eating a balanced diet that includes five or more servings a day of vegetables and fruit, choosing whole grains over processed and refined foods, and limiting red meats and animal fats. It is best to choose foods from a variety of fruits, vegetables and other plant sources such as nuts, seeds, whole grain cereals, and beans to take in all needed nutrients.

Are there any possible problems or complications?

One of the earlier macrobiotic diets, which called for eating all grains, is severely deficient and has been linked to severe malnutrition and even death. Strict macrobiotic diets that include no animal products may result in nutritional deficiencies unless they are carefully planned. The danger may be worse for people with cancer, who may have to contend with unwanted weight loss and often have increased nutritional and caloric requirements. Children may also be particularly prone to nutritional deficiencies resulting from a macrobiotic diet. Macrobiotic diets have not been tested in women who are pregnant or breastfeeding, and some versions may not include enough of certain nutrients for normal fetal growth. Relying on this type of treatment alone and avoiding or delaying conventional medical care for cancer may have serious health consequences.

References

Associated Press. AP World Stream. *Cancer Research News*. Dutch authorities prosecuting a macrobiotic diet practitioner. March 1, 2000.

Barrett S, Herbert V. Questionable cancer therapies. Quackwatch Web site. http://www.quackwatch.org/01 QuackeryRelatedTopics/cancer.html. Updated July 6, 2001. Accessed June 10, 2008.

Cassileth B. *The Alternative Medicine Handbook: The Complete Reference Guide to Alternative and Complementary Therapies*. New York: W.W. Norton; 1998.

Doyle C, Kushi LH, Byers T, Courneya KS, Demark-Wahnefried W, Grant B, McTiernan A, Rock CL, Thompson C, Gansler T, Andrews KS, The 2006 Nutrition, Physical Activity and Cancer Survivorship Advisory Committee; American Cancer Society. Nutrition and physical activity during and after cancer treatment: an American Cancer Society guide for informed choices. *CA Cancer J Clin*. 2006;56:323-353.

Ernst E, ed. *The Desktop Guide to Complementary and Alternative Medicine: An Evidence-Based Approach*. New York: Mosby; 2001.

Kushi LH, Byers T, Doyle C, Bandera EV, McCullough M, McTiernan A, Gansler T, Andrews KS, Thun MJ; American Cancer Society 2006 Nutrition and Physical Activity Guidelines Advisory Committee. American Cancer Society guidelines on nutrition and physical activity for cancer prevention: reducing the risk of cancer with healthy food choices and physical activity. *CA Cancer J Clin*. 2006;56:254-281.

Kushi LH, Cunningham JE, Hebert JR, Lerman RH, Bandera EV, Teas J. The macrobiotic diet in cancer. *J Nutr*. 2001;131:3056S-3064S.

Maritess C, Small S, Waltz-Hill M. Alternative nutrition therapies in cancer patients. *Semin Oncol Nurs*. 2005;21:173-176.

Murphy GP, Morris LB, Lange D, American Cancer Society. *Informed Decisions: The Complete Book of Cancer Diagnosis, Treatment, and Recovery.* New York: Viking; 1997.

National Institutes of Health. *Alternative Medicine: Expanding Medical Horizons: A Report to the National Institutes of Health on Alternative Medical Systems and Practices in the United States.* Washington, DC: US Government Printing Office; 1994. NIH publication 94-066.

Nutrition & special diets: macrobiotics detailed scientific review. Complementary/Integrative Medicine Education Resources, The University of Texas M. D. Anderson Cancer Center Web site. http://www.mdanderson.org/departments/cimer/display.cfm?id=ADFAB15F-16E9-11D5-811000508B603A14&method=displayFull. Accessed June 10, 2008.

US Congress, Office of Technology Assessment. *Unconventional Cancer Treatments: OTA-H-405.* Washington, DC: US Government Printing Office; 1990.

MAITAKE MUSHROOM

Other common name(s): maitake D-fraction, maitake, maitake extract, beta glucan
Scientific/medical name(s): *Grifola frondosa*

Description

Maitake is an edible mushroom from the species *Grifola frondosa* that is native to the mountains of northeastern Japan. Maitake D-fraction is an extract of this large mushroom. The maitake mushroom is eaten as a food, and maitake-D fraction is marketed as a dietary supplement in the United States and Japan. The substance in the maitake mushroom that is thought to be active in humans is called beta glucan.

Overview

Research has shown that maitake D-fraction has effects on the immune system in animal and laboratory studies. There is no convincing clinical evidence to date in peer-reviewed medical journals reporting that the maitake mushroom is effective in treating or preventing cancer in humans, although some human research is now under way.

How is it promoted for use?

Promoters claim that maitake mushroom extract boosts the immune system and limits or reverses tumor growth. It is also said to enhance the benefits of chemotherapy and lessen some side effects of anticancer drugs, such as hair loss, pain, and nausea.

What does it involve?

Maitake D-fraction is available as a liquid extract, tablet, and capsule in health food stores, although the amount of beta glucan contained in each form may vary. The usual dosage of dried mushroom is between 3 and 7 grams daily. Maitake mushrooms are also available in grocery stores and can be eaten as food or made into tea.

What is the history behind it?

For thousands of years, Asian healers have used certain edible mushrooms in tonics, soups, teas, prepared foods, and herbal formulas to promote health and long life. Until recently, the healing properties of mushrooms have been the subject of folklore only. In the past few decades, however, researchers in Japan have been studying the medicinal effects of mushrooms on the immune system, cancer, blood pressure, and cholesterol levels.

The Japanese word "maitake" means "dancing mushroom," called this because people in ancient times were said to dance for joy when they found these mushrooms, which were literally worth their weight in silver. Modern research on the maitake mushroom and its D-fraction extract began in Japan in the mid-1980s and has only recently spread to the United States.

As of the early twenty-first century, much has been written about maitake and its purported magical healing qualities. This increased visibility has sparked a great deal of interest in its use for various human illnesses.

What is the evidence?

Maitake mushrooms and the maitake D-fraction prepared from them contain a type of polysaccharide (a large complex molecule formed by multiple linked sugar molecules) called beta glucan (sometimes called beta glycan). Beta glucan is found in several mushrooms, yeasts, and other foods. Beta glucan is believed to stimulate the immune system and activate certain cells and proteins that attack cancer, including macrophages, T-cells, natural killer cells, and interleukin-1 and -2. In laboratory studies, it appears to slow the growth of cancer in some cell cultures and in mice.

Most of the research on maitake D-fraction has been done in Japan using an injectable form of the extract. A 1997 study published in the *Annals of the New York Academy of Science* found that maitake D-fraction was able to enhance the immune system and inhibit the spread of tumors in mice implanted with breast cancer. In a 1995 report published in the same journal, researchers concluded that maitake D-fraction was able to activate the immune systems of mice that had been injected with liver cancer cells. The extract seemed to prevent the spread of tumors to the liver and prevent the development of cancer in normal cells. A nonrandomized study of fifteen dogs with lymphoma did not find any evidence of benefit from the use of maitake extract.

While animal and laboratory studies may show a certain compound holds promise as a beneficial treatment, further studies are necessary to determine whether the results apply to humans. In 2002, a group of Japanese people with different types of cancer were given maitake D-fraction and maitake powder in addition to standard cancer treatment. Although the researchers thought some patients showed improvement, the study did not include a control group. Because of limitations in the study design, no reliable conclusions can be drawn. It is impossible to say for certain whether any effect was caused by the maitake treatments or standard cancer treatments the patients also received. More scientifically designed studies are needed to determine maitake's potential usefulness in preventing or treating cancer.

The National Cancer Institute is sponsoring a very early (phase I) study at Memorial Sloan-Kettering Cancer Center to learn whether beta glucan can increase the effectiveness of rituximab (a drug used for treating some types of lymphoma and leukemia) by increasing cancer cells' sensitivity to it. This clinical trial is studying the side effects and best dose of beta glucan when given with rituximab. It will look at young patients with relapsed or progressive lymphoma, leukemia, or similar disorders.

In another clinical trial, beta glucan is being tested together with other drugs to learn whether they increase the effectiveness of a monoclonal antibody (3F8). Combining different types of biological therapy may kill more tumor cells. This study is a small open-label trial (so called because both patients and researchers know which treatment is being administered) in patients with neuroblastoma that has not responded to treatment. A trial of maitake extract as treatment for breast cancer is also in progress.

Are there any possible problems or complications?

The maitake mushroom itself has been used as food for centuries and is generally presumed to be safe. So far, studies have not shown any adverse effects from maitake D-fraction or beta glucan, but human studies of their effectiveness in treating cancer have not yet been completed.

In animal studies, beta glucans of the type in maitake mushrooms lowered blood sugar and should be used with caution in people with low blood sugar (hypoglycemia) or those who are on medicines to reduce or control blood sugar. Beta glucans also reduced blood pressure in animals and may have a similar effect in people. Additional studies are needed to find out whether these effects occur in humans.

Allergies to many types of mushrooms, including maitake, have been reported. Relying on this type of treatment alone and avoiding or delaying conventional medical care for cancer may have serious health consequences.

This product is sold as a dietary supplement in the United States. Unlike companies that produce drugs (which must provide the FDA with results of detailed testing showing their product is safe and effective before the drug is approved for sale), the companies that make supplements do not have to show evidence of safety or health benefits to the FDA before selling their products. Supplement products without any reliable scientific evidence of health benefits may still be sold as long as the companies selling them do not claim the supplements can prevent, treat, or cure any specific disease. Some such products may not contain the amount of the herb or substance that is written on the label, and some may include other substances (contaminants). Though the FDA has written new rules to improve the quality of manufacturing processes for dietary supplements and the accurate listing of supplement ingredients, these rules do not take full effect until 2010. The new rules also do not address the safety of supplement ingredients or their effects on health when proper manufacturing techniques are used.

Most such supplements have not been tested to find out if they interact with medicines, foods, or other herbs and supplements. Even though some reports of interactions and harmful effects may be published, full studies of interactions and effects are not often available. Because of these limitations, any information on ill effects and interactions should be considered incomplete.

References

Cunningham-Rundles S, Lin H, Cassileth B. Are botanical glucans effective in enhancing tumoricidal cell activity? American Society for Nutrition. *J Nutr.* 2005;135: 2919S.

Griessmayr PC, Gauthier M, Barber LG, Cotter SM. Mushroom-derived maitake PETfraction as single agent for the treatment of lymphoma in dogs. *J Vet Intern Med.* 2007;21:1409-1412.

Hong F, Yan J, Baran JT, Allendorf DJ, Hansen RD, Ostroff GR, Xing PX, Cheung NK, Ross GD. Mechanism by which orally administered beta-1,3-glucans enhance the tumoricidal activity of antitumor monoclonal antibodies in murine tumor models. *J Immunol.* 2004;173:797-806.

Kodama N, Komuta K, Nanba H. Can maitake MD-fraction aid cancer patients? *Altern Med Rev.* 2002;7(3):236-239.
Comment in:
Altern Med Rev. 2002; 7(6):451; author reply 452-454.

Kodama N, Murata Y, Asakawa A, Inui A, Hayashi M, Sakai N, Nanba H. Maitake D-fraction enhances antitumor effects and reduces immunosuppression by mitomycin-C in tumor-bearing mice. *Nutrition.* 2005;21:624-629.

Konno S. Potential growth inhibitory effect of maitake D-fraction on canine cancer cells. *Vet Ther.* 2004;5:263-271.

Ko YT, Lin YL. 1,3-beta-glucan quantification by a fluorescence microassay and analysis of its distribution in foods. *J Agric Food Chem.* 2004;52:3313-3318.

Maitake. Memorial Sloan-Kettering Cancer Center Web site. http://www.mskcc.org/mskcc/html/69294.cfm. Accessed June 10, 2008.

Maitake. PDRhealth Web site. http://www.pdrhealth.com/drug_info/nmdrugprofiles/herbaldrugs/101810.shtml. Accessed June 10, 2008.

Nanba H. Activity of maitake D-fraction to inhibit carcinogenesis and metastasis. *Ann N Y Acad Sci.* 1995;768:243-245.

Nanba H, Kubo K. Effect of maitake D-fraction on cancer prevention. *Ann N Y Acad Sci.* 1997;833:204-207.

Talpur NA, Echard BW, Fan AY, Jaffari O, Bagchi D, Preuss HG. Antihypertensive and metabolic effects of whole Maitake mushroom powder and its fractions in two rat strains. *Mol Cell Biochem.* 2002;237:129-136.

Tanaka H, Tsunematsu K, Nakamura N, Suzuki K, Tanaka N, Takeya I, Saikai T, Abe S. Successful treatment of hypersensitivity pneumonitis caused by *Grifola frondosa* (Maitake) mushroom using a HFA-BDP extra-fine aerosol. *Intern Med.* 2004;43:737-740.

US National Institutes of Health. Beta-glucan and monoclonal antibody 3F8 in treating patients with metastatic neuroblastoma. ClinicalTrials.gov Web site. http://www.clinicaltrials.gov/ct2/show/NCT00492167. Accessed September 8, 2008.

US National Institutes of Health. Beta-glucan and rituximab in treating young patients with relapsed or progressive lymphoma or leukemia, or lymphoproliferative disorder related to donor stem cell transplantation. Clinical Trials Web site. http://www.clinicaltrials.gov/ct2/show/NCT00087009. Accessed September 8, 2008.

METABOLIC THERAPY

Other common name(s): Kelley's treatment, Gonzalez treatment, Issel's whole body therapy, Gerson therapy

Scientific/medical name(s): none

Description

Metabolic therapy uses a combination of special diets, enzymes, nutritional supplements, and other measures in an attempt to remove "toxins" from the body and strengthen the body's defenses against disease.

Overview

There is no convincing scientific evidence that metabolic therapy is effective in treating cancer. However, there are many different practices that make up metabolic therapy. Some of these practices may be harmful.

How is it promoted for use?

Metabolic therapy is based on the belief that toxic substances in food and the environment build up in the body and create chemical imbalances that lead to diseases such as cancer, arthritis, and multiple sclerosis. Some proponents of this approach say that metabolic therapy rids the body of these toxins and strengthens its resistance to disease. Some claim that a special diet can cure serious illnesses, including cancer. Others claim that they can evaluate a patient's metabolism and diagnose cancer before symptoms appear and that they can locate tumors and learn the tumor's size and growth rate.

What does it involve?

Metabolic therapies vary a great deal depending on the practitioner, but all are based on special diets and detoxification, usually involving natural, whole foods such as fresh fruits and vegetables, as well as vitamins and mineral supplements. Other measures may include colonic irrigation with coffee or hydrogen peroxide enemas, juicing, enzyme supplements, visualization, and stress-reduction exercises. At least one metabolic therapy system also includes the drug laetrile (see "Colon Therapy," page 184, "Enzyme Therapy," page 740, "Imagery," page 97, "Juicing," page 628, and "Laetrile," page 776).

Among the better known types of metabolic therapy are Kelley's treatment, the Gonzalez treatment, Issel's whole body therapy, and Gerson therapy (see "Gerson Therapy," page 616).

Kelley's treatment includes dietary supplements (such as enzymes and large doses of vitamins, minerals, and amino acids), detoxification (such as fasting, exercising, and using laxatives and coffee enemas), a restricted diet, chiropractic adjustments, and prayer. Practitioners classify people into different metabolic types that form the basis for individual dietary and supplement recommendations.

The Gonzalez treatment is similar to Kelley's treatment and includes extracts or concentrates from animal organs such as thymus and liver (taken from beef or lamb) and digestive enzymes as part of the plan (see "Cell Therapy," page 714).

Another form of metabolic therapy is Issel's whole body therapy. Patients are asked to remove teeth that contain mercury dental fillings, follow a strict diet, and eliminate the use of tobacco, coffee, tea, and other substances that are considered harmful (see "Biological Dentistry," page 164). Some patients are encouraged to undergo psychotherapy to relieve stress and deal with anger and emotional distress.

Gerson therapy involves a strict dietary program, coffee enemas, and various mineral or chemical supplements.

What is the history behind it?

Gerson therapy was introduced by Max Gerson, MD, a German-born physician who immigrated to the United States in 1936. Gerson initially used the therapy for treating migraine headaches and tuberculosis and began using it for cancer in 1928. Kelley's treatment was developed in the 1960s by American orthodontist William Donald Kelley, DDS, MS. Nicholas Gonzalez, MD, became interested in metabolic therapy as a medical student in 1981 when he was asked to review Dr. Kelley's work.

In the 1970s and 1980s, Harold Manner, PhD, a biology professor, was also a major proponent of metabolic therapy. He claimed to have cured cancer in mice with injections of laetrile, enzymes, and vitamin A. In his version of metabolic cancer therapy, patients often received another unproven alternative substance, a chemical compound called dimethyl sulfoxide (see "DMSO," page 737). In the early 1980s, Dr. Manner moved to Tijuana, Mexico, to treat patients (see "Questionable Cancer Practices in Mexico," page 810). His clinic in Mexico is still open despite his death in 1988.

What is the evidence?

There is general agreement among scientists that there are differences in the metabolism of certain cells in people who have cancer compared with people who do not have cancer. There is also general agreement regarding the importance of attention to optimal nutrition as a component of conventional oncology care. Otherwise, there is no convincing clinical evidence that supports the claims made for metabolic therapy or any of its components. Some aspects of metabolic therapy may, in fact, be harmful.

An article on metabolic therapies on the Memorial Sloan-Kettering Cancer Center Web site concludes that "Retrospective analyses of the Gerson and Kelley therapies show no evidence of therapeutic efficacy" (2008). And a review article in the *Journal of Clinical Gastroenterology* concludes that "[c]offee enemas are a hazardous derivative of colon therapy.... Its proponents claim that caffeine is absorbed in the colon and leads to a vasodilatation in the liver, which in turn enhances the process of elimination of toxins. None of this is proved, nor is there any evidence of the clinical efficacy of coffee enemas. Coffee enemas are associated with severe adverse reactions" (*J Clin Gastroenterol.* 1997;24:197).

In a 1990 report from the United States Congressional Office of Technology Assessment, three oncologists reviewed the "best cases" collected by Dr. Gonzalez. In the vast majority of these cases, they found claims of benefit from metabolic therapy to be unconvincing. In addition, they found a few cases to be "unusual" at best, meaning that these patients lived longer than typical people with the same type and stage of cancer, but concluded that this difference was probably due to statistical variation that occurs when "best cases" are selected from a large group of patients. A group of physicians who practiced alternative medicine (none of whom were cancer specialists) concluded that the alternative regimen was beneficial in some cases.

A small study of patients with pancreatic cancer—conducted by Dr. Gonzalez, who published the results in *Nutrition and Cancer* in 1999—found that patients treated with pancreatic enzymes survived longer than typical patients with pancreatic cancer. In a recent review of alternative cancer cures, an expert in integrative oncology research methods noted that "The study was small and obviously prone to several biases. Not only is the comparison with national averages unadjusted for confounders (other factors that can affect outcome), but the principal results are based on patient selection; 12 patients who did not comply with treatment were excluded from analysis" (*CA Cancer J Clin.* 2004;54:115). A randomized clinical trial has been sponsored by the National Cancer Institute to evaluate the Gonzalez regimen for treating pancreatic cancer, but no results of this trial have yet been published in any peer-reviewed medical journal.

Are there any possible problems or complications?

Some aspects of metabolic therapy are considered dangerous. There are reports of complications related to liver cell injections, as well as nutritional deficiencies due to restricted diets. Several deaths have been directly linked to injecting live cells from animals (a practice called cell therapy). The drug laetrile may cause nausea, vomiting, headache, dizziness, and even cyanide poisoning, which can be fatal. Care should be taken to make sure that any diet containing raw meat or juices from raw meat is free from contamination, given the increasing number of diseases that are known to be transmitted from animals to people.

Reports of illness and even deaths linked to colonic irrigation have been published in several medical journals. People with diverticulitis, ulcerative colitis, Crohn's disease, severe hemorrhoids, or rectal or colon tumors or who are recovering from bowel surgery, may be at higher risk for bowel injury when using enemas. People with kidney or heart failure may be more likely to experience fluid overload or electrolyte imbalances. Enemas can also cause discomfort and cramps.

Women who are pregnant or breastfeeding should not use this method. Relying on this type of treatment alone and avoiding or delaying conventional medical care may have serious health consequences.

These substances may have not been thoroughly tested to find out how they interact with medicines, foods, or dietary supplements. Even though some reports of interactions and harmful effects may be published, full studies of interactions and effects are not often available. Because of these limitations, any information on ill effects and interactions should be considered incomplete.

References

American Cancer Society. Questionable methods of cancer management: 'nutritional' therapies. *CA Cancer J Clin.* 1993;43:309-319.

American Cancer Society. Unproven methods of cancer management. The metabolic cancer therapy of Harold W. Manner, Ph.D. *CA Cancer J Clin.* 1986;36:185-189.

Barrett S, Herbert V. Manner metabolic therapy. Quackwatch Web site. http://www.quackwatch.org/01QuackeryRelatedTopics/Cancer/manner.html. Accessed June 10, 2008.

Barrett S, Herbert V. Questionable cancer therapies. Quackwatch Web site. http://www.quackwatch.org/01QuackeryRelatedTopics/cancer.html. Updated July 6, 2001. Accessed June 10, 2008.

Centers for Disease Control (CDC). Amebiasis associated with colonic irrigation—Colorado. *MMWR Morb Mortal Wkly Rep.* 1981;30:101-102.

Colonic irrigation. Aetna InteliHealth Web site. http://www.intelihealth.com/IH/ihtIH?d=dmtContent&c=358752. Accessed June 10, 2008.

Eisele JW, Reay DT. Deaths related to coffee enemas. *JAMA.* 1980;244:1608-1609.

Ernst E. Colonic irrigation and the theory of autointoxication: a triumph of ignorance over science. *J Clin Gastroenterol.* 1997;24:196-198.

Eyre HJ, Lange DP, Morris LB. *Informed Decisions: The Complete Book of Cancer Diagnosis, Treatment, and Recovery.* 2nd ed. Atlanta, GA: American Cancer Society; 2001.

Gemcitabine compared with pancreatic enzyme therapy plus specialized diet (Gonzalez Regimen) in treating patients who have stage II, stage III, or stage IV pancreatic cancer. National Institutes of Health, ClincialTrials.gov Web site. http://clinicaltrials.gov/ct/show/NCT00003851. Accessed June 10, 2008.

Gonzalez NJ, Isaacs LL. Evaluation of pancreatic proteolytic enzyme treatment of adenocarcinoma of the pancreas, with nutrition and detoxification support. *Nutr Cancer.* 1999;33:117-124.

Green S. A critique of the rationale for cancer treatment with coffee enemas and diet. *JAMA.* 1992;268:3224-3227.

Green S. Nicolas Gonzalez treatment for cancer: gland extracts, coffee enemas, vitamin megadoses, and diets. Quackwatch Web site. http://www.quackwatch.org/01QuackeryRelatedTopics/Cancer/kg.html. Updated April 20, 2000. Accessed June 10, 2008.

Istre GR, Kreiss K, Hopkins RS, Healy GR, Benziger M, Canfield TM, Dickinson P, Englert TR, Compton RC, Mathews HM, Simmons RA. An outbreak of amebiasis spread by colonic irrigation at a chiropractic clinic. *N Engl J Med.* 1982;307:339-342.

Metabolic therapies. Memorial Sloan-Kettering Cancer Center Web site. http://www.mskcc.org/mskcc/html/69299.cfm. Updated July 21, 2008. Accessed October 10, 2008.

US Congress, Office of Technology Assessment. *Unconventional Cancer Treatments: OTA-H-405.* Washington, DC: US Government Printing Office; 1990.

Vickers A. Alternative cancer cures: "unproven" or "disproven"? *CA Cancer J Clin.* 2004;54:110-118.

MODIFIED CITRUS PECTIN

Other common name(s): citrus pectin, Pecta-Sol, MCP
Scientific/medical name(s): none

Description

Modified citrus pectin (MCP) is a form of pectin that has been altered so that it can be more easily absorbed by the digestive tract. Pectin is a carbohydrate that is made of hundreds or thousands of sugar molecules chemically linked together. It is found in most plants and is particularly plentiful in the peels of apples, citrus fruits, and plums. In modified citrus pectin, the pectin has been chemically altered to break its molecules into smaller pieces. Pectin in its natural form cannot be absorbed by the body and is considered a type of soluble dietary fiber, whereas modified citrus pectin can be absorbed into the bloodstream.

Overview

Animal studies and a couple of uncontrolled human studies have found that MCP may inhibit the spread of prostate cancer and melanoma to other organs. However, there have been no controlled clinical studies to prove this effect in humans.

How is it promoted for use?

Proponents claim that modified citrus pectin slows or stops the growth of melanoma and metastatic prostate cancer. Some also claim that a compound found in MCP strengthens the cancer cell–killing ability of T-cells, cells that also protect against germs.

What does it involve?

Modified citrus pectin is available as a capsule or powder. The dose suggested by manufacturers for the powder is 5 grams (nearly a fifth of an ounce) mixed with water or juice taken three times a day with meals. For capsules, the suggested dose is 800 milligrams three times a day with meals.

What is the history behind it?

Pectin is commonly used as a gelling agent for canning foods and making jellies. It is also used widely in the production of food and cosmetics and as an ingredient in some anti-diarrhea medicines. In the past ten years, the modified form of pectin has been investigated for anticancer properties.

What is the evidence?

Several animal studies found that MCP helped reduce the spread of prostate, breast, and skin cancer. Animals with these types of cancer that were fed MCP had much lower risk for the tumor spreading to the lungs. For example, one study examined the effects of MCP on lung metastases from melanoma cells. Researchers injected mice with melanoma cells. In the mice that were also given MCP, significantly fewer tumors spread to the lungs than in the mice that did not receive the drug. When lung tumors did develop in the mice treated with MCP, the tumors tended to be smaller than those that formed in untreated animals.

These studies appear to show that MCP makes it difficult for cancer cells that break off from the main tumor to join together and grow in other organs. However, in most animal studies, MCP had no effect on the main tumor, suggesting that it may only be useful for preventing or slowing the growth of metastatic tumors in very early stages of development.

Recent laboratory studies of human and animal cells have provided information on how MCP might slow the spread of cancer. MCP appears to attach to galectin-3, a common chemical in many cells. Galectin-3 is present in abnormally high levels in many cancers and plays an important role in the growth, survival, and spread of cancer cells.

Although animal and cell studies are quite encouraging, very little information is available about whether MCP is effective in humans. In one published clinical trial, ten men with prostate cancer were treated with MCP after standard treatment failed. In seven of these men, blood tests found prostate-specific antigen (PSA, a marker of prostate cancer growth). Their PSA doubling time (a measure of how fast PSA goes up) improved in comparison with measurements done before taking MCP, indicating that MCP may have a slowing effect on the cancer's growth. This study had no control group (in this case, a group of men who did not take MCP), which limits the strength of its conclusions on MCP's effectiveness. It also did not measure survival or other important endpoints. However, taken with the information gained from animal studies, it suggests that MCP may have a role in reducing the growth and spread of cancer. Randomized controlled trials looking at larger groups of people must be done before any firmer conclusions can be reached.

Are there any possible problems or complications?

Citrus pectin is categorized as "generally regarded as safe" by the U.S. Food and Drug Administration. When MCP is used as intended, side effects rarely occur. However, some people may experience stomach discomfort after taking MCP. There have been a few case reports in which asthma developed in people after exposure to powdered pectin. Modified citrus pectin may cause serious allergic reactions in those who are allergic to citrus fruits. Relying on this type of treatment alone and avoiding or delaying conventional medical care for cancer may have serious health consequences.

This product is sold as a dietary supplement in the United States. Unlike companies that produce drugs (which must provide the FDA with results of detailed testing showing their product is safe and effective before the drug is approved for sale), the companies that make supplements do not have to show evidence of safety or health benefits to the FDA before selling their products. Supplement products without any reliable scientific evidence of health benefits may still be sold as long as the companies selling them do not claim the supplements can prevent, treat, or cure any specific disease. Some such products may not contain the amount of the herb or substance that is written on the label, and some may include other substances (contaminants). Though the FDA has written new rules to improve the quality of manufacturing processes for dietary supplements and the accurate listing of supplement ingredients, these rules do not take full effect until 2010. The new rules also do not address the safety of supplement ingredients or their effects on health when proper manufacturing techniques are used.

Most such supplements have not been tested to find out if they interact with medicines, foods, or other herbs and supplements. Even though some reports of interactions and harmful effects may be published, full studies of interactions and effects are not often available. Because of these limitations, any information on ill effects and interactions should be considered incomplete.

References

Baldwin JL, Shah AC. Pectin-induced occupational asthma. *Chest.* 1993;104:1936-1937.

Cohen AJ, Forse MS, Tarlo SM. Occupational asthma caused by pectin inhalation during the manufacture of jam. *Chest.* 1993;103:309-311.

Ferdman RM, Ong PY, Church JA. Pectin anaphylaxis and possible association with cashew allergy. *Ann Allergy Asthma Immunol.* 2006;97:759-760.

Guess BW, Scholz MC, Strum SB, Lam RY, Johnson HJ, Jennrich RI. Modified citrus pectin (MCP) increases the prostate-specific antigen doubling time in men with prostate cancer: a phase II pilot study. *Prostate Cancer Prostatic Dis.* 2003;6:301-304.

Herbal/plant therapies: modified citrus pectin. Complementary/Integrative Medicine Education Resources, The University of Texas M.D. Anderson Cancer Center Web site. http://www.mdanderson.org/departments/CIMER/display.cfm?id=89391394-4477-426D-B2BE4320C6952470&method=displayFull. Accessed June 10, 2008.

MCP. PDRhealth Web site. http://www.pdrhealth.com/drug_info/nmdrugprofiles/nutsupdrugs/mod_0175.shtml. Accessed June 10, 2008.

Nangia-Makker P, Hogan V, Honjo Y, Baccarini S, Tait L, Bresalier R, Raz A. Inhibition of human cancer cell growth and metastasis in nude mice by oral intake of modified citrus pectin. *J Natl Cancer Inst.* 2002;94:1854-1862.

Pectin. Memorial Sloan-Kettering Cancer Center Web site. http://www.mskcc.org/mskcc/html/69327.cfm. Accessed June 10, 2008.

Pienta KJ, Naik H, Akhtar A, Yamazaki K, Replogle TS, Lehr J, Donat TL, Tait L, Hogan V, Raz A. Inhibition of spontaneous metastasis in a rat prostate cancer model by oral administration of modified citrus pectin. *J Natl Cancer Inst.* 1995;87:348-353.

Platt D, Raz A. Modulation of the lung colonization of B16-F1 melanoma cells by citrus pectin. *J Natl Cancer Inst.* 1992;84:438-442.

Yu LG, Andrews N, Zhao Q, McKean D, Williams JF, Connor LJ, Gerasimenko OV, Hilkens J, Hirabayashi J, Kasai K, Rhodes JM. Galectin-3 interaction with Thomsen-Friedenreich disaccharide on cancer-associated MUC1 causes increased cancer cell endothelial adhesion. *J Biol Chem.* 2007;282:773-781.

NONI PLANT

Other common name(s): noni fruit, noni juice, Indian mulberry, morinda, hog apple, meng koedoe, mora de la India, ruibarbo caribe, wild pine

Scientific/medical name(s): *Morinda citrifolia*

Description

The noni or morinda plant is a tropical evergreen tree that grows in Tahiti and other Pacific islands, as well as in parts of Asia, Australia, South America, and the Caribbean. The tree can grow to as tall as ten feet and bears a fruit about the size of a potato, which starts out green and ripens into yellow or white. The juice, fruit, bark, and leaves are used in herbal remedies and Polynesian folk medicine.

Overview

There is no reliable clinical evidence that noni juice is effective in preventing or treating cancer or any other disease in humans. Although animal and laboratory studies have shown some positive effects, human studies are just beginning. Research is under way to isolate various compounds in the noni plant so that further testing can be done to learn whether they may be useful in humans.

How is it promoted for use?

Proponents claim the noni fruit and its juice can be used to treat cancer, diabetes, heart disease, cholesterol problems, high blood pressure, human immunodeficiency virus (HIV), rheumatism, psoriasis, allergies, infection, and inflammation. Some believe that the fruit can relieve sinus infections, menstrual cramps, arthritis, ulcers, sprains, injuries, depression, senility, poor digestion, atherosclerosis, addiction, colds, flu, and headaches. It is further claimed that the juice can heal scratches on the cornea of the eye.

In India, proponents use noni as a remedy for asthma and dysentery, and folk healers in the Pacific islands use it for many types of illness. In the United States, some noni juice distributors promote it as a general tonic, stress reliever, facial and body cleanser, and dietary and nutritional supplement.

What does it involve?

Parts of the noni plant are used as a juice, a tonic, a poultice, and in tea. The juice, which has an unpleasant taste and odor, is used on the scalp as a treatment for head lice. Some proponents also advise drinking the juice, mixed with other juices and flavorings to mask its unpleasant taste. The leaves and bark are sometimes made into a liquid tonic for urinary complaints and muscle or joint pain. The unripe noni fruit is mashed together with salt and applied on cuts and broken bones. Ripe fruit is used as a poultice for facial blemishes or as a remedy for skin sores, boils, or infections. Tea made from leaves of the plant is used as a remedy for tuberculosis, arthritis, rheumatism, and as an anti-aging treatment.

In the United States, noni products are sold in various forms including juice, extract, powder, capsules (nutritional supplements and diet aids), facial cleansers, bath gels, and soaps. Noni distributors and Internet sites selling the juice or supplements often recommend that they be taken on an empty stomach.

Noni fruit juice and supplements contain various amounts of vitamin C and A, as well as trace minerals.

What is the history behind it?

The noni fruit has been popular for centuries among Polynesians, who introduced the noni plant to Hawaii. During World War II, soldiers stationed in the South Pacific ate the fruit for added sustenance. Over the past few years, products from the noni plant have become available in health food stores and online in the United States.

In 1998, a company that manufactures noni juice and other noni products for distribution was charged with making unfounded claims by the Attorneys General of Arizona, California, New Jersey, and Texas. The company claimed that the juice could treat, cure, or prevent many diseases including cancer, HIV, diabetes, rheumatism, high blood pressure, cholesterol problems, psoriasis, allergies, heart rhythm abnormality, chronic inflammation, and joint pain. The company was ordered to stop advertising these health claims until it could provide scientific evidence of its claims and receive approval from the U.S. Food and Drug Administration (FDA). That same year, juice marketed under the name of "Noni" was banned in Finland until claims of the juice's ability to prevent, treat, or cure illness were removed from advertising brochures.

Between 2002 and late 2006, the FDA again warned several companies to stop making claims that noni could cure, treat, or prevent disease, since proof of such abilities had still not been submitted to the FDA. However, these claims are still widely made on Web sites and elsewhere.

What is the evidence?

Several animal and laboratory experiments have been done on different compounds taken from the noni plant. A group of Hawaiian researchers caused tumors to grow in mice and then injected specially prepared noni juice into their abdomens. Mice who received the treatment survived twice as long as the untreated mice. Other scientists studying freeze-dried extract from the roots of the plant found that the substance appeared to prevent pain and induce sleep in mice.

Another team of investigators reported that damnacanthal, a compound removed from the root of the noni plant, may inhibit a chemical process that turns normal cells into cancer cells. However, since extracted chemicals or substances are different from the raw plant, a study of an extract might not produce the same result as a study using the whole plant. In addition, while animal and laboratory studies may show a certain substance holds promise as a helpful treatment, further studies are necessary to learn whether the results apply to humans.

An early (phase I) clinical trial of freeze-dried noni fruit extract was done on twenty-nine patients at the University of Hawaii to learn about its actions and toxicities in people with cancer. This study found no toxic effects on patients even at daily doses of 10 grams, but also found that there was no significant effect on quality of life. It was noted, however, that those who got higher doses reported feeling somewhat better. In addition, researchers at Louisiana State University are working to isolate and purify any compounds in the juice that may be active in humans so that further testing can be done.

More research is needed before it can be determined what role, if any, noni plant compounds may play in the treatment of cancer or other health conditions.

Are there any possible problems or complications?

The safety and long-term effects of noni juice and other noni products are not well known. A few cases of liver problems have been reported in people taking noni in European countries. One of these patients had previous liver damage and required a liver transplant, but the others recovered when noni was stopped. Three cases of acute liver inflammation (hepatitis) in people using noni products have been reported, although other herbal products they were using may have been responsible or may have interacted with noni ingredients. Further information is needed to find out the cause of these problems.

The juice has a significant amount of potassium, equivalent to a similar amount of tomato juice or orange juice, and may pose problems for people with kidney disease and others who must restrict their potassium intake. It is also high in sugar, which must be considered for people with diabetes and others restricting their calorie intake. It may cause the urine to turn a pink or reddish color. Noni juice and supplements have not been studied in pregnant or breastfeeding women. Relying on this type of treatment alone and avoiding or delaying conventional medical care for cancer may have serious health consequences.

This product is sold as a dietary supplement in the United States. Unlike companies that produce drugs (which must provide the FDA with results of detailed testing showing their product is safe and effective before the drug is approved for sale), the companies that make supplements do not have to show evidence of safety or health benefits to the FDA before selling their products. Supplement products without any reliable scientific evidence of health benefits may still be sold as long as the companies selling them do not claim the supplements can prevent, treat, or cure any specific disease. Some such products may not contain the amount of the herb or substance that is written on the label, and some may include other substances (contaminants). Though the FDA has written new rules to improve the quality of manufacturing processes for dietary supplements and the accurate listing of supplement ingredients, these rules do not take full effect until 2010. And, the new rules do not address the safety of supplement ingredients or their effects on health when proper manufacturing techniques are used.

Most such supplements have not been tested to find out if they interact with medicines, foods, or other herbs and supplements. Even though some reports of interactions and harmful effects may be published, full studies of interactions and effects are not often available. Because of these limitations, any information on ill effects and interactions should be considered incomplete.

References

Attorneys general curb claims for "tahitian noni." Quackwatch Web site. http://www.quackwatch.org/04ConsumerEducation/News/noni.html. Updated September 12, 2002. Accessed June 10, 2008.

FDA Center for Drug Evaluation and Research. Cyber Letters. US Food and Drug Administration Web site. http://www.fda.gov. Accessed June 15, 2007.

Hiramatsu T, Imoto M, Koyano T, Umezawa K. Induction of normal phenotypes in ras-transformed cells by damnacanthal from Morinda citrifolia. *Cancer Lett.* 1993;73:161-166.

Hirazumi A, Furusawa E. An immunomodulatory polysaccharide-rich substance from the fruit juice of *Morinda citrifolia* (noni) with antitumor activity. *Phytother Res.* 1999;13:380-387.

Hirazumi A, Furusawa E, Chou SC, Hokama Y. Anticancer activity of Morinda citrifolia (noni) on intraperitoneally implanted Lewis lung carcinoma in syngeneic mice. *Proc West Pharmacol Soc.* 1994;37:145-146.

Issell BF, Gotay C, Pagano I, Franke A. Quality of life measures in a phase I trial of noni. *J Clin Oncol.* 2005;23(June 1 Suppl):8217.

Johansen R. The health food product Noni—does marketing harmonize with the current status of research? [in Norwegian]. *Tidsskrift for Den Norske Laegeforening.* 2008;128:694-697.

Liu Z, Hornick C, Woltering E. Noni tree: potential cancer preventative, therapy. LSU Agricultural Center Web site. http://www.lsuagcenter.com/en/communications/publications/agmag/Archive/2005/Winter/Noni+Tree+Potential+Cancer+Preventative+Therapy.htm. Posted April 27, 2005. Accessed June 10, 2008.

Millonig G, Stadlmann S, Vogel W. Herbal hepatotoxicity: acute hepatitis caused by a Noni preparation (Morinda citrifolia). *Eur J Gastroenterol Hepatol.* 2005;17:445-447.

Mueller BA, Scott MK, Sowinski KM, Prag KA. Noni juice (*Morinda citrifolia*): hidden potential for hyperkalemia? *Am J Kidney Dis.* 2000;35:310-312.
Comment in:
Am J Kidney Dis. 2000;35:330-332.

Nelson S. Chemical constituents of noni (*Morinda citrifolia*). College of Tropical Agriculture and Human Resources, University of Hawaii at Mānoa Web site. http://www.ctahr.hawaii.edu/noni/chemical_constituents.asp. Updated December 7, 2006. Accessed June 10, 2008.

Noni. Memorial Sloan-Kettering Cancer Center Web site. http://www.mskcc.org/mskcc/html/69312.cfm. Updated August 2, 2007. Accessed June 10, 2008.

Noni. WholeHealthMD Web site. http://www.wholehealthmd.com/ME2/irmod.asp?sid=17E09E7CFFF640448FFB0B4FC1B7FEF0&nm=Reference+Library&type=AWHN_Supplements&mod=Supplements&mid=&id=5B78D2210C824CBF90BA823C8D2D7086&tier=2. Updated September 14, 2005. Accessed June 10, 2008.

Stadlbauer V, Fickert P, Lackner C, Schmerlaib J, Krisper P, Trauner M, Stauber RE. Hepatotoxicity of NONI juice: report of two cases. *World J Gastroenterol.* 2005;11:4758-4760.

Su BN, Pawlus AD, Jung HA, Keller WJ, McLaughlin JL, Kinghorn AD. Chemical constituents of the fruits of *Morinda citrifolia* (Noni) and their antioxidant activity. *J Nat Prod.* 2005;68:592-595.

West BJ, Jensen CJ, Westendorf J. Noni juice is not hepatotoxic. *World J Gastroenterol.* 2006;12:3616-3619.

Younos C, Rolland A, Fleurentin J, Lanhers MC, Misslin R, Mortier F. Analgesic and behavioral effects of *Morinda citrifolia. Planta Med.* 1990;56:430-434.

Yüce B, Gülberg V, Diebold J, Gerbes AL. Hepatitis induced by Noni juice from *Morinda citrifolia*: a rare cause of hepatotoxicity or the tip of the iceberg? *Digestion.* 2006;73:167-170.

OMEGA-3 FATTY ACIDS

Other common name(s): fish oil, fish oil supplements, marine oil, cod liver oil
Scientific/medical name(s): alpha-linolenic acid, eicosapentaenoic acid, docosahexaenoic acid; also called n-3 fatty acids or n-3 polyunsaturated fatty acids

Description

Omega-3 fatty acids are important nutrients that are involved in many bodily processes. The body cannot make these fatty acids and must obtain them from food sources or from supplements. Three fatty acids compose the omega-3 family: alpha-linolenic acid, eicosapentaenoic acid, and docosahexaenoic acid. Alpha-linolenic acid (ALA) is found in English walnuts, in some types of beans, and in canola, soybean, flaxseed/linseed, and olive oils. The other two, eicosapentaenoic acid (EPA) and docosahexaenoic acid (DHA), are found in fish, including fish oil and supplements.

Overview

Some studies in animals have found that fish oils rich in omega-3 fatty acids suppress the formation and growth of some types of cancer. Studies in humans have produced conflicting results. A recent reanalysis of forty years of research suggests that omega-3 fatty acid supplements do not reduce cancer risk. Evidence is mixed as to whether fish oil supplements improve cancer-related weight loss.

How is it promoted for use?

Some people believe that omega-3 fatty acids protect against the spread of solid-tumor cancers (those that form solid masses) that are related to hormone production, particularly breast cancer. Some also believe that omega-3 fatty acids inhibit the growth of colon, pancreatic, and prostate cancer. Some people and groups advocate use of omega-3 fatty acids to protect against cardiovascular disease and fatal heart attacks. Others believe that omega-3 fatty acids help rheumatoid arthritis, Crohn's disease, eczema, asthma, kidney failure, depression, and more.

What does it involve?

Oils from some cold-water fish such as sardines, salmon, herring, mackerel, halibut, striped bass, tuna, shark, and cod have high concentrations of the omega-3 fatty acids DHA and EPA. Oil from flaxseed contains more alpha-linolenic acid than any other known plant source (see "Flaxseed," page 349). Other plant sources of ALA include Great Northern beans, kidney beans, navy beans, and soybeans (see "Soybean," page 679).

Omega-3 supplements, such as fish oil, fish oil capsules, and cod liver oil (also called marine oils), are available at pharmacies and natural food stores.

Some nutritionists recommend eating a diet rich in fish containing omega-3 fatty acids, eating 1 to 2 teaspoons of flaxseed or flaxseed oil daily, or taking daily supplements containing 1 to 2 grams of omega-3s. Omega-3 fatty acids are unstable and spoil easily, so food manufacturers often remove them from foods to increase shelf life.

What is the history behind it?

Cod liver oil became popular in nineteenth-century England as a vitamin D supplement for sun-deprived children. In the 1950s, a German scientist named Johanna Budwig, PhD, discovered essential fatty acids and developed a diet that she said would fight cancer. Dr. Budwig claimed that many of her patients experienced tumor reduction within three months, and she stated that some experienced even more dramatic results. Dr. Budwig has reportedly used omega-3 fatty acids in combination with other nutrients to treat thousands of people with cancer and other diseases.

In 1996, the American Heart Association released a report stating that eating foods containing omega-3 fatty acids is reasonable and possibly helpful in reducing risk for heart disease. More recent recommendations have suggested eating two or more servings of fatty fish per week and eating foods that are high in alpha-linolenic acid such as flaxseed, canola oil, soybeans, and walnuts to reduce cardiovascular disease risk. People who already have cardiovascular disease are advised to eat more of these products or take supplements.

What is the evidence?

Although some research supports the anticancer claims made for omega-3 fatty acids, some does not. Some studies even show an increase in disease when omega-3 supplements are used. The strongest evidence for the health benefits of fatty acids from fish is in the area of heart disease and its risk factors. The relationship between omega-3 fatty acids, cancer, and other diseases is not as well known.

In 2006, researchers reviewed thirty-eight studies conducted over the past forty years on the effects of omega-3 fatty acids. Researchers looked at studies that showed positive effects, no effects, and negative effects of omega-3 fatty acids on the development of cancer. In the final analysis, it appeared that there was no effect overall. Researchers concluded that omega-3 supplements are unlikely to prevent cancer.

A clinical study published in the journal *Cancer* concluded that omega-3 fatty acids seemed to prolong the survival of cancer patients who were also severely malnourished. An earlier small study looked at patients with advanced pancreatic cancer and severe weight loss. It compared use of EPA mixed with a high-protein, high-calorie supplement with use of the supplement without EPA. After eight weeks, the study found that EPA did not help the patients gain weight. A more recent review of all research on the use of EPA for cancer-related weight loss found only five studies. The reviewers concluded that there was not enough information to determine whether EPA helped people with cancer-related weight loss.

Studies have shown that the fatty acids in fish oil help protect against heart disease and reduce risk factors such as high blood levels of triglycerides. In one study, fish oils appeared to help improve heart rhythm problems that can cause sudden death. However, they may also increase cholesterol and reduce blood clotting. Alpha-linolenic acid (ALA), the omega-3 fatty acid from vegetable oils, has not shown as strong an effect in studies to date, although it may reduce risk for fatal heart disease.

Research is also focusing on the role of omega-3 fatty acids in relation to omega-6 fatty acids. Omega-6 is another type of essential fatty acid that is found in many vegetable oils (such as corn, safflower, and sunflower oils), cereals, snack foods, and baked goods. Unlike omega-3s, omega-6s are plentiful in the typical American diet. Some researchers believe one cause of Americans' high rates of cardiovascular disease may be an imbalance in the ratio of omega-3 to omega-6 fatty acids. Ideally, the ratio of omega-3 to omega-6 fatty acids in the human body is 1-to-1. However, the typical American diet is low in omega-3s and high in omega-6s. Many people have ten to twenty times more omega-6 fatty acids than omega-3 fatty acids in their systems.

A large study followed more than thirty-four thousand women from 1980 to 1998, observing their fish intake and the ratio of fish fatty acids to omega-6 fatty acids in their diets to determine how the ratio affected their colorectal cancer risk. Women who took in more omega-3 fatty acids did not have a lower colorectal cancer risk, but they had fewer large benign colorectal tumors, or adenomas. This study suggests that omega-3 fatty acids may not reduce colorectal cancer risk but may slow its growth. More research is needed to find out whether this possibility holds true.

The American Cancer Society's most recent nutrition guidelines recommend eating a balanced diet that includes five or more servings a day of vegetables and fruit and choosing whole grains over processed and refined foods. Limiting intake of red meats and animal fats (including dairy fats) is also recommended in order to help reduce cancer risk. A good way to do this is to choose fish, poultry, or beans for some meals rather than beef, pork, or lamb. The guidelines note that although a diet high in fish can help lower heart disease risk, the clinical evidence regarding cancer is uncertain.

Are there any possible problems or complications?

Not enough is known about omega-3 fatty acids to determine whether they are safe in large quantities or when taken with other drugs. Omega-3s may increase total blood cholesterol and inhibit blood clotting. People who take blood-thinning medications (anticoagulants) or aspirin should not take extra omega-3 because of the risk for excessive bleeding.

The source of some omega-3 fatty acids may also be a health concern. Many large predatory fish contain toxic chemicals absorbed from pollution. Swordfish, shark, and tilefish (golden bass or golden snapper), for instance, are high in omega-3 fatty acids but may also contain high levels of mercury. King mackerel, a lesser source of omega-3s, may also have high mercury levels. Grouper, red snapper, and fresh or frozen tuna may have more moderate amounts of mercury. Other large fish, such as tuna and salmon, may contain other chemicals such as dioxin and polychlorinated biphenyls or PCBs, although fresh or frozen salmon usually has low mercury levels and large amounts of omega-3 fatty acids. Some studies have shown that farm-raised fish may carry more toxins than fish caught in the wild. Unfortunately, there is no way for a consumer to know what might be present in any particular fish, although some fish are inclined to have higher levels of contamination than others.

The precise risks and benefits of eating these fish are not known at this time. Experts recommend that adults vary the type of fish they eat as part of a healthy, balanced diet to reduce the chances of getting too many contaminants. Mercury poses the greatest risk to young children and unborn babies. Young children and women who are pregnant, trying to get pregnant, or nursing should not eat fish likely to be highly contaminated. They should also limit their intake of fish likely to be moderately contaminated.

For men and middle-aged or older postmenopausal women, the benefits of eating fish may outweigh the risks of mercury or other contaminants. Even so, experts suggest limiting intake of the most-contaminated fish to one serving per week. Most refined fish oil supplements have few or none of these contaminants.

Prolonged use of fish oil supplements can cause vitamin E deficiency, which is why vitamin E is added to many supplements. Fish liver oils (such as cod liver oil) can cause toxic levels of vitamins A and D if overused. Supplements may also cause fishy breath odor, belching, or abdominal bloating. They may also increase a tendency toward anemia in menstruating women. Women who are pregnant or breastfeeding should talk to their doctors before adding extra omega-3 to their diets.

People who are allergic to fish may have serious reactions to fish oil or supplements made from fish and should avoid them. People who are allergic to nuts should avoid supplements that are made of the type of nuts to which they react. Relying on this type of treatment alone and avoiding or delaying conventional medical care for cancer may have serious health consequences.

This product is sold as a dietary supplement in the United States. Unlike companies that produce drugs (which must provide the FDA with results of detailed testing showing their product is safe and effective before the drug is approved for sale), the companies that make supplements do not have to show evidence of safety or health benefits to the FDA before selling their products. Supplement products without any reliable scientific evidence of health benefits may still be sold as long as the companies selling them do not claim the supplements can prevent, treat, or cure any specific disease. Some such products may not contain the amount of the herb or substance that is written on the label, and some may include other substances (contaminants). Though the FDA has written new rules to improve the quality of manufacturing processes for dietary supplements and the accurate listing of supplement ingredients, these rules do not take full effect until 2010. The new rules also do not address the safety of supplement ingredients or their effects on health when proper manufacturing techniques are used.

Most such supplements have not been tested to find out if they interact with medicines, foods, or other herbs and supplements. Even though some reports of interactions and harmful effects may be published, full studies of interactions and effects are not often available. Because of these limitations, any information on ill effects and interactions should be considered incomplete.

References

Bagga D, Capone S, Wang HJ, Heber D, Lill M, Chap L, Glaspy JA. Dietary modulation of omega-3/omega-6 polyunsaturated fatty acid ratios in patients with breast cancer. *J Natl Cancer Inst.* 1997;89:1123-1131.

Burns CP, Halabi S, Clamon G, Kaplan E, Hohl RJ, Atkins JN, Schwartz MA, Wagner BA, Paskett E. Phase II study of high-dose fish oil capsules for patients with cancer-related cachexia. *Cancer.* 2005;103:651-652.

Covington MB. Omega-3 fatty acids. *Am Fam Physician.* 2004;70:133-140.

de Lorgeril M, Salen P, Martin JL, Monjaud I, Boucher P, Mamelle N. Mediterranean dietary pattern in a randomized trial: prolonged survival and possible reduced cancer rate. *Arch Intern Med.* 1998;158:1181-1187.

Dewey A, Baughan C, Dean T, Higgins B, Johnson I. Eicosapentaenoic acid (EPA, an omega-3 fatty acid from fish oils) for the treatment of cancer cachexia. *Cochrane Database Syst Rev.* 2007;(1):CD004597.

Doyle C, Kushi LH, Byers T, Courneya KS, Demark-Wahnefried W, Grant B, McTiernan A, Rock CL, Thompson C, Gansler T, Andrews KS, The 2006 Nutrition, Physical Activity and Cancer Survivorship Advisory Committee; American Cancer Society. Nutrition and physical activity during and after cancer treatment: an American Cancer Society guide for informed choices. *CA Cancer J Clin.* 2006;56:323-353.

Fish and omega-3 fatty acids. American Heart Association Web site. http://www.americanheart.org/presenter.jhtml?identifier=4632. Accessed June 10, 2008.

Fish, levels of mercury and omega-3 fatty acids. American Heart Association Web site. http://www.americanheart.org/presenter.jhtml?identifier=3013797. Accessed June 10, 2008.

Godley PA, Campbell MK, Gallagher P, Martinson FE, Mohler JL, Sandler RS. Biomarkers of essential fatty acid consumption and risk of prostatic carcinoma. *Cancer Epidemiol Biomarkers Prev.* 1996;5:889-895.

Gogos CA, Ginopoulos P, Salsa B, Apostolidou E, Zoumbos NC, Kalfarentzos F. Dietary omega-3 polyunsaturated fatty acids plus vitamin E restore immunodeficiency and prolong survival for severely ill patients with generalized malignancy. *Cancer.* 1998;82:395-402.

Hites RA, Foran JA, Carpenter DO, Hamilton MC, Knuth BA, Schwager SJ. Global assessment of organic contaminants in farmed salmon. *Science.* 2004;303:226-229.

Huang YC, Jessup JM, Forse RA, Flickner S, Pleskow D, Anastopoulos HT, Ritter V, Blackburn GL. n-3 fatty acids decrease colonic epithelial cell proliferation in high-risk bowel mucosa. *Lipids.* 1996;31 Suppl:S313-S317.

Kushi LH, Byers T, Doyle C, Bandera EV, McCullough M, McTiernan A, Gansler T, Andrews KS, Thun MJ; American Cancer Society 2006 Nutrition and Physical Activity Guidelines Advisory Committee. American Cancer Society guidelines on nutrition and physical activity for cancer prevention: reducing the risk of cancer with healthy food choices and physical activity. *CA Cancer J Clin.* 2006;56:254-281.

MacLean CH, Newberry SJ, Mojica WA, Khanna P, Issa AM, Suttorp MJ, Lim YW, Traina SB, Hilton L, Garland R, Morton SC. Effects of omega-3 fatty acids on cancer risk: a systematic review. *JAMA.* 2006;295:403-415.
Erratum in:
JAMA. 2006;295:1900.

Moses AW, Slater C, Preston T, Barber MD, Fearon KC. Reduced total energy expenditure and physical activity in cachectic patients with pancreatic cancer can be modulated by an energy and protein dense oral supplement enriched with n-3 fatty acids. *Br J Cancer.* 2004;90:996-1002.

Norman PE, Powell JT. Vitamin D, shedding light on the development of disease in peripheral arteries. *Arterioscler Thromb Vasc Biol.* 2005;25:39-46. Epub 2004 Oct 21.

Oh K, Willett WC, Fuchs CS, Giovannucci E. Dietary marine n-3 fatty acids in relation to risk of distal colorectal adenoma in women. *Cancer Epidemiol Biomarkers Prev.* 2005;14:835-841.

Omega-3. Memorial Sloan-Kettering Cancer Center Web site. http://www.mskcc.org/mskcc/html/69316.cfm. Accessed June 10, 2008.

Rajakumar K. Vitamin D, cod-liver oil, sunlight, and rickets: a historical perspective. *Pediatrics.* 2003;112:e132-e135.

Yetiv JZ. Clinical applications of fish oils. *JAMA.* 1988;260:665-670.

QUERCETIN

Other common name(s): quercetine, sophretin, meletin
Scientific/medical name(s): 3,3',4',5,7-pentahydroxyflavone

Description

Quercetin is a type of plant-based chemical, or phytochemical, known as a flavonoid (see also "Phytochemicals," page 458). Good sources include apples, onions, teas, red wines, and many other foods. Quercetin is also available as a dietary supplement.

Overview

Quercetin appears to have anti-inflammatory and antioxidant properties. It has been promoted as being effective against a wide variety of diseases, including cancer. While some early laboratory results appear promising, as of yet there is no reliable clinical evidence that quercetin can prevent or treat cancer in humans.

How is it promoted for use?

Quercetin is said to have a number of uses, but most of these are based on early findings from laboratory studies. Some early studies have suggested quercetin has antihistamine properties, and it is often promoted to help control allergies and asthma. Some proponents claim it can help stabilize small blood vessels and may help protect against heart attacks and strokes.

Quercetin is sometimes promoted to help prevent or treat different types of cancer. It has also been promoted to help with the symptoms of chronic prostatitis (swelling of the prostate gland) and to relieve some of the neurologic complications of diabetes.

What does it involve?

Quercetin is a common chemical pigment in the rinds and barks of a wide variety of plants. It is one of the main flavonoids in the diet and is found in large amounts in apple skins, onions, tea, and red wine. It is also found in leafy green vegetables, berries, and in herbs such as ginkgo and St. John's wort.

Quercetin is available in higher amounts in dietary supplements than would typically be found in food sources. Supplements are sold as capsules or tablets ranging in doses from 50 to 500 milligrams. There is no recommended standard dose for quercetin.

What is the history behind it?

Plants containing flavonoids have a long history of use in traditional medicine in many cultures, but flavonoids themselves were not discovered until the 1930s. Quercetin first gained attention several decades ago when it was found to cause DNA mutations in bacteria, a sign that it might actually contribute to causing cancer. Animal research done since that time has been inconclusive, and what little evidence there is in humans does not seem to support this idea. Research in recent years has focused on several possible helpful effects of quercetin, including its potential role in preventing cancer.

What is the evidence?

Most of the research on quercetin and cancer has been done in cell culture or animal studies. These types of studies can suggest possible helpful effects, but they do not provide proof that such effects can be achieved in humans. Controlled clinical trials are needed to show whether quercetin has helpful properties in humans.

Studies done in cell cultures have shown that quercetin has activity against some types of cancer cells. This activity may be due to its antioxidant or anti-inflammatory properties, or it may be due to other mechanisms. Recent studies suggest that quercetin can slow the growth of cancer cells and can help foster apoptosis, a form of natural cell death that does not happen in most cancer cells. Some studies in animals have shown that quercetin may help protect against certain types of cancer, particularly colon cancer.

Studies in humans have mainly been observational epidemiologic ones and have focused on the role of flavonoids in the diet as a group as opposed to quercetin in particular. These types of studies are not as conclusive as clinical trials. They cannot prove cause and effect, but often suggest links that can then be tested in clinical trials. While some of these observational epidemiologic studies have found that people with diets high in flavonoids may have lower risk for breast, lung, pancreatic, and other types of cancer, it is not clear what role quercetin played in their findings. One clinical study of people with a strong inherited tendency to develop colorectal cancer found that the combination of quercetin and curcumin (see "Turmeric," page 514) supplements decreased the number and size of precancerous rectal tumors. No other clinical trials testing quercetin's ability to prevent or treat cancer have been reported in the medical literature. Clinical trials are needed to further clarify quercetin's possible benefits.

In addition to cancer prevention and treatment, preliminary studies have also suggested potential value for quercetin in prostatitis (inflamed prostate) and heart disease. Further studies are needed before any recommendations can be made.

Until conclusive clinical research findings emerge, it is reasonable to include foods that contain quercetin as part of a balanced diet with an emphasis on fruits, vegetables, legumes, and whole grains. The interaction between certain phytochemicals and the other compounds in foods is not well understood, but it is unlikely that any single compound offers the best protection against cancer. A balanced diet that includes five or more servings a day of fruits and vegetables, along with foods from a variety of other plant sources such as nuts, seeds, whole grain cereals, and beans, is likely to be more effective in reducing cancer risk than eating one particular phytochemical in large amounts.

Are there any possible problems or complications?

Quercetin in the amounts consumed in a healthy diet is unlikely to cause any major problems. There have been occasional reports of nausea when supplements are taken in high doses. Quercetin supplements have not been studied for safety in women who are pregnant or breastfeeding. Relying on this type of treatment alone and avoiding or delaying conventional medical care for cancer may have serious health consequences.

This product is sold as a dietary supplement in the United States. Unlike companies that produce drugs (which must provide the FDA with results of detailed testing showing their product is safe and effective before the drug is approved for sale), the companies that make supplements do not have to show evidence of safety or health benefits to the FDA before selling their products. Supplement products without any reliable scientific evidence of health benefits may still be sold as long as the companies selling them do not claim the supplements can prevent, treat, or cure any specific disease. Some such products may not contain the amount of the herb or substance that is written on the label, and some may include other substances (contaminants). Though the FDA has written new rules to improve the quality of manufacturing processes for dietary supplements and the accurate listing of supplement ingredients, these rules do not take full effect until 2010. The new rules also do not address the safety of supplement ingredients or their effects on health when proper manufacturing techniques are used.

Most such supplements have not been tested to find out if they interact with medicines, foods, or other herbs and supplements. Even though some reports of interactions and harmful effects may be published, full studies of interactions and effects are not often available. Because of these limitations, any information on ill effects and interactions should be considered incomplete.

References

Adebamowo CA, Cho E, Sampson L, Katan MB, Spiegelman D, Willett WC, Holmes MD. Dietary flavonols and flavonol-rich foods intake and the risk of breast cancer. *Int J Cancer.* 2005;114:628-633.

Bosetti C, Spertini L, Parpinel M, Gnagnarella P, Lagiou P, Negri E, Franceschi S, Montella M, Peterson J, Dwyer J, Giacosa A, La Vecchia C. Flavonoids and breast cancer risk in Italy. *Cancer Epidemiol Biomarkers Prev.* 2005;14:805-808.

Cruz-Correa M, Shoskes DA, Sanchez P, Zhao R, Hylind LM, Wexner SD, Giardiello FM. Combination treatment with curcumin and quercetin of adenomas in familial adenomatous polyposis. *Clin Gastroenterol Hepatol.* 2006;4:1035-1038.

Hubbard GP, Wolffram S, de Vos R, Bovy A, Gibbins JM, Lovegrove JA. Ingestion of onion soup high in quercetin inhibits platelet aggregation and essential components of the collagen-stimulated platelet activation pathway in man: a pilot study. *Br J Nutr.* 2006;96:482-488.

Kim YH, Lee YJ. TRAIL apoptosis is enhanced by quercetin through Akt dephosphorylation. *J Cell Biochem.* 2007;100:998-1009.

Nöthlings U, Murphy SP, Wilkens LR, Henderson BE, Kolonel LN. Flavonols and pancreatic cancer risk: the Multiethnic Cohort Study. *Am J Epidemiol.* 2007;166:924-931.

Quercetin. Memorial Sloan-Kettering Cancer Center Web site. http://www.mskcc.org/mskcc/html/69346.cfm. Accessed June 10, 2008.

Quercetin. PDRhealth Web site. http://www.pdrhealth.com/drugs/altmed/altmed-mono.aspx?contentFileName=ame0326.xml&contentName=Quercetin. Accessed June 10, 2008.

Schabath MB, Hernandez LM, Wu X, Pillow PC, Spitz MR. Dietary phytoestrogens and lung cancer risk. *JAMA.* 2005;294:1493-1504.
Erratum in:
JAMA. 2005;294:2700.

Shoskes DA, Zeitlin SI, Shahed A, Rajfer J. Quercetin in men with category III chronic prostatitis: a preliminary prospective double-blind, placebo-controlled trial. *Urology.* 1999;54:960-963.

Volate SR, Davenport DM, Muga SJ, Wargovich MJ. Modulation of aberrant crypt foci and apoptosis by dietary herbal supplements (quercetin, curcumin, silymarin, ginseng and rutin). *Carcinogenesis.* 2005;26:1450-1456. Epub 2005 Apr 14.

SEA VEGETABLES

Other common name(s): seaweed, sea veg or sea vegg, sealogica, algae, red algae, green algae, brown algae, kelp, kombu, bladderwrack, wakami, nori, dulse, and others

Scientific/medical name(s): *Fucus vesiculosus*, *Laminaria digitata*, *Macrocystis pyrifera*, *Porphyra tenera*, and others

Description

Seaweed is a type of algae that grows in or near the sea. Certain types of seaweed and other algae have been eaten as food for thousands of years. Several companies sell seaweed and other algae as food supplements, either individually or in combinations, and call them sea vegetables. They have some special uses in medicine and as food additives.

Overview

Despite claims that sea vegetables are super-rich in nutrients that can prevent cancer and help numerous diseases, there is no reliable clinical evidence that this claim is true. Most seaweed does contain iodine, which is also available in iodized salt. However, amounts of iodine in seaweed vary widely, and getting too much iodine can cause thyroid and skin problems for some people. Early laboratory and animal studies of seaweed extracts suggest that certain compounds may one day be used in medicine.

How is it promoted for use?

Proponents claim that sea vegetables contain nutrients that "regenerate" the body. They maintain that sea vegetables are concentrated, containing several times more nutrients than land vegetables. Marketers often claim that seaweed will normalize the thyroid and regulate body weight and that seaweed supplements will reduce food cravings. Infomercials set up to look like interviews have claimed that "degenerative diseases," including tuberculosis, fibromyalgia, cancer, asthma, and diabetes, are due to nutritional deficiencies. They claim that these problems can be prevented or helped by sea vegetables, which they say offer nutrients that cannot be found elsewhere. For example, some proponents say that the iodine added to salt cannot be used by the body, while organic iodine from seaweed is easily absorbed.

What does it involve?

Most sea vegetables are dried after being harvested. If they are to be used as supplements, they are ground up and sold as powders, tablets, or capsules. The marketers of some blends recommend 3 or more capsules per day. Other sellers suggest different amounts of the dried plant in capsule form or suggest blending the dried powders into soups or other foods. Supplements are sold in health food stores, by phone, and over the Internet. Some are even recommended for pets as both vitamin supplements and immune system boosters.

Dried sea vegetables are also sold in Asian and specialty markets to be prepared as food. Most of these plants must be rehydrated before use. Some kinds of seaweed, such as nori, are common ingredients in sushi.

What is the history behind it?

Algae such as kelp (called *kombu* in Japan), *nori,* and *wakami* have been used in Asian cooking for thousands of years. Many types of seaweed are known in the United States by their Japanese names. Seaweed has been used medicinally in China for centuries to treat liver problems, swelling, phlegm, cysts, and enlarged thyroid glands.

In the eighteenth century, kelp was discovered as a source of iodine in the diet and used to treat enlarged thyroid. Called goiter, this condition is often caused by not getting enough iodine in food. Iodine was later added to salt to prevent iodine deficiency in the United States, and the rate of goiter declined dramatically.

Several types of algae have been marketed for use as supplements since the early 1980s. At that time, spirulina and other types of blue-green algae that grow in ponds and lakes became popular. Since then, an ever-increasing variety of seaweeds from ocean sources have been sold as dietary supplements in the United States.

In conventional medicine, stems from kelp were at one time used to enlarge the cervix of the womb for medical procedures, although there are now manmade devices that can be used. Purified compounds from seaweed are approved for use in many types of food. Carrageenan gum, a seaweed extract, is used in foodstuffs to create gels, stabilize mixtures, and thicken liquids. It is a common ingredient in ice cream, jelly, and infant formula. Agar, which is made from red algae, is used to add texture and thickness to foods. It is also a purely vegetable gelatin, unlike the more commonly used type that is made from animal protein. Agar has many uses, from clarifying wine to growing bacteria in the laboratory.

What is the evidence?

Observational studies of people who eat seafood and algae regularly tend to show that they have less breast cancer than those whose diets rely more on meat. Women in Japan, for example, have a lower risk for breast cancer than women in the United States. However, women who move from Japan to the United States are at the same risk as U.S. women within a few generations. This change suggests that the difference is not genetic. Even though there are many factors that may be responsible for the differences in risk—such as other foods, exposures, or lifestyle—scientists have focused on foods, such as omega-3 fatty acids in fish, as one possible explanation. The differences between typical Asian and North American diets and lifestyles are so numerous, however, that it is unlikely that seaweed is the only or even the main factor responsible for differences in cancer risk. For example, soy foods and green tea are also being studied to see whether they influence cancer risk. There are many other possible explanations yet to be explored.

In laboratory studies and some animal studies, compounds from several types of algae have slowed the growth of cancer cells and caused cancer cells to die, often by a process of natural cell death called apoptosis. However, clinical studies in humans have not been done using seaweed supplements. It is also important to note that extracted compounds are not the same as whole algae, and study results are not likely to show the same effects.

Dried seaweed contains large amounts of some nutrients by weight because the water is removed. The standard nutritional analysis is for 3.5 ounces, or 100 grams, which in some cases, would be more than 6 cups of dried seaweed. Actual serving sizes are very small when using seaweed supplements, and nutrient amounts are not guaranteed.

The American Cancer Society's nutrition guidelines recommend eating a balanced diet that includes five or more servings a day of vegetables and fruit, choosing whole grains over processed and refined foods, and limiting red meats and animal fats in order to help reduce cancer risk. Eating whole seaweed rather than supplements can be a way to include a larger variety of plant-based foods. It is best to choose foods from many kinds of fruits, vegetables, and other plant sources such as nuts, seeds, whole grain cereals, and beans.

Are there any possible problems or complications?

Since most seaweeds have varying amounts of iodine and other nutrients, it is difficult to know how much is in any one supplement. Edible seaweeds are generally safe for those who are not allergic. In some people, however, large amounts of iodine can cause goiter (enlargement of or growths on the thyroid) or other serious health problems. In people with known thyroid disorders, their conditions may be made worse by eating kelp or taking seaweed supplements. Eating a lot of seaweed or getting too much iodine from other sources can cause skin outbreaks that look like acne.

Some seaweed also contains large amounts of sodium, which may worsen high blood pressure or heart failure. Depending on where it is grown, some algae can contain concentrated amounts of heavy metals, including arsenic. These contaminated supplements have caused serious toxic effects in the past. Many types of algae are toxic or even fatal when eaten, so it is important to get supplements from trustworthy sources. Early or mild symptoms of toxicity may include nausea, diarrhea, weakness, numbness, and tingling. A recent analysis of dried seaweed samples purchased in London and over the Internet found that some contained worrisome levels of arsenic. Relying on this type of treatment alone and avoiding or delaying conventional medical care for cancer may have serious health consequences.

This product is sold as a dietary supplement in the United States. Unlike companies that produce drugs (which must provide the FDA with results of detailed testing showing their product is safe and effective before the drug is approved for sale), the companies that make supplements do not have to show evidence of safety or health benefits to the FDA before selling their products. Supplement products without any reliable scientific evidence of health benefits may still be sold as long as the companies selling them do not claim the supplements can prevent, treat, or cure any specific disease. Some such products may not contain the amount of the herb or substance that is written on the label, and some

may include other substances (contaminants). Though the FDA has written new rules to improve the quality of manufacturing processes for dietary supplements and the accurate listing of supplement ingredients, these rules do not take full effect until 2010. The new rules also do not address the safety of supplement ingredients or their effects on health when proper manufacturing techniques are used.

Most such supplements have not been tested to find out if they interact with medicines, foods, or other herbs and supplements. Even though some reports of interactions and harmful effects may be published, full studies of interactions and effects are not often available. Because of these limitations, any information on ill effects and interactions should be considered incomplete.

References

Bae SJ, Choi YH. Methanol extract of the seaweed *Gloiopeltis furcata* induces G2/M arrest and inhibits cyclooxygenase-2 activity in human hepatocarcinoma HepG2 cells. *Phytother Res.* 2007;21:52-57.

Barrett S. Algae: false claims and hype. Quackwatch Web site. http://www.quackwatch.org/01QuackeryRelated Topics/algae.html. Updated January 14, 2007. Accessed June 10, 2008.

Branger B, Cadudal JL, Delobel M, Ouoba H, Yameogo P, Ouedraogo D, Guerin D, Valea A, Zombre C, Ancel P; personnels des CREN. Spiruline as a food supplement in case of infant malnutrition in Burkina-Faso [in French] [Abstract]. *Arch Pediatr.* 2003;10:424-431.

Clark CD, Bassett B, Burge MR. Effects of kelp supplementation on thyroid function in euthyroid subjects. *Endocr Pract.* 2003;9:363-369.

Dharmananda S. The nutritional and medicinal value of seaweeds used in Chinese medicine. Institute for Traditional Medicine Web site. http://www.itmonline.org/arts/seaweed.htm. Updated December 2002. Accessed June 10, 2008.

Growing concerns over blue-green algae. *NCAHF News.* March-April 1996;19(2). http://www.ncahf.org/nl/1996/3-4.html. National Council Against Health Fraud Web site. Accessed June 10, 2008.

Gruenwald J. *PDR for Herbal Medicines.* 3rd ed. Montvale, NJ: Thomson PDR; 2004.

Humbert P. Induced acne [in French] [Abstract only]. *Rev Prat.* 2002;52:838-840.

Kushi LH, Byers T, Doyle C, Bandera EV, McCullough M, McTiernan A, Gansler T, Andrews KS, Thun MJ; American Cancer Society 2006 Nutrition and Physical Activity Guidelines Advisory Committee. American Cancer Society guidelines on nutrition and physical activity for cancer prevention: reducing the risk of cancer with healthy food choices and physical activity. *CA Cancer J Clin.* 2006;56:254-281.

Müssig K, Thamer C, Bares R, Lipp HP, Häring HU, Gallwitz B. Iodine-induced thyrotoxicosis after ingestion of kelp-containing tea. *J Gen Intern Med.* 2006;21:C11-C14.

Ostrzenski A. Resectocopic cervical trauma minimized by inserting Laminaria digitata preoperatively. *Int J Fertil Menopausal Stud.* 1994;39:111-113.

Rose M, Lewis J, Langford N, Baxter M, Origgi S, Barber M, MacBain H, Thomas K. Arsenic in seaweed—forms, concentration and dietary exposure. *Food Chem Toxicol.* 2007;45:1263-1267.

Seaweed, kelp, bladderwrack (*Fucus vesiculosus*). Medline Plus Web site. http://www.nlm.nih.gov/medlineplus/druginfo/natural/patient-bladderwrack.html. Accessed June 10, 2008.

Sekiya M, Funahashi H, Tsukamura K, Imai T, Hayakawa A, Kiuchi T, Nakao A. Intracellular signaling in the induction of apoptosis in a human breast cancer cell line by water extract of Mekabu. *Int J Clin Oncol.* 2005;10:122-126.

Teas J, Pino S, Critchley A, Braverman LE. Variability of iodine content in common commercially available edible seaweeds. *Thyroid.* 2004;14:836-841.

USDA national nutrient database for standard reference. National Agriculture Library Web site. http://www.nal.usda.gov/fnic/foodcomp/search/. Accessed June 10, 2008.

Walkiw O, Douglas DE. Health food supplements prepared from kelp—a source of elevated urinary arsenic. *Clin Toxicol.* 1975;8:325-331.

Yuan YV, Walsh NA. Antioxidant and antiproliferative activities of extracts from a variety of edible seaweeds. *Food Chem Toxicol.* 2006;44:1144-1150.

Zhuang C, Itoh H, Mizuno T, Ito H. Antitumor active fucoidan from the brown seaweed, umitoranoo (*Sargassum thunbergii*). *Biosci Biotechnol Biochem.* 1995;59:563-567.

Ziegler RG, Hoover RN, Nomura AM, West DW, Wu AH, Pike MC, Lake AJ, Horn-Ross PL, Kolonel LN, Siiteri PK, Fraumeni JF Jr. Relative weight, weight change, height, and breast cancer risk in Asian-American women. *J Natl Cancer Inst.* 1996;88:650-660.

SELECTED VEGETABLE SOUP

Other common name(s): Selected Vegetables, Sun's Soup, SV, sun soup, Frozen SV, FSV
Scientific/medical name(s): none

Description

Selected Vegetable Soup (SV), also called Sun's Soup, is promoted as a treatment for cancer. There have been several formulas of the soup, two of which are marketed in the United States as dietary supplements.

Overview

Available scientific evidence does not support claims that Selected Vegetable Soup can help treat cancer.

How is it promoted for use?

Selected Vegetable Soup (SV), also called Sun's Soup, is promoted as a treatment for cancer and other medical conditions.

What does it involve?

There have been several formulas of the soup, two of which are marketed in the United States as dietary supplements. One type, called Selected Vegetables, is a freeze-dried vegetable and herb product that reportedly contains vegetables and herbs including soybean, shiitake mushroom, red date, scallion, garlic, lentil bean, leek, mung bean, hawthorn fruit, onion, American ginseng, angelica root, licorice, dandelion root, senegal root, ginger, olive, sesame seed, and parsley. The second formula is called Frozen Selected Vegetables (FSV or Frozen SV). Either type of Selected Vegetable Soup is taken as part of the diet. About an ounce of the freeze-dried formula is usually eaten every day, mixed with water or other kinds of soups. When using the frozen soup, about 10 ounces are usually eaten each day.

What is the history behind it?

Selected Vegetable Soup was first conceived as a treatment for cancer in the mid-1980s. In an effort to help a relative with advanced lung cancer, Alexander Sun, PhD, created a mixture of plant materials he believed had anticancer and immune system–stimulating properties. He patented this product in 1995.

What is the evidence?

Two studies have been published, both of which were conducted by the soup's developer, Alexander Sun, PhD. One of these clinical trials found daily consumption of SV, taken along with conventional cancer treatment, to be nontoxic and associated with improvement in weight maintenance and survival of patients with advanced non–small cell lung cancer. The study involved a very small sample size (fewer than twenty patients). The patients received different types of conventional treatment (surgery, chemotherapy, and radiation therapy) while taking SV, and the study was not randomized or blinded.

The second study, conducted in 2001, looked at sixteen people with non–small cell lung cancer, twelve of whom took FSV while undergoing standard medical treatment. Again, the patients were not randomly assigned to the group receiving or not receiving FSV, and the study was not blinded. Also, patients who received FSV were compared with "historical controls," referring to a group of patients treated in the past. Because historical controls often differ in relevant characteristics from the experimental group, studies using this design are not considered as reliable as randomized, controlled clinical trials.

These design flaws mean that neither of the two studies can yield strong or reliable evidence. More research is needed to determine whether SV is helpful. Information was posted in 2005 regarding a large randomized, blinded clinical trial to look at the use of SV with patients with advanced small cell lung cancer. As of mid-2007, the study is enrolling patients.

Are there any possible problems or complications?

Overall, use of Selected Vegetable Soup is considered safe when it is used as part of a healthy diet. The only problem reported with the use of Selected Vegetable Soup is a feeling of fullness or bloatedness. Relying on this type of treatment alone and avoiding or delaying conventional medical care for cancer may have serious health consequences.

References

Selected vegetables/Sun's soup (PDQ®). National Cancer Institute Web site. http://www.cancer.gov/cancertopics/pdq/cam/vegetables-sun-soup/HealthProfessional. Accessed June 10, 2008.

Sun Farms vegetable soup. Memorial Sloan-Kettering Cancer Center Web site. http://www.mskcc.org/mskcc/html/69391.cfm. Accessed June 10, 2008.

US National Institutes of Health. Effects of selected vegetable and herb mix (SV) on advanced non-small cell lung cancer. ClinicalTrials.gov Web site. http://clinicaltrials.gov/show/NCT00246727. Updated April 10, 2006. Accessed June 10, 2008.

SHIITAKE MUSHROOM

Other common name(s): Japanese mushroom, Black Forest mushroom, golden oak mushroom, oakwood mushroom

Scientific/medical name(s): *Lentinus edodes*, *Lentinula edodes*

Description

A shiitake mushroom is an edible fungus native to Asia and grown in forests. Shiitake mushrooms are the second most commonly cultivated edible mushrooms in the world. Extracts from the mushroom and sometimes the whole dried mushroom are used in herbal remedies.

Overview

Studies in animals have found antitumor, cholesterol-lowering, and virus-inhibiting effects in compounds in shiitake mushrooms. However, clinical studies are needed to determine whether these properties can help people with cancer and other diseases. It is reasonable to include shiitake mushrooms as part of a balanced diet.

How is it promoted for use?

Shiitake mushrooms are promoted to fight the development and progression of cancer and AIDS by boosting the body's immune system. These mushrooms are also said to help prevent heart disease by lowering cholesterol levels and to help treat infections such as hepatitis by producing interferon, a group of natural proteins that stops viruses from multiplying. Promoters claim that eating both the cap and stem of the mushroom may be helpful, but they do not say how much must be eaten to have an effect. They say the strength and effects of the mushroom depend on how it is prepared and consumed.

Promoters claim that shiitake mushrooms contain several compounds with health benefits. A compound called lentinan is believed to stop or slow tumor growth. Another component, activated hexose-containing compound (also known as 1,3-beta glucan), is also said to reduce tumor activity and lessen the side effects of cancer treatment. The mushrooms also contain the compound eritadenine, which is thought to lower cholesterol by blocking the way cholesterol is absorbed into the bloodstream. These claims are currently being studied.

What does it involve?

The fresh or dried whole mushroom is widely available in grocery stores, while extracts of the mushroom are sold in capsule form in health food stores and on the Internet. Kits for growing shiitake mushrooms indoors at home are available from some Internet sellers.

For medicinal purposes, the extracts of compounds in shiitake mushrooms would usually be recommended, rather than the mushroom itself. For example, some Japanese researchers give lentinan along with chemotherapy to treat patients with lung, nose, throat, and stomach cancer. Extracts of the active compounds, such as lentinan and eritadenine, are mainly sold in Japan. Activated hexose-containing compound is sold as a nutritional supplement in the United States, Europe, and Japan.

What is the history behind it?

Medicinal use of shiitake mushrooms dates at least to 100 AD in China. The mushrooms have been widely consumed as a food for thousands of years in the East and more recently in the West. Today, shiitake mushrooms are very popular in the United States as well. Research into the anticancer properties of shiitake mushrooms has been going on since at least the 1960s.

What is the evidence?

Animal studies have shown some positive results regarding the antitumor, cholesterol-lowering, and virus-inhibiting effects of several active compounds in shiitake mushrooms.

There have been some studies in humans. At least one randomized clinical trial of lentinan has shown it to prolong life of patients with advanced and recurrent stomach and colorectal cancer who were also given chemotherapy. Lentinan is a beta glucan (sometimes called beta glycan) that is found in several mushrooms, yeasts, and other foods. Beta glucan is a polysaccharide, a large and complex molecule made up of smaller sugar molecules. The beta glucan polysaccharide is believed to stimulate the immune system and activate certain cells and proteins that attack cancer, including macrophages, T-cells, and natural killer cells. In laboratory studies, beta glucan appears to slow the growth of cancer in some cell cultures.

Several potential cancer-fighting substances have been found in shiitake mushrooms, and purified forms of these compounds are being studied as treatments for stomach and colorectal cancer. It is not known whether any of these results will apply to the mushrooms bought in supermarkets or the extracts that are sold as supplements. One nonrandomized study published in 2002 looked at use of shiitake mushroom extract by men with prostate cancer but did not find any positive effect. Sixty-two men took the extract three times a day. After six months, they did not have any significant decrease in their level of prostate-specific antigen (PSA), a protein in the body that typically increases as prostate cancer grows, and nearly a quarter of them had increases in their PSA level. More human clinical trials are under way to understand which, if any, compounds in shiitake mushrooms may be effective for which types of cancers.

To reduce cancer risk, the American Cancer Society's nutrition guidelines recommend eating a balanced diet that includes five or more servings a day of vegetables and fruit, choosing whole grains over processed and refined foods, and limiting red meats and animal fats. Choosing foods from a variety of fruits, vegetables, and other plant sources such as nuts, seeds, whole grain cereals, and beans is healthier than consuming large amounts of one particular food.

Are there any possible problems or complications?

Shiitake mushrooms and their extracts are generally considered safe, although there are reports of diarrhea or bloating. In some people, allergic reactions have developed affecting the skin, nose, throat, or lungs. Relying on this type of treatment alone and avoiding or delaying conventional medical care for cancer may have serious health consequences.

This product is sold as a dietary supplement in the United States. Unlike companies that produce drugs (which must provide the FDA with results of detailed testing showing their product is safe and effective before the drug is approved for sale), the companies that make supplements do not have to show

evidence of safety or health benefits to the FDA before selling their products. Supplement products without any reliable scientific evidence of health benefits may still be sold as long as the companies selling them do not claim the supplements can prevent, treat, or cure any specific disease. Some such products may not contain the amount of the herb or substance that is written on the label, and some may include other substances (contaminants). Though the FDA has written new rules to improve the quality of manufacturing processes for dietary supplements and the accurate listing of supplement ingredients, these rules do not take full effect until 2010. The new rules also do not address the safety of supplement ingredients or their effects on health when proper manufacturing techniques are used.

Most such supplements have not been tested to find out if they interact with medicines, foods, or other herbs and supplements. Even though some reports of interactions and harmful effects may be published, full studies of interactions and effects are not often available. Because of these limitations, any information on ill effects and interactions should be considered incomplete.

References

Borchers AT, Stern JS, Hackman RM, Keen CL, Gershwin ME. Mushrooms, tumors, and immunity. *Proc Soc Exp Biol Med.* 1999;221:281-293.

Chihara G, Hamuro J, Maeda Y, Shiio T, Suga T, Takasuka N, Sasaki T. Antitumor and metastasis-inhibitory activities of lentinan as an immunomodulator: an overview. *Cancer Detect Prev Suppl.* 1987;1:423-443.

Chung R. Functional properties of edible mushrooms. *Nutr Rev.* 1996;54:S91-S93.

Cunningham-Rundles S, Lin H, Cassileth B; American Society for Nutrition. Are botanical glucans effective in enhancing tumoricidal cell activity? *J Nutr.* 2005;135: 2919S.

deVere White RW, Hackman RM, Soares SE, Beckett LA, Sun B. Effects of a mushroom mycelium extract on the treatment of prostate cancer. *Urology.* 2002;60:640-644.

Fang N, Li Q, Yu S, Zhang J, He L, Ronis MJ, Badger TM. Inhibition of growth and induction of apoptosis in human cancer cell lines by an ethyl acetate fraction from shiitake mushrooms. *J Altern Complement Med.* 2006;12:125-132.

Ikekawa T, Uehara N, Maeda Y, Nakanishi M, Fukuoka F. Antitumor activity of aqueous extracts of edible mushrooms. *Cancer Res.* 1969;29:734-735.

Kawaoka T, Yoshino S, Kondo H, Yamamoto K, Hazama S, Oka M. Clinical evaluation of intrapleural or peritoneal repetitive administration of Lentinan and OK-432 for malignant effusion [in Japanese]. *Gan to Kagaku Ryoho.* 2005;32:1565-1567.

Kodoma N, Komuta K, Nanba H. Can maitake MD-fraction aid cancer patients? *Altern Med Rev.* 2002;7:236-239.
Comment in:
Altern Med Rev. 2002;7:236-451; author reply 452-454.

Konno S. Potential growth inhibitory effect of maitake D-fraction on canine cancer cells. *Vet Ther.* 2004;5:263-271.

Ko YT, Lin YL. 1,3-beta-glucan quantification by a fluorescence microassay and analysis of its distribution in foods. *J Agric Food Chem.* 2004;52:3313-3318.

Kushi LH, Byers T, Doyle C, Bandera EV, McCullough M, McTiernan A, Gansler T, Andrews KS, Thun MJ; American Cancer Society 2006 Nutrition and Physical Activity Guidelines Advisory Committee. American Cancer Society guidelines on nutrition and physical activity for cancer prevention: reducing the risk of cancer with healthy food choices and physical activity. *CA Cancer J Clin.* 2006;56:254-281.

Matsushita K, Kuramitsu Y, Ohiro Y, Obara M, Kobayashi M, Li YQ, Hosokawa M. Combination therapy of active hexose correlated compound plus UFT significantly reduces the metastasis of rat mammary adenocarcinoma. *Anticancer Drugs.* 1998;9:343-350.

Nagahashi S, Suzuki H, Nishiwaki M, Okuda K, Kurosawa Y, Terada S, Sugihara T, Andou K, Hibi T. TS-1/CDDP/Lentinan combination chemotherapy for inoperable advanced gastric cancer [in Japanese]. *Gan to Kagaku Ryoho.* 2004;31:1999-2003.

Shiitake mushroom. Memorial Sloan-Kettering Cancer Center Web site. http://www.mskcc.org/mskcc/html/69377.cfm. Accessed June 10, 2008.

Taguchi T. Clinical efficacy of lentinan on patients with stomach cancer: end-point results of a four-year follow-up survey. *Cancer Detect Prev Suppl.* 1987;1:333-349.

SOYBEAN

Other common name(s): soy, soya, soy protein, soy powder, glycine soja
Scientific/medical name(s): *Glycine max*

Description

The soybean plant is an annual plant native to southeast Asia. It has oblong pods that contain two to four seeds or beans. Soybeans are legumes, a member of the pea family, and are a source of high-quality protein. They are processed to make various foods and food additives.

Overview

In laboratory studies, animal studies, and research looking at groups of people and their dietary habits, certain chemical components of soy have appeared to show protective effects against breast and prostate cancer. Randomized clinical trials are needed to understand how these findings apply to cancer prevention in humans.

Results of research on the effects of consuming isoflavones (a soy component) on colon cancer risk have been mixed. Some human studies on individual soy components have been conducted and others are still under way. Most studies that have shown benefit have used whole soy protein rather than soy components and extracts.

How is it promoted for use?

Soybean products are promoted for their protective properties against breast, prostate, colon, and lung cancer. The effects of soy are thought to be due to substances called isoflavones, although other substances may also contribute. Isoflavones are sometimes called plant estrogens or phytoestrogens because they mimic (although weakly) estrogen that is produced in humans and animals. Genistein, daidzein, and glycitein are isoflavones that are present in small amounts in other foods but are most abundant in soy.

As a protein source, soybean products are promoted as a healthier alternative to meat and as an aid to weight loss. Soy products are also used to lower cholesterol and blood pressure and to relieve symptoms of menopause and osteoporosis. Proponents also suggest that including soy protein in a diet low in saturated fat and cholesterol may help reduce the risk for heart disease.

What does it involve?

Soy can be consumed in many forms, with tofu, soy milk, soy powder, and textured vegetable protein being some of the more popular. The amount of isoflavone varies by type of soy product. Soy is also available as a dietary supplement or pill. Soy protein powders and bars are available in nutrition stores and health food markets. The powder can be added to drinks or used in cooking. Isoflavone supplements are also available, although most tests that show benefit have used whole soy protein.

What is the history behind it?

The soybean has been used as a food source for more than five thousand years. Today, there are more than twenty-five hundred varieties of soybeans grown throughout the world. It was not until relatively recently that studies began on the potential health-promoting properties of the soybean.

Plant estrogens were first identified in the early 1930s, when it was discovered that soybeans, willows, dates, and pomegranates contained compounds similar in structure to estrogens. Scientists began studying the role isoflavones play in reducing breast cancer risk in the 1960s. In a 1981 prospective study in Japan, researchers found that daily intake of miso, a soybean paste, was linked to lower death rates from stomach cancer in more than 260,000 men and women. Around that time, other studies on soy began to be published in the United States. In October 1999, the U.S. Food and Drug Administration (FDA) agreed to allow health claims about soy's role in reducing heart disease on food products containing soy protein.

What is the evidence?

Researchers believe that the isoflavones in soy, such as genistein, daidzein, and glycitein, may play a role in reducing cancer risk. A number of laboratory and animal experiments and human observational studies have found that soy isoflavones may reduce the risk for several types of cancer, including breast, prostate, and colon cancer. However, these results have not yet been reflected in human clinical trials, so no definite conclusions can be made.

There is enough evidence, scientists believe, for phytoestrogens to be studied in clinical trials as an addition to conventional breast or prostate cancer treatment. Human studies sponsored by the National Cancer Institute are under way. Large studies that looked at groups of women with a high soy intake showed a lower risk for breast cancer and endometrial cancer, but there are many possible explanations other than the soy. Further studies that control for these factors are needed. It is also possible that the weak estrogen-like effect of soy might be helpful in prostate cancer prevention, but large human studies are needed.

Some studies have suggested that the effect of soy foods on breast cancer risk depends on the age of the person consuming them. It is thought that high soy intake by young women at a time when breast tissue is developing and estrogen levels are relatively high may offer some protection. However, it is unclear whether soy intake after menopause, when estrogen levels are naturally low, is of any benefit or could even be harmful.

Several clinical studies of women with breast cancer have been done to determine whether soy capsules help with symptoms of menopause. The results have not shown any consistent improvement of symptoms such as hot flashes.

Several studies of men with prostate cancer have suggested that soy foods and/or supplements may reduce levels of prostate-specific antigen (PSA), a substance that typically increases as prostate cancer grows. In another study, while PSA levels did not decrease during soy treatment, they increased less rapidly than they had before the study began. Although these results are encouraging, further research is needed to learn whether soy products help men with prostate cancer to live longer.

Soybeans and soy foods have been shown in clinical trials to lower cholesterol and reduce blood pressure.

The American Cancer Society's nutrition guidelines recommend eating a balanced diet that includes five or more servings a day of vegetables and fruit, choosing whole grains over processed and refined foods, and limiting red meats and animal fats in order to help reduce cancer risk. Using soy foods as a substitute for some servings of animal protein is one way to reduce red meat and animal fat intake. It is best to choose foods from a variety of fruits, vegetables, and other plant sources such as nuts, seeds, whole grain cereals, and beans.

Are there any possible problems or complications?

Eating soybeans is generally considered safe for those who are not allergic to them. Side effects are rare but may include occasional gastrointestinal problems such as stomach pain, loose stools, and diarrhea.

The isoflavones in soy have weak estrogen-like activity, and it remains uncertain how they could affect the growth of estrogen receptor–positive breast cancers. Some researchers suggest they may act as anti-estrogens and reduce cancer growth, while others suggest their estrogen-like activity could cause cancer to grow faster. Until this issue is resolved, many oncologists recommend that people taking tamoxifen or aromatase inhibitors and people with estrogen-sensitive breast tumors should avoid adding large amounts of soy, including soy supplements or isoflavones, to their diets.

Soy isoflavone supplements appear to be safe for most people, although it is possible that there may be risks not yet identified. Isoflavone supplements have not been studied in pregnant women, and these concentrated sources may not be healthy for the fetus. Soy products are considered safe in pregnancy.

A few people are allergic to soy proteins and may have serious or life-threatening reactions to soy-containing foods. These people should avoid all forms of soy and supplements made from it. Soy ingredients may also be listed as soya.

Relying on this type of diet alone and avoiding or delaying conventional medical care for cancer may have serious health consequences.

This product is sold as a dietary supplement in the United States. Unlike companies that produce drugs (which must provide the FDA with results of detailed testing showing their product is safe and effective before the drug is approved for sale), the companies that make supplements do not have to show evidence of safety or health benefits to the FDA before selling their products. Supplement products without any reliable scientific evidence of health benefits may still be sold as long as the companies selling them do not claim the supplements can prevent, treat, or cure any specific disease. Some such products may not contain the amount of the herb or substance that is written on the label, and some may include other substances (contaminants). Though the FDA has written new rules to improve the quality of manufacturing processes for dietary supplements and the accurate listing of supplement ingredients, these rules do not take full effect until 2010. The new rules also do not address the safety of supplement ingredients or their effects on health when proper manufacturing techniques are used.

Most such supplements have not been tested to find out if they interact with medicines, foods, or other herbs and supplements. Even though some reports of interactions and harmful effects may be published, full studies of interactions and effects are not often available. Because of these limitations, any information on ill effects and interactions should be considered incomplete.

References

Dalais FS, Meliala A, Wattanapenpaiboon N, Frydenberg M, Suter DA, Thomson WK, Wahlqvist ML. Effects of a diet rich in phytoestrogens on prostate-specific antigen and sex hormones in men diagnosed with prostate cancer. *Urology.* 2004;64:510-515.

Fournier DB, Erdman JW Jr, Gordon GB. Soy, its components, and cancer prevention: a review of the in vitro, animal, and human data. *Cancer Epidemiol Biomarkers Prev.* 1998;7:1055-1065.

Gruenwald J. *PDR for Herbal Medicines.* 3rd ed. Montvale, NJ: Thomson PDR; 2004.

Henkel J. Soy: health claims for soy protein, questions about other components. *FDA Consumer: The Magazine of the US Food and Drug Administration.* May-June 2000. US Food and Drug Administration Web site. http://www.fda.gov/fdac/features/2000/300_soy.html. Accessed June 10, 2008.

Jacobsen BK, Knutsen SF, Fraser GE. Does high soy milk intake reduce prostate cancer incidence? The Adventist Health Study (United States). *Cancer Causes Control.* 1998;9:553-557.

MacGregor CA, Canney PA, Patterson G, McDonald R, Paul J. A randomised double-blind controlled trial of oral soy supplements versus placebo for treatment of menopausal symptoms in patients with early breast cancer. *Eur J Cancer.* 2005;41:708-714.

Messina M, Bennink M. Soyfoods, isoflavones and risk of colonic cancer: a review of the in vitro and in vivo data. *Baillieres Clin Endocrinol Metab.* 1998;12:707-728.

Messina M. Soy, soy phytoestrogens (isoflavones), and breast cancer. *Am J Clin Nutr.* 1999;70:574-575.

Moyad MA. Soy, disease prevention, and prostate cancer. *Semin Urol Oncol.* 1999;17:97-102.

Natural Standard. Herbal/plant therapies: soy (Glycine max[L.] Merr.) Complementary/Integrative Medicine Education Resources, The University of Texas M. D. Anderson Cancer Center Web site. http://www.mdanderson.org/departments/cimer/display.cfm?id=4B0FB06E-7655-4487-9146CCE58AA7D403&method=displayFull. Accessed June 10, 2008.

Nikander E, Kilkkinen A, Metsä-Heikkilä M, Adlercreutz H, Pietinen P, Tiitinen A, Ylikorkala O. A randomized placebo-controlled crossover trial with phytoestrogens in treatment of menopause in breast cancer patients. *Obstet Gynecol.* 2003;101:1213-1220.

Pendleton JM, Tan WW, Anai S, Chang M, Hou W, Shiverick KT, Rosser CJ. Phase II trial of isoflavone in prostate-specific antigen recurrent prostate cancer after previous local therapy. *BMC Cancer.* 2008;8:132.

Quella SK, Loprinzi CL, Barton DL, Knost JA, Sloan JA, LaVasseur BI, Swan D, Krupp KR, Miller KD, Novotny PJ. Evaluation of soy phytoestrogens for the treatment of hot flashes in breast cancer survivors: a North Central Cancer Treatment Group Trial. *J Clin Oncol.* 2000;18:1068-1074.

Soy. Memorial Sloan-Kettering Cancer Center Web site. http://www.mskcc.org/mskcc/html/69383.cfm. Accessed June 10, 2008.

Soy. PDRhealth Web site. http://www.pdrhealth.com/drugs/altmed/altmed-mono.aspx?contentFileName=ame0457.xml&contentName=Soy. Accessed June 10, 2008.

Schröder FH, Roobol MJ, Boevé ER, de Mutsert R, Zuijdgeest-van Leeuwen SD, Kersten I, Wildhagen MF, van Helvoort A. Randomized, double-blind, placebo-controlled crossover study in men with prostate cancer and rising PSA: effectiveness of a dietary supplement. *Eur Urol.* 2005;48:922-930; discussion 930-931. Epub 2005 Oct 17.

Thanos J, Cotterchio M, Boucher BA, Kreiger N, Thompson LU. Adolescent dietary phytoestrogen intake and breast cancer risk (Canada). *Cancer Causes Control.* 2006;17:1253-1261.

US Food and Drug Administration. FDA Talk Paper: FDA approves new health claim for soy protein and coronary heart disease. Rockville, MD: National Press Office; October 20, 1999. Talk Paper T99-48.

Van Patten CL, Olivotto IA, Chambers GK, Gelmon KA, Hislop TG, Templeton E, Wattie A, Prior JC. Effect of soy phytoestrogens on hot flashes in postmenopausal women with breast cancer: a randomized, controlled clinical trial. *J Clin Oncol.* 2002;20:1449-1455.

Wu AH, Wan P, Hankin J, Tseng CC, Yu MC, Pike MC. Adolescent and adult soy intake and risk of breast cancer in Asian-Americans. *Carcinogenesis.* 2002;23:1491-1496.

VEGETARIANISM

Other common name(s): semi-vegetarian, pesci-vegetarian, lacto-ovo-vegetarian, ovo-vegetarian, lacto-vegetarian, vegan, fruitarian
Scientific/medical name(s): none

Description

Vegetarianism is the practice of eating a diet consisting mainly or entirely of food that comes from plant sources such as fruits and vegetables. Vegetarian diets vary widely. Some people use no animal products, while others who describe themselves as vegetarian may consume dairy products, eggs, fish, and even poultry.

Overview

Some studies have linked vegetarian diets to lower risk for heart disease, diabetes, high blood pressure, obesity, and certain types of cancer, such as colon cancer. A vegetarian diet should be properly planned to ensure it provides all the required nutrients.

How is it promoted for use?

Many proponents of vegetarianism believe a vegetarian diet promotes health because it contains less saturated fat, protein, and cholesterol than omnivorous diets (those in which both plant and animal foods are eaten). Vegetarian diets also provide more fiber, vitamins, minerals, antioxidants, and other phytochemicals (plant chemicals) than diets containing meat (see "Phytochemicals," page 458). Some vegetarians believe it is more natural for humans to consume plant-based foods. Still others choose to eliminate or reduce their consumption of animal products because of religious, cultural, moral, or philosophical reasons.

What does it involve?

All vegetarian diets include plant-based foods such as grains, legumes, seeds, nuts, vegetables, and fruits, but they vary according to whether any animal products are consumed and what kinds. For example, a vegan diet excludes all animal products including meat, fowl, fish, dairy, and eggs. A lacto-ovo-vegetarian diet adds dairy products and eggs; a lacto-vegetarian diet adds only dairy products; and ovo-vegetarian diets add only eggs. A semi-vegetarian may eat mostly plant-based food with small amounts of fish and poultry; and a pesci-vegetarian adds only fish.

One small group of vegetarians called fruitarians eat only raw or dried fruits and fruit vegetables (like tomatoes) because they believe that cooking fruit damages its nutritional properties. They advocate all types of fruits, nuts, and seeds, including non-sweet fruits such as olives, cucumbers, and avocados.

The macrobiotic diet, which is discussed on pages 638–642, includes an emphasis on whole organic grains. It is also mainly vegetarian, although certain fruits and vegetables are excluded. Some types of fish may be allowed.

What is the history behind it?

Vegetarianism has long been a part of many cultures. In the United States, the vegetarian movement began in the mid-1800s. The American Vegetarian Society was founded in 1850. Today, vegetarianism is very popular in the United States and abroad because it is thought to be a healthier approach to diet and nutrition.

The American Cancer Society's most recent nutrition guidelines recommend eating a balanced diet that includes five or more servings a day of vegetables and fruit, choosing whole grains over processed and refined foods, and limiting red meats and animal fats. The National Cancer Institute (NCI) also recommends a diet low in fat and high in plant foods such as fruits and vegetables in order to decrease cancer risk.

Because vegetarianism is becoming more common, the American Dietetic Association created a food guide for the North American vegetarian in 2003. The Association estimated that, as of 2004, there were about six million U.S. adults who followed vegetarian eating plans.

What is the evidence?

Observational epidemiologic studies have linked vegetarian diets with a decreased risk for heart disease, diabetes, high blood pressure, obesity, and colon cancer. A review of research on the effects of vegetarian diets among Seventh-Day Adventists, whose religious doctrine advises against eating animal flesh, found that Seventh-Day Adventists experienced less heart disease and fewer cases of some types of cancer than the general population. On average, Seventh-Day Adventist males had lower-than-average serum cholesterol levels and blood pressure and their overall cancer death rate was about half that of the general population. The overall cancer death rate of females was also lower. A couple of studies indicated an increased risk for colon and prostate cancer with increased animal fat intake. An increase in the consumption of beans and lentils appeared to decrease the risk for colon cancer and prostate cancer. The report cautioned that abstinence from tobacco and alcohol may have contributed to some of the health effects associated with vegetarian diets in the Seventh-Day Adventist community.

An observational epidemiologic study in Germany found the death rate for colon cancer was lower among moderate and strict vegetarians compared with that of the general population. However, the authors of the study also noted vegetarians tend to be more health conscious than average. In Great Britain, a seventeen-year population study that followed eleven thousand vegetarians and health-conscious people concluded that the daily consumption of fresh fruit was linked to a significant reduction in deaths from ischemic heart disease, stroke, and all causes of death combined. Another population study found men who ate a diet rich in grains, cereals, and nuts had a lower risk for prostate cancer.

In 1991, two nutritionists studying the benefits and risks of vegetarian diets reported that vegetarians are not necessarily healthier than nonvegetarians and that well-planned omnivorous diets can provide health benefits as well. They also pointed out that many vegetarians adopt a healthier lifestyle, including more physical exercise and no smoking, which would likely improve their overall health and account for part of the health benefit that was first thought to be due to their diet.

A study published in 2005 compared more than one thousand German vegetarians with nearly seven hundred health-conscious nonvegetarians over a twenty-one-year period, and found that there were no major differences between the groups in terms of death and disease, although the vegetarians had slightly less heart disease. Both groups were healthier than the general population, in part due to less smoking and more physical activity.

The majority of human evidence regarding vegetarianism consists of observational studies of the risk for various diseases such as cancer. Very few clinical studies of people with cancer have been reported. A few studies of men with prostate cancer have reported that comprehensive lifestyle changes including vegetarianism, exercise, and stress reduction can slow the rate increases in blood levels of prostate-specific antigen (PSA). The contribution of maintaining a vegetarian diet to these benefits remains unproven.

Are there any possible problems or complications?

Strict vegetarians, such as vegans, who eat no animal products at all, must be careful to consume adequate amounts of protein. Other nutrients that may be missing from a vegetarian diet include vitamin B12, vitamin D, calcium, zinc, and iron. Some health care professionals consider vegan diets potentially risky, especially for infants, toddlers, and pregnant women. Vegan diets must be carefully planned to ensure adequate amounts of required nutrients are consumed.

Vegan women who breastfeed their infants may want to take supplements containing sufficient vitamin B12. Severe B12 deficiencies in breastfed infants of vegan mothers have caused failure to thrive, poor brain development, and other serious problems.

Switching to a vegetarian diet may increase the amount of dietary fiber consumed, which can cause temporary problems such as bloating, discomfort, and gas. Dietitians suggest a gradual rather than quick change in diet. Relying on this type of diet alone and avoiding or delaying conventional medical care for cancer may have serious health consequences.

References

Centers for Disease Control and Prevention (CDC). Neurologic impairment in children associated with maternal dietary deficiency of cobalamin—Georgia, 2001. *MMWR.* 2003;52;61-64.

Chang-Claude J, Hermann S, Eiber U, Steindorf K. Lifestyle determinants and mortality in German vegetarians and health-conscious persons: results of a 21-year follow-up. *Cancer Epidemiol Biomarkers Prev.* 2005;14:963-968.

Dingott S, Dwyer J. Vegetarianism: healthful but unnecessary. Quackwatch Web site. http://www.quackwatch.org/03HealthPromotion/vegetarian.html. Updated March 17, 2000. Accessed June 10, 2008.

Frentzl-Beyme R, Chang-Claude J. Vegetarian diets and colon cancer: the German experience. *Am J Clin Nutr.* 1994;59:1143S-1152S.

Hebert JR, Hurley TG, Olendzki BC, Teas J, Ma Y, Hampl JS. Nutritional and socioeconomic factors in relation to prostate cancer mortality: a cross-national study. *J Natl Cancer Inst.* 1998;90:1637-1647.

Key TJ, Thorogood M, Appleby PN, Burr ML. Dietary habits and mortality in 11,000 vegetarians and health conscious people: results of a 17 year follow up. *BMJ.* 1996;313:775-779.

Kushi LH, Byers T, Doyle C, Bandera EV, McCullough M, McTiernan A, Gansler T, Andrews KS, Thun MJ; American Cancer Society 2006 Nutrition and Physical Activity Guidelines Advisory Committee. American Cancer Society guidelines on nutrition and physical activity for cancer prevention: reducing the risk of cancer with healthy food choices and physical activity. *CA Cancer J Clin.* 2006;56:254-281.

National Institutes of Health. *Alternative Medicine: Expanding Medical Horizons: A Report to the National Institutes of Health on Alternative Medical Systems and Practices in the United States.* Washington, DC: US Government Printing Office; 1994. NIH publication 94-066.

A new food guide for North American Vegetarians. American Dietetic Association Web site. 2003. http://www.eatright.org/cps/rde/xchg/ada/hs.xsl/governance_5105_ENU_HTML.htm. Accessed June 10, 2008.

Ornish D, Weidner G, Fair WR, Marlin R, Pettengill EB, Raisin CJ, Dunn-Emke S, Crutchfield L, Jacobs FN, Barnard RJ, Aronson WJ, McCormac P, McKnight DJ, Fein JD, Dnistrian AM, Weinstein J, Ngo TH, Mendell NR, Carroll PR. Intensive lifestyle changes may affect the progression of prostate cancer. *J Urol.* 2005;174:1065-1069.

Saxe GA, Major JM, Nguyen JY, Freeman KM, Downs TM, Salem CE. Potential attenuation of disease progression in recurrent prostate cancer with plant-based diet and stress reduction. *Integr Cancer Ther.* 2006;5:206-213.

Singh PN, Fraser GE. Dietary risk factors for colon cancer in a low-risk population. *Am J Epidemiol.* 1998;148:761-764.

WHEATGRASS

Other common name(s): couch grass, wheatgrass diet, agropyron
Scientific/medical name(s): *Triticum aestivum* (subspecies of the family *Poaceae*)

Description

Wheatgrass is a member of the family *Poaceae*, which includes a wide variety of wheat-like grasses. Wheatgrass is commonly found in temperate regions of Europe and the United States. It can be grown outdoors or indoors. The roots and underground stems may be used in herbal remedies.

Overview

There have been almost no clinical studies in humans to support claims made for wheatgrass or wheatgrass diet programs. One very small study suggested that it may help people with colitis, a bowel problem.

How is it promoted for use?

Wheatgrass is promoted to treat a number of conditions including the common cold, coughs, bronchitis, fevers, infections, and inflammation of the mouth and throat. In folk medicine, practitioners used wheatgrass to treat cystitis, gout, rheumatic pain, chronic skin disorders, and constipation. Some proponents equate chlorophyll (the component that makes wheatgrass and other plants green) with hemoglobin, which carries oxygen in the blood, saying that wheatgrass raises the body's oxygen levels.

Although most people use wheatgrass juice as a dietary supplement or as a serving of vegetables, some proponents claim that a dietary program commonly called "the wheatgrass diet" can cause cancer to regress or "shrink" and can extend the lives of people with cancer. They believe that the wheatgrass diet strengthens the immune system, kills harmful bacteria in the digestive system, and rids the body of toxins and waste matter.

What does it involve?

Wheatgrass is available planted in trays of soil and in tablets, capsules, liquid extracts, tinctures, and juices. Some people buy seeds or kits and grow it at home, either indoors or outside. It is most often made into juice, but can also be used to make tea. People generally drink the juice, although a few mix it with water and use it as an enema to "cleanse the liver." It is also mixed into smoothies and other drinks.

The wheatgrass diet, which is used by a small number of wheatgrass enthusiasts, avoids all meat, dairy products, and cooked foods. This diet emphasizes "live foods," such as uncooked sprouts, raw vegetables and fruits, nuts, and seeds.

What is the history behind it?

The wheatgrass diet was developed by Boston resident Ann Wigmore, who immigrated to the United States from Lithuania. Wigmore believed strongly in the healing power of nature. Wigmore's notion that fresh wheatgrass had value came from her interpretation of the Bible and observations that dogs and cats eat grass when they feel ill. Wigmore claimed that the wheatgrass diet could cure disease.

In 1982, the Massachusetts Attorney General sued Wigmore for claiming that her program could reduce or eliminate the need for insulin in diabetics. She later retracted her claims. In 1988, the Massachusetts Attorney General sued Wigmore again, this time for claiming that an "energy enzyme soup" she invented could cure AIDS. Wigmore was ordered to stop representing herself as a physician or person licensed to treat disease. Although Wigmore died in 1993, her Creative Health Institute is still active. Wheatgrass is readily available, and her diet is still in use.

What is the evidence?

Wheatgrass is a natural source of vitamins and minerals. However, available scientific evidence does not support the idea that wheatgrass or the wheatgrass diet can cure or prevent disease. One small early study found that wheatgrass juice, when used along with standard medical care, seemed to help control symptoms of chronic inflammation of the large intestine, a condition called ulcerative colitis. This 2002 study tested fresh wheatgrass juice against a sham drink in a group of people with ulcerative colitis. All of them received regular medical care, including their usual diet. Those who drank about three ounces of the juice every day for a month had less pain, diarrhea, and rectal bleeding than those in the group drinking the placebo.

Although there are individual reports that describe tumor shrinkage and extended survival among people with cancer who followed the wheatgrass diet, there are no clinical trials in the available scientific literature that support this claim.

The American Cancer Society's nutrition guidelines recommend eating a balanced diet that includes five or more servings a day of vegetables and fruit, choosing whole grains over processed and refined foods, and limiting red meats and animal fats. Choosing foods from a variety of fruits, vegetables, and other plant sources such as nuts, seeds, whole grain cereals, and beans is healthier than consuming large amounts of one particular food.

Are there any possible problems or complications?

Wheatgrass is generally considered safe, although a few individuals have reported nausea, headaches, hives, or swelling in the throat within minutes of drinking its juice. Hives and swollen throat are often signs of a serious allergic reaction and should be handled as an emergency. Anyone having these kinds of symptoms after ingesting wheatgrass may have even more severe reactions to it later.

Because it is grown in soils or water and consumed raw, contamination with bacteria, molds, or other substances may be a concern. Women who are pregnant or breastfeeding should not use wheatgrass. Relying on this type of diet alone and avoiding or delaying conventional medical care for cancer may have serious health consequences.

This product is sold as a dietary supplement in the United States. Unlike companies that produce drugs (which must provide the FDA with results of detailed testing showing their product is safe and effective before the drug is approved for sale), the companies that make supplements do not have to show evidence of safety or health benefits to the FDA before selling their products. Supplement products without any reliable scientific evidence of health benefits may still be sold as long as the companies selling them do not claim the supplements can prevent, treat, or cure any specific disease. Some such products may not contain the amount of the herb or substance that is written on the label, and some may include other substances (contaminants). Though the FDA has written new rules to improve the quality of manufacturing processes for dietary supplements and the accurate listing of supplement ingredients, these rules do not take full effect until 2010. The new rules also do not address the safety of supplement ingredients or their effects on health when proper manufacturing techniques are used.

Most such supplements have not been tested to find out if they interact with medicines, foods, or other herbs and supplements. Even though some reports of interactions and harmful effects may be published,

full studies of interactions and effects are not often available. Because of these limitations, any information on ill effects and interactions should be considered incomplete.

References

Ben-Arye E, Goldin E, Wengrower D, Stamper A, Kohn R, Berry E. Wheat grass juice in the treatment of active distal ulcerative colitis: a randomized double-blind placebo-controlled trial. *Scand J Gastroenterol.* 2002;37:444-449.

Blumenthal M, ed. *The Complete German Commission E Monographs: Therapeutic Guide to Herbal Medicines.* Austin, TX: American Botanical Council; 1998.

Byers T, Nestle M, McTiernan A, Doyle C, Currie-Williams A, Gansler T, Thun M; American Cancer Society 2001 Nutrition and Physical Activity Guidelines Advisory Committee. American Cancer Society guidelines on nutrition and physical activity for cancer prevention: reducing the risk of cancer with healthy food choices and physical activity. *CA Cancer J Clin.* 2002;52:92-119.

Fetrow CW, Avila JR. *Professional's Handbook of Complementary & Alternative Medicines.* Philadelphia, PA: Lippincott Williams & Wilkins; 2004.

Gruenwald J. *PDR for Herbal Medicines.* 3rd ed. Montvale, NJ: Thomson PDR; 2004.

Jarvis WT. Wheatgrass therapy. National Council Against Health Fraud Web site. Available at: http://www.ncahf.org/articles/s-z/wheatgrass.html. Posted January 15, 2001. Accessed June 20, 2007.

MacIntosh CJ. Wheatgrass and mold. Urban Agriculture Notes. Canada's Office of Urban Agriculture Web site. http://www.cityfarmer.org/wheatgrass.html. Updated February 23, 2003. Accessed June 10, 2008.

US Congress, Office of Technology Assessment. *Unconventional Cancer Treatments: OTA-H-405.* Washington, DC: US Government Printing Office; 1990.

Wheat grass. Memorial Sloan-Kettering Cancer Center Web site. http://www.mskcc.org/mskcc/html/69419.cfm. Accessed June 10, 2008.

WILLARD WATER

Other common name(s): catalyst altered water

Scientific/medical name(s): none

Description

Manufacturers describe Willard Water as "catalyst altered water." It is supposed to contain calcium, magnesium, a small amount of castor oil, and an electrical (ionic) charge.

Overview

No scientific studies have been conducted on Willard Water, and so there is no evidence to support claims of health benefits. It has not been proven useful for any medical condition and its exact contents are not known. Not enough is known about Willard Water to know whether it is safe.

How is it promoted for use?

Proponents claim that Willard Water eases the burning caused by radiation therapy, relieves sores in the mouth and on the lips, eliminates bad breath, removes plaque from teeth, heals minor skin irritations (such as scrapes, bruises, cuts, insect bites, and burns), prevents hangovers, and eases pain from arthritis and muscle sprains. It is also supposed to help the body absorb and use nutrients, increase enzyme activity, and strengthen the immune system.

What does it involve?

Manufacturers describe Willard Water as "catalyst altered water," which reportedly contains calcium, magnesium, a small amount of castor oil, and an electrical (ionic) charge. It is sold as a concentrate, which is diluted with filtered or bottled water. The liquid can be swallowed, sprayed directly on the skin or in the mouth, added to herbal remedies or bath water, or used as an ointment.

What is the history behind it?

Willard Water was reportedly created around 1970 by Dr. John Willard, a professor at the South Dakota School of Mining and Technology.

What is the evidence?

Since no scientific studies have been conducted on Willard Water, there is no evidence to support these claims. It has not been proven useful for any medical condition and the exact contents are not known.

Are there any possible problems or complications?

Not enough is known about Willard Water to know whether it is safe. Relying on this type of treatment alone and avoiding or delaying conventional medical care for cancer may have serious health consequences.

This product is sold as a dietary supplement in the United States. Unlike companies that produce drugs (which must provide the FDA with results of detailed testing showing their product is safe and effective before the drug is approved for sale), the companies that make supplements do not have to show

evidence of safety or health benefits to the FDA before selling their products. Supplement products without any reliable scientific evidence of health benefits may still be sold as long as the companies selling them do not claim the supplements can prevent, treat, or cure any specific disease. Some such products may not contain the amount of the herb or substance that is written on the label, and some may include other substances (contaminants). Though the FDA has written new rules to improve the quality of manufacturing processes for dietary supplements and the accurate listing of supplement ingredients, these rules do not take full effect until 2010. The new rules also do not address the safety of supplement ingredients or their effects on health when proper manufacturing techniques are used.

Most such supplements have not been tested to find out if they interact with medicines, foods, or other herbs and supplements. Even though some reports of interactions and harmful effects may be published, full studies of interactions and effects are not often available. Because of these limitations, any information on ill effects and interactions should be considered incomplete.

References

What is Willard Water? The Official Willard Water Web site. http://www.dr-willardswater.com/whatis.html. Accessed June 24, 2008.

Chapter Nine

Pharmacologic and Biologic Therapies

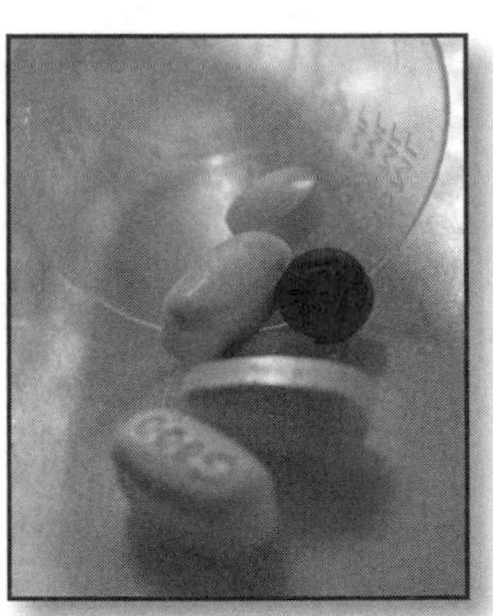

714-X

Other common name(s): 714X
Scientific/medical name(s): trimethylbicyclonitramineoheptane chloride

Description

714-X is used as a complementary/alternative method in Canada, Western Europe, and Mexico to treat cancer, AIDS, and other diseases. It is not legally available in the United States. The ingredient of 714-X claimed by supporters to have anticancer activity is camphor that has been chemically modified by the addition of an extra nitrogen atom. Chemical analysis of 714-X by the U.S. Food and Drug Administration (FDA) found that it consists of 94 percent water; about 5 percent nitrate; 1.4 percent ammonium; less than 1 percent each ethanol, sodium, and chloride; and less than (0.01) percent camphor.

Overview

Available scientific evidence does not support claims that 714-X is effective in treating any type of cancer or other illness. It does not appear to be harmful, but no studies have been done to confirm its safety.

How is it promoted for use?

According to proponents of 714-X, people with serious illnesses such as cancer carry tiny living particles in their bloodstream called somatids. Proponents claim that disease can be diagnosed and monitored by noting the number and forms of somatids in a person's blood. 714-X is said to cure cancer and AIDS by interfering with the flow of somatids through the bloodstream. This interference is said to cause the immune system to grow stronger and cause diseases to regress.

Proponents claim that cancer cells produce a substance called co-cancerogenic K factor (CKF), which protects the cells from the immune system. 714-X supposedly supplies the body with nitrogen, which strips this protective substance and leaves tumor cells vulnerable to attack by the immune system.

What does it involve?

714-X is prepared as a sterile solution and injected into a lymph node in the groin. Ice packs are used to cool the area of injection both before and after. A course of treatment involves daily injections for twenty-one days, followed by two or three days of rest. The cycle is typically repeated several times. 714-X can also be given nasally using a nebulizer. This route is more commonly used for lung or oral cancers.

The FDA has not approved 714-X for use in the United States, and it is illegal to import it into the country. In Canada, 714-X is available only on a compassionate-use basis. While it is not approved for general therapeutic use, doctors may request it under the Emergency Drug Release Program of Health Canada. In October 2004, Health Canada instructed CERBE, the company that sells 714-X, to remove statements concerning 714-X from its Web site.

What is the history behind it?

Early in his career, French-born scientist Gaston Naessens developed the somatoscope, a special microscope that he used to examine blood at extremely high magnifications. Using the somatoscope, Naessens claimed to have discovered tiny living organisms called somatids in the blood of people with serious diseases, including cancer. He believed that somatids were different from bacteria, fungi, viruses, or other microbes previously identified by other scientists and that they were responsible for the development of disease.

In 1956, a French court convicted and fined Naessens for practicing medicine without a license. Naessens moved to Quebec and later developed 714-X. Naessens claimed that 714-X interfered with somatids and could stop or reverse the growth of tumors. The drug's name is derived from the alphabetical position of Naessen's initials. "G" is the 7th letter of the alphabet, and "N" is 14th. "X" is the 24th letter and represents 1924, the year Naessens was born.

In the 1980s, while living in Quebec, Naessens was prosecuted for health fraud and threatened with life imprisonment. He was acquitted after testimony from many 714-X users who claimed that the drug had helped them. In 1992, a U.S. distributor of 714-X was warned by the FDA that claims he was making were illegal because the product was not proven to be safe and effective in treating disease. That same year, the FDA put out an import alert that banned 714-X from being brought into the United States. In 1996, after continuing to sell 714-X, the distributor was convicted of numerous charges, including introducing an unapproved drug into interstate commerce.

What is the evidence?

According to the National Cancer Institute, "No laboratory study of the safety and/or effectiveness of 714-X has been published in scientific literature. A few animal experiments have been conducted, but the results of these experiments have not been reported in peer-reviewed scientific journals...714-X was not found to be effective as an anticancer treatment in these studies" (National Cancer Institute Web site, 2008). Although some patients have reported helpful effects after taking 714-X, available scientific evidence does not support any claims about the existence of somatids or that 714-X can cure cancer, AIDS, or other diseases in humans. No formal clinical studies have been conducted on 714-X. Unlike some other alternative therapies, even a best case series has not been published. A best case series allows an independent review of the medical records of patients treated with unconventional cancer therapies to determine whether the patients actually had cancer, which standard treatments they received, and whether the unconventional treatment may have helped. This information provides a basis for further study of the treatment.

One component of 714-X, camphor, is being researched in animals for potential anticancer activity; however, research is still at a very early stage.

Are there any possible problems or complications?

714-X appears to cause few side effects, but no formal studies of safety have been done. The injections can result in local redness, tenderness, and swelling at the injection site.

It is not known whether 714-X might interact with standard cancer treatment or other drugs. The manufacturers of 714-X state that it can be used along with conventional therapies. However, they believe that it is most likely to be effective in patients who have not had chemotherapy or radiation therapy, and they recommend it be given as early as possible after diagnosis.

Relying on this type of treatment alone and avoiding or delaying conventional medical care for cancer may have serious health consequences.

These substances may have not been thoroughly tested to find out how they interact with medicines, foods, or dietary supplements. Even though some reports of interactions and harmful effects may be published, full studies of interactions and effects are not often available. Because of these limitations, any information on ill effects and interactions should be considered incomplete.

References

714-X (PDQ®). National Cancer Institute Web site. http://www.cancer.gov/cancertopics/pdq/cam/714-X/healthprofessional. Accessed June 11, 2008.

714-X information package. 1996. Canadian Breast Cancer Research Alliance Web site. http://www.breast.cancer.ca/media_news_resource_centre/resources/literature_reviews/714-X/. Accessed June 21, 2007. Site discontinued.

Barrett S. Fanciful claims for 714X. Quackwatch Web site. http://www.quackwatch.org/01QuackeryRelatedTopics/Cancer/714x.html. Updated March 22, 2002. Accessed June 11, 2008.

Ernst E, Cassileth BR. How useful are unconventional cancer treatments? *Eur J Cancer.* 1999;35:1608-1613.

Kaegi E. Unconventional therapies for cancer: 6. 714-X. Task Force on Alternative Therapies of the Canadian Breast Cancer Research Initiative. *CMAJ.* 1998;158:1621-1624.

Kurtzweil P. Investigators' reports: promoter of 714X cure-all faces prison for selling unapproved drug. *FDA Consumer: The Magazine of the US Food and Drug Administration.* November 1996. US Food and Drug Administration Web site. http://www.fda.gov/fdac/departs/996_irs.html. Accessed June 21, 2007.

ANTINEOPLASTON THERAPY

Other common name(s): antineoplastons, A10 (Atengenal, Cengenal), AS2-1 (Astugenal, Fengenal)

Scientific/medical name(s): 3-phenylacetylamino-2,6-piperidinedione, phenylacetic acid, phenylacetylglutamine, phenylacetylisoglutamine

Description

Antineoplaston therapy is a complementary/alternative cancer treatment that involves using a group of synthetic chemicals called antineoplastons, which are intended to protect the body from disease. Antineoplastons are made up mostly of peptides and amino acids originally taken from human blood and urine.

Overview

Thousands of patients have been treated with antineoplastons, mostly at a single clinic, and clinical trials are under way there for many types of cancer. Published clinical trial results are available for a relatively small number of patients, and the effectiveness of antineoplastons as a cancer therapy remains uncertain. Most cancer specialists believe there is insufficient evidence to recommend use of antineoplastons except perhaps in the context of clinical trials that will provide reliable information on the safety and effectiveness of this treatment.

How is it promoted for use?

Supporters have claimed antineoplastons are a part of something called the body's natural biochemical defense system. This system is said to act independently of the body's immune system and to protect against diseases like cancer, which involve a breakdown in the information processing of the body's cells.

Proponents claim antineoplaston therapy has been successful in treating many forms of cancer. They claim people with cancer don't have enough naturally occurring antineoplastons and that this therapy replenishes the body's supply, allowing the biochemical defense system of the body to induce cancer cells to stop growing and to develop features that resemble normal cells (cell differentiation).

What does it involve?

Antineoplastons are given orally or by injection into a vein. The duration of treatment usually ranges from eight to twelve months. A year of treatment can cost from $30,000 to $60,000, depending on the type of treatment, number of consultations, and the need for surgery to implant a catheter for drug delivery.

Antineoplaston therapy was developed by Stanislaw Burzynski, MD, PhD. Initial treatments are given over the course of one to three weeks at a clinic in Houston, founded by Dr. Burzynski. (Other U.S. centers are participating in studies to evaluate this treatment, as well as some centers in other countries.) Further treatments may be given "at home" but require monthly visits to a doctor, either at the Houston clinic or elsewhere with one of Dr. Burzynski's research colleagues. In the past, many of the patients who received antineoplaston treatment also were treated with surgery, radiation, chemotherapy, or combinations of these standard treatments at other centers, and some received chemotherapy prescribed by Dr. Burzynski. Currently, antineoplaston treatment is available in the United States only through participation in clinical trials led by Dr. Burzynski and his colleagues. To be eligible for these clinical studies, patients must have cancer that is growing despite conventional treatments. Patients cannot receive conventional anticancer treatments while they are participating in these antineoplaston studies.

What is the history behind it?

According to the Burzynski Patient Group Web site, "In 1967, Dr. Burzynski identified naturally occurring peptides in the human body that he concluded control the growth of cancer." That same year, he graduated from the Medical Academy in Lublin, Poland. His first article published in the medical literature, which discussed an effect of urinary peptides on growth of cancer cells in laboratory dishes (tissue culture), was published in 1973 while he was working as a researcher at Baylor College of Medicine in Houston. Although Burzynski initially isolated the chemicals that he named antineoplastons from human blood and urine, he later produced these naturally occurring substances in his laboratory.

In 1977, Dr. Burzynski opened his own clinic, where he has used antineoplaston therapy to treat patients for a variety of cancers. He claims that the therapy has cured many patients of their illnesses. However, his methods for conducting and reporting clinical research have been criticized for not following appropriate scientific standards.

In the United States today, antineoplaston therapy can be given only to patients who go to Dr. Burzynski's clinic and enroll in his clinical trials approved by the U.S. Food and Drug Administration (FDA).

What is the evidence?

Some patients claim to have been helped by antineoplaston therapy, but these anecdotal reports are not considered evidence of effectiveness by the medical community, either for this or for any other type of therapy. Some promising results for the use of antineoplaston therapy have been reported in small studies. Most of these studies were directed by Dr. Burzynski himself. Results from a few small studies conducted by one group of researchers in Japan have also been published. However, the available clinical evidence consists of early-phase clinical trials and best case series.

During the 1980s, the United States Congressional Office of Technology Assessment (OTA) reviewed medical journal articles describing cases of cancer patients whom Dr. Burzynski had treated with antineoplaston therapy. Its report, published in 1990, concludes that, "Despite a substantial number of preliminary clinical studies published by Burzynski and his associates describing outcomes among the patients he treated with Antineoplastons and an attempt at a 'best case' review, there is still a lack of valid information to judge whether this treatment is likely to be beneficial to cancer patients" (*Unconventional Cancer Treatments: OTA-H-405*;1990:97). The OTA report criticized Burzynski's research process and noted that his definitions of advanced cancer and of complete and partial cancer remission were not used in accordance with generally accepted definitions. One example they pointed to was a patient said to have had a complete remission after treatment with antineoplastons. The report concluded, however, that this claim was inappropriate because the cancer had been removed by surgery before the antineoplaston treatment was started.

In 1982, consultants to the Ontario (Canada) Ministry of Health visited Burzynski's clinic and reviewed records of twelve patients selected by Burzynski from among the thousands he had treated. According to the OTA report, the Canadian doctors "found no examples of objective response to Antineoplastons" (*OTA-H-405*;1990:96). In 1985, the Canadian Bureau of Prescription Drugs examined the records of Canadian doctors who had treated patients at Dr. Burzynski's clinic in Houston. Of thirty-six patients, thirty-two had died without showing signs of improvement. Of the remaining four, one patient died after slight improvement, while one patient died after stabilizing for a year. The two remaining patients had widespread cancer.

In 1991, the National Cancer Institute (NCI) reviewed several "best cases" (involving patients with brain tumors) chosen by Burzynski. According to a 1992 article in the *Journal of the National Cancer Institute*, "two NCI extramural investigators independently reviewed the case histories of some patients treated with antineoplastons. At the investigators' recommendation, the NCI examined the case histories, pathology slides, and imaging studies from seven patients with primary brain tumors ....[T]he site visit team and, subsequently, the [NCI] Division of Cancer Treatment's Decision Network Committee believed that evidence of possible antitumor effect was demonstrated" (*J Natl Cancer Inst.* 1992;84:1701). The NCI concluded that these results warranted further investigation through clinical trials at other medical centers. But because of disagreement between NCI researchers and Burzynski, the clinical trials were terminated in 1995. By 1999, the researchers concluded that only six of the nine patients treated in that study could be evaluated according to the study's initial requirements. None of the six showed evidence of tumor shrinkage. The researchers noted, however, that the small number of patients participating limited their ability to say with confidence that antineoplaston treatment had no benefit. Side effects of antineoplaston treatment included temporary sleepiness and confusion, and worsening of epilepsy (seizures) in patients who already had that problem (as a result of the tumors).

Dr. Burzynski currently has permission from the FDA to conduct clinical trials of antineoplaston therapy at his clinic. The NCI and researchers at several cancer centers are also conducting laboratory experiments on the peptides involved in antineoplaston therapy.

While many articles have been published and dozens of clinical trials against many types of cancer have been ongoing at Dr. Burzynski's clinic for several years, there have not been any randomized controlled trials—the type of study that is required for new anticancer drugs to be approved by the FDA and recommended by conventional oncologists.

Although some proponents of antineoplaston therapy have suggested that the reviews of this treatment by conventional cancer specialists are biased by mistrust of alternative therapies, even some prominent figures in the field of alternative medicine have reservations about antineoplastons. According to Dr. Andrew Weil, "Over the years, Dr. Burzynski claims to have treated more than 8,000 patients, but his success rates are unknown. His Web site states only that he has helped 'many' people. If antineoplaston therapy works, we should have scientific studies showing what percentage of patients treated have survived and for how long, as well as evidence showing how Dr. Burzynski's method stacks up against conventional cancer treatment.... Until we have credible scientific evidence showing what antineoplastons are, how they act in the body, and what realistic expectations of treatment with them might be, I see no reason for any cancer patient to take this route" (Andrew Weil MD Web site, 2006).

Are there any possible problems or complications?

Proponents claim that antineoplaston therapy is "nontoxic." However, reported side effects include stomach gas, slight rashes, chills, fever, change in blood pressure, unpleasant body odor during treatment, sleepiness, confusion, and seizures. High levels of blood sodium can also be a significant problem with this therapy.

It is not known whether antineoplastons would cause any problems due to interactions with other medications. Relying on this type of treatment alone and avoiding or delaying conventional medical care for cancer may have serious health consequences.

These substances may have not been thoroughly tested to find out how they interact with medicines, foods, or dietary supplements. Even though some reports of interactions and harmful effects may be

published, full studies of interactions and effects are not often available. Because of these limitations, any information on ill effects and interactions should be considered incomplete.

References

The antineoplaston anomaly: how a drug was used for decades in thousands of patients, with no safety, efficacy data. *Cancer Lett.* 1998;24(36).

Antineoplastons. National Cancer Institute Web site. http://cis.nci.nih.gov/fact/7_43.htm. Updated May 20, 2002. Accessed June 11, 2008.

Antineoplaston therapy. Burzynski Patient Group Web site. http://burzynskipatientgroup.org/antitherapy.html Accessed June 11, 2008.

Buckner JC, Malkin MG, Reed E, Cascino TL, Reid JM, Ames MM, Tong WP, Lim S, Figg WD. Phase II study of antineoplastons A10 (NSC 648539) and AS2-1 (NSC 620261) in patients with recurrent glioma. *Mayo Clin Proc.* 1999;74:137-145.

Burzynski SR. Biologically active peptides in human urine. I. Isolation of a group of medium-sized peptides. *Physiol Chem Phys.* 1973;5:437-447.

Cassileth BR. *The Alternative Medicine Handbook: The Complete Reference Guide to Alternative and Complementary Therapies.* New York, NY: W.W. Norton & Co; 1998.

Green S. 'Antineoplastons'. An unproved cancer therapy. *JAMA.* 1992;267:2924-2928.

Hawkins MJ, Friedman MA. National Cancer Institute's evaluation of unconventional cancer treatments. *J Natl Cancer Inst.* 1992;84:1699-1702.

US Congress, Office of Technology Assessment. Pharmacologic and Biologic Treatments. In: *Unconventional Cancer Treatments: OTA-H-405.* Washington, DC: US Government Printing Office; 1990.

Weil A. Antineoplastons: a bogus cancer treatment? Andrew Weil MD Web site. http://www.drweil.com/drw/u/id/QAA400003. Published July 28, 2006. Accessed June 11, 2008.

APITHERAPY

Other common name(s): bee venom therapy (BVT), bee venom, venom immunotherapy, bee pollen
Scientific/medical name(s): none

Description

Apitherapy refers to the use of various products of the common honeybee in alternative remedies. These include venom, propolis (a substance made by bees that is used to coat the inside of hives), raw honey, royal jelly, and pollen.

Overview

Although antitumor properties of some of the ingredients in bee products have been studied in the laboratory, there have been no clinical studies in humans showing that bee venom or other honeybee products are effective in preventing or treating cancer.

How is it promoted for use?

Practitioners claim bee venom contains an anti-inflammatory agent that relieves chronic pain and can be used to treat various diseases, including several types of arthritis; neurological problems such as multiple sclerosis, lower back pain, and migraine headaches; and skin conditions such as eczema, psoriasis, and herpes.

Others claim that raw honey is an energy-building source containing minerals and B-complex vitamins. Proponents claim it has antifungal, antibacterial, anti-inflammatory, and antitumor properties.

Proponents claim bee pollen contains many nutrients required by the human body and that it has five to seven times more protein than beef. Pieces of honeycomb containing pollen are said to be effective for treating allergies. Ingesting bee pollen is also claimed to increase endurance, energy, and overall performance. Some people believe some of the active ingredients in bee products may have possible anticancer effects.

What does it involve?

The usual bee venom treatment uses live bees that sting the patient at a specific site, with the procedure repeated over a period of time. Injections can also be used. For example, for arthritis patients, proponents suggest that the venom be injected at trigger points daily for four to six weeks.

Besides bee venom, the other most popular forms of apitherapy treatments are honey and pollen. They are most commonly taken as pills, powders, and injections. In China, raw honey is applied directly to burns as an antiseptic and painkiller. Other methods may also be used.

Bee products are widely available in pharmacies, health food stores, shops that specialize in bee products, and over the Internet.

What is the history behind it?

Various forms of apitherapy have been used by many cultures since ancient times. There is even a reference in the Koran about the medicinal properties of the liquid ("liquor") produced by bees.

The cultivation of the hive was written about as early as 800 BC. Charlemagne (742–814 AD) is said to have been treated with bee stings. In 1888, Austrian physician Phillip Terc advocated the deliberate use of bee stings as a treatment for rheumatism.

Apitherapy continues to be a popular form of alternative therapy. Studies on the use of bee products or their components to treat various conditions have appeared in the medical literature for at least the past seventy years.

What is the evidence?

Most research on bee venom has focused on the use of immunotherapy to prevent allergic reactions to bee stings. However, several animal and laboratory studies have looked at the anticancer effects of some ingredients of bee products, such as propolis and melittin.

Propolis is a natural compound made by honeybees to coat the inside of their hives. Some of its ingredients have shown antioxidant and antitumor properties in early laboratory and animal studies, but it has not been tested in people.

Melittin is a main component of bee venom. It is thought to kill cells it contacts by breaking them open. It also appears to have anti-inflammatory properties. According to some researchers, melittin shows activity against cancer cells grown in laboratory dishes. Scientists in Australia have changed the structure of the melittin molecule by removing the part that causes allergic reactions in some patients, keeping its cell-killing ability, and combining the molecule with an antibody to target cancer cells. Using this approach, they have been able to show some anticancer activity in studies using mice. Studies in people have not been reported in the available medical literature.

Some early studies have also looked at possible anticancer properties of honey. A study from Japan found that solutions containing honey had some effect against bladder cancer cells in the laboratory and against bladder tumors in mice. No studies have been reported in humans in the medical literature.

While the results from laboratory studies are encouraging, many substances, both natural and manmade, show anticancer activity in the laboratory but turn out not to work in people. Further studies are needed to determine whether these promising but early results with bee products will apply to humans.

Are there any possible problems or complications?

Some people have extreme allergic reactions to bee stings, the most severe of which can prove fatal. Asthma attacks and one death have been attributed to the use of royal jelly. People with weakened immune systems should be cautious about consuming honey, as it may contain bacteria or fungi.

The possible effects of bee venom on pregnancy have not been well studied. Women who are pregnant or breastfeeding should speak with their doctors before using this treatment. Relying on this type of treatment alone and avoiding or delaying conventional medical care for cancer may have serious health consequences.

This product is sold as a dietary supplement in the United States. Unlike companies that produce drugs (which must provide the FDA with results of detailed testing showing their product is safe and effective before the drug is approved for sale), the companies that make supplements do not have to show evidence of safety or health benefits to the FDA before selling their products. Supplement products without any reliable scientific evidence of health benefits may still be sold as long as the companies selling them do not claim the supplements can prevent, treat, or cure any specific disease. Some such products may not contain the amount of the herb or substance that is written on the label, and some may include other substances (contaminants). Though the FDA has written new rules to improve the quality of manufacturing processes for dietary supplements and the accurate listing of supplement ingredients, these rules do not take full effect until 2010. The new rules also do not address the safety of supplement ingredients or their effects on health when proper manufacturing techniques are used.

Most such supplements have not been tested to find out if they interact with medicines, foods, or other herbs and supplements. Even though some reports of interactions and harmful effects may be published, full studies of interactions and effects are not often available. Because of these limitations, any information on ill effects and interactions should be considered incomplete.

References

Cassileth B. *The Alternative Medicine Handbook: The Complete Reference Guide to Alternative and Complementary Therapies.* New York: W.W. Norton; 1998.

Chen CN, Wu CL, Lin JK. Apoptosis of human melanoma cells induced by the novel compounds propolin A and propolin B from Taiwenese propolis. *Cancer Lett.* 2007;245:218-231.

Chen CN, Wu CL, Lin JK. Propolin C from propolis induces apoptosis through activating caspases, Bid and cytochrome *c* release in human melanoma cells. *Biochem Pharmacol.* 2004;67:53-66.

Li H, Kapur A, Yang JX, Srivastava S, McLeod DG, Paredes-Guzman JF, Daugsch A, Park YK, Rhim JS. Antiproliferation of human prostate cancer cells by ethanolic extracts of Brazilian propolis and its botanical origin. *Int J Oncol.* 2007;31:601-606.

Rao CV, Desai D, Simi B, Kulkarni N, Amin S, Reddy BS. Inhibitory effect of caffeic acid esters on azoxymethane-induced biochemical changes and aberrant crypt foci formation in rat colon. *Cancer Res.* 1993;53:4182-4188.

Russell PJ, Hewish D, Carter T, Sterling-Levis K, Ow K, Hattarki M, Doughty L, Guthrie R, Shapira D, Molloy PL, Werkmeister JA, Kortt AA. Cytotoxic properties of immunoconjugates containing melittin-like peptide 101 against prostate cancer: in vitro and in vivo studies. *Cancer Immunol Immunother.* 2004;53:411-421.

Shimizu K, Das SK, Hashimoto T, Sowa Y, Yoshida T, Sakai T, Matsuura Y, Kanazawa K. Artepillin C in Brazilian propolis induces G(0)/G(1) arrest via stimulation of Cip1/p21 expression in human colon cancer cells. *Mol Carcinog.* 2005;44:293-299.

Swellam T, Miyanaga N, Onozawa M, Hattori K, Kawai K, Shimazui T, Akaza H. Antineoplastic activity of honey in an experimental bladder cancer implantation model: in vivo and in vitro studies. *Int J Urol.* 2003;10:213-219.

Winder D, Günzburg WH, Erfle V, Salmons B. Expression of antimicrobial peptides has an antitumour effect in human cells. *Biochem Biophys Res Commun.* 1998;242:608-612.

BOVINE CARTILAGE

Other common name(s): bovine tracheal cartilage (BTC)
Scientific/medical name(s): none

Description

Bovine cartilage is promoted as an alternative treatment for cancer. The cartilage is extracted from various parts of a cow, but usually comes from the trachea (windpipe). Cartilage is a type of connective tissue that is found in the skeletal systems of many animals, including humans. The major compounds in bovine cartilage are proteoglycans, that large molecules form when proteins and complex sugars are chemically linked together.

Overview

Although some laboratory and animal studies have shown that components isolated from bovine cartilage have some ability to halt the growth of cancer cells, these effects have not been studied in humans. No well-controlled clinical studies have been published in the available medical literature.

How is it promoted for use?

Bovine cartilage is promoted as a dietary supplement for the treatment of cancer, osteoporosis, and other conditions. Supporters claim that bovine cartilage may act in several ways: by directly stopping or slowing cancer cell growth, by boosting the immune system and reducing inflammation, and by preventing tumors from forming new blood vessels.

What does it involve?

Bovine cartilage is available as a dietary supplement in pill or powder form. It has also been used in an injectable form. It is usually taken daily, but there are no widely agreed-upon standard doses.

What is the history behind it?

The therapeutic potential of various types of cartilage has been studied for more than forty years. The first reported use of bovine cartilage to treat a person with cancer was in 1972. John F. Prudden, MD, a New York surgeon, treated thirty-one patients with various types of cancer over several years. He published the results of this treatment in 1985. While his initial report showed a high response rate, it was not a formal clinical trial, and some patients also received conventional treatment along with bovine cartilage. Clinical trials done since then have not been able to duplicate these results.

While bovine cartilage is still available as a dietary supplement, interest in its use to treat cancer has dwindled in recent years as a result of the increased popularity of shark cartilage for this same purpose (see "Shark Cartilage," page 824).

What is the evidence?

There is some evidence from laboratory and animal studies that substances in cartilage may have an effect on the immune system and on angiogenesis. However, few studies have been done in humans.

Dr. Prudden's initial 1985 report claimed that more than half of his patients had a complete response to treatment, with all signs of cancer disappearing. However, as mentioned, this was a report of cases and not a preplanned study, and some patients received mainstream treatment at the same time.

Two small studies were conducted after Dr. Prudden's report. In the first study of nine patients with various cancers (reported in 1985), one patient with advanced kidney cancer was said to have had a complete response. In the other eight patients, the cancer continued to grow. This led to a second study of twenty-two patients with kidney cancer. Three of these patients supposedly had a partial response, with the tumor shrinking by more than half. Although the results were presented in an abstract at a 1994 conference, they were never fully reported in a peer-reviewed medical journal. Compared with medical journal articles, conference presentations typically contain relatively sparse details about methods of the study and are not scrutinized as thoroughly by other experts in the same field of research, so it is difficult to evaluate the design of the study or the validity of its conclusions. No further studies of bovine cartilage have been published in the available medical literature.

The forms of bovine cartilage given by injection are regulated as experimental drugs. The products taken by mouth are classified as dietary supplements.

Are there any possible problems or complications?

Side effects of bovine cartilage are reportedly mild and may include fever, nausea, and upset stomach. Those allergic to beef products should avoid it. It is not known whether interactions between bovine cartilage and other medicines would cause any problems. Relying on this type of treatment alone and avoiding or delaying conventional medical care for cancer could have serious health consequences.

This product is sold as a dietary supplement in the United States. Unlike companies that produce drugs (which must provide the FDA with results of detailed testing showing their product is safe and effective before the drug is approved for sale), the companies that make supplements do not have to show evidence of safety or health benefits to the FDA before selling their products. Supplement products without any reliable scientific evidence of health benefits may still be sold as long as the companies selling them do not claim the supplements can prevent, treat, or cure any specific disease. Some such products may not contain the amount of the herb or substance that is written on the label, and some may include other substances (contaminants). Though the FDA has written new rules to improve the quality of manufacturing processes for dietary supplements and the accurate listing of supplement ingredients, these rules do not take full effect until 2010. The new rules also do not address the safety of supplement ingredients or their effects on health when proper manufacturing techniques are used.

Most such supplements have not been tested to find out if they interact with medicines, foods, or other herbs and supplements. Even though some reports of interactions and harmful effects may be published, full studies of interactions and effects are not often available. Because of these limitations, any information on ill effects and interactions should be considered incomplete.

References

Cartilage (bovine and shark) (PDQ®). National Cancer Institute Web site. http://www.cancer.gov/cancertopics/pdq/cam/cartilage/healthprofessional. Accessed June 11, 2008.

Prudden JF. The treatment of human cancer with agents prepared from bovine cartilage. *J Biol Response Mod.* 1985;4:551-584.

Puccio C, Mittelman A, Chun H, Baskind P, Ahmed T. Treatment of metastatic renal cell carcinoma with Catrix [Abstract]. *Proc Amer Soc Clin Oncol.* 1994;13:A-769, 246.

Romano CF, Lipton A, Harvey HA, Simmonds MA, Romano PJ, Imboden SL. A phase II study of Catrix-S in solid tumors. *J Biol Response Mod.* 1985;4:585-589.

CANCELL

Other common name(s): Cantron, Protocel, Entelev, Quantrol, Sheridan's Formula, Jim's Juice, Crocinic Acid, Radic
Scientific/medical name(s): none

Description

Cancell is a substance that has been sold or given to cancer patients under a variety of names as an alternative to conventional treatment. A dark liquid, the exact makeup of Cancell is unknown and may have changed over time and varied between manufacturers. In 1989, a U.S. Food and Drug Administration (FDA) review found it was made up of common chemicals, including nitric acid, sodium sulfite, potassium hydroxide, sulfuric acid, inositol, and catechol.

Overview

Available scientific evidence does not support claims that Cancell has any effect on cancer or any other disease. Because it was marketed as a drug without FDA approval, the FDA received a permanent injunction against its manufacturers in 1989, making it illegal to sell Cancell or Entelev across state lines. However, several similar formulas are now available as dietary supplements, which are not regulated as stringently as drugs.

How is it promoted for use?

Cancell has been promoted as a cure for all forms of cancer and a wide variety of other diseases. According to its manufacturers, it is supposed to cause cancer cells to self-destruct by depriving them of the ability to receive energy. Two theories have been proposed for this activity. The original theory was that the proteins in cancer cells are different from proteins in normal cells and that Cancell causes cells with these different proteins to revert to the "primitive state" where they self-destruct. A later theory held that all cancerous tumors are due to an altered anaerobic cell (a cell that does not require oxygen). This theory claimed that Cancell changes the "vibrational frequency" and energy of the cancer cell, which then causes the cancer cell to self-digest.

Cancell has also been promoted to be effective against AIDS, herpes, chronic fatigue syndrome, lupus, endometriosis, Crohn's disease, fibromyalgia, diabetes, emphysema, scleroderma, Lou Gehrig's disease, multiple sclerosis, cystic fibrosis, muscular dystrophy, Parkinson's disease, Alzheimer's disease, hemophilia, high and low blood pressure, mental illness, and some forms of epilepsy.

What does it involve?

Cancell was promoted for both internal and external use. Although the Cancell brand name is no longer used, similar products, such as Cantron and Protocel, are available for purchase in some health food stores or on the Internet.

The manufacturers recommend taking these products by mouth. Usually, ¼ teaspoon of the liquid is held under the tongue for several minutes before swallowing. The liquid can also be diluted in water or other liquids before taking. This is repeated several times a day. If the patient cannot take the product by mouth, the manufacturer recommends taking it rectally. It also notes that during the first month of treatment, tumors may increase in size, and those with prostate cancer may notice their level of prostate-specific antigen (PSA) goes up instead of down.

Promoters of these products also recommend lifestyle and dietary changes including quitting smoking and avoiding high concentrations of certain vitamins, which reportedly could interfere with treatment.

What is the history behind it?

The formula was first developed in 1936 by James Sheridan, a chemist working for Dow Chemical. Sheridan reported that the formula was a cure for all forms of cancer and a wide variety of diseases and came to him in a dream from God. Sheridan called his product "Entelev." In 1984, Sheridan gave the formula to Edward Sopcak for manufacturing and distribution. The name of the product was changed to Cancell. In 1989, the FDA received a permanent injunction against Sheridan and Sopcak, prohibiting them or their agents from distributing Entelev or Cancell across state lines on the basis that they were adulterated, misbranded, and unapproved new drugs.

Supporters today claim that Sopcak changed the formula for Sheridan's original product to a homeopathic mixture (see "Homeopathy," page 753). However, they claim that for a period of time the name Cancell was used for both the original product and the homeopathic formulation, which led to some confusion. The name of this homeopathic formula was later changed to Quantrol.

Cancell-like products (Cantron, Protocel) continue to be sold in the United States as dietary supplements.

What is the evidence?

Available scientific evidence does not support claims that Cancell or similar products are effective in treating cancer. None of the theories used to support claims made by promoters are compatible with modern scientific data about the molecular basis of cancer. Animal studies of Entelev and Cancell by the National Cancer Institute (NCI) in 1978 and 1980 found they lacked anticancer activity. The NCI performed another series of tests in 1990 and 1991 using human cancer cells and again did not find enough anticancer activity to warrant further testing.

None of the claims of these products' effectiveness against other diseases have been documented through scientific testing and published in peer-reviewed medical journals. Although manufacturers claim the products have helped more than half of the cancer patients who took them, no clinical trials have ever been reported in the peer-reviewed medical literature.

Are there any possible problems or complications?

People may feel temporary, moderate fatigue and flu-like symptoms after taking these products. Ingredients and strength of the mixtures may vary. It is not known whether these products would cause any problems due to interactions with other medications. The manufacturer claims that chemotherapy interferes with the effectiveness of these products. Relying on this type of treatment alone and avoiding or delaying conventional medical care for cancer may have serious health consequences.

This product is sold as a dietary supplement in the United States. Unlike companies that produce drugs (which must provide the FDA with results of detailed testing showing their product is safe and effective before the drug is approved for sale), the companies that make supplements do not have to show evidence of safety or health benefits to the FDA before selling their products. Supplement products without any reliable scientific evidence of health benefits may still be sold as long as the companies selling them do not claim the supplements can prevent, treat, or cure any specific disease. Some such products may not contain the amount of the herb or substance that is written on the label, and some may include other substances (contaminants). Though the FDA has written new rules to improve the quality of manufacturing processes for dietary supplements and the accurate listing of supplement ingredients, these rules do not take full effect until 2010. The new rules also do not address the safety of supplement ingredients or their effects on health when proper manufacturing techniques are used.

Most such supplements have not been tested to find out if they interact with medicines, foods, or other herbs and supplements. Even though some reports of interactions and harmful effects may be published, full studies of interactions and effects are not often available. Because of these limitations, any information on ill effects and interactions should be considered incomplete.

References

American Cancer Society. Questionable methods of cancer management: Cancell/Entelev. *CA Cancer J Clin.* 1993;43:57-62.

CanCell®. Memorial Sloan-Kettering Cancer Center Web site. http://www.mskcc.org/mskcc/html/69160.cfm. Accessed July 21, 2007.

Cancell/Cantron/Protocel (PDQ®). National Cancer Institute Web site. http://www.cancer.gov/cancertopics/pdq/cam/cancell/healthprofessional. Accessed June 11, 2008.

Cassileth B. *The Alternative Medicine Handbook: The Complete Reference Guide to Alternative and Complementary Therapies.* New York: W.W. Norton; 1998.

CELL THERAPY

Other common name(s): cellular therapy, fresh cell therapy, live cell therapy, glandular therapy, xenotransplant therapy
Scientific/medical name(s): none

Description

In cell therapy, processed tissue from the organs, embryos, or fetuses of animals such as sheep or cows is injected into patients. Cell therapy is promoted as an alternative form of cancer treatment.

Overview

Available scientific evidence does not support claims that cell therapy is effective in treating cancer or any other disease. Serious side effects can result from cell therapy. It may in fact be lethal—several deaths have been reported. It is important to distinguish between this alternative method involving animal cells and mainstream cancer treatments that use human cells, such as bone marrow transplantation.

How is it promoted for use?

In cell therapy, live or freeze-dried cells or pieces of cells from the healthy organs, fetuses, or embryos of animals such as sheep or cows are injected into patients. This is supposed to repair cellular damage and heal sick or failing organs. Cell therapy is promoted as an alternative therapy for cancer, arthritis, heart disease, Down syndrome, and Parkinson's disease.

Cell therapy is also marketed to counter the effects of aging, reverse degenerative diseases, improve general health, increase vitality and stamina, and enhance sexual function. Some practitioners have proposed using cell therapy to treat AIDS patients.

The theory behind cell therapy is that the healthy animal cells injected into the body can find their way to weak or damaged organs of the same type and stimulate the body's own healing process. The choice of the type of cells to use depends on which organ is having the problem.

For instance, a patient with a diseased liver may receive injections of animal liver cells. Most cell therapists today use cells taken from the tissue of animal embryos.

Supporters assert that after the cells are injected into the body, they are transported directly to where they are most needed. They claim that embryonic and fetal animal tissue contains therapeutic agents that can repair damage and stimulate the immune system, thereby helping cells in the body heal.

The alternative treatment cell therapy is very different from some forms of proven therapy that use live human cells. Bone marrow transplants infuse blood stem cells—from the patient or a carefully matched donor—after the patient's own bone marrow cells have been destroyed. Studies have shown that bone marrow transplants are effective in helping to treat several types of cancer. In another accepted procedure, damaged knee cartilage can be repaired by taking cartilage cells from the patient's knee, carefully growing them in the laboratory, and then injecting them back into the joint. Approaches involving transplants of other types of human stem cells are being studied as a possible way to replace damaged nerve or heart muscle cells, but these approaches are still experimental.

What does it involve?

First, healthy live cells are harvested from the organs of juvenile or adult live animals, animal embryos, or animal fetuses. These cells may be taken from the brain, pituitary gland, thyroid gland, thymus gland, liver, kidney, pancreas, spleen, heart, ovaries, or testicles or even from whole embryos. Patients might receive one or several types of animal cells. Some cell therapists inject fresh cells into their patients. Others freeze them first, which kills the cells, and they may filter out some of the cell components. Frozen cell extracts have a longer "shelf life" and can be screened for disease. Fresh cells cannot be screened. A course of cell therapy to address a specific disease might require several injections over a short period of time, whereas cell therapy designed to treat the effects of aging and "increase vitality" may involve injections received over many months.

Animal cell extracts are also sold in pill form as dietary supplements, usually called glandular supplements. These, too, allegedly travel to organs of the same kind in the body to promote healing.

What is the history behind it?

The Swiss physician Paul Niehans, MD, invented cell therapy in 1931. During a medical emergency, Dr. Niehans injected a solution containing ground-up parathyroid cells from a calf into a patient who had damaged parathyroid glands. The patient recovered, and Dr. Niehans attributed the improvement to the injection. He went on to apply the idea of animal–human cellular transfer to other diseases.

Dr. Niehans claimed that he treated more than thirty thousand patients with cell therapy. He also claimed that the death rate from cancer among his patients who received cell therapy was five times less than that of the average population. He believed that injections of cells from animals resistant to cancer would increase cancer resistance in humans. A second physician announced similar findings thirty years later. Neither claim has ever been supported by research studies published in medical journals.

Cell therapy may be harmful and is not legally available in the United States. Because of safety concerns and lack of proof of its effectiveness, the U.S. Food and Drug Administration (FDA) has banned the import of cell therapy products into the country. The treatment is provided in clinics and spas in Europe, Mexico, and the Bahamas.

What is the evidence?

None of the therapeutic success claimed by cell therapists has been documented through scientific testing and published in peer-reviewed medical journals. Claims of the therapy's success take the form of individual cases, testimonials, and publicity issued by practitioners of the therapy. Even supporters of cell therapy admit they do not know how cell therapy works in the body. No reliable evidence has been published in medical journals to support the claims of cell therapy.

Are there any possible problems or complications?

Cell therapy may be dangerous, and several patient deaths linked to the therapy have been reported in the medical literature. Patients can contract bacterial and viral infections carried by the animal cells, and some have had life-threatening and even fatal allergic reactions. Other reports list complications such as brain swelling or the immune system attacking blood vessels or nerves following cellular treatment. Serious immune system reactions resulting in death have also been reported. Women who are pregnant or breastfeeding should not use this method, as its possible effects on a fetus are unknown. Relying on this type of treatment alone and avoiding or delaying conventional medical care for cancer may have serious health consequences.

These substances may have not been thoroughly tested to find out how they interact with medicines, foods, or dietary supplements. Even though some reports of interactions and harmful effects may be published, full studies of interactions and effects are not often available. Because of these limitations, any information on ill effects and interactions should be considered incomplete.

References

American Cancer Society. Unproven methods of cancer management: fresh cell therapy. *CA Cancer J Clin.* 1991;41:126-128.

Barrett S. Cellular therapy. Quackwatch Web site. http://www.quackwatch.org/01QuackeryRelatedTopics/Cancer/cellular.html. Updated August 21, 2003. Accessed June 11, 2008.

Cassileth B. *The Alternative Medicine Handbook: The Complete Reference Guide to Alternative and Complementary Therapies*. New York: W.W. Norton; 1998.

Gage FH. Cell therapy. *Nature*. 1998;392:18-24.

US Congress, Office of Technology Assessment. *Unconventional Cancer Treatments: OTA-H-405*. Washington, DC: US Government Printing Office; 1990.

CHELATION THERAPY

Other common name(s): none
Scientific/medical name(s): ethylene diamine tetraacetic acid (EDTA), edetate sodium

Description

Chelation therapy is a mainstream treatment used to treat heavy metal poisoning. However, the term is also used to promote an alternative therapy that is supposed to treat heart disease, cancer, and other conditions. It most often involves the injection of ethylene diamine tetraacetic acid (EDTA), a chemical that binds, or chelates, heavy metals, including iron, lead, mercury, cadmium, and zinc. The term "chelation" comes from the Greek word *chele*, which means "claw," referring to the way the chemical grabs onto metals.

Overview

Chelation therapy is one of several effective treatments for lead poisoning. However, available scientific evidence does not support claims that it is effective for treating other conditions such as cancer. Chelation therapy can be toxic and has the potential to cause kidney damage, irregular heartbeat, and even death.

How is it promoted for use?

Chelation therapy using EDTA has been approved by the U.S. Food and Drug Administration (FDA) as a treatment for lead poisoning for more than forty years. The human body cannot break down heavy metals, which can build up to toxic levels in the body and interfere with normal functioning. EDTA and other chelating drugs lower the blood levels of metals such as lead, mercury, cadmium, and zinc by attaching to the heavy metal molecules, allowing the body to remove them through urination.

Because EDTA can reduce the amount of calcium in the bloodstream, some practitioners suggest chelation therapy may help reopen arteries blocked by mineral deposits, a condition called atherosclerosis or hardening of the arteries. They claim it is an effective and less expensive alternative to coronary bypass surgery, angioplasty, and other techniques designed to unclog blocked arteries.

Chelation therapy has also been promoted as an alternative treatment for many unrelated conditions, such as gangrene, thyroid disorders, multiple sclerosis, muscular dystrophy, psoriasis, diabetes, arthritis, Alzheimer's disease, and the improvement of memory, sight, hearing, and smell.

Some alternative practitioners further claim chelation therapy can be used as a cancer treatment. They claim it can remove "environmental toxins" from the body and block the production of harmful molecules called free radicals that can cause cell damage.

What does it involve?

Chelation therapy is most often given into a vein, either as a short injection or over a period of two to four hours. A typical treatment cycle may include twenty injections or infusions spread over ten to twelve weeks. Chelation therapy can also be given by mouth. Practitioners recommend at least twenty to forty treatments to start; however, some may recommend continued therapy for up to a hundred treatments over a period of several years. Because the therapy removes some important minerals from the body, patients often receive high-dose vitamin and mineral supplements during treatment.

What is the history behind it?

The chemical solution most often used in chelation therapy, EDTA, was first made in Germany in the 1930s. It is now widely accepted as an effective treatment for heavy metal poisoning.

In the 1950s, some scientists theorized that EDTA could remove calcium from the body. Calcium can build up on artery walls, eventually causing heart disease, and it was theorized that use of EDTA could unclog blocked arteries. In some early studies, researchers reported positive results among patients with heart disease who received EDTA. Some said that chelation therapy relieved chest pain caused by blocked arteries. These first observations have not been confirmed by larger, more rigorous studies, but they led some practitioners to begin using chelation therapy for heart and circulatory problems and, later, for several other illnesses. It is estimated that tens of thousands of Americans currently undergo chelation therapy for heart disease.

In 1998, the Federal Trade Commission charged the American College of Advancement in Medicine (ACAM), the principal group promoting chelation therapy, with presenting false advertising and unsubstantiated statements about its benefits. The ACAM agreed to stop publishing any claims that were not based on reliable scientific evidence.

What is the evidence?

Chelation therapy is a proven treatment for lead poisoning and poisoning from other heavy metals. However, available scientific evidence does not support claims that the treatment benefits patients with cancer, heart disease, or any medical problems other than heavy metal poisoning.

There are no published studies that reliably show benefit from using chelation therapy with EDTA against cancer. Some laboratory studies have suggested that agents other than EDTA that chelate copper or iron may affect cancer cells or the formation of tumor blood vessels. In a small study using mice, researchers studied iron-chelating agents to see if they would reduce the growth of neuroblastoma, a type of cancer that occurs in infants and young children. The results, published in 1998, concluded that chelation therapy did not shrink tumors. Few studies of the use of chelation therapy against cancer in humans have been published in peer-reviewed medical journals. These few studies have been small and have not shown a significant level of effectiveness. Research is continuing in this area. A 2006 study found that a new iron chelator called di-2-pyridylketone-4,4,-dimethyl-3-thiosemicarbazone reduced growth of skin cancer cells in mice. However, this experimental treatment has not been tested in humans and is very different from the chelation agents used by alternative practitioners.

Available research does not yet support claims that chelation therapy can treat heart disease. Randomized clinical trials have found that chelation therapy drugs did not benefit patients with impaired circulation in their legs. In 1993, a review of all chelation therapy studies reported during the previous thirty-seven years concluded that scientific data did not support claims that the treatment was useful for treating heart problems. Studies published since then have generally reached the same conclusion. A very large, placebo-controlled study sponsored by the National Center for Complementary and Alternative Medicine is now under way and should provide a more definitive answer as to whether chelation therapy has any effects on heart disease.

According to a number of well-respected organizations, including the American Heart Association, the American Medical Association, the Centers for Disease Control and Prevention, the American Osteopathic Association, the American Academy of Family Physicians, and the FDA, there is no scientific evidence that chelation therapy is an effective treatment for any medical condition except heavy metal poisoning.

Are there any possible problems or complications?

Available scientific evidence does not support claims that chelation therapy is a safe treatment for any type of cancer. Chelation therapy may produce toxic effects, including kidney damage, irregular heartbeat, and swelling of the veins. It may also cause nausea, vomiting, diarrhea, and temporary lowering of blood pressure. Since the therapy removes minerals from the body, there is a risk for developing low calcium levels (hypocalcemia) and bone damage. Chelation therapy may also impair the immune system and decrease the body's ability to produce insulin. People may also feel pain at the site of the EDTA injection. Chelation therapy may be dangerous in people with kidney disease, liver disease, or bleeding disorders. Women who are pregnant or breastfeeding should not use this method.

Chelation therapy is often given along with large doses of vitamins and other minerals, which may actually contribute to the processes that produce dangerous free radicals in the body. Loss of zinc can also lead to mutations in cells. For this reason, chelation therapy may actually increase the risk for cancer.

The possible interactions between chelation therapy and prescription or over-the-counter medicines are not entirely known. Relying on this type of treatment alone and avoiding or delaying conventional medical care for cancer may have serious health consequences.

This substance has not been thoroughly tested to find out how it interacts with medicines, foods, or dietary supplements. Even though some reports of interactions and harmful effects may be published, full studies of interactions and effects are not often available. Because of these limitations, any information on ill effects and interactions should be considered incomplete.

References

Cassileth B. *The Alternative Medicine Handbook: The Complete Reference Guide to Alternative and Complementary Therapies.* New York: W.W. Norton; 1998.

Ernst E, ed. *The Desktop Guide to Complementary and Alternative Medicine: An Evidence-Based Approach.* New York: Mosby; 2001.

Green S. Chelation therapy: unproven claims and unsound theories. Quackwatch Web site. http://www.quackwatch.org/01QuackeryRelatedTopics/chelation.html. Accessed June 11, 2008.

Grier MT, Meyers DG. So much writing, so little science: a review of 37 years of literature on edetate sodium chelation therapy. *Ann Pharmacother.* 1993;27:1504-1509.

Guldager B, Jelnes R, Jørgensen SJ, Nielsen JS, Klaerke A, Mogensen K, Larsen KE, Reimer E, Holm J, Ottesen S. EDTA treatment of intermittent claudication: a double-blind placebo-controlled study. *J Intern Med.* 1992;231:261-267.

Knudtson ML, Wyse DG, Galbraith PD, Brant R, Hildebrand K, Paterson D, Richardson D, Burkart C, Burgess E; Program to Assess Alternative Treatment Strategies to Achieve Cardiac Health (PATCH) Investigators. Chelation therapy for ischemic heart disease: a randomized controlled trial. *JAMA.* 2002;287:481-486.

Natural Standard. Complementary practice: chelation (EDTA) therapy. Complementary/Integrative Medicine Education Resources, The University of Texas M. D. Anderson Cancer Center Web site. http://www.mdanderson.org/departments/cimer/display.cfm?id=4230febd-e954-4025-86affa94c7a8fc71&method=displayfull. Accessed June 11, 2008.

Redman BG, Esper P, Pan Q, Dunn RL, Hussain HK, Chenevert T, Brewer GJ, Merajver SD. Phase II trial of tetrathiomolybdate in patients with advanced kidney cancer. *Clin Cancer Res.* 2003;9:1666-1672.

Selig RA, White L, Gramacho C, Sterling-Levis K, Fraser IW, Naidoo D. Failure of iron chelators to reduce tumor growth in human neuroblastoma xenografts. *Cancer Res.* 1998;58:473-478.

van Rij AM, Solomon C, Packer SG, Hopkins WG. Chelation therapy for intermittent claudication. A double-blind, randomized, controlled trial. *Circulation.* 1994;90:1194-1199.

Whitnall M, Howard J, Ponka P, Richardson DR. A class of iron chelators with a wide spectrum of potent antitumor activity that overcomes resistance to chemotherapeutics. *Proc Natl Acad Sci U S A.* 2006;103:14901-14906.

COENZYME Q10

Other common name(s): CoQ10, Co-Q10, CoQ-10, vitamin Q10
Scientific/medical name(s): ubiquinone, ubidecarenone

Description

Coenzyme Q10 (CoQ10) is part of an enzyme complex that affects certain chemical reactions in the body. It occurs naturally in the body and can also be found in a number of foods, such as mackerel, salmon, sardines, beef, soybeans, peanuts, and spinach, as well as in dietary supplements.

Overview

CoQ10 may promote health and fight some diseases, but more research is needed to find out the role of this substance. Some small studies have suggested that CoQ10 may help treat cancer or reduce chemotherapy-related heart damage, but these results need to be confirmed by larger randomized clinical trials. CoQ10 may reduce the effectiveness of chemotherapy, so most oncologists would recommend avoiding it during chemotherapy.

How is it promoted for use?

Scientists believe CoQ10 is an antioxidant, a compound that blocks the actions of free radicals, activated oxygen molecules that can damage cells. Scientists also believe that CoQ10 may have an effect on the immune system. Some studies have suggested that deficiencies of CoQ10 may contribute to certain diseases such as cancer.

CoQ10 is sometimes promoted as a treatment for cancer (most commonly breast cancer), often in combination with other vitamins. Supporters also claim CoQ10 supplements may protect the heart from the damaging effects of certain chemotherapy drugs, such as doxorubicin

(Adriamycin). CoQ10 supplements have also been promoted for heart disease, stroke, gum disease, and immune deficiencies. Some claim that CoQ10 can reduce pain and weight loss in people with cancer.

What does it involve?

Coenzyme Q10 occurs naturally in the body and can also be obtained from a number of foods or as a supplement. The usual supplement dose used in clinical studies is 90 to 400 milligrams per day. Supplements are available as tablets, capsules, and gelcaps.

What is the history behind it?

Coenzyme Q10 was first identified in 1957. Particularly high amounts were found in heart tissue, which is why researchers became interested in the connection between CoQ10 and heart disease. Studies in the 1960s found a possible connection between cancer (especially breast cancer) and low levels of CoQ10 in the blood. Some laboratory studies have suggested that CoQ10 may have a role as an immune system booster. Since then, researchers have been testing CoQ10 supplements for treating heart disease, cancer, and other conditions. However, no firm conclusions have been reached about its usefulness in treating any disease.

What is the evidence?

Some laboratory and animal studies indicate that CoQ10 could theoretically have an effect on cancer. In addition to its ability to act as an antioxidant, CoQ10 has effects on cellular energy and on the immune system. Some laboratory and animal studies have supported this idea. However, evidence from human studies is still minimal. Early studies involving small numbers of patients have suggested certain CoQ10 supplements may have some anticancer benefits. The studies of CoQ10 for cancer done thus far have been fairly small and did not have scientifically strong designs. More studies are needed with larger groups of patients to determine what effect, if any, it has on cancer.

In a Danish study, thirty-two women with breast cancer that had spread to the lymph nodes were treated with a nutritional supplement program of vitamins, minerals, essential fatty acids, and CoQ10, in addition to standard therapy. Six patients were reported to have some tumor shrinkage, and all survived at least two years. However, there was no comparison group in this study, and it was not clear whether the effects were due to the CoQ10 or to the standard treatments. The study was published in 1994 and has not been duplicated since.

In a Canadian study, ninety women with breast cancer that had not spread to distant organs were given high doses of different combinations of vitamins, minerals, and CoQ10 along with standard treatment. They were compared with women not taking the supplements on the basis of the type of conventional therapy they received and by several breast cancer predictive factors, such as patient age, how far the cancer had spread, and whether cancer cells contained estrogen receptors. Patients receiving only mainstream therapy tended to remain disease-free longer and live longer, although the difference was not quite statistically significant. One weak point of the study was that since the women received a combination of supplements, it was not possible to know how they might have responded to CoQ10 alone.

One clinical trial looked at 142 male smokers randomly chosen to receive antioxidants including CoQ10 or a placebo for two months. The study found no difference in a chemical indicator of DNA damage, suggesting that CoQ10 is not likely to be useful in preventing cancer. However, no long-term clinical studies of CoQ10 and cancer occurrence have been published.

Low levels of CoQ10 have been linked to heart damage from chemotherapy treatment for cancer, especially from drugs called anthracyclines. A recent review looked at six clinical trials that tested the use of CoQ10 to protect the heart against damage from chemotherapy. The overall results suggested that CoQ10 may provide some protection for the heart, but the study designs were weak in several areas. The review concluded that further studies were needed to confirm the results.

No scientific research has been published in available medical journals concerning the possible effects of CoQ10 on pain, weight loss, or increased appetite.

Are there any possible problems or complications?

Few serious reactions to CoQ10 have been reported. Side effects may include headache, heartburn, trouble sleeping, and fatigue. Very high doses may cause involuntary muscle movements. Some users report mild diarrhea and skin reactions. Little is known about dosage or consequences of long-term use of CoQ10 supplements. There have been reports that CoQ10 may interact with blood-thinning medications and could pose a risk for prolonged bleeding.

Because CoQ10 is a strong antioxidant, there are theoretical reasons to suspect that it might interfere with the effectiveness of chemotherapy and radiation therapy. This question has not been adequately studied in clinical trials. Many oncologists would recommend avoiding CoQ10 and other antioxidant supplements during chemotherapy and radiation therapy, as well as for a few weeks before and after these treatments.

Relying on this type of treatment alone and avoiding or delaying conventional medical care for cancer may have serious health consequences.

This product is sold as a dietary supplement in the United States. Unlike companies that produce drugs (which must provide the FDA with results of detailed testing showing their product is safe and effective before the drug is approved for sale), the companies that make supplements do not have to show evidence of safety or health benefits to the FDA before selling their products. Supplement products

without any reliable scientific evidence of health benefits may still be sold as long as the companies selling them do not claim the supplements can prevent, treat, or cure any specific disease. Some such products may not contain the amount of the herb or substance that is written on the label, and some may include other substances (contaminants). Though the FDA has written new rules to improve the quality of manufacturing processes for dietary supplements and the accurate listing of supplement ingredients, these rules do not take full effect until 2010. The new rules also do not address the safety of supplement ingredients or their effects on health when proper manufacturing techniques are used.

Most such supplements have not been tested to find out if they interact with medicines, foods, or other herbs and supplements. Even though some reports of interactions and harmful effects may be published, full studies of interactions and effects are not often available. Because of these limitations, any information on ill effects and interactions should be considered incomplete.

References

Coenzyme Q10. Memorial Sloan-Kettering Cancer Center Web site. http://www.mskcc.org/mskcc/html/69186.cfm. Accessed June 11, 2008.

Coenzyme Q10 (PDQ®). National Cancer Institute Web site. http://www.cancer.gov/cancertopics/pdq/cam/coenzymeQ10/healthprofessional. Accessed June 11, 2008.

Fetrow CW, Avila JR. *Professional's Handbook of Complementary & Alternative Medicines.* Springhouse, PA: Springhouse Corp; 1999.

Folkers K, Brown R, Judy WV, Morita M. Survival of cancer patients on therapy with coenzyme Q10. *Biochem Biophys Res Commun.* 1993;192:241-245.

Hodges S, Hertz N, Lockwood K, Lister R. CoQ10: could it have a role in cancer management? *Biofactors.* 1999;9:365-370.

Lesperance ML, Olivotto IA, Forde N, Zhao Y, Speers C, Foster H, Tsao M, MacPherson N, Hoffer A. Mega-dose vitamins and minerals in the treatment of non-metastatic breast cancer: an historical cohort study. *Breast Cancer Res Treat.* 2002;76:137-143.

Lockwood K, Moesgaard S, Hanioka T, Folkers K. Apparent partial remission of breast cancer in 'high risk' patients supplemented with nutritional antioxidants, essential fatty acids and coenzyme Q10. *Mol Aspects Med.* 1994;15(suppl):S231-S240.

Priemé H, Loft S, Nyyssönen K, Salonen JT, Poulsen HE. No effect of supplementation with vitamin E, ascorbic acid, or coenzyme Q10 on oxidative DNA damage estimated by 8-oxo-7,8-dihydro-2'-deoxyguanosine excretion in smokers. *Am J Clin Nutr.* 1997;65:503-507.

Roffe L, Schmidt K, Ernst E. Efficacy of coenzyme Q10 for improved tolerability of cancer treatments: a systematic review. *J Clin Oncol.* 2004;22:4418-4424.

Spigset O. Reduced effect of warfarin caused by ubidecarenone. *Lancet.* 1994;344:1372-1373.

COLEY TOXINS

Other common name(s): Coley's toxins, mixed bacterial vaccines (MBVs), Issel's fever therapy
Scientific/medical name(s): none

Description

Use of Coley toxins is an early form of immunotherapy, a method of treatment in which a person receives substances designed to boost the immune system and help the body fight off diseases such as cancer. The use of Coley toxins as a cancer treatment involves injecting killed bacterial cultures (*Streptococcus pyogenes* and *Serratia marcescens*) directly into the tumor or bloodstream.

Overview

Modern forms of immunotherapy are based on a better understanding of the effects of the immune system on cancer and are likely to be more effective. Although some practitioners continue to recommend and give Coley toxins, this treatment fell out of use decades ago by most oncologists in favor of more modern treatments. To most mainstream oncologists, the value of Coley's research was as a foundation for much of modern cancer immunotherapy. Some clinical research has been done on this very early form of cancer immunotherapy, but the strength of evidence is limited by the small number of cases and the fact that most research was done in the early part of the twentieth century, when research methods were less rigorous than they are now. Some studies found that Coley toxins improved survival for people with certain forms of cancer, while other studies did not find a significant benefit.

How is it promoted for use?

Supporters claim Coley toxins stimulate the immune system in people with cancer, which helps to fight off disease. Some supporters also believe that tumor cells are more sensitive to heat than normal cells and that the high fever caused by Coley toxins helps to rid the body of cancer.

What does it involve?

Coley toxins are injected directly into the tumor or into the bloodstream in increasing daily doses until a fairly constant state of fever is reached. Treatment is often continued for several months. Patients are monitored closely for side effects and to control fevers as they develop.

The original formula for Coley toxins is no longer used in the United States, although similar formulas are used in at least one clinic. Coley toxins are used in Central America,

Germany, and China, but it is not clear whether they are using the original Coley toxins or a combination of Coley toxins and other bacteria.

What is the history behind it?

Coley toxins were first used in the 1890s by William B. Coley, MD, a bone surgeon at Memorial Hospital in New York City (now Memorial Sloan-Kettering Cancer Center). After his attempt to save a young woman from bone cancer failed, Dr. Coley began reviewing bone cancer cases. He noted that cancer patients in whom bacterial infections developed after surgery seemed to have better outcomes than those who did not have infections. He believed the bacterial infection helped to stimulate the immune system, causing it to fight off cancer cells. At first, Coley injected live bacteria into cancer patients, but because of the danger of serious or even fatal infection with that approach, he began using bacteria that had been killed. His treatment was controversial, despite some reports of cancer regression with its use. Dr. Coley passed away in 1936.

Different formulas of Coley toxins were made by several drug companies in the United States in the first half of the twentieth century. They were used to treat patients with a variety of types of cancer up until the early 1950s, when other forms of cancer treatment became more widely used.

Dr. Coley's daughter, Helen Coley Nauts, published several papers documenting her father's results. She also founded the Cancer Research Institute in New York in 1953, which continues to study how immunology can help diagnose and treat cancer.

Combinations of Coley toxins and other strains of bacteria are still being used at the Waisbren Clinic in Milwaukee, although the clinic recommends that patients try conventional treatments first. Coley toxins or similar treatments are also used in clinics in several other countries. There does not appear to be any active clinical research at this time into the use of the original Coley toxin formula. At least one pharmaceutical company is studying the use of pieces of DNA that may have contributed to the effectiveness of Coley toxins.

Dr. Coley is credited with pioneering the field of cancer immunotherapy. Immunotherapy is sometimes used alone but is more commonly combined with standard cancer treatments or used after conventional treatment. At this time, immunotherapy has a relatively small role in treating people with the most common types of cancer. However, researchers are optimistic that more effective immunotherapies can be developed that will have a greater impact on the outlook for people with cancer.

What is the evidence?

Scientific evidence suggests Coley toxins or other mixed bacterial vaccines may have a role in treating cancer when combined with other treatments. Coley reported his results as case series, which was the way most research was done in the early twentieth century. This format limits the ability of modern researchers to evaluate his findings. A retrospective review by researchers at the former University of Texas Center for Alternative Medicine compared 128 patients treated with surgery and Coley toxins between 1890 and 1960 with 1,675 similar patients treated in 1983 with conventional methods. The review found that survival rates for Coley's patients were about the same as those treated with more modern conventional methods. The University of Texas researchers point out that the study was limited by small sample size, short duration, and selection bias. More research would be needed to determine what benefit, if any, this therapy might have for people with cancer.

Results of three randomized clinical trials of Coley toxins or mixed bacterial vaccines have been published or presented. A 1962 article reported that more than one of four patients treated with Coley toxin showed objective improvement, whereas none of the patients who received a control vaccine made from different bacteria did.

A randomized trial of patients with nodular lymphoma (now known as follicular lymphoma) was discussed at a 1983 conference. Of the patients who received Coley toxins and chemotherapy, 85 percent had a complete response, in which all signs of cancer disappeared. This was compared with a 44 percent complete response rate in the patients who did not receive Coley toxins. Nodular lymphoma is among the cancer types that respond well to modern immunotherapy with monoclonal antibodies, however, so the relevance of this study to modern oncology practice is uncertain. The study was never reported in full in a journal, which has led some researchers to wonder whether long-term follow-up confirmed this degree of benefit.

Results of a Chinese study of patients with advanced liver cancer (hepatocellular carcinoma) were published in 1991. The study reported a significant benefit for patients with liver cancer that was too advanced for surgery, but no significant benefit in those who had surgery. Dr. Coley's earlier reports noted greatest success with sarcomas and lymphomas, and he eventually stopped treating patients with carcinomas. Reasons for the discrepancy between the older results and this more recent study are not clear.

Although Coley toxins are often regarded as an historic key step to modern immunotherapy, much has been learned about the immune system since that time. Modern immunotherapy is likely to be of greater value, especially in treating certain cancers, such as lymphoma, renal cell (kidney) cancer, and melanoma. Several recent laboratory and animal studies have been done to find out how Coley toxins might have worked, why they seemed useful for some cancer types and not others, and how modern methods could be used to develop immunotherapies that are more consistently effective and less toxic. Some immunologists believe that Coley toxins stimulated production of interleukin (IL)-12, a substance that can activate the immune system to attack cancer cells. Laboratory and clinical studies of IL-12 are currently in progress.

Are there any possible problems or complications?

The killed bacteria in Coley toxins can produce fever and nausea. Less common side effects can include headache, back pain, chills, chest pain, and shock-like reactions. There may be a danger that Coley toxins could produce serious infections among patients with weakened immune systems.

Women who are pregnant or breastfeeding should not use these toxins. Relying on this type of treatment alone and avoiding or delaying conventional medical care for cancer may have serious health consequences.

These substances may have not been thoroughly tested to find out how they interact with medicines, foods, or dietary supplements. Even though some reports of interactions and harmful effects may be published, full studies of interactions and effects are not often available. Because of these limitations, any information on ill effects and interactions should be considered incomplete.

References

Biologic/organic/pharmacologic therapies: Coley toxins detailed scientific review. Complementary/Integrative Medicine Education Resources, The University of Texas M. D. Anderson Cancer Center Web site. http://www.mdanderson.org/departments/cimer/display.cfm?id=35F66009-F06A-11D4-810200508B603A14&method=displayFull. Accessed June 11, 2008.

Hoption Cann SA, van Netten JP, van Netten C. Dr William Coley and tumour regression: a place in history or in the future? *Postgrad Med J.* 2003;79:672-680.

Johnston BJ. Clinical effects of Coley's toxin. I. A controlled study. *Cancer Chemother Rep.* 1962;21:19-41.

Johnston BJ. Clinical effects of Coley's toxin. II. A seven-year study. *Cancer Chemother Rep.* 1962;21:43-68.

Kempin S, Cirrincone C, Myers J, Lee III B, Straus D, Koziner B, Arlin Z, Gee T, Mertelsmann R, Pinsky C, Comacho E, Nisce L, Old L, Clarkson B, Oettgen H. Combined modality therapy of advanced nodular lymphomas (NL): the role of nonspecific immunotherapy (MBV) as an important determinant of responses and survival [Meeting abstract]. *Proc Am Soc Clin Oncol.* 1983;24:56.

McCarthy EF. The toxins of William B. Coley and the treatment of bone and soft-tissue sarcomas. *Iowa Orthop J.* 2006;26:154-158.

National Institutes of Health. *Alternative Medicine: Expanding Medical Horizons: A Report to the National Institutes of Health on Alternative Medical Systems and Practices in the United States.* Washington, DC: US Government Printing Office; 1994. NIH publication 94-066.

Richardson MA, Ramirez T, Russell NC, Moye LA. Coley toxins immunotherapy: a retrospective review. *Altern Ther Health Med.* 1999;5:42-47.

Starnes CO. Coley's toxins in perspective. *Nature.* 1992;357:11-12.

Tang ZY, Zhou HY, Zhao G, Chai LM, Zhou M, Lu JZ, Liu KD, Havas HF, Nauts HC. Preliminary result of mixed bacterial vaccine as adjuvant treatment of hepatocellular carcinoma. *Med Oncol Tumor Pharmacother.* 1991;8:23-28.

Tsung K, Norton JA. Lessons from Coley's Toxin. *Surg Oncol.* 2006;15:25-28.

DHEA

Other common name(s): none
Scientific/medical name(s): dehydroepiandrosterone, prasterone

Description

Dehydroepiandrosterone (DHEA) is a steroid hormone produced by the adrenal gland. The body converts it into other important hormones, including the sex hormones estrogen and testosterone. It is normally found in humans, plants, and animals and is available as a dietary supplement.

Wild yam plant extract, also available as a dietary supplement, is thought by some to contain substances from which the body can make DHEA. However, there is no scientific evidence available to suggest that the body can convert any part of the wild yam or its extract into hormones such as DHEA.

Overview

Available scientific evidence does not support claims that DHEA supplements are safe or effective for treating cancer. Caution is advised in their use in people who have cancer, especially types of cancer that respond to hormones, such as certain types of breast cancer, prostate cancer, and uterine cancer. People younger than thirty may run the risk of suppressing the body's natural production of DHEA if they take DHEA supplements. While there are hints that DHEA may have some use in treating certain hormone deficiencies, autoimmune diseases, and mood and memory problems of older age, more research is needed to determine its long-term safety and effectiveness.

How is it promoted for use?

Supporters suggest that DHEA supplements may prevent the growth and recurrence of some types of cancer, protect against heart disease, improve memory, reduce the risk for osteoporosis in women, and help prevent other diseases such as diabetes, Parkinson's disease, and Alzheimer's disease. Some say that DHEA may be an effective treatment for lupus, colitis, and depression.

Since the body's natural levels of DHEA usually begin to decline after a person reaches thirty years of age, some claim that the supplements can help slow the aging process. Some supporters also contend that DHEA boosts the immune system, reduces fat, builds muscle, promotes sleep, increases a person's overall sense of well-being, and increases sex drive.

What does it involve?

DHEA is taken by mouth or applied to the skin. It is made into tablets, capsules, and creams and can also be made into a tea. There are no widely accepted dosage guidelines for DHEA.

What is the history behind it?

DHEA was first discovered in the 1930s. Over the next fifty years, researchers learned that it was made by the adrenal glands and that it was a precursor to other steroid hormones in the body. Some early research in laboratory animals hinted that it might be helpful in certain conditions, although it now appears that the role of DHEA in humans is different from its role in rodents and other animals. No large studies were reported in humans before the 1990s.

DHEA was banned by the U.S. Food and Drug Administration (FDA) in 1985 because of its unproven safety and effectiveness. This ban was removed by the 1994 Dietary Supplement Health & Education Act, and DHEA supplements became available to the public soon after. The National Football League (NFL), the National Basketball Association (NBA), and some other sports groups do not allow players to use DHEA because of the concern that its effects may be similar to those of anabolic (muscle-building) steroids.

What is the evidence?

Very few valid clinical research studies have been done on the link between DHEA supplements and improved health. Some studies have looked at the relationship between DHEA levels in the body and certain diseases, with mixed and sometimes conflicting results.

Available scientific evidence does not support claims that DHEA can slow down or prevent the growth of cancer in humans. Some early laboratory studies found that DHEA can slow the growth of certain types of cancer cells. Others, however, found that DHEA causes some types of cancer cells, such as prostate cancer cells, to grow more quickly. One animal study concluded that DHEA had no influence on either cancer or life span.

One study found no relationship between DHEA levels in the blood and the risk for breast cancer in postmenopausal women, whereas another found that a high level of DHEA in the blood was linked to a higher risk for breast cancer among women older than forty-five years. Although this second study observed a statistical correlation (but did not test the effect of DHEA supplements on breast cancer risk), it does raise concern that intentionally increasing a woman's DHEA levels may be unsafe.

Some studies have also looked the relationship between DHEA and heart disease. One early study showed that men who had high levels of DHEA in their blood were less likely to have died of heart disease, but women who had high DHEA levels were at greater risk for dying of heart disease. A recent analysis of the research found that there was little association between levels of DHEA and heart disease in men or women.

In addition, DHEA has been studied for any possible benefit for other health conditions. No clinical research has convincingly shown that DHEA supplements increase muscle mass, reduce fat, or prevent disease. A study of humans taking DHEA supplements suggested that it may help treat lupus, an autoimmune disease. DHEA's ability to stimulate the immune system is being studied in clinical trials. A 2005 double-blind clinical trial of older women with fibromyalgia found that, although DHEA supplements raised blood levels of DHEA, they did not help with pain, tiredness, mood, brain function, or other quality of life measures.

A small pilot study suggested that DHEA may improve mood, energy, libido, and, in some cases, memory performance in the elderly. However, an analysis of studies available to date showed no convincing evidence that DHEA improved memory in older adults. Some early test results raise the possibility of DHEA being useful in older people with depression, although larger, double-blind clinical trials are needed. DHEA may help some people with adrenal insufficiency (poorly working adrenal glands).

Are there any possible problems or complications?

It is not known whether DHEA is safe for long-term use. Some researchers believe DHEA supplements might actually raise the risk for breast cancer, prostate cancer, heart disease, diabetes, and stroke. DHEA may stimulate tumor growth in types of cancer that are sensitive to hormones, such as some types of breast, uterine, and prostate cancer. DHEA may increase prostate swelling in men with benign prostatic hyperplasia, or BPH, an enlarged prostate gland.

DHEA is a steroid hormone. High doses may cause aggressiveness, irritability, trouble sleeping, and the growth of body or facial hair on women. It also may stop menstruation and lower the levels of HDL, or "good," cholesterol, which could raise the risk for heart disease. Other reported side effects include acne, heart rhythm problems, liver problems, hair loss (from the scalp), and oily skin. It may also alter the body's regulation of blood sugar.

DHEA should not be used with tamoxifen, as it may promote tamoxifen resistance. Patients on hormone replacement therapy may have more estrogen-related side effects when taking DHEA. This supplement may also interfere with other medicines, and potential interactions between it and drugs and herbs should be considered. Always tell your doctor and pharmacist about any supplements and herbs you are taking.

Women who are pregnant or breastfeeding should not use DHEA. Relying on this type of treatment alone and avoiding or delaying conventional medical care for cancer may have serious health consequences.

This product is sold as a dietary supplement in the United States. Unlike companies that produce drugs (which must provide the FDA with results of detailed testing showing their product is safe and effective before the drug is approved for sale), the companies that make supplements do not have to show evidence of safety or health benefits to the FDA before selling their products. Supplement products without any reliable scientific evidence of health benefits may still be sold as long as the companies selling them do not claim the supplements can prevent, treat, or cure any specific disease. Some such products may not contain the amount of the herb or substance that is written on the label, and some may include other substances (contaminants). Though the FDA has written new rules to improve the quality of manufacturing processes for dietary supplements and the accurate listing of supplement ingredients, these rules do not take full effect until 2010. The new rules also do not address the safety of supplement ingredients or their effects on health when proper manufacturing techniques are used.

Most such supplements have not been tested to find out if they interact with medicines, foods, or other herbs and supplements. Even though some reports of interactions and harmful effects may be published, full studies of interactions and effects are not often available. Because of these limitations, any information on ill effects and interactions should be considered incomplete.

References

Arnold JT, Le H, McFann KK, Blackman MR. Comparative effects of DHEA vs. testosterone, dihydrotestosterone, and estradiol on proliferation and gene expression in human LNCaP prostate cancer cells. *Am J Physiol Endocrinol Metab.* 2005;288:E573-E584. Epub 2004 Nov 9.

Dehydroepiandrosterone. Memorial Sloan-Kettering Cancer Center Web site. http://www.mskcc.org/mskcc/html/69201.cfm. Accessed June 11, 2008.

DHEA. PDRhealth Web site. http://www.pdrhealth.com/drug_info/nmdrugprofiles/nutsupdrugs/dhe_0094.shtml. Accessed June 11, 2008.

Finckh A, Berner IC, Aubry-Rozier B, So AK. A randomized controlled trial of dehydroepiandrosterone in postmenopausal women with fibromyalgia. *J Rheumatol.* 2005;32:1336-1340.

Grimley Evans J, Malouf R, Huppert F, van Niekerk JK. Dehydroepiandrosterone (DHEA) supplementation for cognitive function in healthy elderly people. *Cochrane Database Syst Rev.* 2006;(4):CD006221.

Igwebuike A, Irving BA, Bigelow ML, Short KR, McConnell JP, Nair KS. Lack of dehydroepiandrosterone effect on a combined endurance and resistance exercise program in postmenopausal women. *J Clin Endocrinol Metab.* 2008;93:534-538.

Kaaks R, Berrino F, Key T, Rinaldi S, Dossus L, Biessy C, Secreto G, Amiano P, Bingham S, Boeing H, Bueno de Mesquita HB, Chang-Claude J, Clavel-Chapelon F, Fournier A, van Gils CH, Gonzalez CA, Gurrea AB, Critselis E, Khaw KT, Krough V, Lahmann PH, Nagel G, Olsen A, Onland-Moret NC, Overvad K, Palli D, Panico S, Peeters P, Quirós JR, Roddam A, Thiebaut A, Tjønneland A, Chirlaque MD, Trichopoulou A, Trichopoulos D, Tumino R, Vineis P, Norat T, Ferrari O, Slimani N, Riboli E. Serum sex steroids in premenopausal women and breast cancer risk within the European Prospective Investigation into Cancer and Nutrition (EPIC). *J Natl Cancer Inst.* 2005;97:755-765.

Pugh TD, Oberley TD, Weindruch R. Dietary intervention at middle age: caloric restriction but not dehydroepiandrosterone sulfate increases lifespan and lifetime cancer incidence in mice. *Cancer Res.* 1999;59:1642-1648.

Schardt D. Remembering gingko & DHEA: claims of dietary supplement have not been proven. *Nutr Action Health Lett.* 1998;25:9.

Tworoger SS, Missmer SA, Eliassen AH, Spiegelman D, Folkerd E, Dowsett M, Barbieri RL, Hankinson SE. The association of plasma DHEA and DHEA sulfate with breast cancer risk in predominantly premenopausal women. *Cancer Epidemiol Biomarkers Prev.* 2006;15:967-971.

DI BELLA THERAPY

Other common name(s): Di Bella multitherapy, DBM, MDB
Scientific/medical name(s): none

Description

Di Bella therapy is an alternative cancer treatment developed by an Italian physiologist. It is a mixture of the drugs somatostatin and bromocriptine, as well as vitamins, melatonin, and, sometimes, low doses of chemotherapy drugs or other substances combined in varying amounts. Therapy is tailored to the type of cancer and the results of blood tests.

Overview

Available scientific evidence does not support claims that Di Bella therapy is effective in treating cancer. It can cause serious and harmful side effects.

How is it promoted for use?

Supporters of Di Bella therapy claim the drug mixture stimulates the body's self-healing properties and can shrink tumors or even cure cancer. It is partly based on the idea that two of the body's natural hormones—growth hormone and prolactin—may stimulate cancer growth. One component of the therapy (somatostatin) works against growth hormone, while another (bromocriptine) acts against prolactin. Bromocriptine is a drug approved by the U.S. Food and Drug Administration (FDA) for treating pituitary tumors, Parkinson's disease, and fertility problems. Somatostatin is naturally produced in the body, but a similar manmade substance (Octreotide) is sometimes used instead in Di Bella therapy. The inventor claimed he had treated and cured thousands of people who had a variety of cancers and that his formula caused no side effects.

What does it involve?

Patients having Di Bella therapy take the custom-made drug mixture daily. The potency of the mixture and the drugs involved depend on the type of cancer being treated and on the results of blood tests.

What is the history behind it?

Di Bella therapy was invented by Professor Luigi Di Bella, a retired physiologist from Modena, Italy. For several months during 1997 and 1998, Di Bella therapy caused an uproar throughout Italy when a judge in the southern city of Maglie ruled that the government had to pay for Di Bella therapy to treat a two-year-old boy with brain cancer. The child's parents had filed a lawsuit against the Italian Ministry of Health, which had refused to fund the treatment because Di Bella therapy was untested and expensive. A number of similar legal actions followed.

Even though there was no scientific evidence available to prove the benefits of Di Bella therapy, the therapy still had many supporters, and the Italian media quickly spread news about Di Bella's claims and about the lawsuits. Di Bella appeared in many television interviews and was written about in several hundred newspaper articles. Demand for Di Bella's formula depleted the supply of some of its components in many pharmacies, and people with cancer flooded Italian hospitals asking to take part in clinical trials. Thousands of supporters even held rallies in Rome to support government funding of Di Bella therapy.

Finally, bowing to public pressure, the Ministry of Health ordered a clinical study of Di Bella therapy. Some cancer specialists refused to participate for ethical reasons. The results of the clinical trial showed that Di Bella therapy was largely ineffective against cancer. The clinical trial is discussed in greater detail below.

Before the study began, researchers at the University of Parma surveyed more than 1,100 Italian citizens. Of those, 42 percent believed that Di Bella therapy worked, 53 percent were unsure, and only 1 percent thought it was a sham. Of those who responded, 90 percent had learned about the treatment from television, and only 5 percent had asked a doctor about it.

After the study results were published, public interest in the treatment decreased, but Di

Bella therapy still has many supporters despite lack of evidence of its effectiveness. Di Bella passed away in 2003, but his therapy and variations of it are still available in several countries.

What is the evidence?

Di Bella claimed to have cured thousands of patients, but most of the records he kept could not confirm this claim. There is evidence from laboratory studies that some components of Di Bella therapy, such as melatonin and somatostatin, may have some effect on cancer cells, but it is not clear whether they would have the same effect in the human body. Bromocriptine is approved in the United States for use with mainstream treatment to reduce the size of some pituitary tumors before surgery and during radiation therapy. However, studies have not shown that combining these agents, as is done in Di Bella therapy, is effective in treating cancer.

Italy's Health Ministry conducted a study in twenty-six medical centers involving nearly four hundred patients with different forms of advanced cancer. The final report, which included 395 patients, showed that no tumors went into complete remission (meaning they disappeared completely) and only three (less than 1 percent) went into partial remission (meaning they shrank by at least half). A quarter of the subjects died, and more than half got worse. The researchers concluded that Di Bella therapy did not deserve further clinical testing in patients with advanced cancer. Di Bella and his supporters criticized this study for selecting patients with advanced disease and for varying from his protocols.

A study was also published on the survival rates of cancer patients treated by Di Bella from 1971 to 1997. A review of 248 of his records (the 16 percent of his patients for whom good records were kept) showed that the treatment did not improve their survival, and it may have had a negative effect compared with the outcome for similar patients receiving standard treatment.

In a small uncontrolled study published in 2001, Italian researchers treated twenty low-grade non-Hodgkin's lymphoma patients with a regimen similar to that used in Di Bella therapy. It included cyclophosphamide, a drug often used in conventional chemotherapy regimens for lymphomas. After almost two years, seven of the patients had a complete response, while in five patients the tumors advanced. In the other eight patients, the lymphoma shrank slightly or stayed the same. It is not clear how much of a role the cyclophosphamide played in this study. The study did not include any control group, so it is uncertain whether patients receiving the standard treatment would have fared better. In addition, the results have not been duplicated by further research. Further, because of substantial advances in mainstream treatment of low-grade lymphoma during the past few years, few, if any, oncologists would now consider Di Bella therapy to be a reasonable treatment choice for this type of cancer.

Another small uncontrolled study of Di Bella therapy was published in 2006. This study of twenty-eight patients with advanced lung cancer reported an improvement in cough, shortness of breath, pain, fatigue, and insomnia. However, results were based on notes from doctor-patient consultations, rather than standardized measures of patient-reported outcomes. Notably, the article does not mention the number of patients with partial or complete tumor responses or whose disease remained stable, and therefore provides minimal information about the effectiveness of this regimen.

Are there any possible problems or complications?

Side effects of Di Bella therapy may include nausea, vomiting, diarrhea, increased blood sugar levels, low blood pressure, sleepiness, and neurologic symptoms. Some components of Di Bella therapy may interact with pain medications and blood pressure medicines, as well as certain antibiotics or antiviral medicines. People with diabetes and women who are pregnant or breastfeeding should not use this method. Relying on this type of treatment alone and avoiding or delaying conventional medical care for cancer may have serious health consequences.

These substances may have not been thoroughly tested to find out how they interact with medicines, foods, or dietary supplements. Even though some reports of interactions and harmful effects may be published, full studies of interactions and effects are not often available. Because of these limitations, any information on ill effects and interactions should be considered incomplete.

References

Bertelli G. Di Bella therapy was worthless. Quackwatch Web site. http://www.quackwatch.org/01QuackeryRelatedTopics/Cancer/dibella.html. Updated November 21, 2006. Accessed June 11, 2008.

Buiatti E, Arniani S, Verdecchia A, Tomatis L. Results from a historical survey of the survival of cancer patients given Di Bella multitherapy. *Cancer.* 1999;86:2143-2149.

Di bella multitherapy. Memorial Sloan-Kettering Cancer Center Web site. http://www.mskcc.org/mskcc/html/69203.cfm. Accessed August 27, 2008.

Italian Study Group for the Di Bella Multitherapy Trials. Evaluation of an unconventional cancer treatment (the Di Bella multitherapy): results of phase II trials in Italy. *BMJ.* 1999;318:224-228.

Norsa A, Martino V. Somatostatin, retinoids, melatonin, vitamin D, bromocriptine, and cyclophosphamide in advanced non-small-cell lung cancer patients with low performance status. *Cancer Biother Radiopharm.* 2006;21:68-73.

Todisco M, Casaccia P, Rossi N. Cyclophosphamide plus somatostatin, bromocriptin, retinoids, melatonin and ACTH in the treatment of low-grade non-Hodgkin's lymphomas at advanced stage: results of a phase II trial. *Cancer Biother Radiopharm.* 2001;16:171-177.

DMSO

Other common name(s): Rimso-50
Scientific/medical name(s): dimethyl sulfoxide, dimethylsulfoxide

Description

Dimethyl sulfoxide, or DMSO, is an industrial solvent that is a byproduct of making paper. It has been promoted as an alternative cancer treatment since the 1960s.

Overview

Available scientific evidence does not suggest that DMSO is effective in treating cancer in humans. It is being studied as a drug carrier to increase the effectiveness of some chemotherapy drugs currently used to treat bladder cancer. The only use for which DMSO is approved by the U.S. Food and Drug Administration (FDA) is for the treatment of a type of bladder inflammation known as interstitial cystitis.

How is it promoted for use?

Supporters say that DMSO can cause cancerous cells to become noncancerous, or benign, and can slow or stop the progress of cancer in the bladder, colon, ovary, breast, and skin. Some claim that it is useful in treating leukemia, and it has also been used as a part of some metabolic cancer therapies (see "Metabolic Therapy," page 646). Some people have promoted DMSO as preventing cancer. They claim it works by "cleaning" cell membranes and decreasing the effect of cancer-causing substances.

Some researchers believe that DMSO can be used with certain chemotherapy drugs to make them more effective. DMSO is also promoted to reduce the side effects of chemotherapy and radiation treatments in people with cancer. DMSO can supposedly boost the immune system and scavenge free radicals caused by these treatments. In addition, it has been promoted as a way to control the "withdrawal symptoms" felt by cancer patients when taken off conventional cancer treatment.

DMSO is often used as a cream or ointment applied to the skin to reduce pain, decrease swelling, treat autoimmune diseases such as arthritis, and promote healing in wounds and burns.

What does it involve?

DMSO is medically approved in the United States only for the treatment of interstitial cystitis, a type of inflammation of the bladder. When used for this condition, a 50 percent solution of DMSO is instilled into the bladder through a catheter and left there for about fifteen minutes.

As an alternative therapy for cancer, DMSO is available through many health food stores, mail-order outlets, and on the Internet. It is typically applied to the skin in a gel, liquid, or roll-on form. It can also be taken by mouth or as an intravenous injection, in many cases along with other drugs. Strengths and dosages vary widely.

What is the history behind it?

DMSO was first discovered in the mid- to late nineteenth century and has been used as an industrial solvent for more than a hundred years. In the 1950s, it was discovered that DMSO could protect cells from the damage of freezing. In the 1960s, Dr. Stanley Jacob, one of the main proponents of DMSO, began to study other medicinal properties of the substance. In 1965, clinical trials of DMSO were stopped due to questions about its safety. However, in the 1970s, DMSO was approved for use as an anti-inflammatory treatment in dogs and horses and as a prescription drug for a type of bladder inflammation in humans.

What is the evidence?

Tests of DMSO for treating human illness began in the mid-1960s but were stopped because of questions of safety, mainly dealing with a possible ability to cause damage to the eye. Early research did not find that DMSO was useful in the treatment of cancer. However, more recent research in rats has shown that DMSO may deserve further study as a drug carrier to enhance the effectiveness of some chemotherapy drugs for the treatment of bladder cancer.

In a 1988 laboratory study, the addition of 4 percent DMSO to the chemotherapy drugs most often used in the bladder did not kill more cancer cells. However, animal studies done since that time have found that adding DMSO to some chemotherapy drugs helped the bladder to absorb them better. Further studies are needed to learn whether the results apply to humans.

DMSO is a common chemical used in the laboratory. Small amounts of DMSO are sometimes used to dissolve drugs and other chemicals that do not dissolve well in water, so that these substances can be tested in animals or in experiments with cells growing in laboratory dishes. However, in those cases, it is the drug, not DMSO, that acts in the body. DMSO is sometimes used in laboratory studies to help cancer cells mature and/or differentiate (to acquire some characteristics of noncancerous cells). This is one reason that is used to support DMSO as an anti-cancer agent. However, the concentrations typically used in the laboratory would be highly toxic or even fatal to a human. Some researchers have continued laboratory studies to understand how high concentrations of DMSO might influence characteristics of cancer cells. In a 2007 review, the scientists describe how their laboratory studies of DMSO led to discovery of another substance that turned out to be useful as a chemotherapy drug and has already been approved by the FDA.

Research has shown that DMSO appears to have some effect in reducing pain, swelling, and inflammation, as well as having other properties that may make it useful in treating certain conditions. More testing is needed to show it is safe and effective for these uses in people. DMSO is approved by the FDA to treat a single type of bladder disorder (interstitial cystitis) in humans and as a veterinary treatment to reduce swelling in horses and dogs.

Are there any possible problems or complications?

Early clinical trials with DMSO were stopped because of questions about its safety, especially its ability to harm the eye. The most commonly reported side effects include headaches and burning and itching on contact with the skin. It can also cause a powerful garlic-like taste and odor on the breath and skin. Strong allergic reactions have been reported. In high concentrations, DMSO can be fatal to humans. Industrial-grade DMSO is sometimes contaminated with other substances. DMSO can cause contaminants, toxins, and medicines to be absorbed through the skin, which may cause unexpected effects.

DMSO is thought to increase the effects of blood thinners, steroids, heart medicines, sedatives, and other drugs. In some cases this could be harmful or dangerous. Be sure to tell your doctor or pharmacist about all herbs and supplements you are taking, including DMSO.

Women who are pregnant or breastfeeding should not use this treatment. Relying on this type of treatment alone and avoiding or delaying conventional medical care for cancer may have serious health consequences.

This substance has not been thoroughly tested to find out how it interacts with medicines, foods, or dietary supplements. Even though some reports of interactions and harmful effects may be published, full studies of interactions and effects are not often available. Because of these limitations, any information on ill effects and interactions should be considered incomplete.

References

American Cancer Society. Unproven methods of cancer management. Dimethyl sulfoxide (DMSO). *CA Cancer J Clin.* 1983;33:122-125.

Chen D, Song D, Wientjes MG, Au JL. Effect of dimethyl sulfoxide on bladder tissue penetration of intravesical paclitaxel. *Clin Cancer Res.* 2003;9:363-369.

Dimethylsulfoxide. Memorial Sloan-Kettering Cancer Center Web site. http://www.mskcc.org/mskcc/html/69205.cfm. Accessed June 11, 2008.

Hashimoto H, Tokunaka S, Sasaki M, Nishihara M, Yachiku S. Dimethylsulfoxide enhances the absorption of chemotherapeutic drug instilled into the bladder. *Urol Res.* 1992;20:233-236.

Marks PA, Breslow R. Dimethyl sulfoxide to vorinostat: development of this histone deacetylase inhibitor as an anticancer drug. *Nat Biotechnol.* 2007;25:84-90.

Natural Standard. Biologic/organic/pharmacologic therapies: DMSO (dimethyl sulfoxide). Complementary/Integrative Medicine Education Resources, The University of Texas M. D. Anderson Cancer Center Web site. http://www.mdanderson.org/departments/cimer/display.cfm?id=8e9bcb72-f0a0-11d4-810300508b603a14&method=displayfull. Accessed June 11, 2008.

See WA, Xia Q. Regional chemotherapy for bladder neoplasms using continuous intravesical infusion of doxorubicin: impact of concomitant administration of dimethyl sulfoxide on drug absorption and antitumor activity. *J Natl Cancer Inst.* 1992;84:510-515.

Solit DB, Ivy SP, Kopil C, Sikorski R, Morris MJ, Slovin SF, Kelly WK, DeLaCruz A, Curley T, Heller G, Larson S, Schwartz L, Egorin MJ, Rosen N, Scher HI. Phase I trial of 17-allylamino-17-demethoxygeldanamycin in patients with advanced cancer. *Clin Cancer Res.* 2007;13:1775-1782.

US Congress, Office of Technology Assessment. *Unconventional Cancer Treatments: OTA-H-405.* Washington, DC: US Government Printing Office; 1990.

Walker L, Walker MC, Parris CN, Masters JR. Intravesical chemotherapy: combination with dimethyl sulfoxide does not enhance cytotoxicity in vitro. *Urol Res.* 1988;16:329-331.

Windrum P, Morris TC, Drake MB, Niederwieser D, Ruutu T; EBMT Chronic Leukaemia Working Party Complications Subcommittee. Variation in dimethyl sulfoxide use in stem cell transplantation: a survey of EBMT centres. *Bone Marrow Transplant.* 2005;36:601-603.

Yaman O, Ozdiler E, Sözen S, Göğüş O. Transmurally absorbed intravesical chemotherapy with dimethylsulfoxide in an animal model. *Int J Urol.* 1999;6:87-92.

ENZYME THERAPY

Other common name(s): digestive enzyme therapy, pancreatic enzyme therapy, systemic enzyme therapy, proteolytic enzyme therapy

Scientific/medical name(s): none

Description

Enzyme therapy involves taking enzyme supplements as an alternative cancer treatment. Enzymes are natural proteins that stimulate and accelerate biological reactions in the body. Digestive enzymes, many of which are made in the pancreas, break down food and help with the absorption of nutrients into the blood. Metabolic enzymes build new cells and repair damaged ones in the blood, tissues, and organs.

Overview

Available scientific evidence does not support claims that enzyme supplements are effective in treating cancer.

How is it promoted for use?

Enzymes are sometimes used in mainstream medicine. For example, the approved chemotherapy drug asparaginase is an enzyme. Some enzymes are also used for other serious illnesses. Pancreatic enzymes may be given to treat digestive problems resulting from removal of the pancreas or certain diseases of the pancreas.

However, some alternative medicine practitioners claim that digestive enzyme supplements not only relieve digestive problems, such as ulcers and food allergies, but also strengthen the immune system, improve circulation, ease sore throat pain, aid weight loss, and relieve hay fever, ulcers, and rheumatoid arthritis. Proponents also claim that certain enzymes remove a protective coating from cancer cells, allowing white blood cells to identify and attack them.

What does it involve?

Human cells naturally produce about ten thousand different enzymes, which are essential in normal metabolism. Enzyme supplements are extracted from animal organs and some plants such as pineapple and papaya (see "Bromelain," page 281). Among the most popular enzyme supplements are pancreatic enzymes, which come from an animal pancreas.

Enzyme supplements are available as pills, capsules, and powders. Supplements often consist of combinations of several enzymes. Large amounts of the supplements are often taken each day. There is currently no established safe or effective dosage.

Enzyme therapy is a part of some forms of metabolic therapy, including Gerson therapy and the Kelley and Gonzalez programs. (For more detailed information on these regimens, see "Gerson Therapy," page 616, and "Metabolic Therapy," page 646.)

What is the history behind it?

Pancreatic enzymes were reportedly first used to treat cancer in 1902 by John Beard, a Scottish scientist. German researchers later used enzyme therapy to treat patients with multiple sclerosis, cancer, and viral infections. Some enzyme mixtures are still commonly used in several European countries.

Dr. Edward Howell introduced enzyme therapy to the United States in the 1920s. He believed that by eating raw meat, people created an enzyme surplus in the body, which resulted in better health and increased resistance to disease. Other practitioners have advocated the use of enzyme therapy since then, often as part of a larger metabolic therapy regimen. At least one enzyme preparation is currently being studied in the United States for use with chemotherapy in cancer patients.

What is the evidence?

There have been no well-designed studies showing that enzyme supplements are effective in treating cancer. Experts question whether enzymes taken by mouth can reach tumors through the bloodstream, as the enzymes are broken down into amino acids before being absorbed in the intestine.

Studies of enzyme supplements to ease the side effects of cancer treatment have had mixed results. Two studies done in India reported that side effects of radiation therapy in cancer patients taking pancreatic enzyme supplements were less severe than in those taking a placebo. However, these studies were not blinded, meaning patients and their doctors knew whether they were taking the actual enzymes. This means that the results might have been affected by the expectation of improvement, or placebo effect. A blinded German study in which patients did not know whether they were taking the enzymes or placebo pills did not find any benefit.

Several studies done mainly in Eastern Europe have looked at the possible effects of adding enzyme supplements to mainstream cancer treatment. They have generally found that supplements may improve quality of life and could possibly have other benefits. However, these studies are not considered scientifically strong. They looked back in time at patients who were already treated and were not randomized or blinded. A randomized study of the addition of enzyme therapy to standard chemotherapy for multiple myeloma patients is under way in the United States.

A small study of patients with pancreatic cancer—conducted by Dr. Nicholas Gonzalez and published in *Nutrition and Cancer* in 1999—found that patients treated with pancreatic enzymes survived longer than typical patients with pancreatic cancer. However, in a recent review of alternative cancer therapies, an expert in integrative oncology research methods noted that, "The study was small and obviously prone to several biases. Not only is the comparison with national averages unadjusted for confounders, but the principal results are based on patient selection; 12 patients who did not comply with treatment were excluded from analysis" (*CA Cancer J Clin.* 2004;54:115). Well-designed scientific studies control or adjust for confounders, factors besides the method being studied—such as age or cancer stage—that can affect outcome. They have a control group that receives the standard treatment alone, and they generally also include patients who did not complete treatment in the final analysis.

A randomized clinical trial has been sponsored by the National Cancer Institute to evaluate the Gonzalez regimen for treating pancreatic cancer, but no results of this trial have yet been published in a peer-reviewed medical journal.

Are there any possible problems or complications?

There is very little information available on the safety of enzyme supplements. Some manufacturers recommend that people taking blood-thinning medications speak with their doctors before taking enzyme supplements. Care should be taken to make sure that any diet containing raw meat or juices from raw meat is free from bacterial contamination, especially for people with weak immune systems. Some people are allergic to the materials from which the enzymes are made. Be sure to know the source of any enzymes you are considering.

Women who are pregnant or breastfeeding should speak with their doctors before using this method. Relying on this type of treatment alone and avoiding or delaying conventional medical care for cancer may have serious health consequences.

This product is sold as a dietary supplement in the United States. Unlike companies that produce drugs (which must provide the FDA with results of detailed testing showing their product is safe and effective before the drug is approved for sale), the companies that make supplements do not have to show evidence of safety or health benefits to the FDA before selling their products. Supplement products without any reliable scientific evidence of health benefits may still be sold as long as the companies selling them do not claim the supplements can prevent, treat, or cure any specific disease. Some such products may not contain the amount of the herb or substance that is written on the label, and some may include other substances (contaminants). Though the FDA has written new rules to improve the quality of manufacturing processes for dietary supplements and the accurate listing of supplement ingredients, these rules do not take full effect until 2010. The new rules also do not address the safety of supplement ingredients or their effects on health when proper manufacturing techniques are used.

Most such supplements have not been tested to find out if they interact with medicines, foods, or other herbs and supplements. Even though some reports of interactions and harmful effects may be published, full studies of interactions and effects are not often available. Because of these limitations, any information on ill effects and interactions should be considered incomplete.

References

Cassileth B. *The Alternative Medicine Handbook: The Complete Reference Guide to Alternative and Complementary Therapies.* New York: W.W. Norton; 1998.

Dale PS, Tamhankar CP, George D, Daftary GV. Co-medication with hydrolytic enzymes in radiation therapy of uterine cervix: evidence of the reduction of acute side effects. *Cancer Chemother Pharmacol.* 2001;47(suppl):S29-S34.

Ernst E. Complementary therapies in palliative cancer care. *Cancer.* 2001;91:2181-2185.

Gonzalez NJ, Isaacs LL. Evaluation of pancreatic proteolytic enzyme treatment of adenocarcinoma of the pancreas, with nutrition and detoxification support. *Nutr Cancer.* 1999;33:117-124.

Green S. Nicholas Gonzalez treatment for cancer: gland extracts, coffee enemas, vitamin megadoses, and diets. Quackwatch Web site. http://www.quackwatch.org/01QuackeryRelatedTopics/Cancer/kg.html. Revised April 2000. Accessed June 11, 2008.

Gujral MS, Patnaik PM, Kaul R, Parikh HK, Conradt C, Tamhankar CP, Daftary GV. Efficacy of hydrolytic enzymes in preventing radiation therapy-induced side effects in patients with head and neck cancers. *Cancer Chemother Pharmacol.* 2001;47(suppl):S23-S28.

Martin T, Uhder K, Kurek R, Roeddiger S, Schneider L, Vogt HG, Heyd R, Zamboglou N. Does prophylactic treatment with proteolytic enzymes reduce acute toxicity of adjuvant pelvic irradiation? Results of a double-blind randomized trial. *Radiother Oncol.* 2002;65:17-22.

Proteolytic enzymes. Memorial Sloan-Kettering Cancer Center Web site. http://www.mskcc.org/mskcc/html/69342.cfm. Accessed June 11, 2008.

Sakalová A, Bock PR, Dedík L, Hanisch J, Schiess W, Gazová S, Chabronová I, Holomanova D, Mistrík M, Hrubisko M. Retrolective cohort study of an additive therapy with an oral enzyme preparation in patients with multiple myeloma. *Cancer Chemother Pharmacol.* 2001;47(suppl):S38-S44.

Vickers A. Alternative cancer cures: "unproven" or "disproven"? *CA Cancer J Clin.* 2004;54:110-118.

GAMMA LINOLENIC ACID

Other common name(s): evening primrose oil, borage seed oil, black currant oil, GLA
Scientific/medical name(s): gamma linolenic acid

Description

Gamma linolenic acid (GLA) is an omega-6 unsaturated fatty acid made in the human body from linoleic acid, an essential fatty acid found in vegetable oils and egg yolks. The main supplemental sources of GLA are oils of the seeds of evening primrose, borage, and black currant plants. (For more information, see "Evening Primrose," page 345.) Many companies sell these oils as good sources of GLA. It is also found in human breast milk.

Overview

Some studies have shown that GLA can slow or stop the growth of some types of cancer cells in tissue cultures in the laboratory and that it may help some cancer drugs to work better. However, there is very little evidence as yet that GLA supplements are effective in preventing or treating cancer in humans. Human studies are under way to evaluate the role of GLA and other essential fatty acids on the growth of cancer cells.

How is it promoted for use?

Gamma linolenic acid is normally used by the body to make prostaglandins (hormone-like substances). Prostaglandins are believed to be involved in many processes in the body, including regulation of the immune system.

Most GLA in the human body is taken in as linoleic acid and then metabolized to GLA. Most people get plenty of linoleic acid in their diets and can convert it to GLA. Some researchers have suggested that some people (such as those with diabetes or skin allergies) do not make enough GLA from linoleic acid and may therefore benefit from taking GLA supplements.

It has been proposed that GLA supplements may stop or slow the growth of cancer cells. GLA and GLA-rich supplements have also been promoted to help people with breast pain, skin allergies, diabetes, obesity, rheumatoid arthritis, heart disease, high blood pressure, premenstrual syndrome, multiple sclerosis, attention deficit hyperactivity disorder (ADHD), and neurologic problems related to diabetes.

What does it involve?

Gamma linolenic acid is available in liquid and capsule form, usually as a natural ingredient in black currant oil, borage oil, or evening primrose oil. The amount of GLA contained in the different types of supplements varies (for example, evening primrose supplements may contain about 10 percent GLA). Dosages of GLA as a supplement are generally in the range of 500 milligrams to 3,000 milligrams per day. An injectable form of GLA is being studied.

What is the history behind it?

Some of the plants whose seeds contain GLA have been used as folk remedies for hundreds, if not thousands, of years. However, the recognition of GLA and of these seed oils as a source of GLA is much more recent.

Research in the 1980s found that hormone-like substances called prostaglandins played a role in many biological processes. Since GLA was known to be a building block for some prostaglandins, it was reasoned that GLA might be helpful in treating human disease. While GLA is widely touted for its health benefits, research on its effectiveness in human diseases is still at an early stage.

What is the evidence?

Much of the research on GLA has been done using evening primrose oil. This makes it hard to credit any effects specifically to GLA, as the oil has many components, including linoleic acid and vitamin E. Studies of the ability of evening primrose oil and GLA to prevent or treat cancer in humans are still in the earliest stages.

Dietary GLA (most of which is consumed as linoleic acid) contributes to making and regulating prostaglandins; however, the exact role of the different prostaglandins in fighting cancer is still not clear.

Some research in the laboratory has suggested that GLA may prove to be helpful against certain cancers, but this research is still early. In laboratory tests, GLA slowed the growth of several types of human cancer cells. It has also been shown to make certain anticancer drugs better at killing cancer cells in laboratory studies.

There have been fewer clinical trials studying the effect of GLA on tumors. In a small English study of about eighty breast cancer patients, those who took GLA supplements in addition to tamoxifen responded more quickly to treatment than those who took tamoxifen alone. It is not clear if any longer-term benefits were achieved.

An injectable form of GLA was studied in a clinical trial of forty-eight patients with pancreatic cancer. Those who received the highest doses of GLA were reported to live longer. However, a larger study of 278 patients did not find that those receiving GLA (either by mouth or injected into a vein) lived longer than expected. Some researchers have proposed that the injectable form of GLA may be effective only if it is injected directly into the tumor. Future studies may look at GLA combined with chemotherapy drugs.

Some studies have looked at the use of maglumine GLA (which is chemically different from the form sold in dietary supplements) against bladder cancer by infusing it directly into the bladder through a catheter. One small study found that about 43 percent of people with early-stage bladder cancer had their tumors shrink or completely disappear with this therapy. Clearly, more research is needed to learn which method of giving GLA is most effective and whether GLA is useful in treating cancer, either alone or with standard treatments.

Neither GLA nor other GLA-rich supplements (such as evening primrose oil) have been convincingly shown to be useful in preventing or treating any other health conditions.

Are there any possible problems or complications?

Gamma linolenic acid does not appear to be toxic. However, it has been reported to aggravate a type of epilepsy and should not be used by people who take anti-seizure medicines. Long-term use of GLA may lead to inflammation, blood clots, or lowered immune system functioning.

Borage oil, which is sometimes used as a source of GLA, may contain substances that can harm the liver or possibly cause cancer. If you take borage oil, be sure it is certified as free of unsaturated pyrrolizidine alkaloids (UPAs), and do not take more than the recommended dose.

Women who are pregnant or breastfeeding should speak with their doctors before using this treatment. Relying on this type of treatment alone and avoiding or delaying conventional medical care for cancer may have serious health consequences.

This product is sold as a dietary supplement in the United States. Unlike companies that produce drugs (which must provide the FDA with results of detailed testing showing their product is safe and effective before the drug is approved for sale), the companies that make supplements do not have to show evidence of safety or health benefits to the FDA before selling their products. Supplement products without any reliable scientific evidence of health benefits may still be sold as long as the companies selling them do not claim the supplements can prevent, treat, or cure any specific disease. Some such products may not contain the amount of the herb or substance that is written on the label, and some may include other substances (contaminants). Though the FDA has written new rules to improve the quality of manufacturing processes for dietary supplements and the accurate listing of supplement ingredients, these rules do not take full effect until 2010. The new rules also do not address the safety of supplement ingredients or their effects on health when proper manufacturing techniques are used.

Most such supplements have not been tested to find out if they interact with medicines, foods, or other herbs and supplements. Even though some reports of interactions and harmful effects may be published, full studies of interactions and effects are not often available. Because of these limitations, any information on ill effects and interactions should be considered incomplete.

References

Borage. Memorial Sloan-Kettering Cancer Center Web site. http://www.mskcc.org/mskcc/html/69148.cfm. Accessed June 11, 2008.

Evening primrose oil (Oenothera biennis L.). Medline Plus Web site. http://www.nlm.nih.gov/medlineplus/druginfo/natural/patient-primrose.html. Accessed September 8, 2008.

Fearon KC, Falconer JS, Ross JA, Carter DC, Hunter JO, Reynolds PD, Tuffnell Q. An open-label phase I/II dose escalation study of the treatment of pancreatic cancer using lithium gammalinolenate. *Anticancer Res.* 1996;16:867-874.

Fetrow CW, Avila JR. *Professional's Handbook of Complementary & Alternative Medicines.* Springhouse, PA: Springhouse Corp; 1999.

Harris NM, Crook TJ, Dyer JP, Solomon LZ, Bass P, Cooper AJ, Birch BR. Intravesical meglumine gamma-linolenic acid in superficial bladder cancer: an efficacy study. *Eur Urol.* 2002;42:39-42.

Horrobin DF. Essential fatty acid metabolism and its modification in atopic eczema. *Am J Clin Nutr.* 2000;71:367S-372S.

Johnson CD, Puntis M, Davidson N, Todd S, Bryce R. Randomized, dose-finding phase III study of lithium gamolenate in patients with advanced pancreatic adenocarcinoma. *Br J Surg.* 2001;88:662-668.

Kenny FS, Pinder SE, Ellis IO, Gee JM, Nicholson RI, Bryce RP, Robertson JF. Gamma linolenic acid with tamoxifen as primary therapy in breast cancer. *Int J Cancer.* 2000;85:643-648.

Kleijnen J. Evening primrose oil. *BMJ.* 1994;309:824-825.

Menendez JA, Ropero S, Lupu R, Colomer R. Omega-6 polyunsaturated fatty acid gamma-linolenic acid (18:3n-6) enhances docetaxel (Taxotere) cytotoxicity in human breast carcinoma cells: relationship to lipid peroxidation and HER-2/neu expression. *Oncol Rep.* 2004;11:1241-1252.

Menendez JA, Vellon L, Colomer R, Lupu R. Effect of gamma-linolenic acid on the transcriptional activity of the Her-2/neu (erbB-2) oncogene. *J Natl Cancer Inst.* 2005;97:1611-1615.

Phinney S. Potential risk of prolonged gamma-linolenic acid use. *Ann Intern Med.* 1994;120:692.

Whitehouse PA, Cooper AJ, Johnson CD. Synergistic activity of gamma-linolenic acid and cytotoxic drugs against pancreatic adenocarcinoma cell lines. *Pancreatology.* 2003;3:367-373; discussion 373-374. Epub 2003 Sep 24.

Williams HC. Evening primrose oil for atopic dermatitis. *BMJ.* 2003;327:1358-1359.

GLUCARATE

Other common name(s): calcium glucarate, calcium D-glucarate, D-glucarate
Scientific/medical name(s): D-glucaric acid

Description

Glucarate is a phytochemical or plant compound that is found in many fruits and vegetables, including apples, grapefruit, broccoli, brussels sprouts, and bean sprouts. It also occurs naturally in the body in very small amounts.

Overview

Several laboratory and animal studies have found that glucarate seems to have some anticancer effects; however, it has not yet been found to be effective in preventing or treating cancer in humans.

How is it promoted for use?

Proponents claim that glucarate may reduce the risk for colon, lung, liver, skin, prostate, and other types of cancer by increasing the body's ability to eliminate cancer-causing toxins that come from diet and the environment. Supporters also suggest that glucarate may hinder the formation of breast and uterine tumors by helping the body remove excess estrogen and other hormones that promote these diseases.

In dietary supplement form, glucarate is most commonly sold as calcium D-glucarate. Some companies market it as a detoxifying agent or as a supplement for "breast health."

What does it involve?

Glucarate is available as a dietary supplement (most commonly called calcium D-glucarate) in capsule and tablet form. There is no standard dosage.

What is the history behind it?

In the 1980s, cancer researchers found that glucarate supplements showed some anticancer properties in cancer cells and laboratory animals. Research has continued since that time. Some studies in humans are under way, but none have been published as of yet in the peer-reviewed medical literature.

What is the evidence?

Glucarate may have potential as an anticancer agent. However, there is no clinical evidence yet to show that the supplement is effective in treating cancer or lowering cancer risk in humans.

Once in the body, glucarate changes to a substance (d-glucaro-1,4-lactone) that is thought to inhibit a liver enzyme called beta-glucuronidase. This enzyme slows the elimination of certain hormones and chemicals from the body. By acting against beta-glucuronidase, glucarate may allow the body to get rid of these substances more quickly. Several studies have found higher levels of beta-glucuronidase in the tissues of people with cancer than in those without cancer. The significance of this finding is not fully understood. If beta-glucuronidase does play a role in cancer development or progression, the fact that glucarate can affect its activity may be important.

A number of animal studies published in peer-reviewed medical journals have found that fewer breast cancer tumors developed, and existing tumors shrank, in rats that were given dietary glucarate. Animal studies also found that dietary glucarate slowed the development of tumors in the colon, lung, liver, skin, and prostate. These results suggest that dietary glucarate is worthy of further study to evaluate its possible role in preventing and treating cancer in humans. A clinical study was undertaken in 2004, but did not advance beyond preliminary safety data. No clinical trials of glucarate's effectiveness in humans have been published in available medical journals.

Are there any possible problems or complications?

Glucarate seems to be fairly safe; there are no known side effects linked to its use. Glucarate affects beta-glucuronidase, a liver enzyme involved in removing chemicals from the body. It may affect how quickly the liver removes certain drugs from the body, which could change the amount you get when you take medication. It may also affect levels of hormones such as estrogen, which might alter the activity of birth control pills and other hormone-based medicines. Be sure to tell your doctor and pharmacist about any herbs and supplements you are taking. Relying on this type of treatment alone and avoiding or delaying conventional medical care for cancer may have serious health consequences.

This product is sold as a dietary supplement in the United States. Unlike companies that produce drugs (which must provide the FDA with results of detailed testing showing their product is safe and effective before the drug is approved for sale), the companies that make supplements do not have to show evidence of safety or health benefits to the FDA before selling their products. Supplement products without any reliable scientific evidence of health benefits may still be sold as long as the companies selling them do not claim the supplements can prevent, treat, or cure any specific disease. Some such products may not contain the amount of the herb or substance that is written on the label, and some may include other substances (contaminants). Though the FDA has written new rules to improve the quality of manufacturing processes for dietary supplements and the accurate listing of supplement ingredients, these rules do not take full effect until 2010. The new rules also do not address the safety of supplement ingredients or their effects on health when proper manufacturing techniques are used.

Most such supplements have not been tested to find out if they interact with medicines, foods, or other herbs and supplements. Even though some reports of interactions and harmful effects may be published, full studies of interactions and effects are not often available. Because of these limitations, any information on ill effects and interactions should be considered incomplete.

References

Abou-Issa H, Koolemans-Beynen A, Meredith TA, Webb TE. Antitumour synergism between non-toxic dietary combinations of isotretinoin and glucarate. *Eur J Cancer.* 1992;28A:784-788.

Abou-Issa H, Moeschberger M, el-Masry W, Tejwani S, Curley RW Jr, Webb TE. Relative efficacy of glucarate on the initiation and promotion phases of rat mammary carcinogenesis. *Anticancer Res.* 1995;15:805-810.

Calcium glucarate. Memorial Sloan-Kettering Cancer Center Web site. http://www.mskcc.org/mskcc/html/69158.cfm. Accessed June 11, 2008.

Dwivedi C, Oredipe OA, Barth RF, Downie AA, Webb TE. Effects of the experimental chemopreventive agent, glucarate, on intestinal carcinogenesis in rats. *Carcinogenesis.* 1989;10:1539-1541.

Heerdt AS, Young CW, Borgen PI. Calcium glucarate as a chemopreventive agent in breast cancer. *Isr J Med Sci.* 1995;31:101-105.

Walaszek Z, Hanausek M, Narog M, Raich PC, Slaga TJ. Mechanisms of lung cancer chemoprevention by D-glucarate. *Chest.* 2004;125:149S-150S.

Walaszek Z. Potential use of D-glucaric acid derivatives in cancer prevention. *Cancer Lett.* 1990;54:1-8.

Walaszek Z, Szemraj J, Narog M, Adams AK, Kilgore J, Sherman U, Hanausek M. Metabolism, uptake, and excretion of a D-glucaric acid salt and its potential use in cancer prevention. *Cancer Detect Prev.* 1997;21:178-190.

GREEK CANCER CURE

Other common name(s): METBAL, Cellbal, Alivizatos treatment
Scientific/medical name(s): none

Description

The Greek Cancer Cure consists of a blood test reportedly used to diagnose cancer and intravenous therapy designed to cure the disease. The injections are said to contain organic substances such as sugars, vitamins, amino acids, and other ingredients.

Overview

Available scientific evidence does not support claims that the Greek Cancer Cure is effective in preventing, detecting, or treating cancer.

How is it promoted for use?

Practitioners of the Greek Cancer Cure claim the regular use of a special intravenous injection, referred to as a serum, boosts the patient's immune system, enabling it to fight and destroy tumor cells. The inventor of the Greek Cancer Cure claimed to have cured a high percentage of patients who had cancer of the skin, bone, uterus, stomach, and lymphatic system.

What does it involve?

The first stage of the Greek Cancer Cure is a blood test that is said to pinpoint the nature, location, and extent of a patient's cancer. The second stage involves daily intravenous injections of the serum. Treatment lasts from six to thirty days. The secret formula is believed to consist of brown sugar, nicotinic acid (also known as niacin or vitamin B3), vitamin C, and alanine, an amino acid. A supplement that can be taken by mouth is also available.

Patients are advised to limit their intake of salts and acids, limit physical activities, and avoid drugs such as aspirin and laxatives. They are also asked to stop chemotherapy or radiation therapy before beginning the treatment program.

What is the history behind it?

The Greek Cancer Cure was developed in Athens, Greece during the 1970s by microbiologist

Hariton-Tzannis Alivizatos, MD. Dr. Alivizatos was investigated by Greek regulatory officials several times. At one point he lost his license to practice medicine because he failed to submit a sample of his serum to the government for testing. His license was reinstated after he finally agreed, but the Greek government could not establish the serum's effectiveness against cancer and ordered him to stop giving it to patients. In 1983, Dr. Alivizatos again lost his license, this time for two years, following an investigation by the Hellenic Medical Association. He resumed treating patients after the suspension expired.

On several occasions, the American Cancer Society and the National Cancer Institute asked Dr. Alivizatos to provide scientific documentation or information regarding his treatment, but all requests went unanswered. Throughout his career, Dr. Alivizatos closely guarded the details of his blood test and refused to share information with fellow cancer researchers. In 1979, a surgeon from Seattle traveled to Greece, posed as a cancer patient, and underwent treatment by Dr. Alivizatos. He returned with samples of the serum. An analysis conducted at the University of Washington revealed that the formula contained only nicotinic acid (niacin, or vitamin B3) and water.

Dr. Alivizatos died in 1991. Today, his treatment is marketed as METBAL or Cellbal and is reportedly offered in Greece, Poland, and some clinics in North America.

What is the evidence?

Available scientific evidence does not support claims that the Greek Cancer Cure has any effect on cancer. No studies have been published in the available peer-reviewed medical journals to show that the blood tests or the injections used in the Greek Cancer Cure result in any measurable benefit in the treatment of people with cancer.

Are there any possible problems or complications?

The safety of this treatment has not been proven. The intravenous serum can contain levels of nicotinic acid high enough to cause burning at the injection site or flushing of the face and chest. Relying on this type of treatment alone and avoiding or delaying conventional medical care for cancer may have serious health consequences.

These substances may have not been thoroughly tested to find out how they interact with medicines, foods, or dietary supplements. Even though some reports of interactions and harmful effects may be published, full studies of interactions and effects are not often available. Because of these limitations, any information on ill effects and interactions should be considered incomplete.

References

American Cancer Society. Greek cancer cure. *CA Cancer J Clin.* 1990;40:368-371.

Barrett S. Alivazatos Greek cancer cure. Quackwatch Web site. http://www.quackwatch.org/01QuackeryRelatedTopics/Cancer/greek.html. Updated February 14, 2005. Accessed June 11, 2008.

HOMEOPATHY

Other common name(s): homeopathic medicine
Scientific/medical name(s): none

Description

Homeopathy is based on the idea that if large doses of a substance cause a symptom, very small doses of that same substance will cure it. Homeopathic remedies are water-based or alcohol-based solutions containing tiny amounts of naturally occurring plants, minerals, animal products, or chemicals. The term "homeopathy" comes from the Greek words *homoios* (meaning "similar") and *pathos* (meaning "suffering").

Overview

While homeopathy appears to be safe, there is little if any reliable clinical evidence that homeopathic remedies are effective in treating cancer or that they can help with the side effects of cancer or its treatment.

How is it promoted for use?

Homeopathy is most often promoted for use in treating chronic or self-limiting problems such as arthritis, asthma, colds, flu, and allergies. However, some supporters believe that homeopathy can be used to treat and cure cancer.

Some practitioners claim homeopathy can help cancer patients by reducing pain, improving vitality and well-being, stopping the spread of cancer, and strengthening the immune system. Some claim it can lessen certain symptoms and side effects from radiation therapy, chemotherapy, and hormone therapy, such as infections, nausea, vomiting, mouth sores, hot flashes, hair loss, depression, weakness, and ascites (collection of fluid in the abdomen).

Proponents claim that homeopathic solutions, even though they may contain only small quantities (or none) of the original ingredient, contain a "memory" of the substance that somehow interacts with the body to cure illness. It is also believed that shaking or diluting a homeopathic solution releases the essence, or healing life force, of the material.

Some practitioners compare homeopathy to the beliefs of Ayurvedic and traditional Chinese medicine, which claim a need to bring the body into balance in order to restore health and wellness (see "Ayurveda," page 63, and "Chinese Herbal Medicine," page 313). Many supporters of homeopathy admit that they do not know how the treatments work, but insist that future research will unlock the mystery.

What does it involve?

Homeopathy is based largely on the "law of similars," or the notion that "like cures like." In other words, a substance that causes symptoms of illness in a healthy person can relieve those same symptoms in a sick person when given in very small amounts. For example, a patient complaining of vomiting and diarrhea might receive a solution containing tiny amounts of thorn apple, since larger amounts of that herb cause those symptoms.

The second important tenet of homeopathy is the "law of infinitesimals," which states that the more a homeopathic solution is diluted, the more powerful it becomes.

When a patient complains of certain symptoms, the homeopath consults a reference guide that lists thousands of individual symptoms and searches for an entry that matches the patient's description. The remedy, which is determined by the person's health history and symptoms, is called the "simillium." The practitioner then takes this simillium—an extract of the plant, mineral, animal product, or chemical remedy that matches the patient's symptoms—and repeatedly dilutes it, usually in water.

In the terminology of homeopathy, adding one part extract to nine parts water yields a 1X solution (X is the Roman numeral for ten), while adding one part extract to ninety-nine parts water yields a 1C solution (C is the Roman numeral for one hundred). (The 1X and 1C homeopathic dilutions are called 1:10 and 1:100 dilutions, respectively, in conventional chemistry.) The solution is mixed vigorously, and one part of it is diluted again in nine (or ninety-nine) parts water, yielding a 2X (or 2C) solution, and so on. A 6X dilution, for example, would result in one part extract per one million parts water.

Each solution may go through the dilution process as many as thirty to fifty times, to the point where it may be very unlikely that even a single molecule of the original extract remains. Homeopaths believe that even if this is the case, the remaining water retains some type of "memory" of the extract. After the dilution process is complete, the patient is given the remedy to drink or place under the tongue.

What is the history behind it?

Some of the ideas that form the basis of homeopathy go back to the ancient Greeks, but the "modern" version is credited to the German physician Samuel Hahnemann. He developed homeopathy early in the 1800s as a more civilized alternative to some of the harsh medical practices of the time, such as bloodletting and purging. Dr. Hahnemann believed a substance that caused specific symptoms in a healthy person could cure those same symptoms in a sick person, so he gave his patients diluted doses of the offending substances.

To determine the specific effects of each material, Dr. Hahnemann and his assistants conducted "provings," during which they ingested plants, minerals, and other materials, then noted what symptoms resulted. From these experiments, Hahnemann compiled a reference book containing descriptions of the effects of various materials and recommended homeopathic remedies.

In the 1800s, homeopathy may have been better for people than mainstream medicine in some instances, if for no other reason than it did less harm than some of the harsh and ineffective practices used at the time. Homeopathy remained popular through the beginning of the twentieth century, when a better understanding of what caused many diseases and how they could be treated emerged.

The 1938 Food, Drug, and Cosmetic Act required that all drugs be tested for safety before being approved by the U.S. Food and Drug Administration (FDA) and sold to the public. This act also allowed any homeopathic remedy that was included in a standard reference book to be considered a legal drug. However, homeopathic remedies have never been held to the same standards of manufacturing or testing for safety or effectiveness as standard drugs.

Along with the general growth of complementary and alternative methods in recent years, homeopathy has become a more popular alternative form of therapy in the United States.

What is the evidence?

Few laboratory studies of homeopathic remedies have been published, and results are sometimes conflicting. In two 2006 studies, researchers found that homeopathic solutions had no effect on breast or prostate cancer cells growing in laboratory cultures, but that similar solutions slowed the growth of prostate cancer in rats.

There is no reliable clinical evidence showing that homeopathic remedies can treat cancer. The basic premises of homeopathy, developed more than two hundred years ago, are not in agreement with modern scientific principles. Some researchers suggest, however, that homeopathy may result in helpful effects for patients who believe the treatment is working—a phenomenon known as the placebo or expectation effect. One study on the increased use of complementary therapies by people with cancer showed that while certain complementary therapies had no actual antitumor effect, patients reported psychological improvement including increased hope and optimism. The complementary therapies studied included homeopathy.

Some small clinical studies have hinted that homeopathic solutions may have some benefit in reducing certain side effects of cancer or its treatment, but other studies have found them to be no better than a placebo. The number of patients in these studies has usually been small, and few of them have been done. A 2006 review of published studies concluded that "… analysis of published literature on homeopathy found insufficient evidence to support clinical efficacy of homeopathic therapy in cancer care" (*Eur J Cancer.* 2006;42:282). Further research would be needed before homeopathy could be considered likely to be useful for any aspect of cancer care.

Are there any possible problems or complications?

Although some homeopathic solutions contain toxic chemicals, they are typically present in amounts too small to present any danger. Relying on this type of treatment alone and avoiding or delaying conventional medical care for cancer may have serious health consequences.

This product is sold as a dietary supplement in the United States. Unlike companies that produce drugs (which must provide the FDA with results of detailed testing showing their product is safe and effective before the drug is approved for sale), the companies that make supplements do not have to show evidence of safety or health benefits to the FDA before selling their products. Supplement products without any reliable scientific evidence of health benefits may still be sold as long as the companies selling them do not claim the supplements can prevent, treat, or cure any specific disease. Some such products may not contain the amount of the herb or substance that is written on the label, and some may include other substances (contaminants). Though the FDA has written new rules to improve the quality of manufacturing processes for dietary supplements and the accurate listing of supplement ingredients, these rules do not take full effect until 2010. The new rules also do not address the safety of supplement ingredients or their effects on health when proper manufacturing techniques are used.

Most such supplements have not been tested to find out if they interact with medicines, foods, or other herbs and supplements. Even though some reports of interactions and harmful effects may be published, full studies of interactions and effects are not often available. Because of these limitations, any information on ill effects and interactions should be considered incomplete.

References

Alternative medical systems: homeopathy detailed scientific review. Complementary/Integrative Medicine Education Resources, The University of Texas M. D. Anderson Cancer Center Web site. http://www.mdanderson.org/departments/cimer/display.cfm?id=86407E5A-13EE-11D5-811000508B603A14&method=displayFull. Accessed June 11, 2008.

Cassileth B. *The Alternative Medicine Handbook: The Complete Reference Guide to Alternative and Complementary Therapies.* New York: W.W. Norton; 1998.

Downer SM, Cody MM, McCluskey P, Wilson PD, Arnott SJ, Lister TA, Slevin ML. Pursuit and practice of complementary therapies by cancer patients receiving conventional treatment. *BMJ.* 1994;309:86-89.

Holmes OW. Homeopathy and its kindred delusions. Quackwatch Web site. http://www.quackwatch.org/01QuackeryRelatedTopics/holmes.html. Posted March 26, 1999. Accessed June 11, 2008.

Homeopathy. Memorial Sloan-Kettering Cancer Center Web site. http://www.mskcc.org/mskcc/html/69254.cfm. Accessed June 11, 2008.

Jonas WB, Gaddipati J, Rajeshkumar N, Sharma A, Thangapazham RL, Warren J, Singh AK, Ives JA, Olsen C, Mog SR, Maheshwari RK. Can homeopathic treatment slow prostate cancer growth? *Integr Cancer Ther.* 2006;5:343-349.

Milazzo S, Russell N, Ernst E. Efficacy of homeopathic therapy in cancer treatment. *Eur J Cancer.* 2006;42:282-289. Epub 2006 Jan 11.

Oberbaum M, Yaniv I, Ben-Gal Y, Stein J, Ben-Zvi N, Freedman LS, Branski D. A randomized, controlled clinical trial of the homeopathic medication TRAUMEEL S in the treatment of chemotherapy-induced stomatitis in children undergoing stem cell transplantation. *Cancer.* 2001;92:684-690.

Sampson W. Inconsistencies and errors in alternative medicine research. *Skeptical Inquirer.* 1997;21:35-38.

Shang A, Huwiler-Müntener K, Nartey L, Jüni P, Dörig S, Sterne JA, Pewsner D, Egger M. Are the clinical effects of homoeopathy placebo effects? Comparative study of placebo-controlled trials of homoeopathy and allopathy. *Lancet.* 2005;366:726-732.

Shehlin I. Homeopathy: real medicine or empty promises? *FDA Consumer: The Magazine of the US Food and Drug Administration.* December 1996. US Food and Drug Administration Web site. http://www.fda.gov/fdac/features/096_home.html. Accessed June 11, 2008.

Thangapazham RL, Gaddipati JP, Rajeshkumar NV, Sharma A, Singh AK, Ives JA, Maheshwari RK, Jonas WB. Homeopathic medicines do not alter growth and gene expression in prostate and breast cancer cells in vitro. *Integr Cancer Ther.* 2006;5:356-361.

HYDRAZINE SULFATE

Other common name(s): Sehydrin, HS
Scientific/medical name(s): none

Description

Hydrazine sulfate is a chemical commonly used in industrial processes, such as rare metal refining and the making of rocket fuel, rust-prevention products, and insecticides. It is used as an alternative method to treat some symptoms of advanced cancer. Hydrazine sulfate is usually produced in a laboratory but does occur naturally in some plants and mushrooms.

Overview

Most carefully designed clinical studies have not shown that hydrazine sulfate helps people with cancer live longer or feel better. Some, but not all, studies have found it may help reduce weight loss in those with advanced cancer. It may also cause potentially serious side effects.

How is it promoted for use?

Supporters claim hydrazine sulfate may relieve cachexia, a syndrome marked by loss of appetite, weight loss, weakness, and muscle wasting. It is one of the most devastating syndromes resulting from cancer and conditions such as AIDS. Cachexia affects about half of all cancer patients, especially those with advanced cancer of the lung, pancreas, or digestive system. It causes about 10 to 20 percent of all cancer deaths.

According to some theories, cancer cachexia is caused by cancerous tumors using too much energy (in the form of blood sugar), preventing it from being used for normal body functions. For example, energy that should be used to maintain muscle mass is redirected to the tumor. Supporters claim that hydrazine sulfate may block a key enzyme that controls blood sugar levels in the body, restoring the proper energy balance and halting the progressive decline of cachexia.

There are also claims that hydrazine sulfate might affect the cancer itself. By affecting blood sugar levels, it may help prevent tumors from getting more fuel to grow.

What does it involve?

Hydrazine sulfate is usually given as a pill or capsule. It can also be injected. A common dose is 60 milligrams, three times a day for thirty-five to forty days. Treatment is then stopped for two to six weeks. This cycle can be repeated many times.

Hydrazine sulfate is not approved for use with cancer patients in the United States. Doctors can obtain it through the investigational new drug (IND) program of the U.S. Food and Drug Administration (FDA). In Canada, hydrazine sulfate is available by prescription. It is widely used in Europe and in Russia, where it is known as Sehydrin.

What is the history behind it?

Different hydrazine compounds have been studied for more than ninety years as a treatment for cancer and to reduce the symptoms associated with cancer such as weight loss, fatigue, muscle wasting, and decreased appetite. One hydrazine compound, procarbazine, is approved by the FDA for use against cancer.

Hydrazine sulfate was popularized as an unconventional cancer treatment in the mid-1970s by a cancer researcher, Joseph Gold, MD, director of the Syracuse Cancer Research Institute in New York. He based his ideas on the research of Otto Warburg, winner of the Nobel Prize in Medicine in 1931. Dr. Gold reported that hydrazine sulfate inhibited the growth of tumors in rodents as well as in people with advanced cancer. He recommended its use for people with several kinds of cancer, including cancer of the breast, colon, rectum, ovary, lung, and thyroid, Hodgkin's disease and other lymphomas, melanomas, and neuroblastomas. He believed it would be most effective used with conventional cancer treatments.

Hydrazine sulfate was a popular alternative cancer treatment in the United States until the FDA stopped companies from selling it directly to the public in the mid-1970s.

Several studies were conducted in the 1980s and 1990s using hydrazine sulfate with chemotherapy. These studies are discussed in more detail below.

What is the evidence?

Studies show that hydrazine sulfate has many effects in the body. However, research has produced conflicting results. Some studies have found that hydrazine sulfate inhibits the growth of cancerous tumors in laboratory animals, while others report that the chemical can damage DNA and trigger the development of tumors. It also may promote the growth of existing tumors. Some early laboratory studies found that hydrazine sulfate increased the occurrence of tumors in some animals. It is still unclear whether hydrazine sulfate causes or contributes to the development of cancer in humans.

One reason offered to support the use of hydrazine sulfate—that cachexia occurs because cancer cells use too much energy—is inconsistent with the way cachexia is now understood to work. Cachexia is a complex process and is caused largely by cancer cells releasing hormones and other substances that influence the function of normal cells.

Research on hydrazine sulfate in humans has not been encouraging. Several randomized clinical trials found that hydrazine sulfate treatment did not reduce the size of tumors or increase patient survival time. Some patients reported feeling better for brief periods during treatment with hydrazine sulfate, including reports of less pain, lower fever, and increased appetite. Other studies reported that patients treated with the chemical had more normal glucose metabolism, weight gain, and improved appetite. Some patients developed feelings of well-being after nearly six months of therapy.

A 1990 study of sixty-five patients with advanced lung cancer found that adding hydrazine sulfate to their chemotherapy regimen improved their nutritional status. Patients consumed more calories and showed other positive metabolic changes. Patients who started the study in better condition and were given hydrazine sulfate lived longer than those taking a placebo. Among those who started in worse condition, hydrazine sulfate did not improve survival. Based on this study, the National Cancer Institute (NCI) felt that further studies with more patients were needed.

Reports published in 1994 based on three studies sponsored by NCI described outcomes of a total of 636 patients. Two studies looked at advanced lung cancer patients who also were receiving chemotherapy. The third study was limited to patients with advanced colorectal cancer not receiving chemotherapy. In all three studies, patients were randomly chosen to receive hydrazine sulfate or a placebo. None of these well-controlled studies showed that hydrazine sulfate provided a benefit to cancer patients. Nerve damage occurred more often and quality of life was worse among the group receiving hydrazine sulfate. In the colorectal cancer study, survival was shorter in the hydrazine sulfate group. After the studies were published, supporters of hydrazine sulfate claimed that the studies were flawed because some of the patients were getting other drugs (such as tranquilizers) that could alter the drug's effectiveness. A review by the U.S. General Accounting Office found that the studies were done correctly and that their conclusions were valid.

Are there any possible problems or complications?

Side effects are uncommon but can include mild to moderate levels of nausea, vomiting, itching, dizziness, poor motor coordination, and/or tingling or numbness in the hands and feet. Hydrazine sulfate is a moderate monoamine oxidase inhibitor (MAOI). It should not be taken with certain anti-anxiety medicines, cough suppressants (such as dextromethorphan), stimulants (amphetamines), antidepressants, tranquilizers, barbiturates, alcohol, or foods high in tyramine (for example, aged cheeses and fermented products), as it could lead to very high blood pressure levels and other potential harm.

At very high doses, hydrazine sulfate may cause liver damage. People with diabetes should use hydrazine sulfate with caution, as it may affect blood sugar levels. Women who are pregnant or breastfeeding should not use this therapy. Hydrazine sulfate increases development of some forms of cancer in laboratory animals and has been classified as a potential carcinogen by the National Toxicology Program of the U.S. Department of Health and Human Services.

Relying on this type of treatment alone and avoiding or delaying conventional medical care for cancer may have serious health consequences.

This substance has not been thoroughly tested to find out how it interacts with medicines, foods, or dietary supplements. Even though some reports of interactions and harmful effects may be published,

full studies of interactions and effects are not often available. Because of these limitations, any information on ill effects and interactions should be considered incomplete.

References

Biologic/organic/pharmacologic therapies: hydrazine sulfate detailed scientific review. Complementary/Integrative Medicine Education Resources, The University of Texas M. D. Anderson Cancer Center Web site. http://www.mdanderson.org/departments/cimer/display.cfm?id=AD1A435D-17B1-11D5-811000508B603A14&method=displayFull. Accessed June 11, 2008.

Chlebowski RT, Bulcavage L, Grosvenor M, Oktay E, Block JB, Chlebowski JS, Ali I, Elashoff R. Hydrazine sulfate influence on nutritional status and survival in non-small-cell lung cancer. *J Clin Oncol.* 1990;8:9-15.

Hydrazine sulfate. Memorial Sloan-Kettering Cancer Center Web site. http://www.mskcc.org/mskcc/html/69260.cfm. Accessed June 11, 2008.

Hydrazine sulfate (PDQ®). National Cancer Institute Web site. http://www.cancer.gov/cancertopics/pdq/cam/hydrazinesulfate/HealthProfessional/page1. Accessed June 11, 2008.

Kaegi E; Task Force on Alternative Therapies of the Canadian Breast Cancer Research Initiative. Unconventional therapies for cancer: 4. Hydrazine sulfate. *CMAJ.* 1998;158:1327-1330. *CMAJ* Web site. http://www.cmaj.ca/cgi/reprint/158/10/1327. Accessed June 11, 2008.

Kosty MP, Fleishman SB, Herndon JE II, Coughlin K, Kornblith AB, Scalzo A, Morris JC, Mortimer J, Green MR. Cisplatin, vinblastine, and hydrazine sulfate in advanced, non-small-cell lung cancer: a randomized placebo-controlled, double-blind phase III study of the Cancer and Leukemia Group B. *J Clin Oncol.* 1994;12:1113-1120.

Loprinzi CL, Goldberg RM, Su JQ, Mailliard JA, Kuross SA, Maksymiuk AW, Kugler JW, Jett JR, Ghosh C, Pfeifle DM, et al. Placebo-controlled trial of hydrazine sulfate in patients with newly diagnosed non-small-cell lung cancer. *J Clin Oncol.* 1994;12:1126-1129.

Loprinzi CL, Kuross SA, O'Fallon JR, Gesme DH Jr, Gerstner JB, Rospond RM, Cobau CD, Goldberg RM. Randomized placebo-controlled evaluation of hydrazine sulfate in patients with advanced colorectal cancer. *J Clin Oncol.* 1994;12:1121-1125.

Morley JE, Thomas DR, Wilson MM. Cachexia: pathophysiology and clinical relevance. *Am J Clin Nutr.* 2006;83:735-743.

Tisdale MJ. Biology of cachexia. *J Natl Cancer Inst.* 1997;89:1763-1773.

IMMUNO-AUGMENTATIVE THERAPY

Other common name(s): immunoaugmentative therapy, immune augmentative therapy, immune augmentation therapy, immuno-augmentation therapy, IAT

Scientific/medical name(s): none

Description

Immuno-augmentative therapy (IAT) is promoted as an alternative form of cancer treatment. It consists of daily injections of a protein mixture made from human blood with the goal of helping the patient's immune system to attack the cancer. The protein mixture is claimed to contain antitumor antibodies and "deblocking proteins" from healthy donors.

Overview

Available scientific evidence does not support claims that IAT is effective in treating cancer. The existence of "blocking" and "deblocking" proteins has not been verified. In the past, infections have developed in some patients while they were receiving this treatment, although currently this does not seem to be a problem.

IAT should not be confused with immunotherapy, a type of mainstream cancer treatment that uses cytokines (immune system hormones), antibodies, vaccines, and other methods to boost the immune system's attack on cancer cells.

How is it promoted for use?

Proponents claim IAT is a safe, nontoxic, and effective treatment for all types of cancer. They claim IAT causes cancer to stabilize or go into remission. It is not promoted as a cure for cancer, but as a long-term treatment. Like diabetics, IAT patients are told that they can live normal lives as long as they continue to have daily injections.

Practitioners of IAT believe that cancer cells begin to grow and multiply when a person's immune system is out of balance. The components of IAT, which are derived from human blood, consist of antitumor antibodies, which are believed to attack the cancer, and "deblocking proteins," which supposedly remove a "blocking factor" that prevents the patient's immune system from detecting the cancer.

What does it involve?

This therapy involves daily injections under the skin of a protein mixture made from human blood. The first IAT session requires a trip to an IAT clinic. At the clinic, a patient is given a physical exam and blood and urine tests. The results of these tests are fed into a computer program to determine the patient's immune system status. Once this is done, IAT treatment begins. Patients are given daily IAT injections according to their particular situation. Blood tests are done once or twice a day, five days a week, to measure "immune response" and to determine the dose of treatment to be given the next day. Treatment continues until the practitioner believes that the patient's cancer is controlled.

The initial treatments require patients to stay in the area of the clinic for an average of two to three months. The patient is then shown how to self-inject and is sent home to continue treatment, although further clinic visits may be needed.

What is the history behind it?

According to a 1991 review article in *CA: A Cancer Journal for Clinicians*, biologist Lawrence Burton, PhD, developed IAT in the early 1970s, based on his research with fruit flies and mice. He developed a mixture of blood proteins that he believed would slow or stop the growth of cancer cells. He claimed that IAT caused cancer in mice to go into remission. However, a 1990 report from the U.S. Office of Technology Assessment (OTA) said that other researchers questioned the validity of Burton's claims and tried to replicate his experiments but could not achieve the same results.

According to the OTA report, Dr. Burton first offered his treatment to cancer patients in 1973, when he and some sponsors established the Immunology Research Foundation in Great Neck, New York. The *CA* article notes that in 1974, Dr. Burton submitted an investigational new drug application to the U.S. Food and Drug Administration (FDA) to begin human trials with IAT. He later withdrew his application when the FDA asked for further details about his experimental evidence.

In 1977, Dr. Burton closed his New York clinic and opened the Immunology Researching Centre (IRC) in the Bahamas. According to the OTA report, representatives of the Bahamian Ministry of Health and the Pan American Health Organization visited his facility in 1978 and reviewed the charts of several patients. According to their site visit report, "no consistent treatment effect has been achieved when assessed by objective criteria...The material being used to treat patients is similarly a totally unknown quantity. Although the various fractions are referred to by Dr. Burton as 'antibody fractions' and 'complement fractions,' there is in fact no evidence that any of these fractions do contain antibody of any relevance to the tumor involved or that in fact there are any active or even inactive complement components" (Terry and Litvak, 1978).

The OTA report mentioned that the representatives noted that the "[Immunology Researching Centre] was not carrying out its stated intent…to evaluate IAT as a cancer treatment" (*Unconventional Cancer Treatments*: *OTA-H-405*;1990:134). The report concluded that "the present procedures of the Center do not permit any meaningful evaluation" (*OTA-H-405*;1990:134) and recommended that the clinic be closed. The clinic remained open despite these findings. The OTA report stated that Bahamian health authorities closed the clinic in 1985 on charges that the compounds used for IAT injections may have been contaminated with hepatitis B virus and human immunodeficiency virus (HIV), after samples were tested by the state of Washington's Health Department and the CDC. The clinic reopened less than a year later. In the late 1980s, Dr. Burton opened additional clinics in West Germany and Mexico.

The OTA report noted that during the late 1970s and early 1980s, National Cancer Institute officials contacted Dr. Burton asking to evaluate his IAT techniques. No agreement could be reached on research methods and Dr. Burton never disclosed his technique for isolating the blood proteins in IAT, which he had patented. In 1986, the OTA, working with Dr. Burton, developed procedures for a clinical trial of IAT on patients with colon cancer. Communication between Dr. Burton, and the OTA eventually broke down and the OTA's final report stated that "no reliable data are available on which to base a determination of IAT's efficacy" (*OTA-H-405*; 1990:139-140). The OTA report stated that the FDA imposed a ban on the import of IAT drugs in 1986 "due to the direct hazards that have been associated with IAT agents" (Import alert 57-04, 1986).

Dr. Burton died in 1993, but his clinic in the Bahamas continues to operate. Though the clinic has had a different name since 2003, the clinic's Web site notes that it is part of the IRC.

What is the evidence?

The concept that cancer can be treated by enhancing the activity of the immune system is reasonable and is the basis for mainstream immunotherapy. Unlike IAT, however, conventional immunotherapy is founded on scientific principles of immunology and has been tested in clinical trials. It has been shown to be useful in treating melanoma, lymphoma, kidney cancer, bladder cancer, and other types of cancer.

Available scientific evidence does not support claims that IAT is effective in treating people with cancer. Success stories associated with the treatment are based mainly on individual reports provided by Dr. Burton's clinics, and they include little or no supporting evidence.

No outside laboratories or researchers have confirmed the existence of the "blocking" or "deblocking" proteins, which are an essential part of Dr. Burton's theory and treatment. The 1991 *CA* article notes that a contract between Dr. Burton and MetPath (now Quest Diagnostics), a large biomedical laboratory firm, was terminated in December 1980: "According to a 1981 letter from Paul Brown, MD, Chairman of the Board of MetPath at the time of the interaction with Burton, MetPath was unable to develop a reliable test based on Burton's information and "extensive laboratory testing." There were 25 percent false positives in patients without cancer, and 25 percent false negatives in patients with cancer" (*OTA-H-405*;1990:136).

There have been no published reports of randomized controlled clinical trials or of any type of prospective studies of IAT.

Dr. Burton published one best case series of eleven patients with mesothelioma (a cancer of the lining surrounding the lungs or other organs) in 1988. The extent of the patients' cancer was not described. According to the report, the average survival time on IAT was about thirty months, which is longer than is normally seen in these patients. This was a small group of selected patients, and no formal studies have been done to confirm these results.

Another small best case series was conducted for the Agency for Healthcare Research and Quality to determine if IAT warranted further study. Researchers looked at the medical records of sixty cancer patients treated at the IAT clinic in the Bahamas. Of these, nine were found to have had positive outcomes and enough verified data to be considered in the series, although the researchers noted that even some of these records were not complete. While this was a selected best case series and not a predesigned study, the overall suggestion was that there was enough evidence "to recommend that a random controlled trial could be considered" (*AHRQ Publication No.03-E030*, 2003).

Researchers from the University of Kentucky evaluated the results of forty-six cancer patients treated consecutively at an IAT clinic in Mexico during 1989 and published their findings in June 2003. While no significant side effects were noted, none of the patients' tumors shrank. In forty patients (87 percent), the cancer progressed, and twenty-five of these patients died within six months. Quality of life got worse in thirty-five of the forty-six patients during the three months of treatment, although overall, thirty-eight of the patients decided to continue getting IAT. The researchers concluded that the study did not justify the continued use of IAT.

Are there any possible problems and complications?

The safety of IAT has not been established in clinical studies. Based on individual reports from patients who have received IAT, side effects appear to be minor and include fatigue, pain at the injection site, and flu-like symptoms. Some medical professionals fear that infectious agents, such as HIV and hepatitis B virus, may contaminate the unregulated compounds used in IAT, which come from human blood. While there were reports of such exposures in the 1980s, none have been reported in recent years. Relying on this type of treatment and avoiding or delaying conventional medical care for cancer may have serious health consequences.

These substances may have not been thoroughly tested to find out how they interact with medicines, foods, or dietary supplements. Even though some reports of interactions and harmful effects may be

published, full studies of interactions and effects are not often available. Because of these limitations, any information on ill effects and interactions should be considered incomplete.

References

American Cancer Society. Questionable methods of cancer management. Immuno-augmentative therapy (IAT). *CA Cancer J Clin.* 1991;41:357-364.

Barrett S. Immuno-augmentative therapy (IAT). http://www.quackwatch.org/01QuackeryRelatedTopics/Cancer/iat.html. Posted November 9, 1999. Accessed June 11, 2008.

Biologic/organic/pharmacologic therapies: immune augmentation therapy (IAT) detailed scientific review. Complementary/Integrative Medicine Education Resources, The University of Texas M. D. Anderson Cancer Center Web site. http://www.mdanderson.org/departments/cimer/display.cfm?id=ADFAC0FB-16E9-11D5-811000508B603A14&method=displayFull. Accessed June 11, 2008.

Clement RJ, Burton L, Lampe GN. Peritoneal mesothelioma. *Quant Med J Comp Thera.* 1988;1:68-73.

Coulter I, Hardy M, Shekelle P, et al. *Best-Case Series for the Use of Immuno-Augmentation Therapy and Naltrexone for the Treatment of Cancer.* Evidence Report/Technology Assessment No. 78 (Prepared by Southern California-RAND Evidence-based Practice Center under Contract No 290-97-0001). Rockville, MD: Agency for Healthcare Research and Quality. April 2003. AHRQ Publication No. 03-E030.

Green S. Immunoaugmentative therapy. An unproven cancer treatment. *JAMA.* 1993;270:1719-1723.

Pfeifer BL, Jonas WB. Clinical evaluation of "immunoaugmentative therapy (IAT)": an unconventional cancer treatment. *Integr Cancer Ther.* 2003;2:112-119.

Terry W, Litvak J. Report to the Ministry of Health on the site visit to the Immunology Researching Centre, Ltd., Freeport, Grand Bahamas Island, Bahamas. Unpublished document. Pan American Health Organization, Document BdXUTMS-5100, AMRO-1700: January 29-31, 1978. Quoted by: *Unconventional Cancer Treatments: OTA-H-405,*134.

US Congress, Office of Technology Assessment. *Unconventional Cancer Treatments: OTA-H-405.* Washington, DC: US Government Printing Office; 1990.

US Department of Health and Human Services, Public Health Service, Food and Drug Administration. Immuno-Augmentative Therapy (IAT), Import Alert 57-04. In: *Regulatory Procedure Manual,* Part 9, Imports, Chapter 7-79. August 6, 1986. Quoted by: *Unconventional Cancer Treatments: OTA-H-405,* 129.

INOSINE PRANOBEX

Other common name(s): Isoprinosine, Imunovir, methisoprinol, inosiplex, inosinpranobex
Scientific/medical name(s): none

Description

Inosine pranobex is a drug that may mimic the actions of immune-stimulating hormones made in the thymus gland. It is used primarily in European countries, mainly as a treatment for viral infections. It is not used for cancer treatment by conventional oncologists in Europe or anywhere else, but is occasionally recommended on alternative medicine Web sites as an anticancer treatment or for enhancing the immune systems of people living with cancer.

Overview

Available scientific evidence does not support claims that inosine pranobex is effective in treating cancer. The drug is not approved by the U.S. Food and Drug Administration (FDA) and cannot be sold legally in pharmacies in the United States.

How is it promoted for use?

Proponents claim inosine pranobex strengthens the immune system and fights viral infections. They also say it may lower the risk for infection in people being treated for cancer, who often have weakened immune systems. Some assert that it may boost the effects of interferon, which is a drug sometimes used against viral infections and certain types of cancer. Inosine pranobex may also increase the activity of helper T-cells and natural killer cells (types of white blood cells), which may in turn help stop tumors from growing. Some practitioners recommend it as an alternative to conventional cancer therapy. Others suggest that inosine pranobex be used along with mainstream cancer treatment

At one time inosine pranobex was promoted as a way for athletes to improve their endurance and performance, although studies have not borne this out. More recently, it has been promoted for possible use against chronic fatigue syndrome. It is currently used (mostly in European countries) to treat people with AIDS and other viral diseases, including herpes, shingles, warts, influenza, and the common cold and viral infections of the liver (hepatitis) and brain (encephalitis).

What does it involve?

Inosine pranobex is taken as a capsule or tablet. There is no standard dosage, although some studies have used between 1 and 4 grams per day. Some practitioners recommend a maximum of 3 grams per day for autoimmune diseases, with the daily dose divided up and spread evenly throughout the day (for instance, 1 gram every eight hours for a total of 3 grams per day). Some further suggest that the dose be "pulsed," that is, taken for a week or two then stopped for up to a month before restarting.

What is the history behind it?

Inosine pranobex was patented in the late 1960s and has been studied against a number of viral conditions as far back as the early 1970s. In 1981, the FDA refused to allow the drug to be marketed in the United States, citing a lack of evidence that it was effective. Today it is sold in Europe and elsewhere as a treatment for a number of viral diseases, including herpes, influenza, and viral hepatitis.

What is the evidence?

A number of animal and laboratory studies—done mostly in Europe—have found that inosine pranobex increases the activity of helper T-cells and natural killer cells. Although a substantial increase in activity of these immune system cells could slow the growth of tumors, there is no reliable clinical evidence that inosine pranobex is of any clinical value in the treatment of people with cancer. Thus far, very few studies have looked at the effectiveness of inosine pranobex against cancer in people. A French study found no difference in survival or recurrence rates between sixty lung cancer patients treated with surgery alone and another sixty treated with surgery and inosine pranobex. In another, much smaller study, researchers concluded that inosine pranobex combined with the chemotherapy drug 5-fluorouracil was not effective in the treatment of metastatic colorectal cancer. The most recent clinical trial, published in 2003, reported no benefit in patients with melanoma. A 1978 article reported no benefit of inosine pranobex in treating pediatric cancer patients with herpes virus infections. There appears to be little current research on the use of inosine pranobex against cancer.

Based on a large study conducted in Sweden and Denmark, researchers reported in 1990 that inosine pranobex delays the onset of AIDS in people with human immunodeficiency virus (HIV). However, the FDA pointed out several important flaws in the study and noted that other large studies have not found inosine pranobex to be helpful. The FDA concluded that more study was needed before its value for HIV-infected patients could be sufficiently evaluated. There has been substantial progress in treatment of HIV infection and AIDS since 1990, and researchers in this field have since turned their attention to more promising drugs.

Several small studies have suggested that inosine pranobex may be effective, when combined with interferon, to treat subacute sclerosing panencephalitis, a fairly rare brain infection caused by the measles virus. Some studies suggest inosine pranobex may be useful as a treatment for genital warts. More research is needed to confirm these findings.

Are there any possible problems or complications?

The safety of inosine pranobex has not been studied extensively, although it seems to be fairly well tolerated. Some studies have reported possible side effects including dizziness, stomach upset, and heartburn. Inosine pranobex increases blood levels of uric acid, which can increase the risk for gout or kidney stones. Interactions with other drugs are unknown. Talk with your doctor and pharmacist about all the medicines and supplements you are taking before adding inosine pranobex.

Information on the effects of inosine pranobex during pregnancy and breastfeeding is not available. Relying on this type of treatment and avoiding or delaying conventional medical care for cancer may have serious health consequences.

This product is sold as a dietary supplement in the United States. Unlike companies that produce drugs (which must provide the FDA with results of detailed testing showing their product is safe and effective before the drug is approved for sale), the companies that make supplements do not have to show evidence of safety or health benefits to the FDA before selling their products. Supplement products without any reliable scientific evidence of health benefits may still be sold as long as the companies selling them do not claim the supplements can prevent, treat, or cure any specific disease. Some such products may not contain the amount of the herb or substance that is written on the label, and some may include other substances (contaminants). Though the FDA has written new rules to improve the quality of manufacturing processes for dietary supplements and the accurate listing of supplement ingredients, these rules do not take full effect until 2010. The new rules also do not address the safety of supplement ingredients or their effects on health when proper manufacturing techniques are used.

Most such supplements have not been tested to find out if they interact with medicines, foods, or other herbs and supplements. Even though some reports of interactions and harmful effects may be published, full studies of interactions and effects are not often available. Because of these limitations, any information on ill effects and interactions should be considered incomplete.

References

Colozza M, Tonato M, Belsanti V, Mosconi AM, Fiorucci S, Gernini I, Rambotti P, Davis S. 5-Fluorouracil and isoprinosine in the treatment of advanced colorectal cancer. A limited phase I, II evaluation. *Cancer.* 1988;15:1049-1052.

Feldman S, Hayes FA, Chaudhary S, Ossi M. Inosiplex for localized herpes zoster in childhood cancer patients: preliminary controlled study. *Antimicrob Agents Chemother.* 1978;14:495-497.

Gascon GG; International Consortium on Subacute Sclerosing Panencephalitis. Randomized treatment study of inosiplex versus combined inosiplex and intraventricular interferon-alpha in subacute sclerosing panencephalitis (SSPE): international multicenter study. *J Child Neurol.* 2003;18:819-827.
Erratum in:
J Child Neurol. 2004;19:342.

Georgala S, Katoulis AC, Befon A, Georgala C, Rigopoulos D. Oral inosiplex in the treatment of cervical condylomata acuminata: a randomised placebo-controlled trial. *BJOG.* 2006;113;1088-1091.

Imunovir Data Sheet. Medsafe Web site. http://www.medsafe.govt.nz/Profs/Datasheet/i/Imunovirtab.htm. Accessed September 1, 2008.

Khayat D, Rixe O, Martin G, Soubrane C, Banzet M, Bazex JA, Lauret P, Verola O, Auclerc G, Harper P, Banzet P; French Group of Research on Malignant Melanoma. Surgical margins in cutaneous melanoma (2 cm versus 5 cm for lesions measuring less than 2.1-mm thick). *Cancer.* 2003;97:1941-1946.

Kweder SL, Schnur RA, Cooper EC. Inosine pranobex—is a single positive trial enough? *N Engl J Med.* 1990;322:1807-1809.

Pedersen C, Sandström E, Petersen CS, Norkrans G, Gerstoft J, Karlsson A, Christensen KC, Håkansson C, Pehrson PO, Nielsen JO, et al. The efficacy of inosine pranobex in preventing the acquired immunodeficiency syndrome in patients with human immunodeficiency virus infection. The Scandinavian Isoprinosine Study Group. *N Engl J Med.* 1990;322:1757-1763.
Erratum in:
N Engl J Med. 1990;323:1360.

Roeslin N, Dumont P, Morand G, Wihlm JM, Witz JP. Immunotherapy as an adjuvant to surgery in carcinoma of bronchus. Results in three randomised trials. *Eur J Cardiothorac Surg.* 1989;3:430-435.

INSULIN POTENTIATION THERAPY

Other common name(s): IPT, low-dose chemotherapy
Scientific/medical name(s): none

Description

Insulin potentiation therapy (IPT) refers to the use of insulin along with lower doses of chemotherapy to treat cancer. It is also sometimes used with other treatments for chronic diseases.

Overview

Despite individual reports, there are no published scientific studies available showing that IPT is safe or effective in treating cancer in humans. IPT may have serious side effects.

How is it promoted for use?

Insulin potentiation therapy is promoted as a "kinder, gentler" approach to chemotherapy, with "little to none of the negative side effects of chemotherapy." It purports to use about a tenth of the usual dose of cancer treatment medicine. The effect of the chemotherapy is claimed to be magnified, or potentiated, by the use of insulin, which lowers the blood sugar. People who offer this treatment claim that insulin "opens up" the receptors on cancer cells so that more chemotherapy can get in.

IPT has also reportedly been used to treat fibromyalgia, chronic fatigue syndrome, arthritis, and some infections. Some practitioners use IPT along with other complementary or alternative treatments such as cell therapy (see "Cell Therapy," page 714).

What does it involve?

The patient reports to an IPT clinic after having had nothing to eat or drink other than water for six to eight hours. Intravenous (IV) fluids are started, and the patient is given a dose of insulin based on his or her body weight. For people with cancer, low doses of chemotherapy drugs are given a few minutes later so that they reach the bloodstream after the insulin has started to lower the patient's blood sugar. This is called the "therapeutic moment" by some IPT providers.

At this point, the patient usually has some symptoms of low blood sugar (hypoglycemia). These can be quite severe, especially the first time, because people can respond to a standard dose of insulin quite differently. The IV is switched to a high-sugar solution to raise the blood sugar. After the symptoms of low blood sugar begin to improve, the patient may be given food to raise the blood sugar further. During this process, the blood sugar may be checked by fingerstick.

At the next treatment, the insulin dose may be raised or lowered, depending on the patient's response to the first dose. Between treatments, the patient may be given chemotherapy drugs by mouth and may also get vitamins or other supplements. Treatment is usually given twice a week, generally for twelve to eighteen sessions. After the first round of treatment, some people are advised that they need additional "maintenance" sessions.

Some supporters of insulin potentiation therapy recommend using it along with dimethyl sulfoxide (DMSO), a solvent sometimes used to treat a particular bladder problem (see "DMSO," page 737). Other medicines or supplements may be paired with IPT for patients with illnesses other than cancer.

One source was quoted at $15,500 to $17,500 for three to four weeks of "intensive IPT."

What is the history behind it?

Insulin was first isolated from pancreatic tissue in the early 1920s and has been used as a conventional treatment for diabetes since that time. In the early 1930s, insulin was used to produce coma for short periods in patients with schizophrenia in an attempt to cure them or reduce symptoms. About 1 percent of these patients died, however, and survivors often had lifelong complications. This type of treatment for schizophrenia was abandoned in the late 1950s.

IPT was developed in Mexico by Dr. Donato Perez Garcia, Sr., around the same time that insulin had begun to be used in schizophrenics. In fact, some supporters of IPT note that, at this early stage, patients with cancer were also put into insulin comas. Dr. Perez Garcia used this technique to try to treat several types of cancer. His son, Donato Perez Garcia Bellon, and grandson, Donato Perez Garcia, Jr., have followed in his footsteps. A physician from the United States, Dr. Steven G. Ayre, is a supporter of IPT and has published some descriptions of the theory behind it. More recently, books have been published suggesting that IPT can cure cancer, and some alternative clinics have begun to recommend it.

What is the evidence?

One very small published study on IPT was done in Uruguay. It included thirty women with breast cancer that was resistant to mainstream therapies. Of these women, ten received insulin, ten took the chemotherapy drug methotrexate, and ten received IPT using both drugs. After eight weeks, researchers reported that the women in the IPT group had smaller increases in tumor size than either of the other groups. Even though they used lower doses of methotrexate than usual, some side effects (mouth sores) were noted in the IPT group. This study did not look at survival, quality of life, well-being, or lasting effects. No long-term improvements were shown by this study.

Most of the information about insulin potentiation therapy comes from individual reports. Even among those, however, there is no evidence that the people who reported being helped by IPT were followed for long enough to learn whether the treatment worked.

Despite supporters' claims that insulin potentiation therapy has been well researched, no scientific studies that show safety and effectiveness have been published in available peer-reviewed journals. These claims cannot be verified.

There are also concerns about using lower doses of chemotherapy drugs. When chemotherapy drugs are tested in clinical trials, their effects are carefully monitored to learn which dose will best balance the need to kill cancer cells with the goal of keeping side effects at a tolerable level. There is no evidence that chemotherapy at a fraction of the recommended and tested dose can produce the same effect as the full dose if used with insulin.

Are there any possible problems or complications?

Because people respond differently to similar doses of insulin, blood sugar can drop quickly to dangerous levels during IPT. Low blood sugar can cause weakness, shakiness, confusion, rapid heartbeat, sweating, seizures, brain damage, or even death if it is prolonged.

People who are on pills to lower the blood sugar for treatment of diabetes may react more severely to low blood sugar caused by IPT. In addition, several medicines can affect the body's response to blood sugar changes. For example, beta-blocker medicines such as atenolol (Tenormin) and metoprolol (Lopressor) can mask the symptoms of low blood sugar, so the blood sugar may become dangerously low before it is noticed. Sulfa antibiotics (Bactrim and Septra) can make the blood sugar go even lower, as can excessive amounts of alcohol.

The possible effects of insulin potentiation therapy to treat cancer during pregnancy have not been studied. However, chemotherapy drugs are not generally advised during pregnancy. Use of IPT for cancer during pregnancy may harm the fetus.

A few people have severe allergic reactions to certain types of insulin, with reactions including fast heartbeat, low blood pressure, trouble breathing, itching, or rash. Insulin has not been approved by the U.S. Food and Drug Administration (FDA) to lower blood sugar to abnormal levels. Even when used as prescribed, it can be dangerous in some: an estimated 2 to 4 percent of deaths in people with type 1 diabetes are due to low blood sugar. Relying on this type of treatment alone and avoiding or delaying standard medical care for cancer may have serious health consequences.

References

Antidiabetics. Davis's Drug Guide Web site. http://www.drugguide.com/ddo/ub/view/Davis-Drug-Guide/50914/all/antidiabetics. Accessed June 11, 2008.

Ayre SG, Perez Garcia y Bellon D, Perez Garcia D Jr. Insulin potentiation therapy: a new concept in the management of chronic degenerative disease. *Med Hypotheses.* 1986;20:199-210.

Baratz R. Why you should stay away from Insulin Potentiation Therapy (IPT). Quackwatch Web site. http://www.quackwatch.org/01QuackeryRelatedTopics/Cancer/ipt.html. Updated March 10, 2007. Accessed June 11, 2008.

Cryer PE. Hypoglycemia. In: Braunwald E, Fauci AS, Kasper DL, Hauser SL, Longo DL, Jameson JL. eds. *Harrison's Principles of Internal Medicine.* 15th ed. Washington, DC: McGraw Hill; 2001:2138-2143.

Insulin Potentiation Therapy. Memorial Sloan-Kettering Cancer Center Web site. http://www.mskcc.org/mskcc/html/69265.cfm. Updated December 19, 2007. Accessed August 27, 2008.

Lasalvia-Prisco E, Cucchi S, Vázquez J, Lasalvia-Galante E, Golomar W, Gordon W. Insulin-induced enhancement of antitumoral response to methotrexate in breast cancer patients. *Cancer Chemother Pharmacol.* 2004;53:220-224. Epub 2003 Dec 4.

KREBIOZEN

Other common name(s): Carcalon, creatine, lipopolysaccharide C
Scientific/medical name(s): none

Description

Krebiozen was a commercial name for an alternative cancer formula originally prepared from the blood of horses that had been injected with bacteria. An analysis by several federal agencies later found Krebiozen to contain mineral oil and a form of creatine. Creatine is a substance that occurs naturally in the human body and is sold as a dietary supplement.

Overview

Available scientific evidence does not support claims that Krebiozen is effective in treating cancer or any other disease. According to the U.S. Food and Drug Administration (FDA), creatine has been linked to several dangerous side effects.

How is it promoted for use?

Proponents have claimed that Krebiozen cures cancer. They have cited private experiments claiming that Krebiozen stops tumor growth in mice and induces recovery in some people with advanced cancer.

What does it involve?

Krebiozen has been manufactured in powder and liquid forms. The liquid form of Krebiozen was combined with mineral oil and delivered through injection.

What is the history behind it?

Krebiozen was originally developed in Argentina by Stevan Durovic, MD, a Yugoslav physician, and brought to the United States in 1949. It drew the attention of Andrew Ivy, MD, at the University of Illinois, who began making his own version of the drug in 1959, calling it Carcalon. Dr. Ivy privately published two monographs claiming Carcalon's extensive anticancer benefits. Krebiozen therapy grew in popularity during the 1950s and early 1960s.

Durovic claimed his original powder was obtained as an extract from the blood of two thousand Argentinean horses that had been previously injected with *Actinomyces bovis*, a type of bacteria. In an article on Krebiozen, Dr. James Holland describes a 1963 announcement from the U.S. Department of Health, Education, and Welfare that both government and independent scientists had identified the Krebiozen powder given to the FDA by Ivy and Durovic as creatine, a type of amino acid found naturally in muscle tissue. The FDA also found that the Krebiozen solutions for injection contained either mineral oil or a form of creatine dissolved in mineral oil.

Dr. Holland also noted that Drs. Durovic and Ivy and several colleagues were indicted on a number of charges, including fraud, though they were ultimately acquitted. Dr. Durovic left the country a short time later after being indicted for tax evasion. According to William Goodrich, U.S. General Counsel at the time, supporters expressed their enthusiasm vigorously during this period through protests and boycotts, but the Krebiozen boom ultimately collapsed. Krebiozen and Carcalon are rarely used today.

What is the evidence?

A 1973 review reported that a thorough investigation of Krebiozen by federal government agencies found it had no anticancer activity in humans. A committee of twenty-four scientists studied the medical records of 504 "best cases" submitted by the Krebiozen Research Foundation before reaching their conclusion. Following the investigation, the National Cancer Institute (NCI) agreed, saying that it saw no justification for a clinical trial. The NCI director at that time noted that "[t]he committee's report of the 504 case records clearly established that 'Krebiozen' does not possess any anticancer activity in man. The National Cancer Institute has completed its consideration of 'Krebiozen.' There is no justification for a clinical trial, and from a scientific standpoint we regard the case closed" (*CA Cancer J Clin.* 1973:23:114).

Are there any possible problems or complications?

There is no reliable information on the safety of Krebiozen. However, creatine supplements have been linked with some side effects, including vomiting, diarrhea, seizures, anxiety, myopathy (a muscle tissue disorder), irregular heartbeat, blood clots, and even death. Relying on this type of treatment alone and avoiding or delaying conventional medical care for cancer may have serious health consequences.

These substances may have not been thoroughly tested to find out how they interact with medicines, foods, or dietary supplements. Even though some reports of interactions and harmful effects may be published, full studies of interactions and effects are not often available. Because of these limitations, any information on ill effects and interactions should be considered incomplete.

References

American Cancer Society. Unproven methods of cancer management. Krebiozen and carcalon. *CA Cancer J Clin.* 1973;23:111-115.

Creatine. PDRhealth Web site. http://www.pdrhealth.com/drugs/altmed/altmed-mono.aspx?contentFileName=ame0057.xml&contentName=Creatine. Accessed June 11, 2008.

Holland JF. The krebiozen story. Quackwatch Web site. http://www.quackwatch.org/01QuackeryRelatedTopics/Cancer/krebiozen.html. Posted February 29, 2000. Accessed June 11, 2008.

Interview with William W. Goodrich, Office of the General Counsel, 1939-1971, Part 2. October 15, 1986. FDA History: FDA Oral History Program. US Food and Drug Administration Web site. http://www.fda.gov/oc/history/oralhistories/goodrich/part2.html. Accessed June 11, 2008.

Jallut O, Guex P, Barrelet L. Unproven methods in oncology [in French]. *Schweiz Med Wochenschr.* 1984;114:1214-1220.

US Congress, Office of Technology Assessment. *Unconventional Cancer Treatments: OTA-H-405.* Washington, DC: US Government Printing Office; 1990.

LAETRILE

Other common name(s): amygdalin, vitamin B17, Amigdalina B-17
Scientific/medical name(s): mandelonitrile beta-D-gentiobioside, mandelonitrile-beta-glucuronide

Description

Laetrile is a chemically modified form of amygdalin, a naturally-occurring substance found mainly in the kernels of apricots, peaches, and almonds. However, the terms amygdalin and Laetrile are often used interchangeably. Laetrile and amygdalin are promoted as alternative cancer treatments.

Overview

Available scientific evidence does not support claims that Laetrile or amygdalin is effective in treating cancer or any other disease. Both contain a small amount of a substance that can be converted to cyanide in the body, and several cases of cyanide poisoning have been linked to the use of Laetrile. The U.S. Food and Drug Administration (FDA) has not approved Laetrile as a medical treatment in the United States.

How is it promoted for use?

Supporters once called Laetrile "the perfect chemotherapeutic agent," as it was said to kill cancer cells while being nontoxic to normal cells. Promoters claim that societies with diets rich in amygdalin, such as the Hunza and the Karakorum, are "cancer-free peoples." Supporters also say that Laetrile can prevent cancer and can help patients stay in remission. It is also promoted to provide pain relief to people with cancer. Other reported uses for Laetrile have been in the prevention and treatment of high blood pressure and arthritis.

There are several proposed explanations for how Laetrile works. Supporters claim that cancer cells contain more of a certain enzyme that splits the Laetrile molecule and releases the cyanide within it. The cancer cell then supposedly dies from cyanide poisoning. Normal cells supposedly do not have as much of this enzyme and instead contain an enzyme that renders the Laetrile harmless. Supporters claim that normal cells are not affected for this reason.

Another popular theory is that cancer is really a "vitamin deficiency" and that Laetrile is the missing "vitamin B17." Laetrile does not meet the widely accepted scientific definition of a vitamin, in that it has not been proven to be essential to achieving or maintaining good health.

What does it involve?

Amygdalin is most commonly extracted from apricot pits. Laetrile is a related substance and has a slightly different chemical structure. Laetrile or amygdalin is often taken as part of a metabolic therapy that includes a specific diet with high doses of vitamins (see "Metabolic Therapy," page 646). Although no standard treatment plan exists, a typical treatment consists of injecting Laetrile or amygdalin into a vein each day for two to three weeks, followed by taking tablets by mouth as a maintenance therapy. Laetrile and amygdalin are also used in enemas and in solutions applied directly to skin lesions. Chemical analyses of products sold as Laetrile showed that the actual ingredient is often amygdalin rather than Laetrile. For this reason, and because the terms are often used as synonyms, both substances are called Laetrile in the remainder of this document unless otherwise noted.

Laetrile treatments may cost thousands of dollars per week. Laetrile is commonly used in some hospitals and clinics in northern Mexico because it is difficult to get in the United States.

What is the history behind it?

"Bitter almonds" have been used as a medical remedy for thousands of years by cultures as diverse as the ancient Egyptians, Chinese, and Pueblo Indians. In 1802, a chemist discovered that distilling the water from bitter almonds released hydrocyanic acid. In the 1830s, the source of this hydrocyanic acid was purified and called amygdalin. It was thought to be the active ingredient in bitter almonds.

According to a 1991 review, the current use of Laetrile can be directly attributed to the theories of Ernst T. Krebs, Sr., MD, which were first proposed in the 1920s. Krebs tested an extract from apricot pits to treat cancer, but the pills proved too toxic for human use. Around

1952, his son, Ernst T. Krebs, Jr., changed the process of extracting amygdalin and created a chemically modified version, which he named Laetrile. He claimed that the new substance was more potent as an anticancer drug than naturally occurring amygdalin. Despite this chemical distinction, both proponents and skeptics commonly refer to both substances as Laetrile. Adding to this confusion is the fact that many products sold as Laetrile consist mostly of amygdalin.

The same 1991 review notes that, beginning in 1957, Laetrile was repeatedly tested against tumor cells implanted in animals. At least a dozen separate sets of experiments were done at seven institutions. Targets included several different types of cancer. The conclusion was that Laetrile did not have any antitumor activity.

The FDA placed sanctions against the sale of Laetrile. In 1977, the FDA commissioner stated that there was no evidence for the safety or effectiveness of Laetrile. Because of the risk for cyanide poisoning, the government has banned the transport of Laetrile into the United States or across state lines, as well as the use of Laetrile in states without laws specifically allowing it. Since 2000, there have been several instances of prosecution because of Laetrile transport across state lines.

What is the evidence?

From the 1950s through the 1970s, Laetrile grew in popularity in the United States as an alternative treatment for cancer. For this reason, and despite the lack of scientific evidence that Laetrile was effective, the National Cancer Institute (NCI) studied it in 1978 through a retrospective case review (a study that looks back at cases from the past). The NCI sent letters to more than four hundred thousand doctors and other practitioners, asking them to submit positive results from cases involving Laetrile. Whereas an estimated seventy-five thousand people in the United States had taken Laetrile, only ninety-three "positive" cases were submitted, and in only six of those was there evidence of major tumor shrinkage.

A 1991 NCI review of the evidence of Laetrile's effectiveness stated that "[s]cientific studies were conducted for more than 20 years, starting in the mid-1950s, looking for evidence of antitumor efficacy by Laetrile. In no instance was evidence found that treatment with Laetrile results in any benefit against tumors in animals. Despite this negative record, a clinical trial in humans was conducted in 1981. It did not show any anticancer effect of Laetrile" (*CA Cancer J Clin.* 1991;41:188).

The clinical trial of Laetrile on humans was performed between 1979 and 1981 at medical centers around the country. About 175 patients with different types of cancer were treated with a commonly used regimen of Laetrile plus metabolic therapy. Published in 1982, it reported that one patient had major tumor shrinkage (a partial response) at first. Of the patients, 91 percent of their cancers had progressed after three months, and median survival was less than five months. In all patients, the cancer grew within eight months of starting treatment.

In contrast to the NCI's findings, one of the leading proponents of Laetrile claims to have treated nearly thirty thousand cancer patients in several studies of the drug, with promising results. However, these results have not been reviewed or repeated by the scientific medical community.

The consensus of available scientific evidence does not support claims that Laetrile is an effective anticancer treatment, either in animal studies or in human clinical trials. Cancer cells do not seem to be more susceptible to the effects of Laetrile than normal cells. The successes claimed by its supporters are based on individual reports, testimonials, and publicity issued by promoters.

Are there any possible problems or complications?

The use of Laetrile has been linked to cyanide toxicity and death in a few cases. Although drug interactions are unknown, at least one case report suggests that vitamin C may increase the amount of cyanide released from Laetrile in the body. This can increase the risk for cyanide poisoning. This risk is also likely to be increased if the person eats raw almonds or crushed fruit pits while taking Laetrile. Eating fruits and vegetables that contain beta-glucosidase, such as celery, peaches, bean sprouts, and carrots, may increase the risk for cyanide poisoning. Always tell your doctor and pharmacist about any supplements or herbs you are taking.

This treatment should be avoided by children and by women who are pregnant or breastfeeding. Relying on this type of treatment alone and avoiding or delaying conventional medical care for cancer may have serious health consequences.

This substance has not been thoroughly tested to find out how it interacts with medicines, foods, or dietary supplements. Even though some reports of interactions and harmful effects may be published, full studies of interactions and effects are not often available. Because of these limitations, any information on ill effects and interactions should be considered incomplete.

References

American Cancer Society. Unproven methods of cancer management. Laetrile. *CA Cancer J Clin.* 1991;41:187-192.

Amygdalin. Memorial Sloan-Kettering Cancer Center Web site. http://www.mskcc.org/mskcc/html/69118.cfm. Accessed June 11, 2008.

Bromley J, Hughes BG, Leong DC, Buckley NA. Life-threatening interaction between complementary medicines: cyanide toxicity following ingestion of amygdalin and vitamin C. *Ann Pharmacother.* 2005;39:1566-1569. Epub 2005 Jul 12.

Ellison NM, Byar DP, Newell GR. Special report on Laetrile: the NCI Laetrile review. Results of the National Cancer Institute's retrospective Laetrile analysis. *N Engl J Med.* 1978;299:549-552.

Fetrow CW, Avila JR. *Professional's Handbook of Complementary & Alternative Medicines.* Springhouse, PA: Springhouse Corp; 1999.

Herbert V. Laetrile: the cult of cyanide: promoting poison for profit. *Am J Clin Nutr.* 1979;32:1121-1158.

Laetrile/amygdalin (PDQ®). National Cancer Institute Web site. http://www.cancer.gov/cancertopics/pdq/cam/laetrile/healthprofessional. Accessed June 11, 2008.

Lerner IJ. Laetrile: a lesson in cancer quackery. *CA Cancer J Clin.* 1981;31:91-95.

Milazzo S, Lejeune S, Ernst E. Laetrile for cancer: a systematic review of the clinical evidence. *Support Care Cancer.* 2007;15:583-595. Epub 2006 Nov 15.

Moertel CG, Fleming TR, Rubin J, Kvols LK, Sarna G, Koch R, Currie VE, Young CW, Jones SE, Davignon JP. A clinical trial of amygdalin (Laetrile) in the treatment of human cancer. *N Engl J Med.* 1982;306:201-206.

Wilson B. The rise and fall of laetrile. Quackwatch Web site. http://www.quackwatch.org/01QuackeryRelatedTopics/Cancer/laetrile.html/. Updated February 17, 2004. Accessed June 11, 2008.

LIPOIC ACID

Other common name(s): alpha-lipoic acid, thioctic acid
Scientific/medical name(s): 1,2-dithiolane-3-pentanoic acid

Description

Lipoic acid is an antioxidant found in certain foods, including red meat, spinach, broccoli, potatoes, yams, carrots, beets, and yeast. It is also made in small amounts in the human body.

Overview

Lipoic acid plays an important role in metabolism, or the way that cells process chemicals in the body. Recent research has shown it is helpful in treating nerve damage in diabetics. It may have benefit for other conditions as well. There is no reliable scientific evidence at this time that lipoic acid prevents the development or spread of cancer. Its possible role as a complementary therapy to reduce the side effects of radiation therapy or chemotherapy is still unclear.

How is it promoted for use?

Lipoic acid is an antioxidant that is promoted to protect the body against cancer and other diseases. An antioxidant is a compound that blocks the action of free radicals, activated oxygen molecules that can damage cells. Oxidation may also play a role in causing poor health as people age, and some researchers suggest that lipoic acid may be helpful in slowing the aging process.

Lipoic acid has been used to treat diabetic polyneuropathy, a nerve disease affecting many diabetics that causes pain and numbness in the hands and feet. Research suggests lipoic acid may also lower blood sugar levels.

Regarded as a powerful antioxidant, lipoic acid is claimed to strengthen the effects of other antioxidants (such as vitamins C and E) and to regenerate antioxidants used up in the fight against free radicals. It has also been promoted to prevent or treat liver disease and cataracts and to reduce the risk for plaque formation in the arteries.

Some proponents believe that lipoic acid may inhibit genes that trigger cancer cells to grow, and some recommend it as one component of an alternative anticancer regimen or as a complementary therapy to prevent or relieve some side effects of conventional cancer treatments. Researchers have begun to look at whether lipoic acid can help prevent nerve damage from certain chemotherapy drugs.

What does it involve?

Lipoic acid can be obtained from foods, and the body also produces it naturally. As a person ages, his or her body produces less lipoic acid. Supplements are available as capsules and tablets and are sold in health food stores and on the Internet. Many studies have used an injectable form of the nutrient. A safe and effective dosage of this supplement has not been firmly established. Most studies have used doses of 300 to 600 milligrams daily. High doses of any antioxidant supplement may actually cause cell damage.

What is the history behind it?

In 1937, scientists found certain bacteria contained a compound that was later characterized as lipoic acid. The antioxidant activity of lipoic acid has been known and studied since 1939. In 1957, lipoic acid was found in yeast extracts. At one time it was thought to be a vitamin (a substance the body needs but usually cannot make on its own), but it was later discovered that the body does make lipoic acid.

What is the evidence?

There are no studies in humans convincingly showing that lipoic acid supplements prevent the development or progression of cancer. One individual report of a patient receiving an alternative regimen including lipoic acid has been published. However, whereas a number of well-documented case reports with consistent results might suggest value in conducting clinical trials, a single case report is not very helpful in assessing the safety or effectiveness of any treatment.

Early studies of cells grown in the laboratory have suggested that lipoic acid may cause cancer cells to self-destruct, a process known as apoptosis. Much more research will be needed to determine whether it has similar effects in animals and people.

There have been some encouraging results in small animal and human studies on the ability of lipoic acid to reduce some harmful side effects of chemotherapy. Some chemotherapy drugs can damage nerve cells in the body, which can lead to a condition called peripheral neuropathy, in which patients feel pain or other abnormal sensations, usually in the hands or feet. In a small Austrian study, eight of fifteen patients who received lipoic acid after taking the chemotherapy drug oxaliplatin reported improved symptoms. The researchers suggested larger studies should look into this effect. One study of rats suggests that lipoic acid might help reduce heart muscle damage caused by some chemotherapy drugs. A 2006 publication reported that a combination of antioxidants including lipoic acid helped people with advanced cancer regain appetite and body weight.

Studies have also looked at the use of lipoic acid for other conditions. In a recent review article, researchers reported that a number of studies have found lipoic acid to be useful in treating nerve problems in diabetics and that it can improve insulin sensitivity in people with type 2 diabetes. Other studies have suggested that it might be useful in liver disease. Early laboratory and animal studies have also suggested that lipoic acid may be helpful in treating stroke, cataracts, nerve damage from human immunodeficiency virus (HIV) infection, some nervous system diseases (such as Alzheimer's disease), and radiation injury. It may also help people with high cholesterol levels. Studies in people are now under way to determine whether lipoic acid can help with these conditions.

Are there any possible problems or complications?

Lipoic acid found naturally in foods is safe. Research has shown that 300 to 600 milligrams of lipoic acid a day may be safely taken with very few side effects, although some people have reported upset stomach or skin rashes. Diabetics should be aware that high doses of lipoic acid supplements may lower blood sugar levels.

Because it is a powerful antioxidant, there are concerns that lipoic acid could make radiation therapy or chemotherapy less effective. While this concern is based largely on theories of how cancer treatments work, it is supported by some recent studies. For this reason, people being treated for cancer should speak with their doctors before taking this supplement.

The effects of long-term use of this supplement are unknown. Women who are pregnant or breastfeeding should talk with their doctors before taking this supplement. Relying on this type of treatment alone and avoiding or delaying conventional medical care for cancer may have serious health consequences.

This product is sold as a dietary supplement in the United States. Unlike companies that produce drugs (which must provide the FDA with results of detailed testing showing their product is safe and effective before the drug is approved for sale), the companies that make supplements do not have to show evidence of safety or health benefits to the FDA before selling their products. Supplement products without any reliable scientific evidence of health benefits may still be sold as long as the companies selling them do not claim the supplements can prevent, treat, or cure any specific disease. Some such products may not contain the amount of the herb or substance that is written on the label, and some may include other substances (contaminants). Though the FDA has written new rules to improve the quality of manufacturing processes for dietary supplements and the accurate listing of supplement ingredients, these rules do not take full effect until 2010. The new rules also do not address the safety of supplement ingredients or their effects on health when proper manufacturing techniques are used.

Most such supplements have not been tested to find out if they interact with medicines, foods, or other herbs and supplements. Even though some reports of interactions and harmful effects may be published, full studies of interactions and effects are not often available. Because of these limitations, any information on ill effects and interactions should be considered incomplete.

References

Alpha-lipoic acid. Memorial Sloan-Kettering Cancer Center Web site. http://www.mskcc.org/mskcc/html/69117.cfm. Accessed June 11, 2008.

Alpha-lipoic acid. PDRhealth Web site. http://www.pdrhealth.com/drugs/altmed/altmed-mono.aspx?contentFileName=ame0292.xml&contentName=Alpha+Lipoic+Acid. Accessed June 11, 2008.

Berkson BM, Rubin DM, Berkson AJ. The long-term survival of a patient with pancreatic cancer with metastases to the liver after treatment with the intravenous alpha-lipoic acid/low-dose naltrexone protocol. *Integr Cancer Ther.* 2006;5:83-89.

Bustamante J, Lodge JK, Marcocci L, Tritschler HJ, Packer L, Rihn BH. Alpha-lipoic acid in liver metabolism and disease. *Free Radic Biol Med.* 1998;24:1023-1039.

Gedlicka C, Scheithauer W, Schüll B, Kornek GV. Effective treatment of oxaliplatin-induced cumulative polyneuropathy with alpha-lipoic acid. *J Clin Oncol.* 2002;20:3359-3361.

Han D, Sen CK, Roy S, Kobayashi MS, Tritschler HJ, Packer L. Protection against glutamate-induced cytotoxicity in C6 glial cells by thiol antioxidants. *Am J Physiol.* 1997;273:R1771-R1778.

Lawenda BD, Kelly KM, Ladas EJ, Sagar SM, Vickers A, Blumberg JB. Should supplemental antioxidant administration be avoided during chemotherapy and radiation therapy? *J Natl Cancer Inst.* 2008;100:773-783.

Mantovani G, Macciò A, Madeddu C, Gramignano G, Lusso MR, Serpe R, Massa E, Astara G, Deiana L. A phase II study with antioxidants, both in the diet and supplemented, pharmaconutritional support, progestagen, and anti-cyclooxygenase-2 showing efficacy and safety in patients with cancer-related anorexia/cachexia and oxidative stress. *Cancer Epidemiol Biomarkers Prev.* 2006;15:1030-1034.

Moungjaroen J, Nimmannit U, Callery PS, Wang L, Azad N, Lipipun V, Chanvorachote P, Rojanasakul Y. Reactive oxygen species mediate caspase activation and apoptosis induced by lipoic acid in human lung epithelial cancer cells through Bcl-2 down-regulation. *J Pharmacol Exp Ther.* 2006;319:1062-1069. Epub 2006 Sep 21.

Mythili Y, Sudharsan PT, Sudhahar V, Varalakshmi P. Protective effect of DL-alpha-lipoic acid on cyclophosphamide induced hyperlipidemic cardiomyopathy. *Eur J Pharmacol.* 2006;543:92-96. Epub 2006 Jun 9.

Packer L, Witt EH, Tritschler HJ. Alpha-Lipoic acid as a biological antioxidant. *Free Radic Biol Med.* 1995;19:227-250.

van de Mark K, Chen JS, Steliou K, Perrine SP, Faller DV. Alpha-lipoic acid induces p27Kip-dependent cell cycle arrest in non-transformed cell lines and apoptosis in tumor cell lines. *J Cell Physiol.* 2003;194:325-340.

Ziegler D, Nowak H, Kempler P, Vargha P, Low PA. Treatment of symptomatic diabetic polyneuropathy with the antioxidant alpha-lipoic acid: a meta-analysis. *Diabet Med.* 2004;21:114-121.

LIVER FLUSH

Other common name(s): gallbladder flush, liver cleansing
Scientific/medical name(s): none

Description

Liver flushes are recommended by alternative medicine practitioners to detoxify or drive "harmful chemicals and germs" out of the liver and gallbladder. They are often used as part of a larger metabolic treatment regimen (see "Metabolic Therapy," page 646).

Overview

Available scientific evidence does not support claims that liver flushes are useful for preventing or treating cancer or any other diseases.

How is it promoted for use?

Proponents claim that liver flushing rids the organ of unwanted food byproducts, fats, toxins, parasites, and gallstones, thereby preventing or treating a range of diseases, including cancer. They also claim that because the liver is an important hormone regulator, cleansing it will help conditions caused by hormone imbalances. Liver flushes are a key part of several alternative metabolic therapies promoted to treat cancer.

What does it involve?

A liver flush involves eating or drinking a combination of juices, Epsom salts (magnesium sulfate), and oils, often with selected herbs, enzymes, and other components. Liver flush formulas vary widely by practitioner and can also be purchased. The flush is usually done over the course of two or more days and results in several bowel movements. Practitioners often recommend doing a liver flush once or twice a year.

Some practitioners advise combining liver flushes with fasting or other alternative treatments such as coffee enemas. They are often recommended before starting other forms of alternative treatments, as a way to begin with a "clean slate."

What is the evidence?

Promoters of liver flushes and alternative detoxification regimens as a treatment for cancer often cite the belief that cancer is caused by the accumulation of toxins. They say that the process by which cancer develops can be reversed through treatments to remove the toxic substances. This view is not consistent with modern concepts of how DNA mutations cause cancer to develop and grow.

There is no reliable evidence to support any of the claims made for liver flushes. No studies on the use of liver flushes for any condition have been reported in available peer-reviewed medical journals.

Are there any possible problems or complications?

People may have nausea, vomiting, and diarrhea during the flush. Oily or fatty components of liver flushes may cause the gallbladder to contract. This contraction could lead to problems in people with gallstones, which could get stuck in the bile duct. Individual components of the herbal mixtures used in a liver flush may present their own health hazards. Relying on this type of treatment alone and avoiding or delaying conventional medical care for cancer may have serious health consequences.

These substances may have not been thoroughly tested to find out how they interact with medicines, foods, or dietary supplements. Even though some reports of interactions and harmful effects may be published, full studies of interactions and effects are not often available. Because of these limitations, any information on ill effects and interactions should be considered incomplete.

References

American Cancer Society. Questionable cancer practices in Tijuana and other Mexican border clinics. *CA Cancer J Clin.* 1991;41:310-319.

Detoxification therapy. PDRhealth Web site. http://www.pdrhealth.com/content/natural_medicine/chapters/201160.shtml. Accessed July 8, 2005. Content no longer available.

Liver supplements. July 2002. UC Berkeley Wellness Letter Web site. http://www.berkeleywellness.com/html/ds/dsLiverSupps.php. Accessed June 11, 2008.

Moran P. The truth about gallbladder and liver "flushes." Quackwatch Web site. http://www.quackwatch.com/01QuackeryRelatedTopics/flushes.html. Updated March 9, 2007. Accessed June 11, 2008.

LIVINGSTON-WHEELER THERAPY

Other common name(s): Livingston vaccine therapy, Livingston therapy
Scientific/medical name(s): none

Description

Livingston-Wheeler therapy was an alternative cancer method that included vaccines, antibiotics, vitamin and mineral supplements, digestive enzymes, cleansing enemas, support group therapy, and a vegetarian diet. The clinic that offered this therapy is no longer in operation.

Overview

Available scientific evidence does not support claims that Livingston-Wheeler therapy was effective in treating cancer or any other disease.

How is it promoted for use?

Livingston-Wheeler therapy was mainly promoted to treat cancer, but it was also used to treat lupus, arthritis, and other chronic conditions. In the case of cancer, supporters believed that when the body's immune system weakens, it allows a bacterium called *Progenitor cryptocides* to spread and cause cancer. Practitioners claimed Livingston-Wheeler therapy was a form of immunotherapy that could boost the immune system to help a person fight off serious illnesses such as cancer.

What does it involve?

Livingston-Wheeler therapy was given at only one clinic in the United States. Patients entered a ten-day treatment program, which could be expensive, and required home treatment as well.

Follow-up visits to the clinic were also encouraged. At the clinic, patients were evaluated and given standard blood and urine tests. Special hormone, liver function, and tumor marker tests were also done. The patient's immune system was also tested in order to design a personalized immune-enhancement vaccine, which was usually derived from the patient's own urine or blood.

In addition to the vaccine, the patient could be given antibiotics, nutritional supplements, digestive enzymes, bile salts, enemas, laxatives, and blood transfusions. A strict vegetarian diet was enforced and the patient took part in group or support therapy.

What is the history behind it?

During the 1950s, Virginia Livingston, MD (who later remarried and became Livingston-Wheeler), developed a theory that cancer was caused by a bacterium *(Progenitor cryptocides)* that was activated when one's immune system was weakened or under great stress. Based on her theory, she designed a complex treatment to reduce the amount of the bacteria in the body so the immune system could fight the cancer.

She and her husband, Dr. A. M. Livingston, opened the Livingston Clinic in San Diego in 1969. Following her husband's death, she married Dr. Owen Wheeler, one of her former cancer patients. The clinic was renamed the Livingston-Wheeler clinic in 1976. From 1969 to 1984, it is estimated that more than ten thousand people were treated at the clinic. While the clinic specialized in cancer treatment, the therapy was expanded to treat arthritis, lupus, allergies, and AIDS.

In 1990, the California Department of Health Services ordered the clinic to stop giving the immune-enhancement vaccine as part of the treatment program since it was not approved by the U.S. Food and Drug Administration. Dr. Livingston-Wheeler died the same year. The clinic remained open for several years as the Livingston Foundation Medical Center. It is estimated that about five hundred patients with cancer and other problems received treatment there yearly. The clinic is no longer in operation.

What is the evidence?

Available scientific evidence does not support claims that Livingston-Wheeler therapy helps people with cancer. Few studies have evaluated the Livingston-Wheeler therapy. One investigation involving patients with advanced cancer compared survival and quality of life between patients receiving conventional treatment and those undergoing Livingston-Wheeler therapy. According to the 1991 report, there was no difference in survival between the two groups, but the patients treated at Livingston-Wheeler had significantly poorer quality of life. These results refuted the clinic's claim of an 82 percent cure rate, even for people with advanced cancer.

One report found that the bacterium *Progenitor cryptocides*, which Dr. Livingston-Wheeler claimed caused cancer, is actually a mixture of several different types of bacteria incorrectly labeled as one type by Dr. Livingston-Wheeler. The other components of her therapy have also been criticized as lacking scientific evidence.

Are there any possible problems or complications?

The safety of Livingston-Wheeler therapy was never firmly established. Some reported reactions to the vaccine given in the therapy included aching, slight fever, and tenderness at the injection site. Relying on this type of treatment alone and avoiding or delaying conventional medical care for cancer could have serious health consequences.

These substances may have not been thoroughly tested to find out how they interact with medicines, foods, or dietary supplements. Even though some reports of interactions and harmful effects may be published, full studies of interactions and effects are not often available. Because of these limitations, any information on ill effects and interactions should be considered incomplete.

References

American Cancer Society. Unproven methods of cancer management: Livingston-Wheeler therapy. *CA Cancer J Clin.* 1991;41:A7-A12.

Biologic/organic/pharmacologic therapies: Livingston-Wheeler detailed scientific review. Complementary/ Integrative Medicine Education Resources, The University of Texas M. D. Anderson Cancer Center Web site. http://www.mdanderson.org/departments/cimer/display.cfm?id=ADFAB01E-16E9-11D5-811000508B603A14&method=displayFull. Accessed June 11, 2008.

Cassileth BR, Lusk EJ, Guerry D, Blake AD, Walsh WP, Kascius L, Schultz DJ. Survival and quality of life among patients receiving unproven as compared with conventional cancer therapy. *N Engl J Med.* 1991;324:1180-1185.

Livingston-Wheeler therapy. Memorial Sloan-Kettering Cancer Center Web site. http://www.mskcc.org/mskcc/html/69283.cfm. Accessed June 11, 2008.

Vickers A. Alternative cancer cures: "unproven" or "disproven"? *CA Cancer J Clin.* 2004;54:110-118.

LYPRINOL

Other common name(s): green-lipped mussel extract, Lyprinex
Scientific/medical name(s): none

Description

Lyprinol is a fatty acid complex extracted from *Perna canaliculus*, a green-lipped mussel native to New Zealand. It is available in capsule form as a dietary supplement.

Overview

Some early studies have suggested that Lyprinol may be useful against arthritis and other inflammatory conditions, although more research in these areas is needed. Available scientific evidence does not support claims that it can prevent or treat cancer.

How is it promoted for use?

Lyprinol is promoted as a dietary supplement with anti-inflammatory properties. It reportedly works against substances in the body called leukotrienes, which are responsible for some aspects of chronic inflammatory responses. It also is said to contain high levels of some omega-3 fatty acids (see "Omega-3 Fatty Acids," page 659).

Lyprinol is most commonly claimed to be useful against arthritis. It is also promoted for use against other conditions, including asthma, allergies, heart disease, menstrual problems, and inflammatory bowel disease. It received a great deal of media attention in New Zealand for a short time in the late 1990s, when some researchers and manufacturers claimed it could cure cancer. Most of these claims were withdrawn, as there was little evidence to back them up.

What does it involve?

Lyprinol is sold in capsule form in New Zealand and over the Internet. It is usually recommended at doses from 2 to 4 capsules daily. Other extracts of green-lipped mussels are available in capsules, tablets, and as gels for the skin.

What is the history behind it?

The idea that the green-lipped mussel extract could help maintain good health was based on Westerners' observations of Maori tribes in New Zealand in the 1970s and 1980s. Green-lipped mussel powders were marketed as early as the late 1970s as an alternative treatment for arthritis. Lyprinol, a form of mussel extract reported to be more stable than the powders, was first marketed as a dietary supplement in the 1990s and was commonly promoted for use against arthritis and other inflammatory conditions.

In 1999, based on laboratory studies, a researcher announced to the New Zealand media that his data showed that mussel extract kills cancer cells. He claimed that Lyprinol inhibits two cell pathways that may cause inflammation and cancer in animals and humans. Within a few days, two million dollars' worth of Lyprinol was sold in New Zealand. Critics questioned the timing of the announcement, which coincided with the release of a new Lyprinol product on the market. In response to the criticism, the original manufacturer stopped distributing its product, but other makers continued selling it. At the time of the media announcement, another New Zealand researcher warned that Lyprinol might, in fact, contain substances that promote tumor growth rather than kill cancer cells. The manufacturer and distributor of Lyprinol in New Zealand were later convicted and fined for violation of the country's Medicines Act, which states that substances claimed to treat or cure a disease are considered to be medicines and must be proven effective to the Ministry of Health before being sold to the public. Lyprinol and other extracts derived from green-lipped mussels are still available as dietary supplements and are marketed for nonspecific conditions such as "joint health."

What is the evidence?

Despite the initial media hype, available scientific evidence does not support claims that Lyprinol and similar products have any effect on cancer in humans. In 2002, Australian researchers reported on the use of Lyprinol in thirteen patients with advanced prostate and breast cancer. Patients took doses of up to twelve capsules a day, but none had their tumors shrink or noted lower levels of pain. While this study was originally set to enroll up to a hundred patients, no further results have been reported.

Some small studies have reported positive results using Lyprinol against conditions linked to inflammation. A Korean study of sixty patients with osteoarthritis found that most patients noted symptom improvement after eight weeks of treatment with Lyprinol. However, a 2006 review of studies of freeze-dried mussel powder concluded there was little consistent evidence that it helped with any type of arthritis. A Russian study involving forty-six patients found that Lyprinol seemed to reduce asthma symptoms, with no major side effects. Some early studies in mice have also suggested that Lyprinol may be useful against inflammatory bowel disease. According to a 2007 article, Lyprinol inhibits cyclooxygenase, an enzyme involved in inflammation that is also the target of aspirin and related anti-inflammatory drugs. Larger studies in humans are needed to confirm the possible benefits of Lyprinol or other green-lipped mussel extracts for these conditions.

Are there any possible problems or complications?

Lyprinol appears to be relatively nontoxic, although its safety has not been studied extensively in clinical trials. There have been some reports of upset stomach after its use. Some extracts of green-lipped mussels contain proteins that could cause allergic reactions in those with seafood allergies.

Lyprinol has not been studied in pregnancy. Women who are pregnant or breastfeeding should talk to their doctor before use. Relying on this type of treatment alone and avoiding or delaying conventional medical care for cancer may have serious health consequences.

This product is sold as a dietary supplement in the United States. Unlike companies that produce drugs (which must provide the FDA with results of detailed testing showing their product is safe and effective before the drug is approved for sale), the companies that make supplements do not have to show evidence of safety or health benefits to the FDA before selling their products. Supplement products without any reliable scientific evidence of health benefits may still be sold as long as the companies selling them do not claim the supplements can prevent, treat, or cure any specific disease. Some such products may not contain the amount of the herb or substance that is written on the label, and some may include other substances (contaminants). Though the FDA has written new rules to improve the quality of manufacturing processes for dietary supplements and the accurate listing of supplement ingredients, these rules do not take full effect until 2010. The new rules also do not address the safety of supplement ingredients or their effects on health when proper manufacturing techniques are used.

Most such supplements have not been tested to find out if they interact with medicines, foods, or other herbs and supplements. Even though some reports of interactions and harmful effects may be published, full studies of interactions and effects are not often available. Because of these limitations, any information on ill effects and interactions should be considered incomplete.

References

Cho SH, Jung YB, Seong SC, Park HB, Byun KY, Lee DC, Song EK, Son JH. Clinical efficacy and safety of Lyprinol, a patented extract from New Zealand green-lipped mussel (Perna Canaliculus) in patients with osteoarthritis of the hip and knee: a multicenter 2-month clinical trial. *Allerg Immunol* (Paris). 2003;35:212-216.

Cobb CS, Ernst E. Systematic review of a marine nutriceutical supplement in clinical trials for arthritis: the effectiveness of the New Zealand green-lipped mussel *Perna canaliculus. Clin Rheumatol.* 2006;25:275-284. Epub 2005 Oct 12.

Dickson J, Pittman K, Patterson K, Price T, Norman J, Moldovan S, Moretti K, Miller J, Burfield G, Betts H, The Queen Elizabeth Hospital. A phase 1/2 study of Lyprinol in advanced hormone refractory prostate cancer, and hormone and chemotherapy refractory breast cancer. *Proc Am Soc Clin Oncol* 21:2002 (abstract 2154).

Emelyanov A, Fedoseev G, Krasnoschekova O, Abulimity A, Trendeleva T, Barnes PJ. Treatment of asthma with lipid extract of New Zealand green-lipped mussel: a randomised clinical trial. *Eur Respir J.* 2002;20:596-600.

Lyprinol sentence increased. February 19, 2001. New Zealand Ministry of Health Web site. http://www.moh.govt.nz/moh.nsf/aa6c02e6249e7359cc256e7f0005521d/ccd4fe48175fc63ecc2569f8006401f7. Accessed June 30, 2005. Content no longer available.

McPhee S, Hodges LD, Wright PF, Wynne PM, Kalafatis N, Harney DW, Macrides TA. Anti-cyclooxygenase effects of lipid extracts from the New Zealand green-lipped mussel, *Perna canaliculus. Comp Biochem Physiol B Biochem Mol Biol.* 2007;146:346-356.

Taylor J. Claims of media manipulation after NZ diet food frenzy. ABC: AM Archive [Transcript of Australian radio broadcast] Tuesday, 3 August, 1999. http://www.abc.net.au/am/stories/s41055.htm. Accessed September 4, 2008.

Tenikoff D, Murphy KJ, Le M, Howe PR, Howarth GS. Lyprinol (stabilised lipid extract of New Zealand green-lipped mussel): a potential preventative treatment modality for inflammatory bowel disease. *J Gastroenterol.* 2005;40:361-365.

MANGOSTEEN JUICE

Other common name(s): xango, mangostan, queen of fruits, numerous brand names
Scientific/medical name(s): *Garcinia mangostana*

Description

Mangosteen is a tropical fruit native to Southeast Asia that is touted for its antioxidants, especially xanthones, a type of chemical in certain plants. Its fruit, including the rind and pulp, can be purèed and is sometimes sold as a drink. Mangosteen juice products may also be mixed with other types of juice. Its rind may be dried and made into a powder, and substances are also extracted from its bark. Mangosteen products are also available in capsule and tablet form. They are sold in health food stores, on the Internet, and through individual independent distributors.

Despite the name, mangosteen is not related to the mango.

Overview

Although there is no reliable evidence that mangosteen juice, puree, or bark is effective as a treatment for cancer in humans, its fruit has been shown to be rich in antioxidants. Very early laboratory studies suggest it may have promise as a topical treatment for acne. Early small laboratory and animal studies suggest that further research should be done to determine whether it can help to prevent cancer in humans.

How is it promoted for use?

Mangosteen is promoted to support microbiological balance, help the immune system, improve joint flexibility, and provide mental support. Some proponents claim that it can help diarrhea, infections, tuberculosis, and a host of other illnesses. In countries where the tree grows, various parts of the plant are used by native healers.

What does it involve?

In the United States, mangosteen is consumed as a juice or purèe or taken by mouth in capsule or tablet form, often along with other herbs, fruits, or plants. In Asia and the Philippines, the rind may be steeped in water to make tea. Some folk healers prepare an ointment or salve to apply to the skin for conditions such as eczema, injuries, and infections. Others boil the leaves and bark of the tree to make a medicinal drink or to mix with other herbs to apply to wounds. The roots may be boiled to make a drink for women with menstrual problems.

What is the history behind it?

Parts of the mangosteen tree, including the fruit and bark, have been used in folk medicine in Asian countries for many years. In the mid-1800s, a compound in mangosteen, mangostin, was identified as a xanthone, a type of antioxidant. Mangostin was found to have anti-inflammatory effects in rats in the late 1970s. Today, mangosteen is sold in the United States mainly through a network marketing system, in which independent distributors, rather than stores, buy and sell mangosteen juice. Many mangosteen products are also available from health food stores and on the Internet.

In 2006, the U.S. Food and Drug Administration (FDA) warned one mangosteen vendor that the product was being illegally marketed. The FDA observed that the product was being promoted to treat illness, for which it had not been proven safe and effective.

What is the evidence?

Like many other plants, mangosteen extracts have shown in laboratory tests that they can stop certain bacteria and fungi from growing. One laboratory study suggested that mangosteen extract inhibits the growth of acne-causing bacteria. It has not been tested on people to determine whether it can help acne. In the laboratory, it also slowed the growth of certain cancer cells. A small study in rats suggested that the rind of the mangosteen may reduce the risk for cancer cell growth in the bowel. However, the ability of mangosteen to inhibit cancer growth has not been tested in humans.

Are there any possible problems or complications?

Only one case of a serious adverse event possibly related to mangosteen juice has been reported. Doctors described a daily user of mangosteen juice who developed lactic acidosis (acidic blood due to buildup of a byproduct of sugar metabolism). Because mangosteen juice is quite popular and most users do not develop lactic acidosis, the doctors suggest that this problem may have resulted from an interaction of this supplement with other drugs he was taking.

No other ill effects have been reported to date. As with all plants, allergies may be possible. Because of its antioxidant effects, mangosteen supplements may make radiation therapy or chemotherapy less effective. While this concern is based largely on theories of how cancer treatments work, it is supported by some recent studies. For this reason, people being treated for cancer should speak with their doctors before taking this supplement. Other interactions are not well described. Always talk with your doctor and pharmacist about all the supplements and herbs you are taking. Relying on this type of treatment alone and avoiding or delaying conventional medical care for cancer may have serious health consequences.

This product is sold as a dietary supplement in the United States. Unlike companies that produce drugs (which must provide the FDA with results of detailed testing showing their product is safe and effective before the drug is approved for sale), the companies that make supplements do not have to show evidence of safety or health benefits to the FDA before selling their products. Supplement products without any reliable scientific evidence of health benefits may still be sold as long as the companies selling them do not claim the supplements can prevent, treat, or cure any specific disease. Some such products may not contain the amount of the herb or substance that is written on the label, and some may include other substances (contaminants). Though the FDA has written new rules to improve the quality of manufacturing processes for dietary supplements and the accurate listing of supplement ingredients, these rules do not take full effect until 2010. And, the new rules do not address the safety of supplement ingredients or their effects on health when proper manufacturing techniques are used.

Most such supplements have not been tested to find out if they interact with medicines, foods, or other herbs and supplements. Even though some reports of interactions and harmful effects may be published, full studies of interactions and effects are not often available. Because of these limitations, any information on ill effects and interactions should be considered incomplete.

References

Chomnawang MT, Surassmo S, Nukoolkarn VS, Gritsanapan W. Antimicrobial effects of Thai medicinal plants against acne-inducing bacteria. *J Ethnopharmacol.* 2005;101:330-333.

Cyber letters. US Food and Drug Administration Web site. http://www.fda.gov/foi/warning_letters/g6031d.pdf. Accessed July 13, 2007. Content no longer available.

Lawenda BD, Kelly KM, Ladas EJ, Sagar SM, Vickers A, Blumberg JB. Should supplemental antioxidant administration be avoided during chemotherapy and radiation therapy? *J Natl Cancer Inst.* 2008;100:773-783.

Mangosteen. Memorial Sloan-Kettering Cancer Center Web site. http://www.mskcc.org/mskcc/html/69295.cfm. Accessed June 11, 2008.

Mangosteen. Natural Medicines Comprehensive Database. Quackwatch Web site. http://www.quackwatch.org/01QuackeryRelatedTopics/DSH/hm.html. Accessed June 11, 2008.

Moongkarndi P, Kosem N, Luanratana O, Jongsomboonkusol S, Pongpan N. Antiproliferative activity of Thai medicinal plant extracts on human breast adenocarcinoma cell line. *Fitoterapia.* 2004; 75:375-377.

Nabandith V, Suzui M, Morioka T, Kaneshiro T, Kinjo T, Matsumoto K, Akao Y, Iinuma M, Yoshini N. Inhibitory effects of crude alpha-mangostin, a xanthone derivative, on two different categories of colon preneoplastic lesions induced by 1, 2-dimethylhydrazine in the rat. *Asian Pac J Cancer Prev.* 2004;5:433-438.

Wong LP, Klemmer PJ. Severe lactic acidosis associated with juice of the mangosteen fruit *Garcinia mangostana*. *Am J Kidney Dis.* 2008;51:829-833.

MELATONIN

Other common name(s): none
Scientific/medical name(s): N-acetyl-5-methoxytryptamine

Description

Melatonin is a hormone produced naturally by the pineal gland—a pea-sized gland located just beneath the center of the brain—in response to darkness. Melatonin is also available as a manmade supplement.

Overview

Research suggests that the melatonin made by the body plays a large role in the daily rhythms of sleeping and waking. Some recent studies have found that people who work night shifts may be at increased risk for cancer, which could be linked to melatonin levels in the body. Study results regarding the effect of melatonin supplements on survival and quality of life in people with cancer have been mixed, and further research in this area is needed.

How is it promoted for use?

There is some evidence that melatonin may have a role in the regulation of daily body cycles, sleep patterns, mood, and reproduction. Possible effects on tumor growth and aging are also under study.

Melatonin is promoted mainly as a sleep aid. Its production in the body may decrease with age, which, according to proponents, may explain why many older people have trouble sleeping. Melatonin is also promoted to help people adjust to odd or irregular work schedules and to counter the effects of jet lag, as it may restore normal sleeping and waking schedules. Some practitioners also believe that melatonin influences hormones in the body that regulate reproduction, the timing of ovulation, and aging. It is sometimes promoted to prevent Alzheimer's disease and is often sold as an anti-aging hormone.

Proponents also claim that melatonin is a powerful antioxidant, a compound that blocks the action of free radicals, activated oxygen molecules that can damage cells. Because of melatonin's suspected antioxidant properties, some believe it may suppress the growth of some types of cancer cells, especially when combined with certain anticancer drugs. Some supporters suggest that melatonin may also stimulate a type of white blood cell called a natural killer cell, which attacks tumors.

Others suggest that melatonin levels and daily body cycles are abnormal in some people with cancer and that melatonin supplements may help them sleep at night. There are also claims that melatonin may decrease the toxic effects of radiation therapy and chemotherapy.

What does it involve?

Melatonin is sold as a supplement and is available in drugstores, health food stores, and over the Internet. There are no widely accepted recommendations for dosage or duration of use. Melatonin can also be found in many foods, such as milk, peanuts, almonds, turkey, and chicken, but in such small amounts that one would have to eat very large volumes to obtain a measurable dose.

What is the history behind it?

The existence of the pineal gland has been known for thousands of years, although its function remained a mystery until the late twentieth century. In the 1600s, the French philosopher René Descartes called the pineal gland "the seat of the soul," because many people believed emotions originated there.

Researchers at Yale University first discovered melatonin and its connection to the pineal gland in the late 1950s. Its link to sleep and hormonal influences and its possible link to cancer have been studied since that time. Melatonin became available as a dietary supplement in the 1990s.

What is the evidence?

Some recent research has suggested that low melatonin levels in the body may be linked to a higher risk for certain types of cancer. For example, a few studies have found that women who work night shifts for many years (and therefore would be expected to have lower levels of melatonin) seem to have a slightly higher risk for breast and colorectal cancer. Even if these studies are confirmed, however, they do not necessarily mean that melatonin supplements can lower cancer risk.

Melatonin has been shown to slow or stop the growth of several types of cancer cells when studied in the laboratory. Whether this same effect occurs in the body is unknown.

Several studies have looked at the use of melatonin to treat cancer. Melatonin has been used alone and combined with chemotherapy, radiation therapy, hormone therapy (such as tamoxifen), or immunotherapy (such as interleukin-2) in a number of studies involving different types of cancer. Some of the studies have suggested that melatonin may extend survival and improve quality of life for patients with certain types of untreatable cancers such as advanced lung cancer and advanced melanoma. Some studies reported that a small number of cancers went into total or partial remission, while other studies indicated that melatonin caused little or no response in tumors.

In a 2005 clinical trial looking at cancer-related weight loss (cachexia), melatonin was compared with fish oil in a small group of patients with advanced intestinal cancer. Although neither group gained weight on these substances, three of the eleven patients in the melatonin group did not lose additional weight over the four-week trial period. However, this study was limited by its small size and short period of follow-up, and other factors may have accounted for the more stable weight in these patients.

Most of the studies reporting positive results from melatonin were small and conducted by the same group of Italian researchers. Before the results are widely accepted, they will need to be confirmed in larger studies at other centers.

Some early studies have reported that melatonin may improve appetite, blood platelet counts, and mouth sores in people undergoing chemotherapy. But a study of melatonin's ability to ease the effects of chemotherapy on the blood counts of lung cancer patients found that high doses of the hormone had little effect. More research is needed to clarify these results.

There is relatively good evidence that melatonin supplements can influence sleep and fatigue and can help with jet lag and some sleep problems. Research has not yet shown the most effective way to use melatonin supplements for patients with sleep disorders or for people who have trouble sleeping occasionally. Some research shows that melatonin affects not only how quickly people fall asleep but also the duration and quality of sleep.

Are there any possible problems or complications?

There appear to be few short-term side effects from taking melatonin. Some people report headaches or feeling drowsy or confused after taking it. People taking high doses have reported nightmares and trouble sleeping.

The effects of long-term use of melatonin and how it interacts with other medicines or supplements are unknown. Some reports have indicated that melatonin may interact with blood-thinning medicines and with medications for seizures or diabetes. People taking these medicines should speak with their doctors before taking melatonin.

Since melatonin may have an effect on hormone levels, women who are trying to conceive, are pregnant, or are breastfeeding should not use this supplement. The National Institute on Aging has also warned that melatonin may constrict blood vessels, which could be dangerous for people with high blood pressure or heart disease. Some practitioners believe that children and people under the age of forty should not take melatonin because their bodies make enough of the hormone naturally. Some also caution people with severe mental illness and those taking steroid medications against using melatonin.

Because it has antioxidant properties, concerns have been raised that melatonin might interfere with radiation therapy or chemotherapy, possibly making these treatments less effective. While this concern is based largely on theories of how cancer treatments work, it is supported by some recent studies. For this reason, people being treated for cancer should speak with their doctors before taking this supplement.

Some experts also suggest that people with immune system disorders (such as severe allergies, rheumatoid arthritis, or cancers such as lymphoma) should not take melatonin because it may further stimulate the immune system and worsen these conditions. Again, this is based on a theory and not scientific evidence, but people with immune system problems should speak with their doctors before taking this supplement.

Relying on this type of treatment alone and avoiding or delaying conventional medical care for cancer may have serious health consequences.

This product is sold as a dietary supplement in the United States. Unlike companies that produce drugs (which must provide the FDA with results of detailed testing showing their product is safe and effective before the drug is approved for sale), the companies that make supplements do not have to show evidence of safety or health benefits to the FDA before selling their products. Supplement products without any reliable scientific evidence of health benefits may still be sold as long as the companies selling them do not claim the supplements can prevent, treat, or cure any specific disease. Some such products may not contain the amount of the herb or substance that is written on the label, and some may include other substances (contaminants). Though the FDA has written new rules to improve the quality of manufacturing processes for dietary supplements and the accurate listing of supplement ingredients, these rules do not take full effect until 2010. The new rules also do not address the safety of supplement ingredients or their effects on health when proper manufacturing techniques are used.

Most such supplements have not been tested to find out whether they interact with medicines, foods, or other herbs and supplements. Even though some reports of interactions and harmful effects may be published, full studies of interactions and effects are not often available. Because of these limitations, any information on ill effects and interactions should be considered incomplete.

References

Brzezinski A. Melatonin in humans. *N Engl J Med.* 1997;336:186-195.

Cerea G, Vaghi M, Ardizzoia A, Villa S, Bucovec R, Mengo S, Gardani G, Tancini G, Lissoni P. Biomodulation of cancer chemotherapy for metastatic colorectal cancer: a randomized study of weekly low-dose irinotecan alone versus irinotecan plus the oncostatic pineal hormone melatonin in metastatic colorectal cancer patients progressing on 5-fluorouracil-containing combinations. *Anticancer Res.* 2003;23:1951-1954.

Davis S, Mirick DK. Circadian disruption, shift work and the risk of cancer: a summary of the evidence and studies in Seattle. *Cancer Causes Control.* 2006;17:539-545.

Ghielmini M, Pagani O, de Jong J, Pampallona S, Cont A, Maestroni G, Sessa C, Cavalli F. Double-blind randomized study on the myeloprotective effect of melatonin in combination with carboplatin and etoposide in advanced lung cancer. *Br J Cancer.* 1999;80:1058-1061.

Karasek M. Melatonin in humans—where we are 40 years after its discovery. *Neuro Endocrinol Lett.* 1999;20:179-188.

Lawenda BD, Kelly KM, Ladas EJ, Sagar SM, Vickers A, Blumberg JB. Should supplemental antioxidant administration be avoided during chemotherapy and radiation therapy? *J Natl Cancer Inst.* 2008;100:773-783.

Lissoni P. Is there a role for melatonin in supportive care? *Support Care Cancer.* 2002;10:110-116. Epub 2001 Nov 13.

Lissoni P, Barni S, Ardizzoia A, Tancini G, Conti A, Maestroni G. A randomized study with the pineal hormone melatonin versus supportive care alone in patients with brain metastases due to solid neoplasms. *Cancer.* 1994;73:699-701.

Lissoni P, Chilelli M, Villa S, Cerizza L, Tancini G. Five years survival in metastatic non-small cell lung cancer patients treated with chemotherapy alone or chemotherapy and melatonin: a randomized trial. *J Pineal Res.* 2003;35:12-15.

Lissoni P, Paolorossi F, Tancini G, Ardizzoia A, Barni S, Brivio F, Maestroni GJ, Chilelli M. A phase II study of tamoxifen plus melatonin in metastatic solid tumour patients. *Br J Cancer.* 1996;74:1466-1468.

Melatonin. Memorial Sloan-Kettering Cancer Center Web site. http://www.mskcc.org/mskcc/html/69298.cfm. Accessed June 11, 2008.

Natural Standard. Biologic/organic/pharmacologic therapies: melatonin. Complementary/Integrative Medicine Education Resources, The University of Texas M. D. Anderson Cancer Center Web site. http://www.mdanderson.org/departments/cimer/display.cfm?id=90e5bf72-ee9e-463e-bc9ea125d8912312&method=displayfull. Accessed June 11, 2008.

Persson C, Glimelius B, Rönnelid J, Nygren P. Impact of fish oil and melatonin on cachexia in patients with advanced gastrointestinal cancer: a randomized pilot study. *Nutrition.* 2005;21:170-178.

Pills, patches, and shots: can hormones prevent aging? National Institute on Aging Web site. http://www.niapublications.org/tipsheets/pills.asp. Accessed June 11, 2008.

Schernhammer ES, Laden F, Speizer FE, Willett WC, Hunter DJ, Kawachi I, Colditz GA. Rotating night shifts and risk of breast cancer in women participating in the Nurses' Health Study. *J Natl Cancer Inst.* 2001;93:1563-1568.

Schernhammer ES, Laden F, Speizer FE, Willett WC, Hunter DJ, Kawachi I, Fuchs CS, Colditz GA. Night-shift work and risk of colorectal cancer in the Nurses' Health Study. *J Natl Cancer Inst.* 2003;95:825-828.

OXYGEN THERAPY

Other common name(s): oxygenation therapy, hyperoxygenation, bio-oxidative therapy, oxidative therapy, ozone therapy, autohemotherapy, hydrogen peroxide therapy, oxidology, oxymedicine, germanium sesquioxide

Scientific/medical name(s): O_3 (ozone), H_2O_2 (hydrogen peroxide)

Description

Oxygen therapy introduces substances into the body that are supposed to release oxygen. The extra oxygen is believed to increase the body's ability to destroy disease-causing cells. Two of the most common compounds used in oxygen therapy are hydrogen peroxide and ozone—a chemically active form of oxygen. This type of treatment is different from the common medical uses of oxygen, which involve increasing the amount of oxygen gas in inhaled air. It is also different from hyperbaric oxygen, which involves the use of pressurized oxygen gas (see "Hyperbaric Oxygen Therapy," page 206).

Overview

Available scientific evidence does not support claims that putting oxygen-releasing chemicals into a person's body is effective in treating cancer. It may even be dangerous. There have been reports of patient deaths from this method.

How is it promoted for use?

Different varieties of oxygen therapy are promoted as alternative treatments for dozens of diseases, including certain types of cancer, asthma, emphysema, AIDS, arthritis, heart and vascular diseases, multiple sclerosis, and Alzheimer's disease.

Some supporters claim that cancer cells thrive in low-oxygen environments. They believe adding oxygen to the body creates an oxygen-rich condition in which cancer cells cannot survive. Supporters of this type of treatment claim that it increases the efficiency of all cells in the body and increases energy, promotes the production of antioxidants, and enhances the immune system.

What does it involve?

Ozone gas may be mixed with air or liquids and introduced into the body. It may be given under pressure into the rectum, vagina, or other body opening or injected into a muscle or under the skin. In an approach called autohemotherapy, the practitioner uses a special device to force ozone into a pint of blood that has been drawn from the patient. The blood is then returned to the patient's body.

In conventional medicine and first aid, a dilute solution of hydrogen peroxide is applied to skin wounds. As an alternative therapy, hydrogen peroxide is usually taken by mouth or injected into a vein. Some practitioners promote it for use rectally, vaginally, as a nasal spray, and as eardrops. It is often used to soak affected parts of the body. The stronger solutions (about 35 percent) recommended by alternative medicine practitioners are sold in some health food stores.

The frequency of treatments varies widely, from three times a day over several weeks to once a week for several months.

What is the history behind it?

The history of putting oxygen-releasing substances into the body follows several tracks. Interest in ozone dates back to the mid-1800s in Germany, where it was claimed to purify blood. During World War I, doctors used ozone to treat wounds, trench foot, and the effects of poison gas. In the 1920s, ozone and hydrogen peroxide were used experimentally to treat the flu.

One of the earliest accounts of the medical use of hydrogen peroxide was a short article by I. N. Love, MD, in 1888 in the *Journal of the American Medical Association.* Dr. Love described one case in which he felt hydrogen peroxide had been useful in removing pus from the nose and throat of a child with diphtheria, and he also recommended using hydrogen peroxide for "cancer of the womb… as a cleanser, deodorizer, and stimulator of healing." Unlike most current articles in that prestigious journal, the 1888 report did not include details that would be required today, such as whether patients treated with peroxide lived longer than those receiving placebo, or even whether there was any evidence that peroxide caused cancers of the womb to shrink or disappear. In 1920, hydrogen peroxide injections were used to treat patients during an epidemic of viral pneumonia.

In 1919, William F. Koch, MD, a Detroit physician, proposed that cancer was caused by a single toxin and that the disease could be prevented or reversed by removing that toxin. To achieve this goal, Dr. Koch claimed he had developed glyoxylide, an oxygen compound that could be injected into patients' muscles. Dr. Koch and his followers claimed that glyoxylide forced cancer cells to absorb oxygen, which helped to rid the body of the cancer-causing toxin. In 1942, the U.S. Food and Drug Administration (FDA) charged Dr. Koch with making false claims about glyoxylide. The courts upheld the accusations, and in 1963 the California Cancer Advisory Council reported that glyoxylide therapy had "no value in the diagnosis, treatment, alleviation, or cure of cancer." Later researchers were unable to confirm that glyoxylide ever existed, and studies by theoretical physical chemists showed that the chemical structure that Koch claimed to be glyoxylide cannot possibly exist. (Nonetheless, a number of alternative medicine Web sites continue to promote glyoxylide as a cancer cure.)

During the 1930s, Otto Warburg, MD, a winner of the Nobel Prize in 1931 for his research on respiratory enzymes, discovered that cancer cells have a lower respiration rate than normal cells. He reasoned that cancer cells thrived in a low-oxygen environment and that increased oxygen levels might therefore harm and even kill them. Many of the beliefs held by oxygen therapy practitioners are based on Dr. Warburg's theories concerning cancer, even though technical advances have since offered a great deal more information about how cancer cells really use oxygen. Even if more oxygen is available, it does not cause the cancer cell to switch back to normal oxygen use. And, a higher oxygen level does not seem to hurt cancer cells any more than it hurts healthy cells.

Much of the more recent use of hydrogen peroxide can be traced to Father Richard Wilhelm, a retired high school teacher and former Army chaplain. He claimed to have discovered the healing potential of hydrogen peroxide through acquaintance with a doctor who headed the Mayo Clinic's division of experimental bacteriology, Edward Carl Rosenow, MD. Wilhelm promoted drinking hydrogen peroxide for a host of human ailments.

What is the evidence?

Available scientific evidence does not support claims that increasing oxygen levels in the body will harm or kill cancer cells. It is difficult to get the oxygen level around the cancer cells in the middle of a tumor higher because the blood supply tends to be poor. But there are differences in the way cancer cells use oxygen that may allow new treatments to better target cancer cells.

According to Dr. Stephen Barrett, who writes about health fraud, a researcher from the Dominican Republic claimed that his clinic had used ozone gas to cure thirteen people with cancer. An investigative news group later learned that two of the patients had died of cancer, three could not be found, two refused to be interviewed, three were alive but still had cancer, and in three cases it was not clear that the patients had actually ever had cancer.

Some researchers have studied hydrogen peroxide as an addition to radiation therapy. Although some patients appeared to benefit, many did not. Some laboratory tests have looked at the combined effects of hydrogen peroxide and certain chemotherapy drugs against cancer cells, but it is still too early to tell if this will be of any benefit. According to a review article in *CA: A Cancer Journal for Clinicians*, attempts to treat patients by injecting hydrogen peroxide directly into solid tumors or into the blood system have generally been ineffective. In one study, mice were injected with glucose oxidase (an enzyme that breaks down glucose, with one of the byproducts being hydrogen peroxide) bound to microspheres, a technique that caused hydrogen peroxide to be released directly at the tumor site. Mice that received injections lived longer than those that did not. The researchers in this study concluded that more research on the use of hydrogen peroxide with other antitumor drugs was needed.

In one 2008 study, some tumors in rabbits disappeared without any treatment, but more disappeared after treatment with ordinary oxygen, and even more disappeared after ozone treatment. However, the relevance of such tumors to cancer in humans remains unproven.

A 2001 review of ozone therapy concluded that "... few rigorous clinical trials of the treatment exist. Those that have been published demonstrated no evidence of effect... Until more positive evidence emerges, ozone therapy should be avoided" (*Med J Aust.* 2001;174:91).

Are there any possible problems or complications?

The medical literature contains several accounts of patient deaths attributed directly to putting oxygen-releasing substances into the body.

Hydrogen peroxide can be harmful if swallowed, especially the concentrated solutions sold in some health food stores. "Food grade" peroxide is very concentrated. It contains 35 percent hydrogen peroxide, a concentration that is more than ten times stronger than the 3 percent peroxide approved for use on the skin. Food grade hydrogen peroxide is approved by the FDA to clean food surfaces and for certain bleaching tasks in food production. The FDA requires that any peroxide that might remain in food be broken down into oxygen and water before the food reaches the consumer. Drinking food grade hydrogen peroxide can cause vomiting, severe burns of the throat and stomach, and even death. If it gets in the eyes, it can damage the corneas and cause blindness. Direct skin contact with food grade hydrogen peroxide can cause blistering or burns, and breathing its vapors can also be harmful.

Hydrogen peroxide injections can have dangerous side effects. High blood levels of hydrogen peroxide can create oxygen bubbles that block blood flow and can cause gangrene and death. Destruction of blood cells has also been reported after intravenous injection of hydrogen peroxide. Some people can also have serious allergic reactions to hydrogen peroxide. A 1993 review article also found some research evidence that too much oxygen in the body's tissues may damage genetic material and promote abnormal growth.

A 2001 review of ozone therapy warned that, "The risks of ozone therapy are played down by its proponents. Yet, numerous reports of serious complications, including hepatitis, and at least five fatalities have been reported" (*Med J Aust.* 2001;174:91).

Women who are pregnant or breastfeeding should not use this method, as its possible effects on a fetus are unknown. Relying on this type of treatment alone and avoiding or delaying conventional medical care for cancer may have serious health consequences.

References

American Cancer Society. Questionable methods of cancer management: hydrogen peroxide and other 'hyperoxygenation' therapies. *CA Cancer J Clin.* 1993;43:47-56.

Barrett S. "Miraculous recoveries". Quackwatch Web site. http://www.quackwatch.org/01QuackeryRelatedTopics/Cancer/miracles.html. Updated October 18, 2000. Accessed June 11, 2008.

Cassileth B. *The Alternative Medicine Handbook: The Complete Reference Guide to Alternative and Complementary Therapies.* New York: W.W. Norton; 1998.

Cina SJ, Downs JC, Conradi SE. Hydrogen peroxide: a source of lethal oxygen embolism. Case report and review of the literature. *Am J Forensic Med Pathol.* 1994;15:44-50.

Ernst E. A primer of complementary and alternative medicine commonly used by cancer patients. *Med J Aust.* 2001;174:88-92.

FDA warns consumers against drinking high-strength hydrogen peroxide for medicinal use. FDA News. July 27, 2006. US Food and Drug Administration Web site. http://www.fda.gov/bbs/topics/NEWS/2006/NEW01420.html. Accessed June 11, 2008.

Gatenby RA, Gillies RJ. Why do cancers have high aerobic glycolysis? *Nat Rev Cancer.* 2004;4:891-899.

Green S. Oxygenation therapy: unproven treatments for cancer and AIDS. Quackwatch Web site. http://www.quackwatch.org/01QuackeryRelatedTopics/Cancer/oxygen.html. Accessed June 11, 2008.

León OS, Menéndez S, Merino N, Castillo R, Sam S, Pérez L, Cruz E, Bocci V. Ozone oxidative preconditioning: a protection against cellular damage by free radicals. *Mediators Inflamm.* 1998;7:289-294.

Loughlin KR, Manson K, Cragnale D, Wilson L, Ball RA, Bridges KR. The use of hydrogen peroxide to enhance the efficacy of doxorubicin hydrochloride in a murine bladder tumor cell line. *J Urol.* 2001;165:1300-1304.

Oxygen therapies. Memorial Sloan-Kettering Cancer Center Web site. http://www.mskcc.org/mskcc/html/69317.cfm. Accessed June 11, 2008.

Sherman SJ, Boyer LV, Sibley WA. Cerebral infarction immediately after ingestion of hydrogen peroxide solution. *Stroke.* 1994;25:1065-1067.

Schulz S, Häussler U, Mandic R, Heverhagen JT, Neubauer A, Dünne AA, Werner JA, Weihe E, Bette M. Treatment with ozone/oxygen-pneumoperitoneum results in complete remission of rabbit squamous cell carcinomas. *Int J Cancer.* 2008;122:2360-2637.

Watt BE, Proudfoot AT, Vale JA. Hydrogen peroxide poisoning. *Toxicol Rev.* 2004;23:51-57.

POLY-MVA

Other common name(s): Poly MVA, Polydox, lipoic acid-palladium complex (LAPd), palladium lipoic complex, synthetic DNA reductase

Scientific/medical name(s): none

Description

Poly-MVA is a liquid dietary supplement that contains various minerals, B complex vitamins, palladium, amino acids, and lipoic acid (see "Lipoic Acid," page 780, "Vitamin B Complex," page 534). The "MVA" stands for minerals, vitamins, and amino acids.

Overview

Poly-MVA has been promoted as a nontoxic alternative to chemotherapy. Some also promote it to be used alongside mainstream cancer treatment. Available scientific evidence does not support claims that Poly-MVA is effective in preventing or treating cancer.

How is it promoted for use?

The main ingredient of Poly-MVA is said to be the lipoic acid–palladium complex. According to the inventor of Poly-MVA, this complex can alter the electrical charge of DNA molecules and other parts of cells. This activity is said to help repair damaged DNA and cause cancer cells to self-destruct, a process called apoptosis. Proponents have also claimed palladium allows lipoic acid, an antioxidant, to reach cells in the body it could not otherwise reach. The other components of Poly-MVA are said to complement these actions and to help restore nutrients needed for energy.

Poly-MVA has been promoted as a "metallo-vitamin." It is recommended by some practitioners as a way to prevent or treat cancer. Supporters of Poly-MVA have claimed that it is effective against several types of tumors and that it boosts the immune system, reduces pain, and helps people regain energy and appetite. It has been suggested that Poly-MVA may improve quality of life, especially in those undergoing chemotherapy or radiation therapy. Some even claim it may lead to longer survival.

Poly-MVA has also been reported to be useful in other conditions, including asthma, psoriasis, chronic fatigue syndrome, and AIDS.

What does it involve?

Poly-MVA is a reddish-brown liquid that is taken by mouth. No studies have been done to determine safe or effective doses, although the manufacturer recommends doses ranging from ½ teaspoon to 8 teaspoons a day. Poly-MVA is used at some health clinics in the United States and Mexico, and it can be bought on the Internet.

What is the history behind it?

Poly-MVA was created by Merrill Garnett, DDS, a former dentist with some graduate training in biochemistry. He has conducted research in "electrogenetics" since the late 1950s at different laboratories on Long Island, New York. He is the founder and director of the Garnett McKeen Laboratory, which continues to study Poly-MVA and similar compounds.

According to the manufacturer, Poly-MVA has been available in the United States since 1992. In 1995, Garnett patented "palladium complexes and methods for using same in the treatment of tumors and psoriasis." Poly-MVA remains a popular supplement, despite a lack of proof of effectiveness.

What is the evidence?

Available scientific evidence does not support claims that Poly-MVA is effective in preventing or treating cancer. The makers of Poly-MVA claim it has a history of "over forty years of laboratory research and testing and fifteen years of clinical use." However, reports of Poly-MVA's effectiveness are anecdotal or small studies that have not been confirmed or published in scientific journals.

No studies of Poly-MVA in humans have been published in peer-reviewed medical journals. Thus far, the only study published in a peer-reviewed journal was an animal study using gerbils, which explored the possible effects of Poly-MVA in protecting nerve cells from lack of oxygen.

Are there any possible problems or complications?

The potential risks and side effects of Poly-MVA are not known, as no results from human studies have been reported. Palladium compounds have the potential to cause allergic reactions in some people. Because lipoic acid is a powerful antioxidant, Poly-MVA may make radiation therapy or chemotherapy less effective. While this concern is based largely on theories of how cancer treatments work, it is supported by some recent studies. For this reason, people being treated for cancer should speak with their doctors before taking this supplement.

Relying on this type of treatment alone and avoiding or delaying conventional medical care for cancer may have serious health consequences.

This product is sold as a dietary supplement in the United States. Unlike companies that produce drugs (which must provide the FDA with results of detailed testing showing their product is safe and effective before the drug is approved for sale), the companies that make supplements do not have to show evidence of safety or health benefits to the FDA before selling their products. Supplement products without any reliable scientific evidence of health benefits may still be sold as long as the companies selling them do not claim the supplements can prevent, treat, or cure any specific disease. Some such products may not contain the amount of the herb or substance that is written on the label, and some may include other substances (contaminants). Though the FDA has written new rules to improve the quality of manufacturing processes for dietary supplements and the accurate listing of supplement ingredients, these rules do not take full effect until 2010. The new rules also do not address the safety of supplement ingredients or their effects on health when proper manufacturing techniques are used.

Most such supplements have not been tested to find out if they interact with medicines, foods, or other herbs and supplements. Even though some reports of interactions and harmful effects may be published, full studies of interactions and effects are not often available. Because of these limitations, any information on ill effects and interactions should be considered incomplete.

References

Antonawich FJ, Fiore SM, Welicky LM. Regulation of ischemic cell death by the lipoic acid-palladium complex, Poly MVA, in gerbils. *Exp Neurol.* 2004;189:10-15.

Lawenda BD, Kelly KM, Ladas EJ, Sagar SM, Vickers A, Blumberg JB. Should supplemental antioxidant administration be avoided during chemotherapy and radiation therapy? *J Natl Cancer Inst.* 2008;100:773-783.

Moss RW. A friendly skeptic looks at PolyMVA part I. CancerDecisions Newsletter. Oct 18, 2003. The Moss Reports, Cancer Decisions Newsletter Web site. http://www.cancerdecisions.com/101803.html. Accessed June 11, 2008.

Moss RW. A friendly skeptic looks at PolyMVA part II. CancerDecisions Newsletter. Oct 24, 2003. The Moss Reports, Cancer Decisions Newsletter Web site. http://www.cancerdecisions.com/102403.html. Accessed June 11, 2008.

Polydox. Memorial Sloan-Kettering Cancer Center Web site. http://www.mskcc.org/mskcc/html/69336.cfm. Updated September 17, 2007. Accessed June 11, 2008.

PREGNENOLONE

Other common name(s): none
Scientific/medical name(s): 3-hydroxypregn-5-en-20-one

Description

Pregnenolone is a steroid the body makes as a precursor to other steroid hormones, such as progesterone, DHEA (see "DHEA," page 729), mineralocorticoids (which regulate electrolyte balance), corticosteroids (which influence inflammation and metabolism), estrogens, and androgens.

Overview

Available scientific evidence does not support claims that pregnenolone can help treat conditions such as arthritis, multiple sclerosis, and cancer. Some research in animals has suggested that pregnenolone may help improve memory, but no research in humans has been reported.

How is it promoted for use?

Pregnenolone is mainly promoted as an alternative treatment that improves memory and alertness and reduces stress, depression, and fatigue. Some promoters claim pregnenolone also helps treat a variety of other conditions such as arthritis, cancer, osteoporosis, obesity, multiple sclerosis, premenstrual syndrome, and menopause.

What does it involve?

Pregnenolone supplements are sold in tablet and capsule form and as a topical cream. There is no standard dose, although it is available in strengths ranging from 5 to 50 milligrams.

What is the history behind it?

Pregnenolone was the subject of several animal and human studies during the 1940s. Some suggested potential clinical use for arthritis as well as for improving performance by reducing stress. Subsequent research demonstrated that pregnenolone is the precursor used by the body in producing all steroid hormones. As researchers learned more about these other hormones, interest in pregnenolone as a treatment decreased. For example, cortisol (another hormone made from pregnenolone) was found to be useful in treating inflammation as seen in arthritis and other diseases, and doctors felt treatment with cortisol made more sense than treatment with pregnenolone, which was used by the body in producing not only cortisol but also estrogens, androgens, and other hormones. Chemically modified or synthetic versions of natural steroid hormones have been developed and tested as drugs in clinical trials, and those found to be more potent and to have more specific effects are now preferred in clinical medicine.

Interest in pregnenolone as a treatment has increased recently among some alternative practitioners, and a number of Web sites currently advocate its use for arthritis, Alzheimer's disease, athletic training, and cancer.

What is the evidence?

Available clinical evidence does not support claims that pregnenolone helps treat a variety of conditions such as arthritis, cancer, osteoporosis, obesity, multiple sclerosis, premenstrual syndrome, and menopause. Studies in mice suggest possible enhancement of memory, but it is unclear whether this benefit would occur in humans.

Clinical studies done during the 1940s suggested that pregnenolone might enhance attention span and physical and mental performance. These studies have not been replicated with modern clinical research methods, although a small study reported in 1997 as an abstract (but not a full article) found no effect on strength, balance, or memory. Some animal studies have suggested that pregnenolone may help improve memory, but no human studies have been reported in the available peer-reviewed medical literature to confirm this.

Are there any possible problems or complications?

Very little is known about the safety of the supplements or the effects of long-term use. Some laboratory studies in cancer cells and animals have suggested that pregnenolone may stimulate the growth of hormone-responsive cancers such as prostate and breast cancer. The body uses pregnenolone to make steroid hormones such as DHEA and testosterone. High doses may cause aggressiveness, irritability, trouble sleeping, and the growth of body or facial hair on women. It also may stop menstruation and lower the levels of HDL, or "good," cholesterol, which could raise the risk for heart disease. Other possible side effects include acne, heart rhythm problems, liver problems, loss of hair from the scalp, and oily skin.

Little is known about drug interactions, although some studies suggest it may interfere with the action of certain sleeping medicines or calming medicines (benzodiazepines). Always tell your doctor and pharmacist about any supplements or herbs you are taking.

Women who are pregnant or breastfeeding should not use pregnenolone. Relying on this type of treatment alone and avoiding or delaying conventional medical care for cancer may have serious health consequences.

This product is sold as a dietary supplement in the United States. Unlike companies that produce drugs (which must provide the FDA with results of detailed testing showing their product is safe and effective before the drug is approved for sale), the companies that make supplements do not have to show evidence of safety or health benefits to the FDA before selling their products. Supplement products without any reliable scientific evidence of health benefits may still be sold as long as the companies selling them do not claim the supplements can prevent, treat, or cure any specific disease. Some such products may not contain the amount of the herb or substance that is written on the label, and some may include other substances (contaminants). Though the FDA has written new rules to improve the quality of manufacturing processes for dietary supplements and the accurate listing of supplement ingredients, these rules do not take full effect until 2010. The new rules also do not address the safety of supplement ingredients or their effects on health when proper manufacturing techniques are used.

Most such supplements have not been tested to find out if they interact with medicines, foods, or other herbs and supplements. Even though some reports of interactions and harmful effects may be published, full studies of interactions and effects are not often available. Because of these limitations, any information on ill effects and interactions should be considered incomplete.

References

Flood JF, Morley JE, Roberts E. Memory-enhancing effects in male mice of pregnenolone and steroids metabolically derived from it. *Proc Natl Acad Sci U S A.* 1992;89:1567-1571.

Grigoryev DN, Long BJ, Njar VC, Brodie AH. Pregnenolone stimulates LNCaP prostate cancer cell growth via the mutated androgen receptor. *J Steroid Biochem Mol Biol.* 2000;75:1-10.

Meieran SE, Reus VI, Webster R, Shafton R, Wolkowitz OM. Chronic pregnenolone effects in normal humans: attenuation of benzodiazepine-induced sedation. *Psychoneuroendocrinology.* 2004;29:486-500.

Pregnenolone. PDRhealth Web site. http://www.pdrhealth.com/drug_info/nmdrugprofiles/nutsupdrugs/pre_0211.shtml. Accessed June 11, 2008.

Roberts E. Pregnenolone—from Selye to Alzheimer and a model of the pregnenolone sulfate binding site on the $GABA_A$ receptor. *Biochem Pharmacol.* 1995;49:1-16.

Sih R, Morley JE, Kaiser FE, Herning M. Effects of pregnenolone on aging. *J Investig Med.* 1997;45:348A.

Tariq SH, Kamel H, Morley JE. Dehydroepiandrosterone and pregnenolone. In: Meikle AW, ed. *Endocrine Replacement Therapy in Clinical Practice.* Totowa, NJ; Humana Press; 2003: 307-368.

QUESTIONABLE CANCER PRACTICES IN MEXICO

Other common name(s): many possible names
Scientific/medical name(s): none

Description

Some practitioners of alternative medicine who treat cancer using unproven and unapproved therapies—especially those who market their treatment as a "cure"—have moved just across the Mexican border, where they are still able to attract U.S. patients. Although there are many legitimate cancer treatment centers in Mexico, many of these "border clinics" offer treatments that are unproven or simply do not work. Some also have offices in San Diego or other U.S. towns near the Mexican border. These offices are used as contact points to find U.S. patients, who are then referred to the actual clinics in Mexico. Specific information can be difficult to obtain because of secrecy requirements; in some cases the clinics are operating illegally in Mexico and are subject to closure by Mexican authorities if they are caught.

Overview

One estimate is that there are about thirty-five to fifty alternative medicine clinics and hospitals in Mexican border towns, particularly Tijuana. Investigative news reporters offer some accounts of what the clinics do, but getting good information on their actual practices can be difficult. Before entering some of these clinics, patients are reportedly required to sign agreements stating that they will not to talk to the press. Oftentimes, reporters, investigators, and other outside observers are not allowed in.

Despite these secrecy requirements, some family members have come forward to place complaints that their loved ones got worse or died shortly upon returning home, often after being told they were cured. Families have also told tragic stories of loved ones whose cancer was detected early enough to be treated effectively, but who instead sought care in these border clinics. By the time many of these people learned their cancer had progressed during alternative treatment, it was too late for conventional treatment that could cure them.

How is it promoted for use?

Some clinics offer a cure, while others have toned down their advertising and no longer claim to cure cancer. However, most patients who ask are told they "can be helped" or that there is a "good chance" their cancer can be cured. Treatment in these clinics is often advertised as an alternative to traditional medical care, a "natural" or "nontoxic" alternative to cancer treatment.

Treatment may be promoted based on some of the beliefs listed below about how cancer begins and progresses:

- *The belief that a "buildup of toxins" from foods, food additives, and environmental pollution is the main cause of chronic diseases.* While it is true that there is a link between diet and disease, available scientific evidence does not point to food "toxins" or additives as the cause of disease. The idea that sugar feeds cancer cells is often cited as a reason to avoid certain foods. But even the healthiest foods contain some form of sugar or carbohydrate. The body converts these sugars into glucose as a fuel to supply energy to all of its cells, which cannot function without it. For example, whole fruits and vegetables contain sugars, but they have actually been proven to help reduce cancer risk.
- *The belief that removing toxins from the body (a process called detoxification) and dietary changes can reverse cancer after it has developed and spread.* Available scientific evidence does not support claims that removing certain foods or other substances from the diet or environment will change the outcome of cancer once it has been found. While dietary changes may be helpful to a cancer patient, there is no proof that they will cure cancer. Other measures used for detoxification, such as colon cleansing, can be harmful.

- *The belief that tumors can and do thrive without oxygen and are killed by substances that increase the oxygen supply to the tumor.* The idea that cancer cells thrive in low oxygen levels is based on the lower-than-normal rates of respiration in tumors. However, modern researchers attribute the reduced respiration rate and lower oxygen levels in tumors to the poor blood supply and lack of blood vessels in tissue surrounding rapidly growing tumors. Currently, there is no available scientific evidence supporting the use of products that claim to kill tumors by raising levels of oxygen in the blood (also called hyperoxygenation or oxymedicine), such as hydrogen peroxide and ozone (see "Oxygen Therapy," page 800).
- *The belief that food additives, such as artificial colors and preservatives, cause cancer and that "natural" substances are not harmful.* There is no evidence that food additives are a major threat when used properly and in normal amounts. It is known that some types of industrial pollution and hazardous substances in the workplace have been linked with a higher number of some tumors. However, even if these substances could be removed from the body of a person with cancer (and, in most cases, this is not possible), doing so would not influence growth of a cancer that has already formed.

What does it involve?

Border clinics offer a variety of treatments. They often advertise "individualized therapy," which combines different kinds of alternative and complementary treatments. Metabolic therapy is one of the main treatments offered in these clinics (see "Metabolic Therapy," page 646). Metabolic therapy is not well defined and includes many different kinds of treatment. Although some of the individual methods used in metabolic therapy can be found in the United States, border clinics commonly offer a number of those different treatments used in metabolic therapy in each facility. Because the focus in metabolic therapy is more on the body's function or condition than on the specific treatments, an endless variety of activities that are supposed to help the body's function can be included. These treatments are claimed to be for the three purposes described below: detoxification, immune system support, and fighting the cancer.

Detoxification ("detox") refers to removing so-called toxic agents from the body. It can use many methods:

- special diets (see "Macrobiotic Diet," page 638, "Fasting," page 608, "Vegetarianism," page 684)
- large quantities of pressed liver and carrot juice (see "Juicing," page 628)
- removal of mercury-amalgam fillings
- cleansing enemas or colonics, some of which may include coffee, wheat grass, or other substances (see "Colon Therapy," page 184, "Wheatgrass," page 688)
- chelation therapy (see "Chelation Therapy," page 717)

To reduce the risk of fluid and mineral imbalances, small amounts of juices or other foods may be given. Enemas or colonics may be given as often as every two hours to remove "toxic buildup" in the bowel. The claim that colon cleansing improves the body's ability to digest food shows a basic error in understanding of human anatomy and physiology, since almost all nutrients are actually absorbed in the small intestine. The digested material then enters the large intestine (colon), which absorbs only water and a few minerals. The belief that detox will help the large intestine absorb nutrients is false.

Immune system support is another part of metabolic therapy and may include vitamins, special diets, and nutrition treatments, as well as herbs and other practices, that are supposed to help the body fight the cancer. Large amounts of nutritional supplements are included in most metabolic therapies. Supplements are claimed to balance the diet, detoxify the body, help restore the patient's normal metabolic patterns, strengthen the immune system, and destroy tumors. Various "tumor-specific" substances are promoted and sold with the claim that they are effective, natural, and nontoxic.

A number of different supplements may be offered:

- large doses of vitamins, especially vitamins A, C, and B complex (see Chapter 7 for entries on individual vitamins)
- a variety of minerals, including calcium, potassium, magnesium, selenium, and zinc (see Chapter 7 for entries on minerals)
- enzymes to reduce tumor growth and aid digestion (see "Enzyme Therapy," page 740)
- other products including para-aminobenzoic acid, carnitine, lecithin, inositol, RNA, DNA, and a number of herbs and herbal products (see "Inositol Hexaphosphate," page 624, "DHEA," page 729, and listings of individual herbs, Chapter 7)

Some of these treatments have not been studied by scientists. Others have been tested and appear to have no helpful effect. Some are known to cause harm.

Antitumor treatments are supposed to attack the cancer. Various substances and devices are promoted and sold with the claim that they are effective, natural, and nontoxic to normal cells. Although there are many types of treatment available in Mexico, the treatments listed below are some of the most common:

- electronic "zappers"—electromagnetic devices that are supposed to kill cancer cells (see "Electromagnetic Therapy," page 194)
- light therapy, including UV blood irradiation (see page 210)
- bee venom therapy (see "Apitherapy," page 704)
- cancer salves (see page 171)
- enzyme therapy (see page 740)

- shark cartilage (see page 824)
- induced hypoglycemic (insulin) therapy (see "Insulin Potentiation Therapy," page 770)
- homeopathy (see page 753)
- oxygen therapy, such as ozone or hydrogen peroxide (see page 800)
- antineoplaston therapy (see page 700)
- anticancer vaccines (other than those that have been researched by conventional immunologists and oncologists and found to be helpful in carefully controlled clinical trials)
- hydrotherapy (see page 203)
- whole body hyperthermia (see "Heat Therapy," page 199)
- laetrile, often given with massive doses of vitamins, and dimethylsulfoxide (see "Laetrile," page 776, "DMSO," page 737)
- glandular extracts or live cells or blood from animals, promoted to boost the affected organ system (see "Cell Therapy," page 714)
- urea, based on the idea that urine has cleansing powers (see "Urotherapy," page 834)
- cesium chloride, claimed to inhibit cancer growth by making the pH of cancer cells "basic" instead of acidic (see page 303)
- hydrazine sulfate, said to destroy tumors (see page 757)
- germanium sesquioxide (see "Germanium," page 360)
- low-dose chemotherapy (using doses not researched or recommended by mainstream oncologists), sometimes in combination with other types of treatments

Few of the dozens of products promoted as antitumor agents by metabolic therapists have been approved for use or even recognized as experimental drugs by the U.S. Food and Drug Administration. Several products, such as laetrile and germanium sesquioxide, have been tested and found to be toxic and/or ineffective. Hyperoxygenators have no demonstrated benefits, and both hydrogen peroxide (given by mouth and into the vein) and ozone (given rectally) can be harmful. Several clinics use low-dose (also called micro-dose) chemotherapy in combination with other treatments. Available scientific evidence does not support the claim that micro-dose chemotherapy is effective.

What is the history behind it?

According to an article in *Time* magazine, no one is exactly sure when U.S. citizens began going to alternative medicine clinics in Mexico. Since the early 1960s, U.S. regulatory agencies have become increasingly stringent in their requirements for treatments' proof of effectiveness. Ralph Moss, in his brief history of the Tijuana clinics, notes that the clinics were set up mainly by U.S.

citizens in response to stronger regulation of nonstandard treatments, many of which were unproven.

According to Mr. Moss, the number of clinics in Tijuana increased in the 1970s because of interest in laetrile. The popularity of these clinics began to decline after the mid-1980s and many have since closed. This decline was caused partly by the North American Free Trade Agreement (NAFTA), which was passed in the 1990s. Among other things, NAFTA allows the United States, Canada, and Mexico to work together to take action against cross-border health fraud. The three countries banded together in 1994 to form the Mexico-United States-Canada Health Fraud Work Group, or MUCH.

There have been a number of investigations and convictions of fraudulent providers over the past decade. According to an investigative report in the *San Diego Times-Union*, Mexican regulators shut down or restricted about a dozen clinics in 2001 after finding that many of the clinics were unlicensed and that some were offering very dangerous treatments. One clinic founder pleaded guilty to fraud and money laundering in 2002, after he set up a company that offered "magnetic field" therapy. In an article on the Monterrey (Mexico) Wellness Center, Dr. Stephen Barrett noted that the clinic operator advertised a high cure rate for cancer and other serious diseases at his clinic in Monterrey, Mexico. The clinic operator discouraged people from getting standard medical care, and he and other company officers solicited investments in their "new technology." The company reportedly had received $675,000 in payments before it closed. Its owner, who had represented himself as a world-renowned scientist, was sentenced to more than seven years in federal prison. According to the U.S. attorney prosecuting the case, all of the clinic's patients died.

In 2003, the U.S. Federal Trade Commission (FTC) stopped a Canadian company that was marketing treatments with its "zoetron" machine to U.S. consumers. According to an FTC press release, the patients wired $15,000 to Canada, then traveled to Tijuana for treatment with "Cell Specific Cancer Therapy," which was claimed to be a pulsed magnetic field. The company's owners were charged with making false claims about their device. The FTC states that the zoetron machine turned out to be a ring of weak magnets that did nothing for the cancer. Mexican authorities, working with the United States and Canada, shut down the clinic where the "treatment" was offered.

In 2004, United States and Mexican authorities worked together to shut down yet another Tijuana clinic. The owners, who were based in Bonita (in San Diego County), were charged with fraud. In a separate case, the clinic where Coretta Scott King was treated in 2006 was shut down by Mexican authorities. Mrs. King died shortly after being treated there, and Mexican investigators subsequently learned that the clinic providing her treatment was not authorized to do surgery, laboratory tests, or diagnostic procedures, according to an article in the *San Diego*

Union Tribune. This clinic was headed by an American man. According to the *Atlanta Journal-Constitution*, he had been charged with practicing medicine without a license in 1970 in California and had pleaded guilty to charges of smuggling illegal medicines into the United States in 1996. As reported by Dr. Stephen Barrett, the clinic operator had previously obtained a naturopathic license using a forged degree, misrepresented hydrogen peroxide as a treatment for cancer and arthritis, and pleaded guilty to tax evasion as well as the smuggling charge. In this and other cases, clinic operators who have been convicted of crimes in the United States have still been able to open and run clinics in Mexico.

Despite regulatory agencies' attempts to stop illegal or fraudulent activities, many clinics close and then reopen under other names in new locations. According to Mexican official Dr. Alfredo Gruel Culebro, "Even if they are shut down, they can request a new permit altogether and start operating practically next door" (*San Diego Union Tribune;* February 4, 2006).

What is the evidence?

It is impossible to fully and precisely evaluate all of the treatments described in this section in a single discussion. For the most part, the methods promoted in Mexican border clinics are not consistent with scientific understanding of how cancer and its treatment work. On the other hand, there are many medical practitioners in Mexico who use methods based in responsible science. Some practitioners combine scientifically proven methods with other therapies that show no evidence of helping. But because the hundreds of regimens used in clinics change often, any full evaluation would be outdated almost immediately. For information on each treatment, see the description and evidence in this book regarding that particular treatment.

Although these clinics often claim great success in advertisements and books, they have not published convincing evidence in medical journals to support those claims. Attempts by researchers to study results from those clinics have been constrained by incomplete records and limited follow-up with patients, which usually does not allow any comparison with results of mainstream oncology treatment.

Are there any possible problems or complications?

Patients traveling to the Tijuana area for treatment appear to be subjecting themselves to costly and potentially hazardous regimens, especially if they postpone standard medical care. They usually do not know exactly what they are getting, and they do not know whether the treatment is helpful until time and money have been spent. During the treatment, for example, patients are generally told that they are improving. When symptoms worsen, it may be described as a "healing crisis" or "the toxins coming out."

Most of these therapies have not been tested using the safeguards put in place by U.S.

regulatory agencies and the scientific community to ensure treatments are effective and safe. Available scientific evidence does not support claims that they work. Often, only lay literature, such as patient testimonials and books written by those selling the treatments, is provided when promoters are asked for proof that their treatments work.

There are reports of cancer patients leaving these clinics very happy with their care, believing themselves cured. But most clinics offer no proof of their cure rates and rarely follow up with patients over the long term to see whether their conditions were actually improved by treatment. There are many reports of people who have had severe or life-threatening side effects from the treatments. And there are far more who have died needlessly after coming to mainstream oncologists too late to get timely, effective treatment.

Finally, patients at these border clinics can expect to pay $2,500 to $7,000 a week or more for treatment, plus travel expenses. They are often required to pay all or most of the fee before entering the program. Some clinics have additional costs for extra treatments, and companions may be charged up to $300 a week to share a room with the patient. The recommended stay is often several weeks. Outpatient programs often cost $1,000 to $2,000 a week. Insurance programs almost never cover these treatments, although some of the clinics with U.S. offices have tried to file for insurance reimbursement. Some of these offices have been prosecuted for filing false or fraudulent insurance claims. Most programs also recommend follow-up therapy at home for additional fees, and some patients may be urged to return to the clinic for more treatment. Those who look to these border clinics for alternative treatments often bankrupt themselves in search of a cure.

The American Cancer Society urges individuals with cancer to seek treatment from qualified cancer care professionals who can offer cancer treatments that have been proven to be safe and effective or that are currently being studied in carefully monitored clinical trials. If you believe you have experienced fraud at the hands of any Mexican border clinic, you can contact the U.S. Food and Drug Administration at 888-463-6332, or make a report online at www.fda.gov/medwatch.

Relying on this type of treatment and avoiding or delaying conventional medical care for cancer may have serious health consequences.

These substances may have not been thoroughly tested to find out how they interact with medicines, foods, or dietary supplements. Even though some reports of interactions and harmful effects may be published, full studies of interactions and effects are not often available. Because of these limitations, any information on ill effects and interactions below should be considered incomplete.

References

American Cancer Society. The metabolic therapy of Harold W. Manner, PhD. *CA Cancer J Clin.* 1986;36:185-189.

Barrett S, Herbert V. Questionable cancer therapies. Quackwatch Web site. http://www.quackwatch.com/01QuackeryRelatedTopics/cancer.html. Updated July 6, 2001. Accessed June 11, 2008.

Barrett S. James Gary Davidson and the Monterrey Wellness Center. Quackwatch Web site. http://www.quackwatch.org/01QuackeryRelatedTopics/Cancer/davidson.html. Updated September 13, 2002. Accessed June 11, 2008.

Barrett S. The shady activities of Kurt Donsbach. Quackwatch Web site. http://www.quackwatch.org/01QuackeryRelatedTopics/donsbach.html. Updated September 10, 2007. Accessed June 11, 2008.

Canadian company settles FTC charges that it offered bogus cancer therapy to US citizens. Federal Trade Commission Press Release. February 25, 2004. Federal Trade Commission Web site. http://www.ftc.gov/opa/2004/02/csct.htm. Accessed June 11, 2008.

Cearley A, Dibble S. Clinics under the radar no longer. *San Diego Union Tribune.* February 4, 2006. Sign On San Diego Web site. http://www.signonsandiego.com/uniontrib/20060204/news_7m4clinics.html. Accessed June 11, 2008.

Crabtree P, Dibble S. Borderline medicine. Tijuana alternative clinics frustrate regulators. *San Diego Union Tribune.* Feb 24, 2002. Sign On San Diego Web site. http://utawards.signonsandiego.com/borderline_medicine.html. Accessed June 11, 2008.

Crabtree P, Dibble S. High hopes, false promises Even some alternative care allies are leery of Tijuana. *San Diego Union Tribune.* February 25, 2002. http://utawards.signonsandiego.com/borderline_medicine2.html. Accessed July 10, 2007.

FTC, Canada, and Mexico officials crack down on foreign companies that offer bogus cancer treatment. Federal Trade Commission Press Release. February 20, 2003. Federal Trade Commission Web site. http://www.ftc.gov/opa/2003/02/csct.htm. Accessed June 11, 2008.

Gonzalez NJ, Isaacs LL. Evaluation of pancreatic proteolytic enzyme treatment of adenocarcinoma of the pancreas, with nutrition and detoxification support. *Nutr Cancer.* 1999;33:117-124.

Green S. Nicolas Gonzalez treatment for cancer: gland extracts, coffee enemas, vitamin megadoses, and diets. Quackwatch Web site. http://www.quackwatch.com/01QuackeryRelatedTopics/Cancer/kg.html. Updated April 20, 2000. Accessed June 11, 2008.

Judd A, McKenna MAJ, Keefe B. Clinic, founder operate outside the norm. *Atlanta Journal Constitution.* February 1, 2006. http://www.ajc.com. Accessed April 11, 2006. Content no longer available.

Metabolic therapy. American Cancer Society Web site. http://www.cancer.org/docroot/ETO/content/ETO_5_3x_Metabolic_Therapy.asp. Updated July 12, 2007. Accessed June 12, 2008.

Moss RW. Patient perspectives: Tijuana cancer clinics in the post-NAFTA era. *Integr Cancer Ther.* 2005;4:65-86.

Murphy GP, Morris LB, Lange D, American Cancer Society. *Informed Decisions: The Complete Book of Cancer Diagnosis, Treatment, and Recovery*. New York: Viking; 1997.

Richardson MA, Russell NC, Sanders T, Barrett R, Salveson C. Assessment of outcomes at alternative medicine cancer clinics: a feasibility study. *J Altern Complement Med.* 2001;7:19-32.

Underwood J. Mexico's controversial clinics. Feb 3, 2006. Time Magazine Web site. http://www.time.com/time/health/article/0,8599,1156292,00.html. Accessed June 11, 2008.

US Congress, Office of Technology Assessment. *Unconventional Cancer Treatments: OTA-H-405*. Washington, DC: US Government Printing Office; 1990.

REVICI'S GUIDED CHEMOTHERAPY

Other common name(s): biologically guided chemotherapy, Revici cancer control, lipid therapy, Revici's method
Scientific/medical name(s): none

Description

Revici's guided chemotherapy is a chemical therapy promoted as an alternative cancer treatment. The therapy varies for every patient but can include a chemical formula made of varying amounts of lipid alcohols, caffeine, zinc, lithium, and iron or a formula that contains fatty acids, selenium, magnesium, and sulfur. Despite its name, Revici's guided chemotherapy is entirely different from mainstream chemotherapy or the new targeted therapies that are an increasingly important part of standard cancer treatment.

Overview

Available scientific evidence does not support claims that Revici's guided chemotherapy is effective in treating cancer or any other disease. It may also cause potentially serious side effects.

How is it promoted for use?

Revici's guided chemotherapy is promoted for the treatment of various types of cancer, including colon, bone, lung, and brain cancer, as well as heart disease, arthritis, AIDS, chronic pain, drug addiction, injury from radiation, and schizophrenia. Emanuel Revici, MD, the inventor of the therapy, claimed that even advanced cancer could be treated with his method.

The therapy is based on the theory that cancer and other diseases result from an imbalance of lipids (fats or fat-like substances) in the body that is thought to cause abnormal metabolism. Revici believed that the imbalance led to diseases that could be classified as either anabolic (meaning "constructive") or catabolic (meaning "destructive"). The type of imbalance was determined mainly by looking a patient's urine, and from that determination, a lipid-based remedy could be designed to restore the proper balance.

What does it involve?

Revici's therapy uses urine and blood tests to detect lipid imbalances. A chemical formula of lipids and lipid-based substances is then developed that is unique to each patient. The substances may include alcohols (such as glycerol, butanol, and octanol), sterols (such as cholesterol and steroid hormones), compounds containing certain elements (iodine, mercury, lithium, selenium, zinc, and iron), nicotinic acid derivatives, and other substances.

Revici's guided chemotherapy is given by mouth or injection in dosages tailored to each patient. After the first treatment, patients are taught to test their urine at home and monitor the lipid imbalance. If there are changes, the patient is given a new formula. This therapy is available at a few clinics started by Revici associates.

What is the history behind it?

According to a 1989 review article in *CA: A Cancer Journal for Clinicians*, Emanuel Revici was born in Romania in 1896 and received a medical degree from the University of Bucharest in 1920. After graduation, he taught internal medicine and practiced in Bucharest. In the 1920s, he began research into lipids and cellular metabolism. From 1935 to 1941, he conducted clinical research and practiced medicine in Paris, and from 1941 to 1946 in Mexico City. He began experimenting with a variety of drugs and compounds to treat cancer in 1941.

In 1947, he moved to Brooklyn, New York, and started the Institute of Applied Biology to conduct research into cancer and other diseases. In 1955, he moved the Institute to Manhattan along with his medical practice. According to the information in the *CA* article, New York State has challenged Revici's medical license on a number of occasions since 1983. In 1984, the Board of Regents restricted his medical practice, and four years later, it tightened the restrictions when he was found guilty of professional misconduct. Stephen Barrett and Victor Herbert, who investigate medical fraud, report that Revici's license was revoked in 1993.

Revici died in 1998 at the age of 101, but his therapy is still offered by some of his associates in New York City.

What is the evidence?

Most of the cases Revici treated were not well documented. In his 1961 book, Revici listed a large number of case histories of patients whose tumors he claimed had shrunk or disappeared completely. Some of his patients also testified at a congressional hearing in New York that Revici's treatment caused their cancer to go into remission.

The only published clinical study of Revici's guided chemotherapy appeared in the *Journal of the American Medical Association* in 1965. It was done by a group of nine doctors known as the Clinical Appraisal Group. They studied thirty-three cancer patients referred to Revici for treatment after conventional treatment failed. Twenty-two of the patients died from cancer while on Revici's therapy, eight showed no improvement, and the remaining three showed signs of cancer growth. The group concluded that Revici's method was without value. Revici countered that the original protocol he had agreed to had not been followed.

Studies of Revici's chemotherapy are hampered by the fact that each formula is different. According to the 1989 *CA* review article, a number of scientists who have offered to evaluate his methods were not able to reach agreement with Revici about a study protocol. The same article reports that, in 1945, a group of American doctors studied Revici's treatment methods in Mexico and found no positive evidence to support their value in treating cancer. In 1988, the American Cancer Society requested that Revici provide documentation of his work, but never received a reply.

Are there any possible problems or complications?

Revici's guided chemotherapy for cancer has never been proven to be safe or effective. Revici himself said that his treatment might cause the area around a cancerous tumor to become inflamed and the tumor itself to grow larger and more painful before it shrank or disappeared. Selenium compounds, which are sometimes used in this therapy, can be toxic at high doses (see also "Selenium," page 488).

This treatment should be avoided by women who are pregnant or breastfeeding. Relying on this type of treatment alone and avoiding or delaying conventional medical care for cancer may have serious health consequences.

These substances may have not been thoroughly tested to find out how they interact with medicines, foods, or dietary supplements. Even though some reports of interactions and harmful effects may be published, full studies of interactions and effects are not often available. Because of these limitations, any information on ill effects and interactions should be considered incomplete.

References

American Cancer Society. Revici Method. *CA Cancer J Clin.* 1989;39:119-122.

Barrett S, Herbert V. Questionable cancer therapies. Quackwatch Web site. http://www.quackwatch.org/01QuackeryRelatedTopics/cancer.html. Updated July 6, 2001. Accessed June 11, 2008.

Biologic/organic/pharmacologic therapies: Revici guided chemotherapy detailed scientific review. Complementary/Integrative Medicine Education Resources, The University of Texas M. D. Anderson Cancer Center Web site. http://www.mdanderson.org/departments/cimer/display.cfm?id=DDB1CCA0-1711-11D5-811000508B603A14&method=displayFull. Accessed June 11, 2008.

Lyall D, Schwartz M, Herter FP, Hudson PB, Wright JC, Findley CW, Galbraith JM, Stout AP, Haagensen CD. Treatment of cancer by the method of Revici. *JAMA.* 1965;194:279-280.

National Institutes of Health. *Alternative Medicine: Expanding Medical Horizons: A Report to the National Institutes of Health on Alternative Medical Systems and Practices in the United States.* Washington, DC: US Government Printing Office; 1994. NIH publication 94-066.

Revici E. *Research in Physiopathology as a Basis of Guided Chemotherapy; with Special Application to Cancer.* Princeton, NJ: D Van Nostrand for the American Foundation for Cancer Research; 1961.

US Congress, Office of Technology Assessment. *Unconventional Cancer Treatments: OTA-H-405.* Washington, DC: US Government Printing Office; 1990.

SEA CUCUMBER

Other common name(s): beche-de-mer, Holothurian, Haishen
Scientific/medical name(s): Holothuroidea (many different species names)

Description

Sea cucumbers are marine animals that have a soft body with the shape and texture of a cucumber. There are more than one thousand species of sea cucumbers, ranging in size from one inch to several feet long and inhabiting all oceans, especially the Indian and the western Pacific.

Overview

There is little reliable scientific evidence to support claims that sea cucumber is effective in treating cancer, arthritis, and other diseases.

How is it promoted for use?

Some forms of sea cucumber have been used in traditional Asian folk remedies to help heal wounds and for conditions such as joint pain and impotence. They are a regular part of some Asian diets. Modern promoters claim sea cucumbers contain compounds that fight conditions such as cancer, arthritis, sports injuries, tendinitis, and other inflammatory diseases.

What does it involve?

Sea cucumber extract is available as a dietary supplement, either alone or combined with other ingredients (usually in supplements promoted "for joint health"). The supplements contain ground, dried sea cucumber and come in tablet form. Sea cucumbers, like all other animals, are made up of thousands of chemicals, so the exact ingredients of supplements are likely to vary between products. As a regular part of some Asian diets, they are available as a food in some Asian markets in the United States.

What is the history behind it?

It is thought that sea cucumbers have been used as part of the diet in some Asian countries for hundreds of years. Some varieties of sea cucumber have been used in traditional Asian folk remedies.

What is the evidence?

Research is currently under way to learn whether some compounds made by sea cucumbers may be helpful against cancer. Compounds called triterpenoids have shown some promise in laboratory studies in slowing cancer cell growth and in stopping the formation of new blood vessels that tumors need to grow. In another early laboratory study, a fatty acid (12-MTA) that came from a sea cucumber was found to slow the growth of prostate cancer cells. No studies testing these compounds in animals or humans have been reported as of yet in available scientific publications. Results of such studies are needed to find out whether these compounds are useful against cancer in living organisms. It is important to note also that extracted chemicals or substances are different from supplements made of the whole sea cucumber and would not be expected to produce the same results.

Are there any possible problems or complications?

Sea cucumber supplements have not been tested for safety, and the possible side effects are unknown. People who are allergic to seafood may want to avoid sea cucumber. Relying on this type of treatment alone and avoiding or delaying conventional medical care for cancer may have serious health consequences.

This product is sold as a dietary supplement in the United States. Unlike companies that produce drugs (which must provide the FDA with results of detailed testing showing their product is safe and effective before the drug is approved for sale), the companies that make supplements do not have to show evidence of safety or health benefits to the FDA before selling their products. Supplement products without any reliable scientific evidence of health benefits may still be sold as long as the companies selling them do not claim the supplements can prevent, treat, or cure any specific disease. Some such products may not contain the amount of the herb or substance that is written on the label, and some may include other substances (contaminants). Though the FDA has written new rules to improve the quality of manufacturing processes for dietary supplements and the accurate listing of supplement ingredients, these rules do not take full effect until 2010. The new rules also do not address the safety of supplement ingredients or their effects on health when proper manufacturing techniques are used.

Most such supplements have not been tested to find out if they interact with medicines, foods, or other herbs and supplements. Even though some reports of interactions and harmful effects may be published, full studies of interactions and effects are not often available. Because of these limitations, any information on ill effects and interactions should be considered incomplete.

References

Sea cucumber. Memorial Sloan-Kettering Cancer Center Web site. http://www.mskcc.org/mskcc/html/69368.cfm. Accessed June 11, 2008.

Sugawara T, Zaima N, Yamamoto A, Sakai S, Noguchi R, Hirata T. Isolation of sphingoid bases of sea cucumber cerebrosides and their cytotoxicity against human colon cancer cells. *Biosci Biotechnol Biochem.* 2006;70:2906-2912. Epub 2006 Dec 7.

Tong Y, Zhang X, Tian F, Yi Y, Xu Q, Li L, Tong L, Lin L, Ding J. Philinopside A, a novel marine-derived compound possessing dual anti-angiogenic and anti-tumor effects. *Int J Cancer.* 2005;114:843-853.

Yang P, Collin P, Madden T, Chan D, Sweeney-Gotsch B, McConkey D, Newman RA. Inhibition of proliferation of PC3 cells by the branched-chain fatty acid, 12-methyltetradecanoic acid, is associated with inhibition of 5-lipoxygenase. *Prostate.* 2003;55:281-291.

Zou ZR, Yi YH, Wu HM, Wu JH, Liaw CC, Lee KH. Intercedensides A-C, three new cytotoxic triterpene glycosides from the sea cucumber *Mensamaria intercedens* Lampert. *J Nat Prod.* 2003:66:1055-1060.

SHARK CARTILAGE

Other common name(s): Carticin, Cartilade, BeneFin, Neovastat (AE-941)
Scientific/medical name(s): none

Description

Shark cartilage is extracted from the heads and fins of sharks. Cartilage is a type of connective tissue that is found in the skeletal systems of many animals, including humans. Sharks' skeletons are made almost entirely of cartilage. The major compounds in shark cartilage are proteoglycans and glycoproteins (large molecules with protein and carbohydrate components), as well as protein and calcium salts. Shark cartilage is promoted mainly as an alternative to conventional cancer treatment, but some forms are being studied for use along with standard therapies.

Overview

Most shark cartilage products are sold as dietary supplements in the form of pills or powders. Most have not been tested for effectiveness, for safety, or to verify the purity of ingredients. Available scientific evidence does not support claims that shark cartilage supplements are an effective treatment for cancer, osteoporosis, or any other disease. One shark cartilage product, called AE-941, is in the early phases of development as an investigational new drug.

Although some laboratory and animal studies have shown that some components in shark cartilage have the ability to slow the growth of new blood vessels, these effects have not been proven in humans. The few small clinical studies of shark cartilage products published to date have not shown any benefit against cancer. Further clinical trials of the supplements and of a purified cartilage extract are currently under way.

How is it promoted for use?

Supporters believe that shark cartilage supplements or cartilage from other animals, such as cows, can slow or stop the growth of cancer (see also "Bovine Cartilage," page 708). According to its supporters, shark cartilage contains proteins that stop angiogenesis, the process of blood vessel development. Tumors need a network of blood vessels to survive and grow, so cutting off the tumor's blood supply starves it of nutrients, causing it to shrink or disappear. Some supporters also claim that shark cartilage can help against other diseases, such as osteoporosis, arthritis, psoriasis, macular degeneration, and inflammation of the intestinal tract.

What does it involve?

Shark cartilage is usually taken by mouth as a capsule, powder, or liquid extract, but some people have trouble taking it by mouth because of the strong fishy smell and taste. It is sometimes used as an enema. The dose and length of treatment varies widely. Manufacturers often recommend large doses (up to one cup a day). Chondroitin, a supplement often used with glucosamine to help arthritis, is also made from cartilage. Either bovine or shark cartilage may be used to produce chondroitin.

Shark cartilage dietary supplements are different from AE-941, a liquid shark extract known as Neovastat. This extract is regulated by the U.S. Food and Drug Administration (FDA) as an investigational new drug. AE-941 is being used in carefully controlled clinical trials for people who have agreed to be part of the study.

What is the history behind it?

A New York surgeon named John Prudden began investigating the use of animal cartilage as a medical treatment in the early 1950s. He used powdered cow cartilage to help heal the wounds of surgical patients and later used it to treat cancer. He reported that tumors shrank in more than half of the patients he treated, but the results have not been repeated in other studies.

Since then, many kinds of cartilage, from animals such as pigs, sheep, chickens, cows, and sharks, have been studied. After the 1992 publication of a popular book titled *Sharks Don't Get Cancer*, written by I. William Lane, PhD, shark cartilage supplements became very popular among people interested in alternative medicine. The idea was that since cancer does not seem to develop in sharks as much as in humans, there may be something in the sharks' systems that protects them from the disease.

Interest in shark cartilage increased after a television news magazine aired a segment in 1993 showing a study of patients with advanced cancer in Cuba who had gone into remission after being treated with shark cartilage. The results, however, have not been published in a peer-reviewed medical journal. The National Cancer Institute (NCI) later concluded that the results of the Cuban study were "incomplete and unimpressive" (*J Natl Cancer Inst.* 1993;85:1190-1191).

According to the FDA and the Federal Trade Commission, some manufacturers of shark cartilage supplements have been fined and/or forced to remove their products from the market for making unproven claims that they have cancer-fighting abilities. Such claims can be made only for drugs with proven effects.

Finding drugs that halt the spread of cancer by stopping the growth of blood vessels has been the subject of many conventional research studies in recent years. Some researchers believe that this therapy, called anti-angiogenesis therapy, holds a great deal of promise for certain types of cancer. A number of anti-angiogenesis drugs are currently being studied, and one is already approved to treat certain types of cancer. In addition, several drugs that were approved for other uses, including cancer treatment, have anti-angiogenic effects. These are now being studied more carefully for their role in anti-angiogenesis. Some researchers are trying to purify compounds in cartilage that stop the growth of blood vessels. But the most promising anti-angiogenic substances now in existence are those that have been purified from sources other than cartilage or that have been made in laboratories.

What is the evidence?

The consensus of available scientific evidence does not support claims that shark cartilage supplements are an effective treatment for cancer in humans. Although studies using cow and shark cartilage in people with cancer began in the early 1980s, few have been published. The scientific truth of many of these studies is open to question because they do not describe how treatment was given, how patients were assessed, long-term survival outcomes, or information about the cartilage used and its components.

Some experiments have shown that some forms of shark cartilage possess a modest ability to slow the growth of new blood vessels in laboratory cell cultures and in animals, but the effects on humans are not known. According to one review, results from nine clinical series of patients receiving shark cartilage were mixed. None of the series were done under strict scientific controls.

In one clinical trial involving about fifty patients, researchers concluded that shark cartilage supplements had no effect on patients with advanced-stage cancers. When a more recent placebo-controlled clinical trial tested shark cartilage in more than eighty patients with advanced cancer, no benefit was found. "It wasn't well tolerated, there wasn't any suggestion of benefit in terms of quality of life, there wasn't any suggestion of benefit in terms of survival" (*J Natl Cancer Inst.* 2005;97:1562), commented Charles L. Loprinzi, the physician who authored the study report.

Researchers generally agree that the protein molecules in shark cartilage may be too large to be absorbed by the digestive tract and are simply excreted without ever reaching tumors in the body. However, some scientists have suggested that these substances may be more readily absorbed when taken in a liquid form. One study concluded that the liquid shark cartilage extract AE-941 (Neovastat), taken by mouth, effectively slowed the growth of new blood vessels in healthy men, suggesting to the study authors that the active ingredients in liquid shark cartilage were available for use by the body's healing systems. A small study of the extract found that larger doses were better than smaller doses at prolonging survival in patients with advanced kidney cancer. A larger study was then done. While the results of this study have not been published, the manufacturer has stopped testing it against kidney cancer, suggesting that the results may not have been positive. The NCI sponsored a large, placebo-controlled randomized clinical trial using the extract with conventional chemotherapy and radiation therapy for the treatment of advanced (stage III) lung cancer. Preliminary results in this study were reported at the 2007 meeting of the American Society of Clinical Oncology. Based on analysis of outcomes from 379 patients, the researchers concluded that AE-941 did not improve overall survival.

Are there any possible problems or complications?

Shark cartilage is not thought to be toxic, although it has been known to cause nausea, indigestion, fatigue, fever, and dizziness in some people. It may affect liver function, so ask your doctor before taking it if you have any kind of liver disease. It may also slow down the healing process for people recovering from surgery. People with a low white blood cell count should not take shark cartilage enemas, because there is a risk for life-threatening infection. Children should not take it because it could interfere with body growth and development.

Allergic reactions are possible. People with seafood allergies should avoid shark cartilage and chondroitin that is made from it. Women who are pregnant or breastfeeding should also avoid these supplements.

It is not known whether shark cartilage could cause any problems from interactions with other medicines. Relying on this type of treatment alone and avoiding or delaying conventional medical care for cancer may have serious health consequences.

This product is sold as a dietary supplement in the United States. Unlike companies that produce drugs (which must provide the FDA with results of detailed testing showing their product is safe and effective before the drug is approved for sale), the companies that make supplements do not have to show evidence of safety or health benefits to the FDA before selling their products. Supplement products without any reliable scientific evidence of health benefits may still be sold as long as the companies selling them do not claim the supplements can prevent, treat, or cure any specific disease. Some such products may not contain the amount of the herb or substance that is written on the label, and some may include other substances (contaminants). Though the FDA has written new rules to improve the quality of manufacturing processes for dietary supplements and the accurate listing of supplement ingredients, these rules do not take full effect until 2010. The new rules also do not address the safety of supplement ingredients or their effects on health when proper manufacturing techniques are used.

Most such supplements have not been tested to find out if they interact with medicines, foods, or other herbs and supplements. Even though some reports of interactions and harmful effects may be published, full studies of interactions and effects are not often available. Because of these limitations, any information on ill effects and interactions should be considered incomplete.

References

Barrett S. Government action curbs shark cartilage claims. Quackwatch Web site. http://www.quackwatch.org/04ConsumerEducation/News/Shark.html. Revised July 22, 2004. Accessed October 16, 2008.

Batist G, Patenaude F, Champagne P, Croteau D, Levinton C, Harinton C, Escudier B, Dupont E. Neovastat (AE-941) in refractory renal cell carcinoma patients: report of a phase II trial with two dose levels. *Ann Oncol.* 2002;13:1259-1263.

Berbari P, Thibodeau A, Germain L, Saint-Cyr M, Gaudreau P, Elkhouri S, Dupont E, Garrel DR, Elkouri S. Antiangiogenic effects of the oral administration of liquid cartilage extract in humans. *J Surg Res.* 1999;87;108-113.
Erratum in:
J Surg Res. 2000;89;197. El-Khouri S [corrected to Elkhour S].

Cartilage (bovine and shark) (PDQ®). National Cancer Institute Web site. http://www.cancer.gov/cancertopics/pdq/cam/cartilage/healthprofessional. Updated April 17, 2008. Accessed June 11, 2008.

Ebube NK, Mark W, Hahm H. Preformulation studies and characterization of proposed chondroprotective agents: glucosamine HCl and chondroitin sulfate. *Pharm Dev Technol.* 2002;7:457-469.

Ernst E, Cassileth BR. How useful are unconventional cancer treatments? *Eur J Cancer.* 1999;35:1608-1613.

Federal Trade Commission. Complaint. Docket No. C-3826. Federal Trade Commission Web site. http://www.ftc.gov/os/1998/09/9723071.cmp.htm. Accessed July 11, 2007.

Federal Trade Commission. Complaint. Docket No. C-3895. Federal Trade Commission Web site. http://www.ftc.gov/os/1999/09/bodysystemcmp.htm. Accessed July 11, 2007.

Federal Trade Commission. Complaint. Docket No. C-4021. Federal Trade Commission Web site. http://www.ftc.gov/os/2001/08/formorcmp.htm. Accessed July 11, 2007.

Finkelstein JB. Sharks do get cancer: few surprises in cartilage research. *J Natl Cancer Inst.* 2005;97:1562-1563.

FTC v Heritage Health Products Company. Federal Trade Commission Web site. http://www.ftc.gov/os/caselist/heritagehealth/040427stipheritagehealth.pdf. Accessed June 11, 2008.

Herbs and supplements: shark cartilage. Medline Plus Web site. http://www.nlm.nih.gov/medlineplus/druginfo/natural/patient-sharkcartilage.html. Accessed July 11, 2007. Content no longer available.

Loprinzi CL, Levitt R, Barton DL, Sloan JA, Atherton PJ, Smith DJ, Dakhil SR, Moore DF Jr, Krook JE, Rowland KM Jr, Mazurczak MA, Berg AR, Kim GP; North Central Cancer Treatment Group. Evaluation of shark cartilage in patients with advanced cancer: a North Central Cancer Treatment Group trial. *Cancer.* 2005;104:176-182.

Lu C, Lee JJ, Komaki R, Herbst RS, Evans WK, Choy H, Desjardins P, Esparaz BT, Truong M, Fisch MJ. A phase III study of Æ-941 with induction chemotherapy (IC) and concomitant chemoradiotherapy (CRT) for stage III non- small cell lung cancer (NSCLC) (NCI T99-0046, RTOG 02-70, MDA 99-303). *J Clin Oncol,* 2007 ASCO Annual Meeting Proceedings Part I. Vol 25, No. 18S (June 20 Supplement), 2007: 7527

Matthews J. Media feeds frenzy over shark cartilage as cancer treatment. *J Natl Cancer Inst.* 1993;85:1190-1191. Quoted in: Barrett S. Quackwatch Web site.

Miller DR, Anderson GT, Stark JJ, Granick JL, Richardson D. Phase I/II trial of the safety and efficacy of shark cartilage in the treatment of advanced cancer. *J Clin Oncol.* 1998;16:3649-3655.

Ostrander GK, Cheng KC, Wolf JC, Wolfe MJ. Shark cartilage, cancer and the growing threat of pseudoscience. *Cancer Res.* 2004;64:8485-8491.
Erratum in:
Cancer Res. 2005;65:374.

Raloff J. A fishy therapy: a thriving but controversial dietary supplement. *Science News Online.* 2005;167:154. Science News Web site. http://www.sciencenews.org/articles/20050305/bob9.asp. Accessed July 11, 2007. Content no longer available.

Shark cartilage. Memorial Sloan-Kettering Cancer Center Web site. http://www.mskcc.org/mskcc/html/69374.cfm. Updated July 17, 2007. Accessed June 11, 2008.

US Department of Health and Human Services. Company ordered to halt sales of unapproved drugs, reimburse buyers. *FDA Consumer: The Magazine of the US Food and Drug Administration.* September-October 2004. US Food and Drug Administration Web site. http://www.fda.gov/fdac/departs/2004/504_upd.html#sales. Accessed June 11, 2008.

SHARK LIVER OIL

Other common name(s): none
Scientific/medical name(s): alkylglycerols, alkoxyglycerols, squalene, squalamine

Description

Shark liver oil is promoted as a complementary or alternative form of treatment for cancer and other diseases. The oil is taken from the liver of cold-water sharks. Shark liver oil is a rich source of alkylglycerols, chemicals that may have anticancer properties. Alkylglycerols are also found in human bone marrow and in breast milk. Other chemicals in shark liver oil being studied against cancer are squalamine and squalene.

Overview

Shark liver oil is widely used alongside conventional cancer treatment in northern Europe and is sold as a dietary supplement in the United States. Available scientific evidence does not support claims that shark liver oil supplements are effective against cancer in humans. Recent research has focused on certain components of shark liver oil (alkylglycerols, squalamine, and squalene). Early laboratory studies suggest that they may have antitumor effects in animals, but their effects in humans are not yet known. Clinical trials are currently under way.

How is it promoted for use?

Shark liver oil is promoted as a dietary supplement used to boost the immune system, fight off infections, heal wounds, and to treat cancer and lessen the side effects of conventional cancer treatment.

Alkylglycerols, one of the components found in shark liver oil, are thought to be helpful in several ways. It has been suggested that they fight cancer by killing tumor cells indirectly. Proponents claim they activate the immune system in two ways: by stimulating immune system cells called macrophages, which consume invading germs and damaged cells; and by inhibiting protein kinase C, which is a key regulator of cell growth. Proponents also claim that alkylglycerols reduce the side effects of chemotherapy and radiation treatment, supposedly because of their ability to protect cell membranes.

Because of their supposed immune-boosting effects, alkylglycerols are also claimed to help against colds, flu, chronic infections, asthma, psoriasis, arthritis, and AIDS. Since macrophages are also important in wound healing, alkylglycerols are said to have healing effects. These claims have not been studied in controlled clinical trials.

Other compounds in shark liver oil, such as squalamine and squalene, have also been promoted to have anticancer effects. Because some early studies have shown that squalamine can slow the growth of tumor blood vessels, proponents claim it may help to treat cancer, either alone or combined with chemotherapy. It is also being studied for use against macular degeneration, an eye condition that results in loss of vision. Squalene has been promoted as having cell-protecting abilities, which may reduce the side effects of chemotherapy. These claims are currently being studied. Depending on the commercial preparation, shark liver oil may also be rich in omega-3 fatty acids and vitamin A. Shark liver oil has also been used in some moisturizing skin creams and lotions, although several cosmetics companies have recently removed this ingredient because of concern regarding the decline of some shark species.

What does it involve?

Shark liver oil is available as a dietary supplement in capsule and liquid forms. There are no standardized dosages. These supplements are available at health food stores and over the Internet.

What is the history behind it?

Shark liver oil has been used as a folk remedy by people on the coasts of Norway and Sweden for hundreds of years. It was mainly used to promote wound healing and as a general remedy for conditions of the respiratory tract and the digestive system.

In the 1950s, a young Swedish doctor suggested that extracts of bone marrow helped boost the recovery of white blood cells in children undergoing radiation therapy and chemotherapy for leukemia. The active ingredient in the bone marrow extract was identified as alkylglycerols. Shark liver oil was found to be one of the richest sources of alkylglycerols. Around 1986, the first commercially purified shark liver oil with a "standard dose" of alkylglycerols was marketed. It is still widely used in many northern European countries.

What is the evidence?

Available scientific evidence does not support claims that shark liver oil supplements are effective against cancer in humans. Most of the studies on alkylglycerols and cancer have been done in the laboratory. A few studies showed some benefit in women with cervical cancer who were also undergoing radiation therapy. These studies were published by a single group of Scandinavian researchers in the 1970s and 1980s and have not been confirmed by other research groups. There appears to be very little recent research on the benefits of alkylglycerols in preventing or treating cancer.

More recently, research has focused on squalamine, a substance found in shark liver oil that stops the growth of tumor blood vessels. Researchers found that squalamine decreased the number of lung metastases—tumors that spread to the lung from a primary cancer elsewhere in the body—found in laboratory animals. Early studies in people with cancer have shown that squalamine can safely be combined with chemotherapy, but whether it helps shrink tumors or prolongs survival is not clear. It is currently being studied with other treatments for lung and prostate cancer.

Squalene, a substance found in olive oil and some types of shark liver oil, has been studied in the laboratory. One laboratory study found that squalene seemed to protect normal bone marrow cells from the effects of some chemotherapy drugs while still allowing the drugs to affect cancer cells. It is not yet clear whether this protective effect will extend to animals and humans.

Are there any possible problems or complications?

Although many people have taken shark liver oil, the issue of potential toxicity at the usual doses has not been well studied. Some mild digestive problems such as nausea, upset stomach, and diarrhea have been reported. Some animal studies have found that shark liver oil and its components may raise blood cholesterol levels. A Japanese study found some shark liver oil supplements to be contaminated with polychlorinated biphenyls (PCBs) and polybrominated diphenyl ethers (PBDEs). PCBs can have harmful effects in humans and may increase the risk for some types of cancer. People with seafood allergies may also react to shark liver oil.

Relying on this type of treatment alone and avoiding or delaying conventional medical care for cancer may have serious health consequences.

This product is sold as a dietary supplement in the United States. Unlike companies that produce drugs (which must provide the FDA with results of detailed testing showing their product is safe and effective before the drug is approved for sale), the companies that make supplements do not have to show evidence of safety or health benefits to the FDA before selling their products. Supplement products without any reliable scientific evidence of health benefits may still be sold as long as the companies selling them do not claim the supplements can prevent, treat, or cure any specific disease. Some such products may not contain the amount of the herb or substance that is written on the label, and some may include other substances (contaminants). Though the FDA has written new rules to improve the quality of manufacturing processes for dietary supplements and the accurate listing of supplement ingredients, these rules do not take full effect until 2010. The new rules also do not address the safety of supplement ingredients or their effects on health when proper manufacturing techniques are used.

Most such supplements have not been tested to find out if they interact with medicines, foods, or other herbs and supplements. Even though some reports of interactions and harmful effects may be published,

full studies of interactions and effects are not often available. Because of these limitations, any information on ill effects and interactions should be considered incomplete.

References

Akutsu K, Tanaka Y, Hayakawa K. Occurrence of polybrominated diphenyl ethers and polychlorinated biphenyls in shark liver oil supplements. *Food Addit Contam.* 2006;23:1323-1329.

Alkoxyglycerols. PDRhealth Web site. http://www.pdrhealth.com/drug_info/nmdrugprofiles/nutsupdrugs/alk_0018.shtml. Accessed July 11, 2007. Content no longer available.

Bhargava P, Marshall JL, Dahut W, Rizvi N, Trocky N, Williams JI, Hait H, Song S, Holroyd KJ, Hawkins MJ. A phase I and pharmacokinetic study of squalamine, a novel antiangiogenic agent, in patients with advanced cancers. *Clin Cancer Res.* 2001;7:3912-3919.

Brohult A, Brohult J, Brohult S, Joelsson I. Reduced mortality in cancer patients after administration of alkoxyglycerols. *Acta Obstet Gynecol Scand.* 1986;65:779-785.

Das B, Yeger H, Baruchel H, Freedman MH, Koren G, Baruchel S. In vitro cytoprotective activity of squalene on a bone marrow versus neuroblastoma model of cisplatin-induced toxicity. Implications in cancer chemotherapy. *Eur J Cancer.* 2003;39:2556-2565.

Hao D, Hammond LA, Eckhardt SG, Patnaik A, Takimoto CH, Schwartz GH, Goetz AD, Tolcher AW, McCreery HA, Mamun K, Williams JI, Holroyd KJ, Rowinsky EK. A Phase I and pharmacokinetic study of squalamine, an aminosterol angiogenesis inhibitor. *Clin Cancer Res.* 2003;9:2465-2471.

Herbst RS, Hammond LA, Carbone DP, Tran HT, Holroyd KJ, Desai A, Williams JI, Bekele BN, Hait H, Allgood V, Solomon S, Schiller JH. A phase I/IIA trial of continuous five-day infusion of squalamine lactate (MSI-1256F) plus carboplatin and paclitaxel in patients with advanced non-small cell lung cancer. *Clin Cancer Res.* 2003;9:4108-4115.

Pugliese PT, Jordan K, Cederberg H, Brohult J. Some biological actions of alkylglycerols from shark liver oil. *J Altern Complement Med.* 1998;4:87-99.

Sills AK Jr, Williams JI, Tyler BM, Epstein DS, Sipos EP, Davis JD, McLane MP, Pitchford S, Cheshire K, Gannon FH, Kinney WA, Chao TL, Donowitz M, Laterra J, Zasloff M, Brem H. Squalamine inhibits angiogenesis and solid tumor growth in vivo and perturbs embryonic vasculature. *Cancer Res.* 1998;58:2784-2792.

Squalene. PDRhealth Web site. http://www.pdrhealth.com/drug_info/nmdrugprofiles/nutsupdrugs/squ_0240.shtml. Accessed June 11, 2008.

Teicher BA, Williams JI, Takeuchi H, Ara G, Herbst RS, Buxton D. Potential of the aminosterol, squalamine in combination therapy in the rat 13,762 mammary carcinoma and the murine Lewis lung carcinoma. *Anticancer Res.* 1998;18:2567-2573.

US Department of Health and Human Services. Report on carcinogens, 11th edition. National Toxicology Program Web site. http://ntp.niehs.nih.gov/ntp/roc/toc11.html. Accessed June 11, 2008.

UROTHERAPY

Other common name(s): autourotherapy, urine therapy, urea therapy
Scientific/medical name(s): none

Description

Urotherapy is an alternative method that involves the use of a patient's own urine to treat cancer.

Overview

No well-controlled studies published in available scientific literature support the claims that urotherapy can control or reverse the spread of cancer.

How is it promoted for use?

Urotherapy has been promoted for a wide variety of diseases and conditions, including cancer. Advocates of urotherapy propose several ways by which the treatment can slow or stop the growth of cancer. One is that urine can stimulate the body's immune system. Cancer and other diseases release chemicals called antigens into the bloodstream. When the immune system detects them, it responds by making antibodies to fight the invading disease. Some of the antigens made by cancer cells appear in the urine, so practitioners have hypothesized that if they give urine to cancer patients, the immune system would react more vigorously by making a greater number of antibodies, thereby increasing its capacity to kill tumor cells.

Other practitioners have suggested that urine inhibits the ability of cancer cells to crowd together, which disrupts their flow of nutrients and waste excretion. Without any way to nourish themselves or get rid of waste products, the tumor cells die.

One proponent asserts that certain components in urine establish a biochemical defense system that works independently of the body's immune system. It is claimed that these chemicals do not destroy cancer cells, but rather "correct" their defects and prevent them from spreading.

What does it involve?

Patients undergoing urotherapy may drink their own urine (from a few drops to full glasses), use it as an enema, or have it injected directly into the bloodstream or into tumors. In powdered form, urea, the primary component of urine, has been applied directly to tumors appearing on the skin. Urea may also be packed into capsules or dissolved in a flavored drink. There are no established guidelines for how much urine or urea should be used.

What is the history behind it?

The thought of drinking urine may offend the sensibilities of most Westerners, but in fact, human urine has been considered a healing agent in many Asian cultures for centuries. In India, this practice has been a part of traditional medical practices for thousands of years.

In the mid-1950s, a Greek doctor named Evangelos Danopolous, MD, professed that he had identified anticancer properties in urea and had used the compound to successfully treat patients with certain types of skin and liver cancer. Dr. Danopolous claimed that his therapy significantly extended patients' lives. He published several small positive case reports, but later studies by other researchers did not achieve the same results.

Other doctors have also claimed that urea has anticancer characteristics. One of them, Vincent Speckhart, MD, testified about urea's benefits before a House of Representatives committee. A breast cancer patient whom Dr. Speckhart treated with urea reportedly recovered from her disease and was alive ten years after therapy.

Urotherapy is currently offered along with other forms of alternative therapy in some cancer clinics in Mexico.

What is the evidence?

There are some individual reports of urotherapy's ability to stop cancer growth. However, available scientific evidence does not support claims that urine or urea given in any form is helpful for cancer patients. Two small studies done during the 1980s found urea did not cause tumors to shrink in patients with cancer in the liver.

Are there any possible problems or complications?

Individuals have reported that drinking or injecting urine or applying it directly to the skin is safe and not linked to any harmful side effects, but the safety of these practices has not been established by scientific studies. There have been reports of nausea, vomiting, upset stomach, and diarrhea after drinking one's own urine, especially during the first few days. Some medications are excreted into the urine, and by drinking their own urine, patients can accumulate toxic levels of these drugs. Relying on this type of treatment alone and avoiding or delaying conventional medical care for cancer may have serious health consequences.

References

Clark PI, Slevin ML, Webb JA, Osborne RJ, Jones S, Wrigley PF. Oral urea in the treatment of secondary tumours in the liver. *Br J Cancer.* 1988;57:317-318.

Danopoulos ED, Danopoulou IE. Eleven years experience of oral urea treatment in liver malignancies. *Clin Oncol.* 1981;7:281-289.

Danopoulos ED, Danopoulou IE, Besbeas S, Ramantanis G. The effects of urea treatment in combination with curettage in extensive lip cancers. *J Surg Oncol.* 1982;19:127-131.

Eldor J. Urotherapy for patients with cancer. *Med Hypotheses.* 1997;48:309-315.

Gussow L. Take-home lessons from unusual toxicology cases. *Emergency Medicine News;* 2004;26:52,57.

Hooper TL, Rahman M, Magell J. Oral urea in the treatment of colo-rectal liver metastases. *Clin Oncol.* 1984;10:341-344.

Chapter Ten

Resource Guide

HEALTH INFORMATION ON THE INTERNET

This Resource Guide comprises a variety of national organizations that provide useful information about cancer and cancer treatment; many focus on complementary and alternative cancer therapies.

In addition to the resources listed here, a vast array of information about cancer and complementary and alternative therapies can be found on the Internet. Mass communication technology makes it possible for researchers and clinical experts to quickly share new evidence and information quickly, which can be very valuable to the public in making health decisions. Much of the information on the Internet is written by promoters of unproven treatments, and anyone can post material or claims about treatment online. Therefore, one should investigate the credentials and reputation of the organizations or individuals providing the information. Claims or "facts" regarding complementary and alternative therapies found on the Internet should not be a substitute for medical advice, nor should this material be assumed to be valid or accurate.

How then does a consumer know how to evaluate a site's trustworthiness? The Health on the Net Foundation (HON) established a Code of Conduct for medical and health care-related Web sites, providing guidelines for choosing and creating sites that are ethical and contain reliable information. Sites that adhere to the eight principles listed here are considered to demonstrate ethical behavior. So, look for the "HON" logo—it is usually posted on the home page.

HON Code of Conduct *

1. Authoritative

Any medical or health advice provided and hosted on the site will be given only by medically trained and qualified professionals unless a clear statement is made that a piece of advice offered is from a non-medically qualified individual or organization.

2. Complementarity

The information provided on the site is designed to support, not replace, the relationship that exists between a patient/site visitor and his/her existing physician.

3. Privacy

Confidentiality of data relating to individual patients and visitors to a medical/health Web site, including their identity, is respected by the Web site. The Web site owners honor or exceed the legal requirements of medical/health information privacy that apply in the country and state where the Web site and mirror sites are located.

4. Attribution
Where appropriate, information contained on the site will be supported by clear references to source data and, where possible, will have specific HTML links to that data. The date when a clinical page was last modified will be clearly displayed (e.g., at the bottom of the page).

5. Justifiability
Any claims relating to the benefits/performance of a specific treatment, commercial product, or service will be supported by appropriate, balanced evidence in the manner outlined above in Principle 4.

6. Transparency
The designers of the Web site will seek to provide information in the clearest possible manner and provide contact addresses for visitors that seek further information or support. The Webmaster will display his/her e-mail address clearly throughout the Web site.

7. Financial Disclosure
Support for this Web site will be clearly identified, including the identities of commercial and non-commercial organizations that have contributed funding, services, or material for the site.

8. Advertising Policy
If advertising is a source of funding, it will be clearly stated. A brief description of the advertising policy adopted by the Web site owners will be displayed on the site. Advertising and other promotional material will be presented to viewers in a manner and context that facilitates differentiation between it and the original material created by the institution operating the site.

** Reprinted with permission from the Health on the Net Foundation.*

Keep in mind that new Web sites appear daily while old ones expand, move, or disappear entirely. Some of the Web sites or content outlined below may change. Often, a simple Internet search will point to the new link for a given organization.

The American Cancer Society does not necessarily endorse the agencies, organizations, corporations, and publications represented in this resource guide. This guide is provided for assistance in obtaining information only.

American Cancer Society (ACS)

Toll-free: 800-ACS-2345 (800-227-2345)
Web site: http://www.cancer.org

The American Cancer Society is the nationwide community-based volunteer health organization dedicated to eliminating cancer as a major health problem by preventing cancer, saving lives, and diminishing suffering from cancer, through research, education, advocacy, and service. For comprehensive, up-to-date cancer information, visit the Web site or call the National Cancer Information Center, toll-free, 24 hours a day, 7 days a week. ACS offers a wide variety of educational programs, services, and referrals, as well as information related to complementary and alternative methods.

American Botanical Council (ABC)

Telephone: 512-926-4900
Web site: http://abc.herbalgram.org

ABC was founded and incorporated in 1988 as a nonprofit research and education organization. Their journal is called HerbalGram. ABC offers an online herb reference guide and selections from the Commission E monographs. Additional materials are available for members.

Emergency Use Investigational New Drug Program for Oncology Drugs

Toll-free: 888-463-6332

Through this program, patients with severe or life-threatening illnesses who are not eligible for clinical trials and who are in an urgent medical crisis may be able to receive drugs not yet approved by the FDA. The program is also known as the Compassionate Use IND Program. The patient's doctor should contact the FDA with questions regarding compassionate use of an investigational drug. The program allows only doctors to make emergency IND requests. There are two direct lines (again, for doctors' use only):

Division of Drug Oncology Products: 301-796-2330
Division of Biological Oncology Products: 301-796-2320

FDA Center for Food Safety and Applied Nutrition (CFSAN)

Toll-free: 800-FDA-1088
Web site: http://vm.cfsan.fda.gov
Web site (dietary supplement information): http://www.cfsan.fda.gov/~dms/supplmnt.html

CFSAN is an office of the U.S. Food and Drug Administration. The center promotes and protects public health interest by ensuring that food is safe, nutritious, and wholesome and that it is honestly, accurately, and informatively labeled. The center offers information on numerous dietary supplements.

Memorial Sloan-Kettering Cancer Center

Telephone: 212-639-2000
Web site: http://www.mskcc.org/mskcc/html/11570.cfm

Memorial Sloan-Kettering Cancer Center's *About Herbs, Botanicals, & Other Products* database provides information for consumers about herbs, botanicals, supplements, and other aspects of integrative oncology, including details about adverse effects, interactions, and potential benefits or problems.

National Agricultural Library Food and Nutrition Information Center (FNIC)

Telephone: 301-504-5414
Web site: http://fnic.nal.usda.gov

The Food and Nutrition Information Center (FNIC) provides access to a wide range of food and nutrition resources from both governmental and nongovernmental sources to consumers, health professionals, educators, and researchers. FNIC provides information on dietary supplements, including vitamins, minerals, and herbs.

National Cancer Institute (NCI)

Toll-free: 800-4-CANCER (800-422-6237)
Web site: http://www.cancer.gov
Web site (Spanish version): http://www.cancer.gov/espanol

This government agency provides cancer information through several services, including the ones listed below.

Physicians' Data Query (PDQ®) Database

Web site: http://www.cancer.gov/cancertopics/pdq

The Physicians' Data Query (PDQ®) database is NCI's comprehensive cancer database. It contains peer-reviewed summaries on cancer treatment, screening, prevention, genetics, and supportive care, and complementary and alternative medicine, as well as a registry of cancer clinical trials from around the world and other information.

Cancer Topics

Web site: http://cancer.gov/cancerinformation

This comprehensive Web site contains information on diagnosis, treatment, support, resources, literature, clinical trials, prevention and risk factors, and testing. Up to twenty publications can be ordered online. The publications list is searchable.

Clinical Trials

Web site: http://www.cancer.gov/clinicaltrials

Maintained by the NCI, this site offers information about ongoing cancer clinical trials and explanations of what a trial is and what is involved. A link to the PDQ search engine allows users to search for clinical trials by state, city, and type of cancer.

National Institutes of Health (NIH) National Center for Complementary and Alternative Medicine (NCCAM)

Toll-free: 888-644-6226
Web site: http://nccam.nih.gov

The NCCAM, part of the National Institutes of Health (NIH), facilitates research and evaluation of unconventional medical practices and distributes the information to the public. The Web site provides information on some complementary and alternative therapies promoted as treatments for different diseases.

National Institutes of Health (NIH) Office of Dietary Supplements (ODS)

Telephone: 301-435-2920
Web site: http://ods.od.nih.gov/

The ODS works to broaden understanding of dietary supplements by evaluating scientific information, stimulating and supporting research, disseminating research results, and educating the public. The office provides information on dietary supplements, tips for consumers on informed decision-making, consumer safety information, background information, and more.

National Library of Medicine (includes Medline)

Toll-free: 888-FIND-NLM (888-346-3656)
Web site: http://www.nlm.nih.gov

This Web site of the National Institutes of Health provides a search engine for health, medical, and scientific literature and research, as well as links to other government resources. Medline (http://medlineplus.gov/) is a searchable site with health information from the National Library of Medicine about cancer and other conditions. It includes lists of hospitals and physicians, a medical encyclopedia and a medical dictionary, information on prescription and nonprescription drugs, health information from the media, and links to thousands of clinical trials.

PubMed

Web site: http://www.ncbi.nlm.nih.gov/PubMed

As part of the National Library of Medicine (NLM), this web site provides access to literature references in Medline and other databases, with links to online journals. The site is searchable by key word.

Quackwatch

Web site: http://www.quackwatch.com

Quackwatch, Inc. is a nonprofit corporation whose purpose is to combat health-related frauds, myths, fads, and fallacies. The Quackwatch Web site is a comprehensive source of information regarding fraudulent claims. The site is searchable by keyword.

Society for Integrative Oncology

Web site: http://www.integrativeonc.org/

SIO is a nonprofit, multidisciplinary organization of professionals dedicated to studying and facilitating cancer treatment and the recovery process through the use of integrated complementary therapy, including natural and botanical products, nutrition, acupuncture, massage, mind-body therapies, and other complementary therapies. The Society also issues integrative oncology guidelines, available on its Web site.

The University of Texas M. D. Anderson Cancer Center Complementary and Integrative Medicine Education Resources

Toll-free: 800-392-1611

Web site: http://www.mdanderson.org/departments/cimer/index.cfm

M. D. Anderson Cancer Center's Complementary/Integrative Medicine Education Resources (CIMER) Web site is designed to help patients and physicians decide how best to integrate complementary therapies into their care to enhance patients' quality of life and avoid harm. The site contains useful information on a variety of complementary therapies, answers to frequently asked questions, and videos, presentations, recommended reading, and related links.

GLOSSARY

Adequate Intake (AI): the average daily intake of a particular nutrient (such as a vitamin) recommended by the Food and Nutrition Board (FNB) of the United States National Academies of Sciences. AI values are based on observations of the average intake of a group of healthy people. The FNB publishes Recommended Dietary Allowances (RDA) for some nutrients but may provide an AI if there is not enough evidence to establish an RDA.

adjuvant (AJ-uh-vunt) therapy: treatment used in addition to the main treatment. It usually refers to hormone therapy, chemotherapy, radiation therapy, or immunotherapy added after surgery to increase the chances of curing the disease or preventing recurrence. *Compare with* neoadjuvant therapy.

alternative therapy (alternative medicine): an unproven medication or therapy that is recommended instead of standard (proven) therapy. Some alternative therapies have dangerous or even life-threatening side effects. With others, the main danger is that the patient may lose the opportunity to benefit from standard therapy. The American Cancer Society recommends that patients considering the use of any alternative or complementary therapies discuss these therapies with their conventional health care team. *See also* complementary therapy.

amino acid: one of several molecules that join together to form proteins. There are twenty common amino acids.

anecdotal (an-ik-DOHT-uhl) report: a patient or doctor's report of an experience with an illness or treatment. It is different from a case report published in a peer-reviewed, medical journal, because such journals do not publish reports without prior review by experts to confirm that the report is likely to be true and accurate. It is also important to distinguish anecdotal reports from journal articles describing groups of similar patients, because the latter provide information on usual or likely outcomes.

anemia (uh-NEEM-ee-uh): not having enough red blood cells. Symptoms can include shortness of breath, difficulty breathing on exertion, and fatigue. These symptoms occur because there are not enough red blood cells to carry oxygen to the body's tissues.

anesthesia (an-es-THEE-zhuh): the loss of feeling or sensation as a result of drugs or gases. General anesthesia causes loss of consciousness (puts you to sleep). Local or regional anesthesia numbs only a certain area of the body.

angiogenesis (an-jee-o-JEN-uh-sis): the formation of new blood vessels. Some cancer treatments work by blocking angiogenesis, thus preventing blood from reaching the tumor.

antibody: a protein produced by the body's immune system cells and released into the blood. Antibodies defend the body against germs such as bacteria and are also important in the immune system's resistance to cancer. Each antibody recognizes and attaches to specific chemical components of germs and cancer cells called antigens. *See also* antigen.

anticoagulant (an-tee-ko-AG-yuh-lunt): a drug that helps prevent blood clots from forming. Also called a blood thinner.

antigen (AN-tuh-jen): a substance that causes the body's immune system to react. This reaction often involves production of antibodies but may also involve immune system cells that attack germs of cancer cells. For example, the immune system's response to antigens that are part of bacteria and viruses helps people resist infections. Cancer cells have certain antigens that can be found by laboratory tests. Antigens are important in diagnosis of some forms of cancer and in watching a patient's response to treatment. Other cancer cell antigens play a role in immune reactions that may help the body's resistance against cancer. *See also* antibody.

antioxidant (an-tee-OK-sih-dent): a compound that destroys activated oxygen molecules, known as free radicals, that can damage cells. Free radicals can damage important parts of cells such as genes. Depending on how severe the damage is, the cells may die or they may become cancerous. Examples of antioxidants include vitamins C and E and beta carotene. *See also* free radical.

apoptosis (a-pop-TOE-sis): a type of cell death in which a series of molecular steps in a cell lead to its death. This is the body's normal way of getting rid of unneeded or abnormal cells and is different from the process of cell death by decay. Radiation therapy and many drugs used to treat cancer cause apoptosis. Also called programmed cell death.

bacteria: single-cell microorganisms, some of which cause infections and disease in animals and humans.

basic science: laboratory studies that are not aimed at specific problems, but provide the necessary knowledge and background for later applied research. For example, basic science research about how cell growth is regulated has led to discovery of many new anticancer drugs.

behavioral research: research into what motivates people to act as they do. The results of such research can be used to help convince people to adopt healthy lifestyles and to follow lifesaving screening and treatment guidelines. Behavioral research also provides insight into how people cope with cancer and other illnesses and ways to improve the well-being of people living with cancer.

benign tumor: an abnormal growth that is not cancerous and does not spread to other areas of the body. *Compare with* malignant tumor.

best case series: a group of case reports about patients given similar treatments. The reports usually contain demographic information about the patients (such as age and gender) and information on diagnosis, treatment, response to treatment, and follow-up after treatment.

beta carotene: a precursor of vitamin A that is found mainly in yellow and orange vegetables and fruits. It functions as an antioxidant and may play a role in cancer prevention. *See also* antioxidant.

biopsy (BUY-op-see): the removal of a sample of tissue to see whether cancer cells are present.

blinded study: a type of research study in which the patients or the patients and their doctors do not know which drug or treatment is being given. In a single-blinded study, the patient does not know which treatment is being given, whereas in a double-blinded study, neither the patients nor their doctors know which drug they are receiving. The opposite of a blinded study is an open-label study.

bodywork: any of a number of complementary or alternative methods centered on manipulation of the body, such as massage, yoga, and relaxation techniques, aimed at promoting physical and emotional well-being.

botanical: having to do with, or derived from, plants.

cachexia (ka-KEK-see-uh): a profound loss of body weight and muscle mass, weakness, and malnutrition. Cachexia may occur in patients with cancer or other chronic diseases.

cancer: cancer is not just one disease but a group of related diseases. In all forms of cancer, cells in the body change and grow out of control. Most types of cancer cells form a lump or mass called a tumor. The tumor can invade and destroy healthy tissue. Cells from the tumor can break away and travel to other parts of the body. There they can continue to grow. This spreading process is called metastasis. When cancer spreads, it is still named after the part of the body where it started. For example, if breast cancer spreads to the lungs, it is still called breast cancer, not lung cancer.

Some cancers, such as blood cancers, do not form a tumor. Not all tumors are cancer. A tumor that is not cancer is called benign. Benign tumors do not grow and spread the way cancer does. Benign tumors are usually not a threat to life. Another word for cancerous is malignant.

cancer care team: the group of health care professionals who work together to find, treat, and care for people with cancer. The cancer care team may include the following and others: oncology specialists (medical oncologist, radiation oncologist), surgeons (including surgical specialists such as urologists, gynecologists, neurosurgeons, etc.), primary care physicians, radiologists and pathologists, nurses, oncology nurse specialists, and oncology social workers. Complementary care providers (for example, massage therapists, acupuncturists) may be part of the cancer care team. Whether the team is linked formally or informally, there is usually one person who takes the job of coordinating the team.

cancer cell: a cell that divides and reproduces abnormally and has the potential to spread throughout the body, crowding out normal cells and tissue. *See also* metastasis.

carcinogen (kar-SIN-o-jin): a substance that causes cancer or helps cancer grow. For example, tobacco smoke contains many carcinogens that greatly increase the risk for lung cancer and several other types of cancer.

carotenoid (kuh-RAHT-in-oyd): a substance found in certain plants such as dark green, leafy vegetables and yellow and orange fruits and vegetables. Carotenoids may reduce the risk for developing cancer.

case-control study: a study that compares two groups of people: those with the disease or condition under study (cases) and a very similar group of people who do not have the disease or condition (controls). Researchers start by finding cases and controls, and then study the medical and lifestyle histories of the people in each group (usually by surveys asking them to recall their past health-related habits) to learn what factors may be associated with the disease or condition. Both case-control studies and cohort studies are types of observational studies. *See also* cohort study, observational study.

catheter (KATH-it-ur): a thin, flexible tube through which fluids enter or leave the body; for example, a tube to drain urine.

cell: the basic unit of which all living things are made. Cells replace themselves by splitting and forming new cells (mitosis). The processes that control the formation of new cells and the death of old cells are disrupted in cancer.

cell culture: a process during which a human, plant, or animal cell is adapted to grow in the laboratory, often in laboratory dishes or flasks containing a fluid that nourishes the cells. Cultured cancer cells may be used to test the effects of drugs, herbs, vitamins, or other substances. However, it is important to remember that studies of cultured cells do not always accurately predict how a treatment will work in human patients. Only a small fraction of studies that seem promising in cell culture studies turn out to be useful for treating patients with cancer.

cell cycle: the series of steps that a cell must go through to divide; some chemotherapy drugs act by interfering with the cell cycle.

chemoprevention (key-mo-pre-VEN-shun): prevention of disease such as cancer using drugs, chemicals, vitamins, or minerals. While this idea is not ready for widespread use, it is a very promising area of study.

chemotherapy (key-mo-THER-uh-pee): treatment with drugs to destroy cancer cells. Chemotherapy is often used, either alone or with surgery or radiation, to treat cancer that has spread or come back (recurred), or when there is a strong chance that it could recur.

chi (chee): in traditional Chinese medicine, the vital energy or life force that keeps a person's spiritual, emotional, mental, and physical health in balance. Also called qi.

cholesterol (kuh-LESS-tuh-rawl): a fat-like substance found in the blood and in all cells of the body. Cholesterol is needed for many body processes, but too much cholesterol in the blood can increase the risk for heart disease and stroke.

clinical research: studies that involve people as the research subjects and are intended to learn how to more effectively prevent, diagnose, or treat patients. In contrast, preclinical research involves laboratory studies, such as cell culture or animal experiments.

clinical trials: studies in which people volunteer as participants in research to test new ways of preventing, diagnosing, or treating health problems to determine their safety and effectiveness. Before a new treatment is used on people, it is studied in the laboratory. If these studies suggest the treatment will work, the next step is to test its value for patients. The main questions researchers want to answer are the following:

Does this treatment work?
Does it work better than what we're now using?
What side effects does it cause?
Do the benefits outweigh the risks?
Which patients are most likely to find this treatment helpful?

During the course of treatment, the doctor may suggest looking into a clinical trial. This does not mean that the patient is being asked to be a human "guinea pig." A clinical trial is done only when there is some reason to believe that the treatment being studied may be of value and is likely to be as good as the current standard of care. It does not mean that the case is hopeless and the doctor is suggesting a last-ditch effort.

cohort study: a research study that compares a particular outcome (such as getting a particular type of cancer) in groups of individuals who are alike in many ways but differ by a certain characteristic. Information about possible risk factors or protective factors of people in the group being studied (called the cohort) is collected at the start of the study, before the outcome occurs. Then researchers keep in touch with the participants to check information about the outcome. For example, a cohort study might collect information about what people eat and what supplements they use, and then follow their health for many years to see which foods or supplements are statistically linked to lower cancer risk. Both cohort studies and case-control studies are types of observational studies. *See also* case-control study, observational study.

Commission E: the German Federal Institute for Drugs and Medical Devices Commission E. A committee made up of scientists, toxicologists, doctors, and pharmacists formed by the German government in 1978 to evaluate the safety and effectiveness of herbs. The Commission published the Commission E Monographs, a therapeutic guide to herbal medicine including 380 monographs, and it was translated into English in 1998. The commission itself no longer exists.

compassionate use: a way to provide an investigational drug or treatment to a patient who is not eligible to receive the treatment in a clinical trial, but who has a serious illness for which other treatments are not available. Under compassionate use, patients can receive promising but not yet fully studied or approved cancer therapies when no other treatment option exists.

complementary therapy (complementary medicine): supportive methods that are used in addition to conventional treatments. Some complementary therapies may help relieve certain symptoms of cancer, relieve side effects of conventional cancer therapy or improve a patient's sense of well being. Complementary methods are not intended to cure disease, rather they are provided to help control symptoms and improve quality of life. Some methods, such as massage therapy, yoga, and meditation, which are now called complementary, have been previously referred to as "supportive care." *See also* alternative therapy.

complete blood count (CBC): a test to check the level of red blood cells, white blood cells, and platelets in the blood.

controlled clinical trial: a clinical trial, or study of humans, that compares a control, or comparison, group with an experimental group.

control group: in research or clinical trials, the group that does not receive the treatment being tested. The group may get a placebo or sham treatment, or it may receive standard therapy. If a standard treatment is known to be effective, clinical trial ethical guidelines do not permit researchers to withhold such treatment from the control group or to give them only a placebo. Also called the comparison group.

conventional treatment: the currently accepted and widely used treatment for a certain type of disease, based on past research. Also called conventional therapy. *Compare with* unconventional therapies.

curative treatment: treatment aimed at producing a cure. *Compare with* palliative treatment.

cytokine (SY-toe-kine): a substance that is produced by cells of the body's immune system that can affect the immune response. Cytokines can also be produced in the laboratory and given to people to help the body's immune response to cancer.

dermatitis (der-muh-TY-tis): inflammation of the skin.

detection: finding disease. Early detection means that the disease is found at an early stage, before it has increased or spread to other sites. Many forms of cancer can reach an advanced stage without causing symptoms. Examples of early detection tests include mammography to detect breast cancer early, the Pap test to find early cervical cancer or precancerous changes in cervical cells, and colonoscopy to find early colorectal cancer or precancerous polyps.

diagnosis (dy-ug-NOH-sis): identifying a disease by its signs or symptoms and by using imaging procedures and laboratory findings. For some types of cancer, the earlier a diagnosis is made, the better the chance for long-term survival.

Dietary Reference Intakes (DRI): recommendations developed by U.S. and Canadian scientists about the amounts of nutrients to be eaten each day to meet the needs of most healthy people. *See also* Adequate Intake.

dietary supplement: legally defined in the Dietary Supplement Health and Education Act of 1994 as "…a product (other than tobacco) that is intended to supplement the diet that bears or contains one or more of the following dietary ingredients: a vitamin, a mineral, an herb or other botanical, an amino acid [the individual building blocks of protein], a dietary substance for use by man to supplement the diet by increasing the total daily intake, or a concentrate, metabolite, constituent, extract, or combinations of these ingredients." This definition includes ordinary multivitamins that help increase intake of essential substances that are part of a usual diet, as well as products like shark cartilage extract or echinacea (purple coneflower) that are not ordinarily considered essential nutrients or part of a usual diet.

DNA: deoxyribonucleic acid. DNA is the genetic "blueprint" found in the nucleus of each cell. It holds genetic information on cell growth, division, and function.

double-blinded study: a type of study in which neither the doctor nor the patient knows which of several possible therapies the person is receiving.

drug resistance: the ability of cancer cells to become resistant to the effects of the chemotherapy drugs used to treat cancer.

ecologic study: a type of observational study that collects information about risk factors, protective factors, and health outcomes for groups of people. Unlike cohort studies and case-control studies, these studies do not collect information about individual people, but instead use averages for large groups. For example, a cohort study or a case-control study might study the protective effect of a particular food on cancer risk by surveying thousands of people about their diet and looking for differences between those with or without cancer. An ecologic study might correlate cancer rates in two countries with information on overall national consumption of that food. Although ecologic studies can provide some important information, they are generally considered less reliable than cohort studies and case-control studies.

edema (ih-DEE-muh): an unnatural accumulation of watery fluid in tissue.

electrolyte (ee-LEK-troh-lite): a substance that can conduct electrical current when it is dissolved in body fluids or water. Some examples of electrolytes are sodium, potassium, chloride, and calcium.

endorphin (en-DOR-fin): a morphine-like chemical that is made naturally in the brain and relieves pain.

enema: the injection of a liquid through the anus into the rectum.

enzyme: a protein that speeds up chemical reactions in the body.

epidemiologic research: the study of diseases in populations by collecting and analyzing statistical data. In the field of cancer, epidemiologists look at how many people have cancer, who gets specific types of cancer, and what factors (such as environment or personal habits) play a part in the development of cancer. The two main types of epidemiologic research are observational studies (such as ecologic, case-control, and cohort studies) and intervention studies (clinical trials). In typical usage, when people refer to epidemiologic studies, they are usually thinking of observational studies.

etiology (ee-tee-AHL-uh-jee): the cause of a disease. In cancer, there are many causes; research has shown that both genetics and lifestyle are major factors in many cancers.

experimental drug: *see* investigational treatment.

fatigue: a common symptom during cancer treatment, a bone-weary exhaustion that doesn't get better with rest. For some, this condition can last for some time after treatment.

fatty acid: an important component of fats that is used by the body for energy and tissue development.

FDA: *see* U.S. Food and Drug Administration.

fiber: dietary fiber includes a wide variety of plant carbohydrates that are not digested by humans. Fibers are classified as "soluble" (like oat bran) and "insoluble" (like wheat bran).

Soluble fiber helps to reduce blood cholesterol, thereby lowering the risk for heart disease. Good sources of fiber are beans, vegetables, whole grains, and fruits. Links between fiber and cancer risk are inconclusive. Eating these foods is still recommended because they have other health benefits and contain other substances that can help prevent cancer.

five (5)-year survival rate: the percentage of people with a given cancer who are expected to survive five years or longer with the disease. Five-year survival rates have some drawbacks. Although the rates are based on the most recent information available, they must include data from patients treated more than five years earlier. Advances in cancer treatment often occur quickly. Five-year survival rates, while statistically valid, may not reflect these advances. They should not be seen as a predictor in an individual case.

free radical: a highly reactive chemical that has an unpaired electron. Free radicals often contain oxygen and can damage important cellular molecules such as DNA or lipids or other parts of the cell, and this damage can lead to cancer. Free radicals can also be produced when cells are exposed to radiation and chemotherapy and are an important way in which these treatments kill cancer cells.

gene therapy: a new type of treatment in which defective genes are replaced with normal ones. In research on gene therapy as a possible treatment for cancer, researchers are trying to improve the body's ability to fight the disease or to make the cancer cells more responsive to other kinds of therapy.

genetic risk factor: a risk factor that is inherited from a parent. A risk factor is anything that increases a person's chance of getting a disease such as cancer. Risk factors can be lifestyle-related or environmental, or genetic (inherited). Having a risk factor, or several risk factors, does not mean that a person will get the disease. Most cancers are not caused by genetic risk factors. If a patient has several family members with cancer, however, genetic testing may be considered. *See also* risk factor.

hemoglobin (HEE-moh-gloh-bin): the iron-containing respiratory substance inside red blood cells.

hepatitis (heh-puh-TY-tis): inflammation of the liver.

herbal medicine: a type of medicine that uses roots, stems, leaves, flowers, or seeds of plants to improve health, prevent disease, and treat illness.

homeopathic medicine: an alternative medical system based on the belief that natural substances, prepared in a special way and used most often in very small amounts, restore health. According to these beliefs, in order for a remedy to be effective, it must cause in a healthy person the same symptoms being treated in the patient. Also called homeopathy.

hormone: a chemical substance released into the body by endocrine glands, such as the thyroid, adrenal gland, or ovaries. Hormones travel through the bloodstream and set in motion various body functions. Testosterone and estrogen are examples of male and female hormones.

hormone replacement therapy: a therapy in which hormones are given to women after menopause to replace the hormones no longer produced by the body. Also called HRT.

hormone therapy: treatment with hormones, with drugs that either mimic or interfere with hormone action or hormone production, or the surgical removal of hormone-producing glands. Hormone therapy may kill cancer cells or slow their growth.

hospice: a special kind of care for people in the final phase of illness, their families and caregivers. The care may take place in the patient's home or in a home-like facility.

hypercalcemia (hy-per-kal-SEE-mee-uh): abnormally high levels of calcium in the blood.

hypocalcemia (hy-po-kal-SEE-mee-uh): abnormally low levels of calcium in the blood.

imaging tests: methods used to produce pictures of internal body structures. Some imaging methods used to help diagnose or stage cancer are x-rays, computed tomography (CT) scans, magnetic resonance imaging (MRI), and ultrasound.

immune system: the complex system by which the body resists infection by microbes such as bacteria or viruses and rejects transplanted tissues or organs. The immune system may also help the body fight some cancers.

immunology (ih-myoo-NAH-loh-jee): the study of how the body resists infection and certain other diseases. Knowledge gained in this field is important to those developing cancer treatments based on the principles of immunology.

immunotherapy (im-you-no-THER-uh-pee): treatments that promote or support the body's immune system response to a disease such as cancer.

informed consent: a legal document that explains a course of treatment, the risks, benefits, and possible alternatives; the process by which patients agree to treatment.

insulin (IN-suh-lin): a hormone made by the pancreas. Insulin controls the amount of sugar in the blood by moving it into cells, where it can be used by the body for energy.

interferon (in-ter-FEAR-on): a group of natural hormone-like proteins produced by the body that help regulate the immune system, boosting activity when a threat, such as a virus, is found. Interferons are sometimes used in cancer immunotherapy. *See also* cytokine.

interleukin (in-ter-LOO-kin): a group of natural hormone-like proteins produced by the body that regulate the growth and function of certain types of immune system cells. Interleukins are sometimes used in cancer immunotherapy. *See also* cytokine.

intervention study: a kind of epidemiologic study in which a possible cause-and-effect relationship is studied by changing a given factor. Clinical trials are intervention studies in which people volunteer to receive new treatments chosen to be tested by researchers. *See also* epidemiologic research, observational study.

investigational treatment: a treatment that is being studied in a clinical trial. Before a drug or other treatment can be used regularly to treat patients, it is studied and carefully tested, first in a laboratory setting (in vitro) and then in animals (in vivo). After these studies are completed and the therapy is found to be safe and promising, it is then tested to see if it helps patients. After careful testing among patients shows the drug or other treatment is safe and effective, the U.S. Food and Drug Administration (FDA) may approve it for regular use. Only then does the treatment become part of the standard, conventional collection of proven therapies used to treat disease in humans. Also called experimental treatment or experimental drug.

in vitro research: studies conducted in an artificial environment outside a living organism (e.g., cell cultures). In Latin, literally means "in glass," referring to the glass dishes and flasks used before disposable plastic ones became more popular.

in vivo research: studies conducted within a living organism (e.g., animals or humans). In Latin, literally means "in life."

integrative therapy: the combined use of evidence-based proven therapies and complementary therapies.

intravenous (in-tra-VEEN-us) (IV) line: a needle or a thin tube inserted in a vein and used for supplying fluids and medications.

invasive cancer: cancer that has spread beyond the layer of cells where it first developed to involve adjacent tissues.

lipid: a fatty substance.

local or localized cancer: a cancer that is confined to the organ where it started; that is, it has not spread to distant parts of the body. *Compare with* metastatic cancer.

lymph nodes: small bean-shaped collections of immune system tissue such as lymphocytes, found along lymphatic vessels. They remove cell waste, germs, and other harmful substances from lymph. They help fight infections and also have a role in fighting cancer, although cancers sometimes spread through lymph nodes. Also called lymph glands.

lymphatic (lim-FA-tik) system: a network of tissues and organs (including lymph nodes, spleen, thymus, and bone marrow) that produce and store lymphocytes (cells that fight infection) and the channels that carry the lymph fluid. The lymphatic system is an important part of the body's immune system, as its function is to fight infection. Invasive cancers sometimes penetrate the lymphatic vessels (channels) and spread (metastasize) to lymph nodes. *See also* lymph nodes.

lymphoma (lim-FOAM-uh): a cancer of lymphocytes, which are the main cell type of the immune system. Lymphoma involves a type of white blood cells called lymphocytes. The two main types of lymphoma are Hodgkin's disease and non-Hodgkin's lymphoma. *See* lymphatic system.

macrophage (MAK-row-faj): a type of white blood cell that engulfs and destroys germs and damaged cells.

malignant (muh-LIG-nunt): cancerous.

malignant (muh-LIG-nunt) tumor: a mass of cancer cells that may invade surrounding tissues or spread (metastasize) to distant sites in the body. *Compare with* benign tumor.

meridian: in traditional Chinese medicine, one of twenty channels that form a network through which the body's vital energy (chi or qi) flows. The meridians connect the body's acupuncture sites.

metabolism (meh-TA-boh-lih-zom): all of the chemical changes in a cell or organism that produce the energy and basic materials that are needed for important life processes.

metastasis (meh-TAS-teh-sis): cancer cells that have spread to one or more sites elsewhere in the body, often by way of the lymphatic system or bloodstream. Regional metastasis is cancer that has spread to the lymph nodes, tissues, or organs close to the primary site (the site in which the cancer started). Distant metastasis is cancer that has spread to organs or tissues that are farther away. The plural of this word is metastases.

metastasize (meh-TAS-tuh-size): the process in which cancer cells spread to one or more sites elsewhere in the body, often by way of the lymphatic system or bloodstream. *See also* metastasis, lymphatic system.

metastatic (met-uh-STAT-ick) cancer: a description of cancer that has spread from the primary site (where it started) to other structures or organs, nearby or far away (distant). *See also* metastasis, metastasize.

micronutrient: a substance the body needs in very small amounts, such as vitamins and minerals.

mineral: inorganic elements consumed as nutrients and required to maintain health. Some minerals, such as calcium, are needed in relatively large amounts; others, such as iodine, are required in smaller amounts.

monoclonal antibody (mah-no-KLO-nuhl an-tih-BAH-dee): a manmade version of immune system proteins called antibodies. Several monoclonal antibodies are approved for use as drugs for treating cancer and other diseases. Others are used in laboratory tests to help detect cancer cells and to diagnose many other health problems. *See also* antibody.

natural killer cell: a type of white blood cell that attacks tumor cells and cells that have been infected by some kinds of germs. Most other immune system cells recognize abnormal substances such as viruses only after a prior infection or vaccination. In contrast, as their name suggests, natural killer cells can attack abnormal cells without any prior exposure.

naturopathy (nay-chuh-RAHP-uh-thee): a system of disease prevention and treatment that avoids drugs and surgery. Naturopathy is based on the use of natural agents to help the body heal itself. Naturopathic practitioners may also advocate herbal products, nutrition, acupuncture, and aromatherapy as forms of treatment.

neoadjuvant (nee-oh-AJ-uh-vunt) therapy: additional treatment given before the main treatment, especially before surgery. *Compare with* adjuvant therapy.

nonsteroidal anti-inflammatory (non-steh-ROY-dul an-tee-in-FLA-muh-tor-ee) drug: a drug such as aspirin that decreases fever, swelling, pain, and redness. Also called NSAID.

observational study: a type of study in which individuals are observed or certain outcomes (such as survival, presence of various symptoms, or quality of life) are measured. The researchers look for a statistical link between outcomes and factors such as diet, exercise, use of various complementary or alternative methods. No attempt is made by the researchers to affect the outcome (for example, no treatment is given or recommended).

oncologist (on-KAHL-uh-jist): a doctor with special training in the treatment of cancer.

oncology (on-KAHL-oh-jee): the branch of medicine concerned with the diagnosis and treatment of cancer.

osteoporosis (os-tee-oh-puh-ROH-sis): thinning of bone tissue, resulting in less bone mass and weaker bones. Osteoporosis can cause pain, deformity (especially of the spine), and broken bones. This condition is common among postmenopausal women.

palliative (PAL-ee-uh-tiv) treatment: treatment that relieves symptoms, such as pain, but is not expected to cure the disease. Its main purpose is to improve the patient's quality of life. Sometimes chemotherapy and radiation are used as palliative treatments. *Compare with* curative treatment.

peer review: the process by which articles and grants written by researchers are evaluated for technical and scientific quality and correctness by other experts in the same field.

peptide: a compound consisting of two or more amino acids joined together.

phytochemical (fy-toh-KEH-mih-kuhl): a substance found in plants. Some phytochemicals may lower cancer risk.

phytoestrogen (fy-toh-ES-truh-jin): an estrogen-like substance that is found in some plants and plant products. Phytoestrogens may have anticancer effects.

placebo (pluh-SEE-boh): an inert, inactive substance that may be used in studies (clinical trials) to compare the effects of a given treatment with no treatment. In common speech, a "sugar pill." Sometimes called a sham treatment.

placebo (pluh-SEE-boh) effect: a beneficial effect of a particular treatment that comes from the patient's expectations about the treatment rather than from the treatment itself.

poultice: a soft, moist mass of bread, meal, clay, or other adhesive substance, usually heated, spread on cloth, and applied to warm, moisten, or stimulate an aching or inflamed part of the body.

precancerous: *see* premalignant.

premalignant: changes in cells that may, but do not always, become cancerous. Also called precancerous.

prognosis (prog-NO-sis): a prediction of the course of disease; the outlook for the chances of survival.

prospective study: a study in which researchers identify and collect information about potential risk factors and protective factors from a group of people at a specific point (or points) in time and then wait to see who gets what diseases. Results are examined using statistical methods to identify associations between factors (for example, inherited genes, eating a healthy diet, amount of exercise, use of dietary supplements) and risk for illness. Prospective studies generally provide more reliable information than retrospective studies. Cohort studies are an example of prospective studies. *See also* retrospective study, cohort study.

prostate-specific antigen (PSA): a protein made by the prostate gland. Levels of PSA in the blood often go up in men with prostate cancer as well as other conditions. The PSA test is used in early detection of prostate cancer. It is also used to check the results of treatment.

protective factor: something that may decrease the chance of getting a certain disease. Some examples of protective factors for cancer are eating a healthy diet, getting regular physical activity, and maintaining a healthy weight.

protein: a large molecule made up of a chain of smaller units called amino acids. Small chains of amino acids are called peptides, and longer chains (some biochemists say at least fifty amino acids) are called proteins. Proteins such as enzymes and antibodies serve many vital biological functions.

protocol: a formal outline or plan, such as a description of what treatments a patient will receive and exactly when each should be given. *See also* regimen.

psychotherapy: treatment of mental, emotional, personality, and behavioral disorders using methods such as discussion, listening, and counseling.

quackery: the promotion of methods claiming to prevent, diagnose, or cure cancer or other health problems that are known to be false or unproven. These methods are often based on the use of patient testimonials as evidence of their effectiveness and safety. Many times the treatment is claimed to be effective against other diseases as well as cancer.

quality of life: a person's self-reported subjective sense of well-being and ability to do the things that are important to him or her. Quality of life is an important outcome of health care and is a valuable addition to objective clinical measurements (such as survival rates or tumor response rates). Scientific evaluation of quality of life is done with standardized surveys, and such surveys are now often used in evaluating the benefits of conventional or complementary treatments.

questionable treatments: unproven or untested therapies. *Compare with* standard therapy.

radiation therapy: treatment with radiation to destroy cancer cells. This type of treatment may be used to reduce the size of a cancer before surgery, to destroy any remaining cancer cells after surgery, or, as the main treatment for cancer.

randomized or randomization: a process used in clinical trials that uses chance to assign participants to different groups to compare treatments. Randomization means that each person has an equal chance of being in the treatment (experimental) or comparison (control) groups. This helps reduce the chance of bias in the results that might happen if, for example, the healthiest people all were assigned to a particular treatment group. *See also* control group, clinical trials.

Recommended Dietary Allowance (RDA): intake level for a particular nutrient sufficient to meet the nutrient requirement of nearly all (97 to 98 percent) healthy individuals. RDAs are established by the Food and Nutrition Board (FNB) of the United States National Academies of Sciences.

recurrence: cancer that has come back after treatment. *Local recurrence* means that the cancer has come back at the same place as the original cancer. *Regional recurrence* means that the cancer has come back in the lymph nodes near the first site. *Distant recurrence* is when cancer metastasizes after treatment to organs or tissues (such as the lungs, liver, bone marrow, or brain) farther from the original site than the regional lymph nodes.

red blood cells: blood cells that contain hemoglobin, the substance that carries oxygen to all of the cells of the body. *See also* anemia.

regimen: a strict, regulated plan (such as diet, exercise, or other activity) designed to reach certain goals. In cancer treatment, a plan to treat cancer. *See* protocol.

rehabilitation: activities to help a person adjust, heal, and return to a full, productive life after injury or illness. This regimen may involve physical restoration (such as the use of prostheses, exercises, and physical therapy), counseling, and emotional support.

relapse: reappearance of cancer after a disease-free period. *See* recurrence.

remission: complete or partial disappearance of the signs and symptoms of cancer in response to treatment; the period during which a disease is under control. A remission may not be a cure.

retrospective study: a study in which researchers compare people with a disease or other condition with a similar group of people who are not affected and then look back in time to see what differences in risk factors (for example, genetics or their lifestyles) might have contributed to the different health outcomes. Because information about risk factors is usually obtained from surveys that ask people to remember past behavior (for example, their typical diet or exercise levels ten or more years ago), retrospective studies are usually not considered as reliable as prospective studies. Most case-control studies are retrospective studies. *Compare with* prospective study.

review study: a study in which researchers collect and summarize the findings of several other studies. In some review studies, the researchers may use statistical methods to essentially combine past smaller studies into a larger one that provides more reliable information.

risk factor: anything that affects a person's chance of getting a disease such as cancer. Different cancers have different risk factors. For example, unprotected exposure to strong sunlight is a risk factor for skin cancer; smoking is a risk factor for lung, mouth, larynx, and other cancers. Some risk factors can be controlled. Others, like a person's age, can't be changed.

screening: the search for disease, such as cancer, in people without symptoms. Mammography, colonoscopy, and the Pap test are examples of screening tests for cancer. Screening may refer to coordinated programs in large populations.

side effects: unwanted effects of treatment, such as hair loss caused by chemotherapy and fatigue caused by radiation therapy.

sign: an observable physical change caused by an illness. *Compare with* symptom.

staging: the process of finding out whether cancer has spread and, if so, how far. There is more than one system for staging. The TNM system, described below, is the standard for most types of cancer. The TNM system for staging provides three key pieces of information: **T** refers to the size and local spread of the **T**umor; **N** describes how far the cancer has spread to nearby **N**odes; and **M** shows whether the cancer has spread (**M**etastasized) to other organs of the body. Letters or numbers after the T, N, and M give more details about each of these factors. To summarize this information, the TNM descriptions can be grouped together into a simpler set of stages, labeled with Roman numerals. In general, the lower the number, the less the cancer has spread. A higher number means a more serious cancer.

standard therapy: the most commonly used and widely accepted form of treatment for a disease. *Compare with* questionable treatments.

steroid: a class of organic compounds. Many important hormones, such as estrogen and testosterone, are steroids.

survival rate: the percentage of survivors alive within a certain period of time after diagnosis or treatment. For cancer, a five-year survival rate is often given. This *does not* mean that people cannot live more than five years, or that those who live for five years are necessarily permanently cured.

symptom: a change in the body caused by an illness, as described by the person experiencing it. *Compare with* sign.

systemic therapy: treatment that reaches and affects cells throughout the entire body; for example, chemotherapy. *Compare with* targeted therapy.

targeted therapy: treatment that attacks some part of cancer cells that make them different from normal cells, as opposed to treatment that harms all cells or that harms all growing or dividing cells. They tend to have fewer side effects than some standard treatments such as chemotherapy. *Compare with* systemic therapy.

tincture: an alcohol solution of a medicinal substance.

tissue: a collection of cells, united to perform a particular function in the body.

Tolerable Upper Intake Level (UL): highest average daily intake level of a particular nutrient likely to pose no health risk for nearly all individuals. ULs are established by the Food and Nutrition Board (FNB) of the United States National Academies of Sciences. As intake increases above the UL, the potential risk for adverse health effects increases.

toxin: a poison produced by some animals, plants, and bacteria.

tumor: an abnormal lump or mass of tissue. Tumors can be benign (noncancerous) or malignant (cancerous).

tumor marker: a substance produced by cancer cells and sometimes normal cells. Most are not very useful for cancer screening because other body tissues not related to a cancer can produce the substance, too. But tumor markers may be very useful in monitoring for response to treatment when a cancer is diagnosed or for a recurrence. Tumor markers include CA 125 (ovarian cancer), CEA (GI tract cancers), and PSA (prostate cancer).

tumor vaccine: an experimental treatment for cancer, in which cancer cells (from the patient or from other patients) or chemical constituents of cancer cells are injected into the patient, or mixed with the patient's white blood cells in the laboratory and then returned to the patient. The therapy works by causing the immune system to recognize and attack the cancer cells.

ultrasound: an imaging method in which high-frequency sound waves are used to outline a part of the body. The sound wave echoes are picked up and displayed on a screen.

uncontrolled study: a clinical study that does not have a comparison, or control, group.

unconventional therapies: all types of complementary and alternative treatments that fall outside the definition of conventional (proven) therapies. *Compare with* conventional treatment.

unproven therapy: any therapy that has not been scientifically tested and approved. It may also refer to treatments or tests that are under investigation. In general, adequate scientific evidence is not available to support the use of unproven or untested treatments. However, this term is of limited value since it can be applied to some investigational treatments that were effective in animals and early-phase clinical trials and are still under study in randomized clinical trials, as well as to some alternative treatments that have been convincingly shown to be useless or even harmful.

U.S. Food and Drug Administration (FDA): an agency of the United States Department of Health and Human Services. The FDA is responsible for regulating drugs, biological medical products, blood products, medical devices, and radiation-emitting devices, along with several other categories of products.

U.S. Pharmacopeia (USP): an official public standards–setting authority for all prescription and over-the-counter medicines and other health care products manufactured or sold in the United States. USP also sets standards for food ingredients and dietary supplements.

vitamin: an organic compound essential in small amounts for normal functioning of the body.

x-ray: one form of radiation that can be used at low levels to produce an image of the body on film or at high levels to destroy cancer cells.

INDEX

B

C

F

I

O

P

Q

R

T

U

Books Published by the American Cancer Society

Available everywhere books are sold and online at **www.cancer.org/bookstore**

CANCER INFORMATION

General

The Cancer Atlas (available in English, Spanish, French, Chinese)
Cancer: What Causes It, What Doesn't
The Tobacco Atlas, Second Edition (available in English, Spanish, French)

INFORMATION FOR PEOPLE WITH CANCER

Site-Specific

ACS's Complete Guide to Colorectal Cancer
Breast Cancer Clear & Simple: All Your Questions Answered
QuickFACTS™ Advanced Cancer
QuickFACTS™ Bone Metastasis
QuickFACTS™ Colorectal Cancer, Second Edition
QuickFACTS™ Lung Cancer
QuickFACTS™ Thyroid Cancer

Praise for *QuickFACTS™ Lung Cancer*:

"The ACS has achieved its goal of providing overviews that tackle need-to-know issues and supply references for additional follow-up information as desired. **Recommended.**"
—*Library Journal*

Symptoms and Side Effects

ACS's Guide to Pain Control: Understanding and Managing Cancer Pain, Revised Edition
Eating Well, Staying Well During and After Cancer
Lymphedema: Understanding and Managing Lymphedema After Cancer Treatment

EMOTIONAL AND DAY-TO-DAY SUPPORT

Cancer Caregiving A to Z: An At-Home Guide for Patients and Families
Cancer in the Family: Helping Children Cope with a Parent's Illness
Caregiving: A Step-by-Step Resource for Caring for the Person with Cancer at Home, Revised Edition
Couples Confronting Cancer: Keeping Your Relationship Strong
Get Better! Communication Cards for Kids & Adults (bilingual communication cards)
Social Work in Oncology: Supporting Survivors, Families, and Caregivers
What Helped Get Me Through: Cancer Survivors Share Wisdom and Hope
When the Focus Is on Care: Palliative Care and Cancer

HELP FOR CHILDREN

Because... Someone I Love Has Cancer: Kids' Activity Book (5 twist-up crayons included)
Jacob Has Cancer: His Friends Want to Help (coloring book)
Mom and the Polka-Dot Boo-Boo
Our Dad Is Getting Better
Our Mom Has Cancer (available in hardcover and paperback)
Our Mom Is Getting Better

HEALTH BOOKS FOR CHILDREN

Healthy Air: A Read-Along Coloring & Activity Book (25 per pack; Tobacco avoidance)
Healthy Bodies: A Read-Along Coloring & Activity Book (25 per pack; Physical activity)
Healthy Food: A Read-Along Coloring & Activity Book (25 per pack; Nutrition)
Healthy Me: A Read-Along Coloring & Activity Book
Kids' First Cookbook: Delicious-Nutritious Treats to Make Yourself!

TOOLS FOR THE HEALTH CONSCIOUS

ACS's Healthy Eating Cookbook: A celebration of food, friendship, and healthy living, Third Edition

Celebrate! Healthy Entertaining for Any Occasion

Good for You! Reducing Your Risk of Developing Cancer

The Great American Eat-Right Cookbook: 140 Great-Tasting, Good-For-You Recipes

Kicking Butts: Quit Smoking and Take Charge of Your Health

National Health Education Standards: Achieving Excellence, Second Edition (available in paperback and on CD-ROM)

INSPIRATIONAL SURVIVOR STORIES

Angels & Monsters: A child's eye view of cancer

Chemo and Me: My Hair Loss Experience

Crossing Divides: A Couple's Story of Cancer, Hope, and Hiking Montana's Continental Divide

I Can Survive (illustrated)